The Great Instauration

The Great Instauration

Science, Medicine and Reform 1626—1660

CHARLES WEBSTER

HM

HOLMES & MEIER PUBLISHERS
New York

(1975)

First published in the United States of America 1976 by
Holmes & Meier Publishers, Inc.
101 Fifth Avenue
New York, New York 10003

Library of Congress Cataloging in Publication Data
Webster, Charles.
The great instauration.
Bibliography: p.
Includes index.
1. Science—History—England. 2. Medicine—England—History. 3. Great Britain—History—Puritan Revolution, 1642–1660. I. Title.
Q127.G4W4 1976 509'.42 76–4550
ISBN 0–8419–0267–4

PRINTED IN GREAT BRITAIN

In Memory
of
Maurice Henry

Contents

Preface

This book is based on a series of lectures given to my W.E.A. class in Leeds in 1968. The main theme was discussed in a paper prepared for a seminar organised by P. M. Rattansi and R. M. Young in 1968/9; this was subsequently published in *Acta Comeniana* in 1970. It is hoped that the subject of the scientific, medical and social ideas of the English Puritans is of sufficient interest to merit presentation of this material to a wider audience. I firmly believe that it is impossible to understand the scientific outlook of any society without reference to the more general context of prevailing beliefs and values. The present case-study, relating as it does to a period of great intrinsic interest, and to events which are important for our understanding of the growth of the modern scientific movement, will stimulate others to undertake similar investigations. It is only by this means that tenaciously held prejudices about modern science will be broken down and the study of science, technology and medicine placed in proper historical perspective.

Seventeenth-century English history has attracted the attention of many gifted historians and it has been my privilege to have had access to their work and in some cases to have entered into direct correspondence with them on matters relating to this present book. Notes in the text will confirm that I have been generously assisted by colleagues and friends from the time that my historical work was begun, while I was still teaching at the City Grammar School, Sheffield.

I am also deeply indebted to the Wellcome Trustees, who have made funds available to support me during the period of composition of this book. It is owing to the generosity of the Wellcome Trust that research in the history of medicine is now coming to be adequately represented in English academic institutions.

Many hands have contributed to the typing; in particular Mrs. Irene Ashton of Sheffield has shown great expertise in converting my ragged manuscript into polished typescript. I have also received incalculable help from Margaret Pelling, who has patiently checked and corrected the entire manuscript, and subsequently prepared the index. Finally I would like to thank Helena, Charles and above all Carol for their forbearance.

Charles Webster

Abbreviations

The following abbreviations are used in the Notes:

Abbott	W. C. Abbott (ed.), *Writings and Speeches of Oliver Cromwell*, 4 vols. (Cambridge, Mass., 1937-47).
Annals	Annals of the College of Physicians; Royal College of Physicians Library, London.
Aubrey	John Aubrey, *Brief Lives*, ed. A. Clark, 2 vols. (Oxford, 1898).
Bacon *Works*	*The Works of Francis Bacon*, ed. J. Spedding, R. L. Ellis & D. D. Heath, 14 vols. (London, 1857-74). Vols. 8–14 = *Letters & Life*.
Biographia Britannica	*Biographia Britannica*, ed. A. Kippis, 6 vols. (London, 1747-66).
BL	Boyle Letters, Royal Society Library, London.
BM	British Museum (now British Library)
Bodleian	Bodleian Library, Oxford
Boyle *Works*	*The Works of the Honourable Robert Boyle*, ed. T. Birch, 6 vols. (London, 1772).
BP	Boyle Papers, Royal Society Library, London.
Calamy Revised	*Calamy Revised*, ed. A. G. Matthews (Oxford, 1934).
CJ	*Journals of the House of Commons*
CPW	*Complete Prose Works of John Milton*, ed. Don M. Wolfe (New Haven, 1953-).
CSPD	*Calendar of State Papers Domestic*
DNB	*Dictionary of National Biography*
DSB	*Dictionary of Scientific Biography*, ed. C. C. Gillispie (New York, 1970-).
EHR	*English Historical Review*
Ephemerides	Samuel Hartlib, 'Ephemerides', Hartlib Papers, Sheffield University Library.
Firth & Rait	C. H. Firth & R. S. Rait, *Acts and Ordinances of the Interregnum*, 3 vols. (London, 1911).
Harleian Miscellany	W. Oldys (ed.), *A Copious and Exact Catalogue of Pamphlets in the Harleian Library*, 10 vols. (London 1808-12).
HDC	G. H. Turnbull, *Hartlib, Dury and Comenius. Gleanings from Hartlib's Papers* (London, 1947).

HLQ	*The Huntington Library Quarterly*
HP	Hartlib Papers, Sheffield University Library. Quoted by bundle number in roman numerals, followed by the section indicated variously according to the handlists of the Hartlib Papers.
JEGP	*Journal of English and Germanic Philology*
JHI	*Journal of the History of Ideas*
LJ	*Journals of the House of Lords*
Mede *Works*	*Works of the Pious and Profoundly learned Joseph Mede,* ed. John Worthington (London, 1672).
MGP I & II	*Monumenta Germaniae Paedagogica,* vols. xxvi & xxxii (Berlin, 1903-4).
Notes & Records	*Notes and Records of the Royal Society of London*
ODO	J. A. Comenius, *Opera Didactica Omnia* (Amsterdam, 1657; rpt. Prague, 1957).
Oldenburg *Correspondence*	A. R. Hall & M. B. Hall (eds.), *The Correspondence of Henry Oldenburg* (Madison & Milwaukee, 1965-).
Petty Papers	*The Petty Papers. Some unpublished writings of Sir William Petty,* ed. Marquis of Lansdowne, 2 vols. (London, 1927).
Phil. Trans.	*Philosophical Transactions of the Royal Society of London*
Specification of Patent	'Letters Patent and Specification of Letters Patent', 1617-1852. Patent Commissioners (London, 1854-7).
Underwood	*History of the Worshipful Society of Apothecaries of London, abstracted from the notes of C. Wall by H. C. Cameron,* vol. 1, ed. E. A. Underwood (London, 1963).
Univ. Oxon. Arch.	University of Oxford Archives
VCH	*Victoria County History*
Venn	J. Venn & J. A. Venn, *Alumni Cantabrigienses. Part I. From the Earliest Times to 1751,* 4 vols. (Cambridge, 1922-7).
Walker Revised	A. G. Matthews, *Walker Revised* (Oxford, 1948).
Wood *Athenae* & Wood *Fasti*	A. Wood, *Athenae Oxonienses,* ed. P. Bliss, 4 vols. (Oxford, 1813-20).
Wood *Hist. & Antiq.*	A. Wood, *The History and Antiquities of the University of Oxford,* ed. J. Gutch, 2 vols. (Oxford, 1792-96).
Worthington, *Diary*	John Worthington, *Diary and Correspondence,* ed. J. Crossley, 3 vols. (Chetham Soc., Manchester, xiii, xxxvi, cxiv, 1847-86).

Acknowledgments

I have received the assistance of many librarians and I would like to thank particularly Miss J. L. Gilham of Sheffield University Library for her help with the Hartlib Papers which have been extensively utilised in the present study. The Hartlib Papers are quoted with the kind permission of their owner Lord Delamere. I have also had the benefit of access to G. H. Turnbull's transcript of Hartlib's Ephemerides, which I am currently preparing for publication. I should also like to thank the relevant bodies for permission to quote from the manuscripts in the archives of the Royal Society, the Royal College of Physicians, Trinity College Dublin, and the Osborn Collection, Yale University.

Introduction

The history of science has predominantly assumed the character of an index of progress towards our present intellectual condition. By this standard alone, the period considered in the present study is one of almost unparalleled importance. It was distinguished by a spectacular phase of creative work in experimental science, the rapid development of scientific organisation, and a major philosophical reorientation. It is not an exaggeration to claim that between 1626 and 1660, a philosophical revolution was accomplished in England.

It is impossible to avoid noticing that the discoveries which now constitute such an important element in our scientific outlook, and which are basic to our general education, occurred at a time of general intellectual readjustment. The period of spectacular scientific advance coincided with the economic, political and religious changes of the Puritan Revolution. This coincidence inevitably raises the question of the relationship between the various fields of intellectual activity. Although it is increasingly appreciated that there was a considerable degree of interaction between most areas of speculation and that intellectual attitudes were deeply influenced by social and economic circumstances, developments in science have usually been considered without more than incidental reference to other factors in the historical situation. However this is not so much a reflection of the independent character of scientific activity as a distortion in perspective caused by the evaluation of science in terms of the contribution made to a small number of classic problems selected chiefly from the physical sciences. This highly exclusive approach may be satisfactory for certain limited purposes, but it is contended here that the characterisation of many of the most intrinsically interesting scientific, medical and technological developments which occurred during the Puritan Revolution, cannot be undertaken without serious reference to the intellectual and social context in which they occurred. The present study is designed to bring the treatment of the sciences into line with that accorded to other aspects of intellectual and social history.

A work of this kind makes no pretence of providing a detailed guide to discoveries and precursors; rather it aims to contribute towards an understanding of the worldview of a particular society. In this case, it has been decided to concentrate on the Puritans, the group which formed the dominant element in English society in the middle of the seventeenth century. Puritan contributions to science have already attracted some attention because of their relevance to the seventeenth-century intellectual revolution, but the historical study of attitudes towards the natural world has an inherent value which is independent of any proof of affinity with the conventional wisdom of modern western society. Current beliefs must not be allowed to exercise a censorship on the past; the worldview of any cultural group merits attention in its own terms. Only by accepting this scale of values, will the role of scientific ideas within the complex network of beliefs of any society be fully appreciated.

The following chapters survey the scientific activities of the period 1626 to 1660 in terms of priorities which were uppermost at that time. From this perspective the famous discoveries take on a more limited function. They are an integral part of the picture, but they are by no means the most conspicuous element. Work on astronomy, mechanics and physiology of the kind which has subsequently won acclaim was undertaken mainly by small sections of the community of natural philosophers whose circumstances favoured studies of this kind. The majority of investigators approached science from altogether different points of view. Although the work of this larger class has hardly been noticed, it is essential for any apprehension of the general pattern of intellectual change. By such detailed reference to the historical context, we may come to appreciate the ideological factors which allowed particular philosophical attitudes to prevail, or which caused rival groups to apply their resources towards the study of different types of natural phenomena.

Any investigation of the place of science within the conceptual framework of economic, social, political and religious ideas involves a considerable readjustment of perspective. The historian of science cannot afford to ignore the general historical situation, if he is to be concerned with more than superficial description. Equally, the historian must recognise that science (as much as economics or political theory), when viewed in non-anachronistic terms represents an extremely significant aspect of the historical picture.

While the revolutionary decades 1640-1660 have been adopted as the nucleus for the present study, it has also been necessary to pay considerable attention to the years before the Revolution, both for the sake of comparison, and for examination of the genesis of important elements in the puritan ideology. The revolutionary crisis began in 1640, but the foundations of puritan power were laid at a much earlier date. For the sake of convenience, 1626 has been adopted as a starting point; however this date has not been arbitrarily chosen. 1626 was marked by a major phase in the consolidation of the opposition party of puritan laymen and clergy. A leading member of this group was John Preston, the Master of Emmanuel College, Cambridge. Among Preston's protégés was Samuel Hartlib, who came from Elbing to study at Cambridge during 1625 and 1626. He decided to settle permanently in England where he quickly became one of the leading activists in the puritan movement. 1626 is also the year of the death of Francis Bacon, whose philosophical system, the *Instauratio Magna,* came to assume overwhelming significance among puritan intellectuals. Immediately after Bacon's death, other events occurred which were important for the formation of the puritan worldview. These included the publication in late 1626 of Bacon's utopian fragment *New Atlantis,* and the simultaneous publication in 1627 of two major millenarian commentaries, Joseph Mede's *Clavis Apocalyptica* and Johann Heinrich Alsted's *Mille Annis Apocalypticis Diatribe.* Then in 1628, the year of the publication of William Harvey's *De motu cordis,* and of the death of John Preston, the Massachusetts Bay Company was founded. Thus between 1626 and 1628 personal allegiances were settled and intellectual trends set in motion which achieved their full expression at the outset of the Puritan Revolution in 1640. It is also interesting to note that, as the sociological analysis of Merton has demonstrated, this period between 1626 and 1640 is marked by a definite acceleration in the rate of recruitment to the sciences.

In the course of any assessment of the attitude towards the natural world of the Puritans, it is necessary not only to break away from the preoccupation with similarities between past and present science, but also to acknowledge the intellectual gulf which separates the highly-developed professional science of modern industrial societies from its analogue in earlier periods. Even to establish the continuity of present science with that of the nineteenth century is difficult, but social and religious developments since 1700 make it much harder for us to appreciate the modes of thought prevalent before that date. We have been misled by the subtle philosophical reasoning of Hobbes, the rigorous experimentalism of Harvey or Boyle, and the abstract mathematical analysis of Newton, into believing that the natural philosophers before 1700 thought in essentially modern terms, differing merely in lacking our considerable resources of experience and information. Full exploration of the evidence indicates that any understanding of the seventeenth-century worldview necessitates attention to the character of religious motivations, of adherence to philosophical tenets which have subsequently been discarded, and of involvement in contemporary political affairs. In other words, while a number of principles were adopted in the seventeenth century which are congruent with modern scientific knowledge, the general conceptual framework in which these principles were maintained was entirely different.

In order to draw attention to this factor, the present book begins by considering the scientific implications of puritan eschatology. The intellectuals of the mid-seventeenth century were deeply affected by the catastrophic events of the Thirty Years War, which disrupted the life of the entire European continent. England for a time stood apart from this conflict, but in 1641 the Irish Rebellion signalled the onset of a civil war which gradually engulfed the whole nation, Ireland, even the West Indies and the American colonies. In the face of this universal crisis there emerged a growing conviction, particularly among the Puritans, that Christian civilisation was approaching its final age. Millennial eschatology had widespread repercussions, and the search for a mode of life appropriate to the situation inevitably affected attitudes towards the natural world. The unprecedented upheavals of the period were seen, not as a sign of a further fall from grace, but as a prelude to the final judgement and rule of the saints. Puritan theologians were thus able to draw comfort from the omens; parliamentarians projected their policies as having divine sanction and their military forces assumed the character of Christ's army in a holy war. The sciences were employed to add precision to the millennial outline drawn up by theologians; conversely, millennial ideas furnished the natural philosopher with new premises and goals. It seemed that the fateful intellectual decline which had begun with the Fall of Adam might at last be reversed. Some indications of restitution had already occurred, following the Reformation, but to all appearances the tide of history now flowed ever faster and the natural philosopher might dare to look forward to an age of unprecedented achievement. The Puritan Revolution was therefore seen as a period of promise, when God would allow science to become the means to bring about a new paradise on earth. Science accordingly assumed considerable significance in the puritan programme and the puritan intellectuals became committed to a dedicated attempt to procure the return of man's dominion over nature.

Because of its profound implications for science, eschatology provides a natural foundation for the exploration of the ramifications of puritan science and medicine. After an introductory discussion of the philosophical dimension of millenarian eschatology, the later sections of this book will consider the major aspects of puritan science; and in these sections an attempt will be made to estimate the degree to which the Puritans were able to translate their ideas into social action, in accordance with their avowedly utopian commitments.

I

The Great Instauration

> 'So at length, when universal learning has once completed its cycle, the spirit of man, no longer confined within this dark prison-house, will reach out far and wide, till it fills the whole world and the space far beyond with the expansion of its divine greatness. Then at last most of the chances and changes of the world will be so quickly perceived that to him who holds this stronghold of wisdom hardly anything can happen in his life which is unforeseen or fortuitous. He will indeed seem to be one whose rule and dominion the stars obey, to whose command earth and sea hearken, and whom winds and tempests serve; to whom, lastly, Mother Nature herself has surrendered, as if indeed some god had abdicated the throne of the world and entrusted its rights, laws, and administration to him as governor.'
>
> Milton, Prolusion VII, *CPW*, i, p.296.

(i) Providential History

At the inception of the English Revolution two themes were brought together which had come to assume particular importance among English Puritans. The first was millenarian eschatology and the second, belief in the revival of learning. The former was associated with the belief that God had sanctioned the Reformation and would ultimately grant complete victory for the reformed churches over the catholic forces of Antichrist. During the Counter-Reformation, the Thirty Years War, and the period of Laudian suppression in England, the millennial idea was important in reviving the flagging spirits of the entrenched protestants. However bleak the immediate prospects, the saints could look forward to a period of reconciliation and utopian conditions on earth. The revival of learning was a newer concept, but it came to occupy an increasingly important role in the puritan consciousness. The recent reaction against the corrupt philosophy of the heathens and the search for a new philosophy based on experience appeared to seventeenth-century protestants to be thoroughly consistent with the religious reformation. The invention of printing and of gunpowder, and particularly the voyages of discovery, seemed to herald a revival of learning which was seen as thoroughly consistent with the envisaged utopian paradise and indeed capable of providing the means whereby the utopian conditions would be realised.

Upon examination of the prophetic texts, it was immediately appreciated that the advancement of learning and the return of the dominion of man over nature were important elements in the eschatological scheme. In this context, the fourth verse of Daniel 12 was of crucial significance and it will be seen below that this verse became the common denominator of the puritan millennial forecasts. The text was constantly reiterated, and given new connotations; it became central to the writings of the philosophers from whom the Puritans drew their inspiration. Thus the advancement of learning became an important dimension of the general millennial scheme and by this means science, medicine and technology were assured of an integral part in the mentality of the English Puritans throughout the revolutionary decades.

John Milton was not exceptional in believing that 1640 marked a turning point in English history. He was merely giving articulate expression to a view-point which was held by a mounting body of puritan opinion. Indeed this idea became central to Milton's thought and to the whole puritan movement during the revolutionary decades. According to Milton, the long-suffering elect had at last been rescued from the very shores of the Red Sea and were about to be brought in triumph from the wilderness to perform great works. 'Brittains God' had watched over His favoured nation as it suffered under the intolerable yoke of prelates and papal power. Having stubbornly resisted persecution, the saints were at last permitted to take up the offensive and prepare to sweep away the 'remaining dregs of superstition'. This situation provided them with their supreme test. If they succeeded England would once again play an honourable part in world reformation. But if their spirit failed, the nation might never again be permitted to share the benefits of God's grace; it would be condemned to live in darkness into the final age of the world and suffer under the final retribution. Uncompromising exertions were demanded, for 'if we freeze at noone after an earely thaw, let us fear lest the Sunne for ever hide himselfe, and turne his orient steps from our ungratefull Horizon justly condemn'd to be eternally benighted.'[1]

The parliamentarians entered into civil war convinced that their efforts were part of a preordained cosmic plan, which would terminate with the establishment of the Kingdom of God. Puritans of all shades of opinion rationalised their situation; they conveyed to the public the impression that the nation was entering into a holy war, in which the royalist enemy represented the forces of Antichrist.

The public was well-prepared for this analysis, being accustomed since the Reformation to examine events with a view to detecting evidence of God's special providential favours towards England. An authoritative statement of this position was Sir Walter Ralegh's monumental and widely read *History of the World,* which represented history, from

1. *Animadversions upon the Remonstrants Defence Against Smectymnuus* (London, 1641); *CPW,* i, p.705. For Milton's eschatology, see Fixler (100).

the creation to the last judgement, as a progressive manifestation of divine purpose.[2] Ralegh compiled his history of the ancient world with the intention of demonstrating that 'the iudgements of GOD are for ever unchangeable; neither is he wearied by the long process of time, and wont to give his blessing in one age, to that which he hath cursed in another.'[3] Although Ralegh's text made no direct reference to contemporary affairs, his readers were given ample scope for drawing parallels, with respect to sequences of events and personalities, between the ancient and the modern world. In order to underline this point, Ralegh's preface, which was fundamentally a masterly apologia for providential history, cited illustrations from recent French and English history to prove that divine retribution applied as much to the destiny of modern rulers as it had to the ancient monarchies. Ralegh's illustrations served not only an historical, but also a didactic and prophetic function.

Operating from essentially the same standpoint, Bacon recommended the compilation of a 'History of Providence' designed to trace the correspondence between the 'secret' and 'revealed' aspects of God's will. Among the philosopher's unpublished manuscripts was 'an Epitome of the Histories of the Bibel', which might well have related to his scheme for such a history.[4] Detection of rational purpose behind the serpentine windings and intricate mazes of history would serve to console the faithful and convict the consciences of the wicked.

The general appeal of the providential view of history is indicated by a stationer's comment to Hartlib that he 'commended Verulam's writings, above all Raleghs preface to the Historie which hee counted one of the excellentest peeces in the world for matter and eloquence or style.'[5] In more direct terms than Ralegh's sophisticated drama, Foxe's *Acts and Monuments* viewed history as a prolonged and shifting struggle between Christ and Antichrist, with England designated as the setting for the climax which would entail the complete supremacy of the elect. An unbroken line of saints and martyrs, beginning with Wycliffe and the Lollards, bore witness to the continuing outpouring of God's grace in recent times. Puritans under James I and Charles I cherished Foxe's image of Britain as the spearhead of the reformation, as they waited patiently for an opportunity to regain the initiative. Milton's unfulfilled plan for a national heroic epic was perhaps intended to illuminate this ideal, at a time of deep disquiet for the Puritans and when Foxe's book was refused a licence for reprinting.[6]

2. Sir Walter Ralegh, *The History of the World* (London, 1614): other editions —1617, 1621, 1628, 1634, 1652 etc. See J. Racin, 'The Early Editions of Ralegh's History of the World', *Studies in Bibliography*, 1964, *17*: 199–209; C. A. Patrides (ed.), *Sir Walter Ralegh: The History of the World* (London, 1971).

3. Ralegh (ed. Patrides), *op. cit.*, p.50.

4. Bacon, *De Augmentis* (13), p.66; Ephemerides 1639.

5. Ephemerides 1634.

6. William Haller, *Foxe's Book of Martyrs and the Elect Nation* (London, 1963); William M. Lamont, *Godly Rule: Politics and Religion, 1603–60* (London, 1969), *passim*; Fixler (100), pp.68–72.

One predictable consequence of preoccupation with providential history was curiosity about the final stages of human civilisation. Ralegh's history ended prematurely in antiquity, leaving the path to the day of judgement uncharted. Nevertheless, he followed other Christian historians in providing a general structure for future events in terms of a cyclical view of history. Generally, Christian synopses of history were constructed in terms of four or six monarchies, following the six Days of creation or the four Kingdoms of Daniel. But ultimately it had become necessary to postulate release from this cyclical process of generation and corruption, with the last judgement and the establishment of a durable Kingdom of God.[7] Events of the reformation suggested to the Puritans that the 'sad and ceasles revolution' of history was about to terminate in a period of 'Peace and termes of Cov'nant with us', which would raise the 'Britannick Empire to a glorious and enviable heighth with all her Daughter Ilands about her.'[8] Providential history merged with prophecy and eschatology, as the Puritans focused their attention on God's intended final settlement and its chronology. The precise nature of the judgement provided one area for speculation, but there was equal concern with penultimate events and with the prospects for the Kingdom of God on earth. This aspect of eschatology was particularly attractive since it appeared to offer a promise of imminent utopia.

In the search for further enlightenment about their place in the eschatological sequence, the doctrine of the millennium assumed among the Puritans a fundamental importance. As Woodhouse has observed, 'Daniel and Revelation afforded a key to events, past and present, and a vision of the future. From these books the Millenarians derived a view of history and a motive of revolution. And the pattern exhibited coloured the thought of many who could not be described as active adherents, so that one may speak of Millenarian doctrine as in a sense typical.'[9] Recent researches have confirmed the impression that millenarian influence was pervasive during the early years of the Puritan Revolution, although if this movement is to be understood in meaningful terms, it is necessary to heed Woodhouse's warning that the millennium was susceptible to many grades of interpretation.[10] At a

7. For examples of the extensive literature on this subject, see F. Smith Fussner, *The Historical Revolution: English Historical Writings and Thought* (London, 1962), Chapter VII; F. E. Manuel, *Shapes of Philosophical History* (London, 1965), pp.46–69; Herschel Baker, *The Race of Time* (Toronto, 1967); C. A. Patrides, *The Phoenix and the Ladder: The Rise and Fall of the Christian View of History* (Berkeley and Los Angeles, 1964).

8. Milton, *Of Reformation* (London, 1641); *CPW*, i, p.614; J. A. Bryant Jr., 'Milton's Views on Universal and Civil Decay', in J. M. Patick (ed.), *SAMLA Studies in Milton* (Gainesville, Fla., 1953), pp.1–19.

9. Woodhouse (340), p.41.

10. Fixler (100); Tuveson (294); Walzer (304); N. Cohn, *The Pursuit of the Millennium* (London, 1957); P. Toon (ed.), *Puritans the Millennium and the Future of Israel* (Cambridge, 1970).

purely verbal level, Daniel and the Apocalypse provided a rich vocabulary appropriate for describing the terminal struggles between Christ and Antichrist. Apocalyptic imagery had been widely used since the Reformation to rouse protestant vigilance against the encroachment of catholicism. 'Antichrist' and 'Babylon' then became popular epithets in the campaign against the 'novelties' associated with the ecclesiastical order of Archbishop Laud. One influential interpretation of the millennium was expounded in the commentaries of the Presbyterian Thomas Brightman. He modified the Augustinian account of history to locate the onset of the millennium in the fourteenth century, coincident with the first stirrings of the Reformation and the invasion of Europe by the Turks. Brightman regarded the millennium as the period during which the church would grow in authority to defeat Antichrist and ultimately establish the Kingdom of God on earth. This point of view differed substantially from the less orthodox interpretation, which anticipated that the millennium would begin at some date in the future. In this case a thousand-year rule of the elect was expected to follow the defeat of Antichrist. Many variants coexisted along with these two main interpretations, and there was endless room for divergence over points of detail. For instance, it was difficult to establish exactly at what stage the final suppression of Satan would occur, or when Christ would assume personal rule over His people. Some authorities concentrated on the spiritual aspects of the final age, while others speculated about the temporal dimension of His Kingdom.

All varieties of millenarianism found advocates and were openly publicised after 1640. The apocalyptic idea was exploited in a generalised manner to assist the campaign for the removal of abuses within the established church, and then to generate support for the Long Parliament, which was represented as God's agent of reformation. Apocalyptic imagery inspired the nation to resistance, providing consolation in defeat and renewing faith in ultimate victory. Apocalyptic themes came to play a dominating role in sermons, while the unrestricted press poured out a torrent of millennial tracts, including new editions of Brightman's massive works, translations of J. H. Alsted and Joseph Mede, and millenarian sermons, as well as astrological predictions and prophecies for popular consumption. This literature emanated from writers of widely varying education, who represented all facets of puritan opinion, and it was adapted for the tastes of all social classes. The Fast Sermons preached before the Long Parliament, one of the most important baro-

---

W. M. Lamont, *Godly Rule* (London, 1969); *idem,* 'Puritanism as History and Historiography', *Past and Present,* 1969, No. 44: 133–46; *idem,* 'Richard Baxter, the Apocalypse and the Mad Major', *ibid.*, 1972, No. 55: 68–90; B. S. Capp, *The Fifth Monarchy Men* (London, 1972); *idem, 'Godly Rule* and the Millennium', *Past and Present,* 1971, No. 52: 106–17; *idem,* 'The Millennium and Eschatology in England', *ibid.*, 1972, No. 57: 157–62. C. Hill, *Antichrist in Seventeenth Century England* (Oxford, 1971).

meters of informed puritan opinion, rapidly came to reflect the millennial theme.[11]

Millenarianism has always been a latent force in Christianity, but it has rarely received the sanction of the dominant ecclesiastical authorities. But periodically, usually in times of crisis, it has burst into the open and achieved brief but often spectacular phases of expression and wide public appeal. The Puritan Revolution was one of these periods and it was exceptional in the degree of penetration of millennial beliefs at all levels in the puritan community.

The eccentric activities of the Fifth Monarchists are well-known, but it should be remembered that this sect represented a peripheral remnant, exploiting a belief which had been central to puritanism at the outset of the English Revolution. Whether their millenarianism was conceived in terms of the latter-day glory of the church, or the personal reign of Christ, Puritans believed that they were participants in a crucial historical drama in which there would be both acceleration, and unexpected turns in events. They were warned, by Culpeper for example, to be prepared for rapid mutations and radical changes: 'and as we come nearer the center of Spirituall and Civill Truth soe will the motion be quicker and the day, (in any one place or kinde of governmente) will be shorter.' Thomas Goodwin informed his readers that they 'live now in the Extremity of Times, where Motions and Alterations being so near the Centre, become quickest and speediest; and we are at the Verge, and as it were within the Whirle of that great Mystery of Christ's Kingdome.'[12] The great cycles of history would terminate in a spiral of traumatic activity which would destroy the old imperfect order and pave the way for a new age.

(ii) The Chances and Changes of the World

It is apparent from the above remarks that millenarian eschatology would have been an important factor in shaping the worldview of that generation of Puritans which grew up in the decades before the Civil War. It became impossible to approach the future with equanimity, once it was clear that the world was approaching a cosmic watershed. If the nation was about to witness a period of unprecedented change, which would end in either uncompromising retribution, or idyllic rewards, no aspect of life could be free from the consequences. Accord-

11. J. F. Wilson, *Pulpit in Parliament* (London and Princeton, N.J., 1969), p.195.

From an examination of the Thomason Collection Capp estimates that 70 per cent of the ministers publishing new works between 1640 and 1653 subscribed to some form of millenarianism: *The Fifth Monarchy Men*, pp.38–9, 46–9. The reader will have no difficulty in adding to Capp's tentative list of works including millennial references.

12. Letter from Sir Cheney Culpeper to Samuel Hartlib, 11 March 1645/6, HP XIII; Goodwin, *An Exposition upon the Revelation*, quoted from *Works*, 3 vols. (London, 1683), ii, p.190.

ingly it became essential for puritan intellectuals to explore the implications of millennial eschatology, which was no less relevant to science and medicine than to politics and social policy.

The eschatological doctrines dominant among the English Puritans during the first decades of the seventeenth century were appropriate for a period of retrenchment. After a period of militancy and consolidation in the previous century, the tide turned and under the early Stuarts the Anglican church drifted away from the course of reformation. Antichrist appeared to be undergoing one of his periodic revivals. Although the balance was bound to be restored, this situation occasioned deep despondency among the Puritans; the triumph of the true church seemed a prospect too removed—'Sion lies waste and Thy Jerusalem, O Lord is fallen to utter desolation. Against Thy prophets and Thy holy men The sin hath wrought a fatal combination.'[13] In the Valley of Despair, there was a tendency to relapse into scepticism, whether about the western intellectual inheritance or recently contrived philosophies. The Golden Age, which was the subject of considerable literary comment among the English writers of the Renaissance, was seen as a remote ideal inherited from a receding past.

Millennial eschatology called for a more optimistic attitude; God would not permit man to attain his goals without tribulation, but a successful outcome need not be long delayed.

Millenarianism generated a more critical and aggressive attitude towards all agencies which were recognised as obstacles to the Reformation. First, as a political force, but soon in civil war, the Puritans were urged to unremitting exertions, with the assurance that they would be preserved by irresistible Providential forces. Following Brightman, the Anglican church was identified with Laodicea, the lukewarm; with striking uniformity, parliamentary sermons and pamphlets drew upon the resources of messianic language to demand a more zealous approach to reformation. The early prose writings of Milton, quoted from above, were a characteristic expression of this movement.[14]

For most Puritans, the millennium had only a transitory appeal. Once the immediate political and military objectives were attained, the quest for a stable religious and political settlement began; the millennium and messianic imagery were pushed into the background. However, for many reformers the millenarian doctrine had a deeper and more permanent significance. The New Jerusalem was not conceived in terms of minor religious changes, but as a dramatic leap forward which would achieve not only totally successful religious concord, but also social amelioration and intellectual renewal. Thus all social institutions were subjected to critical scrutiny, with a view to securing a higher plane of

13. Fulke Greville, *Caelica,* cix. For a further discussion of this subject, see Hill (149), Introduction.

14. For a brief survey of this subject, see Lamont, *Godly Rule,* Chapter IV; Fixler (100), Chapter III.

perfection. Millenarianism emancipated reformers from any obligation of respect for long-established institutions or of operation within the boundaries imposed by current intellectual values. An iconoclastic approach to conventional beliefs was permissible, if this cleared the way for an ideology more consistent with the gospels and the life of the saints in the New Jerusalem. Reference to this standard encouraged a more receptive attitude to new ideas, providing that these were consistent with puritan ethical tenets. Indeed, there was a positive inducement to think in utopian terms, given the biblical assurance that the saints were guaranteed success even in their most radical experiments. This positive spirit was responsible for the generation of ambitious schemes for the reconciliation of the churches, pressure for an aggressive foreign policy against catholic powers, support for the return of the Jews to England, and various unsuccessful attempts at a godly political settlement. Millenarianism also provided an incentive for idealists to frame social welfare proposals, plans for utopian communities, or proposals for law reform and the 'advancement of learning'. Implementation of these schemes was expected to initiate a gradual improvement in social organisation which would ultimately lead to a replication of the conditions of life associated with the Garden of Eden. In this age of perfection, man himself would recapture the intellectual attributes sacrificed by Adam at the Fall—in Milton's terms,

> 'Nature would surrender to man as its appointed governor, and his rule would extend from command of the earth and seas to dominion over the stars.'

It is apparent that millenarianism was not merely an abstract theological issue, but that its implications extended to the entire puritan social ethic. Accordingly it was inevitable that millenarianism should influence puritan attitudes towards the natural world. In general terms, it induced an increased confidence in the capacity of the human intellect; spectacular advances could be anticipated in all fields of learning. Hence the millennial doctrine promoted a confident, active and exploratory approach to nature in reaction against the sceptical and pessimistic attitude associated with the form of Christian humanism which had dominated the previous generation of puritan intellectuals. This change in temper among English Puritans precisely mirrors the change which had occurred among German intellectuals such as Alsted or Andreae a generation earlier, at the outset of the Thirty Years War.

The extent to which the implications of millenarianism were apparent to leading puritan theologians is well illustrated by the works of Goodwin, Twisse and many of their contemporaries. These writers indicate the degree to which the idea of the revival of knowledge was incorporated into the millennial scheme. The introduction of one of the major works by John Goodwin, the tempestuous vicar of St. Stephen's Coleman Street, was mainly contrived as an apologia for the revival of biblical exegesis. Goodwin argued that it was unreasonable to place a prohibition on new scriptural insights 'only because we never saw the face or heard the name till yesterday'. The parallel which naturally occurred to him was drawn from the results of recent geographical exploration. God had only recently revealed the existence of America, which was thought to equal the rest of the known world in extent. Goodwin predicted that, just as the earth was revealing a rich treasury, there would be an even more 'infinite varietie and endless varietie of the riches and treasures of the Scripture'.[15] He then turned to the prophetic text which provided the classic statement of his position. From the millennial passages of Daniel, it was concluded that the final age would be blessed by an unparalleled increase in knowledge:

> 'Secondly, the Scriptures themselves give us a propheticall intimation of this, that in and towards the latter ages of the world, their foundations (as it were) shall be discovered, and their great depths broken up, and that *knowledge shall abound, as the waters cover the face of the Sea. But thou, oh Daniel* (saith the Angell to him, *Dan* 12, 4) *shut up the words and seale the booke even to the time of the end* [meaning that *Daniel* should so carrie the tenour of this part at least, of his prophecie, that it should not be cleerely understood till the drawing neere of the time wherein it is to be fulfilled: and then] *many shall runne to and fro,* [that is, shall discourse and beate out the secrets of GOD in the scriptures with more libertie and freedome of judgement and understanding, and traverse much ground to and againe, on which no man should set foot, till that time] *and knowledg* [by this meanes] *shall be increased.*'[16]

The voyages of discovery and other achievements were cited to support the conviction that a new age was imminent. The comprehensive survey on the 'Power of Providence' produced by Hakewill, which will be discussed below, supplied ample examples to show that, in divinity, philosophy, ecclesiastical history, civil law, natural history and natural philosophy, even the longest-held opinions had ultimately suffered rejection. This far-ranging catalogue demonstrated that established systems of divinity, arts and sciences rested upon totally unsure foundations.

The text Daniel 12:4 came to play a fundamental role in the puritan faith in an imminent restoration of knowledge and return of man's dominion over nature. The importance attached to this latter belief is manifest in the authorised translation of the *Clavis Apocalyptica* of Joseph Mede, of Christ's College Cambridge, by then deceased. Mede's work had already achieved enormous popularity among puritan divines in the Latin form, originally published in 1627. In view of the wide

15. Goodwin, *Imputatio Fidei* (120), sig. b3v–b4r.
16. *Ibid.*, sig. b4r–v. Brackets as in the original.

public interest in the millennium and the increasing use of millennial texts to buttress the authority of parliament, it is not surprising that the Committee for Printing and Publishing of Books of the Long Parliament took an active interest in the propagation of Mede's work. Richard More, the Member of Parliament for Bishop's Castle produced a translation of the book and this was submitted by the Committee to Arthur Jackson, the minister of St. Michael Wood Street, in February 1642. In April Jackson reported favourably on the quality of the translation, noting that some of Mede's views were unconventional, but that 'the printing would not be perillous'. Accordingly the Committee ordered printing and *The Key of the Revelation* was furnished with a substantial explanatory introduction by Mede's friend William Twisse, vicar of Newbury, Berkshire.

Twisse described the recent rise of millenarianism among orthodox protestant theologians and explained Mede's part in this movement. Mede himself had scrupulously avoided specific predictions about the chronology of the period preceding the millennium, apart from one daring pronouncement that the pouring of the fourth vial signified the reign of Gustavus Adolphus. The defeat of Rome, the collapse of the Turkish Empire and the conversion of the Jews would occur at unascertained dates in the future. Twisse now undertook to explain the relevance of the recent crisis to the millennial sequence. The war, which had gradually engulfed Europe, was now 'amongst us'; an 'antichristian generation' had spread its tentacles of power. But the duration of this influence would be extremely short; indeed, Twisse predicted that after a war lasting for only three and a half years there would emerge a period of unparalleled joy for the saints.

> 'After this strange warre and slaughter of Witnesses which hasteneth to a Period, the continuance of it shall be but three years and a half, in which space of time, they that dwell on earth shall rejoyce over them and make merrie, and send gifts one to another because these prophets tormented them that dwelt upon the earth.'[17]

The successful conclusion of this war would denote the onset of the final events preceding the millennium. Military and political triumphs would be associated with intellectual regeneration.

Twisse actually began his preface by quoting Daniel: 'Many shall runne (or passe) to and from, and knowledge shall be encreased'. In this context he reported having recently read a manuscript which suggested Daniel had prophesied that navigation, commerce, the revival of knowledge, 'should meet in one time or age'. Twisse believed that this 'observation is justified by experience', even if divines questioned its relation to the text of Daniel. Twisse however did not doubt the connection and he regarded Mede's commentary on the 'mysterious booke'

17. Mede, *Key of the Revelation* (187), sig. b2v–3r.

of Revelation as one of the most recent manifestations of the revival of knowledge.[18]

The writings of Goodwin as well as Twisse show a tendency to press Mede's millennial interpretations to a radical extreme. In the interests of political militancy and religious reformation it was necessary for them to emphasise the imminence of the millennium. For this purpose Mede's conception of the future dramatic destruction of Antichrist and the inauguration of a thousand-year reign of Christ with his saints was more appealing than the gradualistic pattern of change sketched out by Brightman. Hence although Brightman's call for militancy captured warm support, Mede came to exercise the greater influence on puritan millenarian speculation.[19] The people were more likely to dedicate themselves to a self-sacrificing struggle with the forces of evil if they could be provided with both an insight into the millennial chronology and an impression of the prospects in store for the victorious saints. For reasons of prudence, doubt and lack of urgency, Mede had avoided describing the millennial kingdom in detail, but in 1640 the transformation of the political situation made it imperative for his followers to amplify this aspect of his commentary. A vision of intellectual progress and social amelioration, as outlined above, gave greater verisimilitude to the millennial ideal. With differing points of emphasis, the ideas about the millennial Kingdom put forward by John Goodwin and Twisse would have been congenial to such activists as Milton, Winstanley, Thomas Goodwin, Burroughes, Hartlib and his correspondents, or to the author of *A Glimpse of Sions Glory*. In each case Daniel 12:4 occasioned particular comment.

A Glimpse of Sions Glory gave a popular exposition of millennial doctrine, but the intellectual implications of Daniel 12:4 nevertheless received considerable emphasis. The anonymous author believed that this chapter of the scriptures had previously been misinterpreted, but that it now stood revealed as the authentic prediction about the times before the day of judgement; it was the book which God had ordered Daniel to close and which would only be understood when the millennium was imminent. From Daniel there emerged a picture of a 'glorious Reformation' in which 'they that are wise shall shine as the Brightness of the Firmament' and 'many shall runne to and fro, and take paines in finding it out, and Knowledge shall be increased'.[20]

Even at a late stage in the Puritan Revolution, John Beale retained an optimistic attitude to the millennial prophecies. The Fifth Monarchist Mary Rand may have been naïve in her predictions about the Philosopher's Stone, but a more sophisticated scholar could interpret this prophecy as justification for the Baconian programme:

18. *Ibid.*, sig. A3r. For the identification of the manuscript consulted by Twisse, see below, pp.21–2.

19. Lamont, *Godly Rule*, pp.94–8, suggests that Brightman was the major influence.

20. *A Glimpse of Sions Glory* (118).

> 'I cannot tell whether the philosophers stone will become soe speedily vulgar, as Mary Rante hath prophesyed but I see many juste grounds of appreciating gold, and of raysing vulgar things to bee more truely excellent, than gold or any Jewells. And of amplifying the dominion of good men over Gods works and of turning curses into blessings. Is it not high time for all that can believe so much as is nowe become obvious and in a manner exposed to their natural eyes, to unite together and joyne their strength and counsayles into the execution, performance, and practise of the best things and for the best ends?'

Through hard, disciplined labour and with the free communication of ideas, man would be restored to the condition foretold by Daniel:

> 'And as Man is thus by Light restord to the dominion over his own house, soe, by Magnalias that are brought to light, Hee is restored to a dominion over all the beasts of the field, over the birds of the ayre and over the fishes of the Sea. Here you must adde the discovery of, or dominion over all the Workes of God; the conversion of Stones into Metalls and backe againe; of poisons into powerful Medicines, of bushes, thornes and thickets into Wine and oyle, and of all the Elements to take such guise as Man by divine Wisdome commands. . . . And let all these Naturale Artificiall and Spiritual Wonders bee allwayes recorded to the prayse of the Most High.'[21]

The authors cited above, whether commenting directly on the text of Daniel or not, were united in believing in an imminent intellectual restoration. This was to be a notable aspect of the promised 'glorious Reformation'. Ideas on the intellectual dimension of the millennium matured very quickly, fed by chronological calculations and the innovatory philosophical ideas of Bacon and Comenius. Beale's letters show that a remarkably full impression of the millennial Kingdom had been achieved by that date. In addition the vocabulary of Bacon had been assimilated into the millenarian ideology; his philosophical programme, the *Instauratio Magna,* came to be regarded by Beale's generation as the authentic guide to intellectual regeneration. Accordingly the fragmentary philosophical system bequeathed by Bacon became for puritan intellectuals both the basis for their conception of philosophical progress and the framework for their utopian social planning.

(iii) Chronology

For the demanding exercise of predicting the millennial sequence, it was necessary to rely on expert witnesses, able both to utilise the evidence of

21. Letter from Beale to Hartlib, 22 March 1658/9, HP LI; for Mary Rand's prophecy, see Hill, *Antichrist* (151), p.119.

history, chronology and astronomy, and to deploy the techniques of computation. Mede was equipped to undertake this synthesis, but his *Clavis Apocalyptica* relied almost exclusively on a scientific and critical comparison of texts, or 'synchronism' between the prophecies of Daniel and St. John. However, certain mathematicians became absorbed with this problem, particularly in England, where a continuous and conspicuous tradition from Napier to Newton commented on biblical chronology, with special reference to the millennium. This demanding work was not merely an expression of disinterested scientific curiosity; it provides further evidence of the deep penetration of the millennial idea. The most detailed repository of information respecting the millennial chronology accessible to the Puritans was Johann Heinrich Alsted's *Diatribe de Mille Annis Apocalypticis* (1627), a commentary on Revelation 20, which was translated into English by William Burton in 1643, 'the yeare of the last expectation of the saints'.[22] Alsted's work represents the culmination of a considerable wave of numerological millennial forecasting in Germany in the first decades of the seventeenth century. Alsted approached his subject in a predictably encyclopaedic manner, and by drawing upon his knowledge of scriptural analysis and cosmology, he was able to reach a precise conclusion. As his translator claimed :

> 'Alstedius the Champion of the late Millenarians, and a maine prop of this new revised Doctrine, names and confidently determines the yeare of Christ 1694 (being 52 yeares hence) for the first yeare of this triumphant Reigne of the Saints on earth.'[23]

Since Alsted's tract, designed 'to comfort the desolation of Germany', telescoped the penultimate stages of history into fifty years, the hard-pressed protestant allies could foresee victory in the not-too-distant future. Alsted described this period as one of 'prostasis' or preparation for the final coming. The same prediction was equally appealing to the English Puritans at the outset of the Civil War, particularly since the German scholar attached particular importance to the conjunctions of Jupiter and Saturn expected in 1642 or 1643. These years were supposed to mark the 'Revolution of some new Government or Empire'.[24] Subsequent events seemed to uphold Alsted's predictions in a remarkable manner.

Alsted's numerological exercises were imitated by various English millenarians. Perhaps the best-known of these exponents was John Archer, the persecuted lecturer at All Hallows Lombard Street. In his extremely widely-read tract, Archer optimistically predicted that the conversion of the Jews would occur in 1650 or 1656; this would be

22. *The Beloved City,* 1643, p.119 (2). For a popular exposition of Alsted's ideas issued at the same time, see *The Worlds proceeding Woes and Succeeding Joyes* (1).

23. Alsted, *The Beloved City* (2), p.XX.

24. Alsted, *The Worlds Proceeding Woes* (1), pp.4–7.

followed in 1666 by the fall of Rome. Thereafter Christ would appear to take up his throne.[25] The number of the beast, 666, had always played an important part in millenarian speculation and the most ingenious English commentator on this theme was the versatile inventor, Francis Potter, rector of Kilmington, Somerset. His tract *Of the Number 666* was widely circulated in manuscript form and ultimately published at Oxford, his own university town, in 1642. Potter's curious work was described by Mede as 'the happiest that ever yet came into the world' on its subject.[26] Potter concentrated on 'the Root and Figure of every number, [which] are those things which are most essentiall and remarkable in it'.[27] By utilising what was then regarded as an advanced technique in arithmetic, the author believed that he could shed fresh light on the problem just as Gilbert in *De magnete* had used new techniques to investigate magnetism. The results of Potter's complex calculations were relatively unremarkable. As a good Anglican he made no comment on the millennium; but the protestant cause was identified with the number 12 (square root of 144), while Rome was characterised by 25 (approximate square root of 666). Hence yet another means was found to associate Rome with Antichrist. On eschatological matters Potter followed Foxe in pressing for a militant attitude against Rome on the part of the protestant princes, but it was left to others to spell out the precise chronology of the millennium. Generally it was expected that a rapid escalation of events would occur between 1641 and 1666. Although as indicated above millenarian ideas gained a wide currency, categorical and precise predictions of the kind just outlined were not universally welcomed. In spite of being an exponent of the latter-day glory of the church, and admirer of the work of Alsted, Hakewill objected 'that hee so precisely and punctually sets downe the very time, (namely the yeare of 1694) for the commencement of his happy and glorious Millenary'.[28] Ultimately only the Fifth Monarchist sects favoured precise predictions, and even they were judicious enough to propose alternative dates. Within these sects apocalyptic importance was attached to almost every year between 1641 and 1666.[29] Moderate millenarians were somewhat more cautious; but while appreciating the dangers of hasty speculation, they agreed that a sense of urgency was imperative. Hence, in the course of an examination of the views of John Tillinghast, the leading systematiser of Fifth Monarchist prophecies, John Beale commented that he was 'old enough to knowe, that noe small number of confident men have beene deluded in their

25. Archer, *The Personall Reigne of Christ upon Earth* (London, 1642).

26. Potter, *An Interpretation of the Number 666* (224); Madan (184), no. 1032. Letter from Mede to Hartlib, 24 January 1637/8, Mede *Works*, p.1077.

27. Potter (224), sig. *1r.

28. Hakewill (126), p.558. For similar reservations see Thomas Hayne, *Christs Kingdom* (London, 1642), Chapter V.

29. Capp, *The Fifth Monarchy Men*, pp.191–4; Hill, *Antichrist* (151), gives much information on millenarian prophecies.

presumptions upon this kind of calculation'. But such failures were not to be an excuse for complacency; the protestant nations should order their affairs in anticipation 'that the judgement will begin amongst us. For our protestants and all those who call themselves reformed, must ere long bee reformed, and bee newe-modelled before wee bee fit to call in the nations'. They should live in constant anticipation of a 'generall reformation' and of the second coming of Christ.[30]

(iv) The Golden Age

It is now necessary to examine the sources which were instrumental in shaping puritan opinion on the millennial kingdom and the promised state of learning. The writers quoted above give a remarkably uniform impression of the anticipated state of nature, suggesting that their views were developed within a well-formulated context. They were acutely conscious that, from an initial state of bliss, western society had entered into a catastrophic decline. For protestants however the Reformation marked a turning-point, and from their consolidated position in the seventeenth century they were able to look forward to a glorious future, which might exceed all past ages, even though its attainment would involve considerable upheavals and personal sacrifice. Thus the Puritans at the outset of the English Revolution were in a position analogous to that of the humanists of the Renaissance; they were totally disenchanted with their immediate intellectual inheritance and they looked back for inspiration to a distant unspoilt age.

Just as much as the humanists, the Puritans sought justification through affiliation with an indisputable, ancient authority. But whereas the former could draw sustenance from the Golden Age of Greek antiquity, the Puritans were obliged to react against this pagan model. Their inspiration came rather from the Fathers of the early church or the patriarchs of Israel. Therefore, although the Puritans became innovatory with respect to the immediate past, they were also deeply committed to the restoration of ancient wisdom. As philosophers and scientists, the Puritans are customarily remembered for their antipathy to ancient authority; they appear to be leading advocates of the 'new science' and the 'new philosophy' which evolved in the fertile climate of the seventeenth century. But as far as the Puritans themselves were concerned, new ideas were as has been indicated acceptable only if these conformed with their basic religious premises. Thus they were pledged to general 'reform' or 'new-modelling', but also just as much to 'revival', 'renewal', 'restitution', 'restoration' or 'instauration'. The language of this movement leaves no doubt that in pushing knowledge forward towards new frontiers, the labourers were convinced that their mission was sanctified by Israel's God. As Beale proclaimed:

30. Letter from Beale to Hartlib, 26 March 1659, HP LI. See also his letter of 15 May 1658, HP LII.

'Can good men think that since the Gospell is published, that Wisdome is extinguished by which Daniel reformed and recovered and agitated the Monarchy of the world and foretold the state of times to come.'[31]

The ultimate inspiration for puritan ideas on the Kingdom of God was of course biblical. The opening chapters of Genesis provided a model of the utopian state of innocence before the Fall; the Pentateuch and Historical Books gave an insight into the intellectual capacities of such patriarchs and rulers as Moses and Solomon; the Prophetic Books provided assurances of the return to an age of bliss. This latter prophecy was confidently reiterated by certain early Fathers, like Papias and Irenaeus, who embellished the account of the future Golden Age with materials drawn from Hellenistic sources.

To the Puritans of the seventeenth century, the Garden of Eden and the New Jerusalem were more than a poorly-authenticated record of man's ancestry, or a confused fantasy about the future. To the author of *Paradise Lost,* the Garden of Eden represented an ideal state of affairs which had an indisputable historical basis. Ralegh conducted his investigation into the location, size, and physical description of the Garden of Eden with scientific precision. To the commentators on the Apocalypse, the New Jerusalem was a concrete and attainable goal for the reformed church. Utopian town planners drew up their schemes with reference to the physical features of the city of Jerusalem.[32] With the amazing virtuosity of practised hands, the puritan exegesists elaborated a comprehensive picture from even the most scanty biblical materials. This was not merely an academic exercise; the reconstructions were presented in such terms as to provide an inducement to action; rewards were described in terms which were congenial to the mentality of the seventeenth century. Thus Milton's Paradise was luxuriant but it was not a steaming tropical jungle. It was fertile and temperate, not unlike the landscape of the south of England. There were no thorns or weeds, but Adam was not permitted to lead a passive and indulgent life. Rather, he was an active tenant farmer, charged by God to 'dress and keep his garden'. Like a dedicated English yeoman, he was committed to 'pleasant paines-taking'. Thus Adam was granted dominion over all other creatures, but only on condition that he displayed a lively scientific curiosity about his environment.[33] Intellectually Adam represented an ideal balance between the active, and the contemplative life. His knowledge was extensive, indeed encyclopaedic, as witnessed by his naming of creatures (Genesis 1:28), which

31. Letter from Beale to Hartlib, 15 September 1657, HP LI.

32. Potter (see note 26); Hermann Bauer, *Kunst und Utopie: Studien über das Kunst-und-Staatsdenken in der Renaissance* (Berlin, 1965); G. Münter, *Idealstädte ihre Geschichte vom 15.–17. Jahrhundert* (Institut für Theorie u. Geschichte der Baukunst, Studien zur Architektur u. Kunstwissenschaft, i, Berlin, 1957).

33. Milton, *Paradise Lost,* IV, 436–9, 625.

was customarily regarded as including an ability to decipher the nature of every creature from its name. Man's return to a state of grace would be rewarded by a restitution of this dominion over nature.

> 'And therefore it is not the pleasure of curiosity, nor the quiet of resolution, nor the raising of the spirit, nor victory or wit, nor faculty of speech, nor lucre of profession, nor ambition of honour or fame, nor inablement for business, that are the true ends of knowledge; some of these being more worthy than other, though all inferior and degenerate: but it is a restitution and reinvesting (in great part) of man to the sovereignty and power (for whensoever he shall be able to call the creatures by their true names he shall again command them) which he had in his first state of creation.'[34]

As Williams has perceptively noted, the description of Adam's intellectual attributes came to resemble the comprehensive tables of the sciences which introduced Bacon's *De Augmentis Scientiarum*.[35] The enterprise of reconstruction undertaken with respect to Adam and the Garden of Eden, was repeated in lesser detail for Moses, Solomon and a whole host of minor biblical figures, including Cain, Aholiab, Bezaleel and Elias the prophet. These figures were presented as an inspiring example of the capacities of the human intellect; they were an illustration of the powers which might be attained by the regenerate souls of the seventeenth century.

Perhaps the most detailed impression of the New Jerusalem based on biblical sources was produced by John Stoughton, the influential minister of St. Mary Aldermanbury. For this subject, Stoughton turned from the unadorned style of his English sermons to a rhapsodic Latin prose style which is often reminiscent of Virgil. He comforted his readers with the assurance that the catastrophic disruptions of the Thirty Years War would end with the fall of Babylon and the establishment of a millennial state (Millennium Optimum resurgentis in illa Luce Gloriae Sionis). Diverse biblical texts were assimilated to give a vivid impression of the new age. This would be a period of perfect harmony, both in the celestial and terrestrial worlds. The harmony of the heavenly spheres would be matched by aesthetic harmonies on the earth. There would be neither night, nor day; the sun and moon would shine simultaneously, both with a more radiant light. The heavens would radiate with an infinity of stars and the earth would be more fruitful. The whole earth would bring forth exotic fruits of a kind which had hitherto been confined to limited regions; all crops would yield more heavily. The mountains would generate gems and precious metals in abundance. Imperfections in the environment would vanish and there would be no limitation on human longevity. The wolf

34. Bacon, *Valerius Terminus,* Works, iii, p.222.
35. Williams, *The Common Expositor* (334), p.81.

and the lamb would live together in peace and no creature would prey upon another. This peaceful coexistence would extend to human society, which would evolve towards a utopian state under the guidance of the saints. The divisions between the protestant churches would be healed and they would unite in the blood of Christ 'in unum universi, in unum Corpus, in unum Spiritum, unum Sensum, qui vere audiunt Christiani'. Besides this return to the state of grace, the general revival of learning, which was already underway, would be pressed to its conclusion. Philosophy and poetry would be purified; voyages of exploration would reveal new and rich lands; technological labours would be rewarded; children would learn efficiently by new and effortless methods. The hard and unrewarding methods of the scholastics would be replaced by a revolutionarily new approach to knowledge, in which the public good would take precedence over individual gain. Philosophers would be guided by a plan for the Great Instauration (Instaurationem Magnam), which would direct both the course of systematic observation and the search for new secrets of nature by means of fructiferous experiments.[36]

Stoughton's predictions, albeit expressed with uncharacteristic floridity, would have been totally acceptable to the puritan intellectuals. Twisse and Goodwin represented the same point of view, but in a more conventional exegetical context. Milton's Paradise and Stoughton's New Jerusalem were essentially similar expressions, derived from a common biblical source. Running throughout their writing was the belief in a Great Instauration, the complete return of man's dominion over nature. Although this doctrine of regeneration could be justified on many grounds, it is clear from the above survey of millenarian writings that the biblical text which provided the main foundation for this belief was the prophetic book of Daniel. Puritan commentators increasingly turned to Daniel, and their attention became particularly focused on its final chapter. Among the thirteen verses of this chapter, verse four contained the justification for the Great Instauration:

> 'But thou, O Daniel, shut up the words, and seal the book, *even* to the time of the end: many shall run to and fro, and knowledge shall be increased.'

This text not only provided the basis for speculations about an intellectual reformation, it also related this event to the millennium. Further, it predicted that the meaning of the verse would not be fully comprehended until the dawn of the final age. At the advent of the Civil War, this verse appeared to relate very much to the English condition, and Daniel 12:4 stands out accordingly as the common factor in all of the millenarian writings cited above. The book of Daniel was unsealed; and its millennial prophecies were deciphered with reference to the Thirty Years War. The catastrophic events of this conflict

36. Stoughton, *Felicitas ultimi saeculi*, 1640 (272).

appeared to signify the irreversible decay of the old political and religious order. On the other hand, Europe seemed to be on the verge of an intellectual rebirth. In scientific and philosophical matters, neither the scholastics, nor the erudite authorities of antiquity or the Renaissance, were capable any longer of giving intellectual satisfaction. The technological discoveries of the Renaissance, particularly those relating to gunpowder, printing and navigation, appeared to represent a movement towards the return of man's dominion over nature. In the wake of technological improvements would come the rise of experimental philosophy, and in accordance with the prophecy of Daniel, communications had been improved in all respects, thus creating the conditions for a dramatic increase in knowledge.

(v) Philosophies of the Millennium

Millenarianism, then, was able to contribute an initial spur to action and an inspiring picture of final rewards. It also defined the ethical standards appropriate for life in the final age. But it offered no detailed and specific programme for the attainment of these ambitious intellectual and moral goals. The Puritans were therefore obliged to look beyond biblical authority in their search for philosophical enlightenment and the means of social improvement.

Their first task was to redress that inclination to philosophical scepticism which had been generated by experience of moral decline and persecution under the early Stuarts. Meditation on the Fall and the corruption of human nature had come to preclude any thoughts of regeneration, which seemed too distant to bear thinking about. This tendency to derogate the human intellect and dwell on the dangers of curiosity had found repeated literary expression. Fulke Greville concluded:

> '*What then are all these humane Arts, and lights, But seas of errors? In whose depths who sound, Of truth finde only shadowes, and no ground.*'[37]

Consistent with this attitude was a tendency to emphasise the intellectual (and indeed physical) superiority of the ancients, which was very liable to pass over into a general defence of scholastic theology and philosophy. In refuting this whole viewpoint, John Goodwin in *Imputatio Fidei* turned to the most energetic defender of the moderns, George Hakewill of Exeter College Oxford. Hakewill's *An Apologie or Declaration of the Power and Providence of God* was first issued in 1627; it was enlarged both in 1630 and 1635, to become the major exposition of the view that the moderns were 'capable of deepe speculations and . . . as *masculine,* and lasting birthes, as any of the ancienter

37. Greville, *A Treatise of Humane Learning,* xxxiv. Italics as in the original.

times have done.'[38] Hakewill's survey provided convenient support for the contention that in all spheres of knowledge there were signs of a return to primitive purity. If the moderns failed to excel, Hakewill maintained, it was not because of any necessary deficiency of wit, nor the world's decay, but because of their own moral decadence. Hakewill wrote too early to be influenced by the full tide of puritan millenarianism. The first edition of his work emphasised the cyclical view of history, and the Kingdom of God was described in Augustinian terms. However in the third edition he commented briefly but favourably on both Mede and Alsted; he had accepted that the church would shortly witness an age of unparalleled lustre and glory and that 'either Elias himselfe, or some other great heroicall spirit . . . is yet to bee sent, for the accomplishing of this great businesse in *restoring of all things*'.[39]

John Jonston, a Scoto-Polish student at Leyden, was prompted by Hakewill's work to produce a similar defence of modern learning.[40] Although it was less well-known at first in England, and dismissed by Hakewill as a plagiarism, Jonston's book is of considerable interest in reflecting the drift of protestant opinion. Ostensibly Jonston covered the same ground as Hakewill, but much more briefly. Although he was indebted to Hakewill with respect to general matters of organisation, much of his illustrative material was original. Indeed he showed a much greater familiarity with contemporary developments in experimental science. This evidence convinced him that 'we may be able to do more than any Age before us. That they should not reflect on former times as to forget that God hath reserved something for them, if they not be wanting in themselves.'[41] Jonston also differed from Hakewill in displaying a far greater receptivity to millenarian ideas. Having begun with Hakewill's premise that the church was about to witness an age of great glory, he assembled chronological evidence from millennial writers to show that the ruin of Antichrist would occur in the near future. He described the opinions of Alsted, but inclined to the estimate made by Matthias Martinus, that the millennium had begun in 1628. In a somewhat ironical vein, Jonston claimed to be hesitant about expressing millenarian opinions, since such beliefs were still regarded as unorthodox in spite of the support of such venerable authorities as Papias, Irenaeus, Apollinarius, Tertullian, and Lactantius.[42]

Hakewill and Jonston undermined the position of the defenders of

38. Hakewill (126), sig. a2v–3r. Hakewill's work is discussed from a slightly different point of view by Jones (163).

39. Hakewill (126), pp.556–7.

40. John Jonston, *Naturae constantia seu diatribe . . . per posterium temporum cum prioris collationem* (Amsterdam, 1634). English translation—*A History of the Constancy of Nature* (165).

41. *Ibid.*, Preface.

42. *Ibid.*, pp.170–80.

ancient authority and helped to consolidate the mood of self-confidence among the Puritans. This was of considerable dialectical value, but their works otherwise provided only vague guidance about a positive philosophical programme. For this latter purpose the millenarians turned primarily to Bacon, but also increasingly to the more recent writings of Comenius. Comenius wrote too late to influence Hakewill, but Jonston made reference to both the synopsis of natural philosophy and the new method of teaching languages of his friend Comenius. John Stoughton emphasised the parallel between the Fathers of the early church and contemporary intellectual reformers in these terms:

> 'Unius Instauratoris Artium Admirator
> Summus, ut Aquila Sublimus:
> Veri Conditoris Templi Pansophiae Amator
> Sincerus ut Phoenici similis:
> Boni Conciliatoris Ecclesiarum Aemulator
> Sanctus ut Columbae Simplicis
> Verbo:
> Amator Polycarpi Pansophi Comenii:
> Aemulator Irenaei Ecclesiastici Duraei:
> Admirator Chrysostomi Organici Verulami.'[43]

The *instauratio magna* of Bacon, the *pansophia* of Comenius and the irenicism of Dury were represented by Stoughton as key manifestations of the approach of the final age.

Although neither Bacon nor Comenius is customarily regarded as sympathising with the millenarian position, it was entirely legitimate for the Puritans to draw attention to this aspect of their philosophies. The modern commentator tends to overlook this factor since he is usually concerned with those aspects of the thought of Bacon and Comenius which are relevant to contemporary philosophy or education, but the Puritans adopted an entirely different perspective. This necessarily involved selective, but not limited, reading. Manuscript writings as well as published works provided the basis for puritan assessments of both Bacon and Comenius.

It has already been observed, that Twisse introduced his Preface to Mede's *Key of the Revelation* by quoting Daniel 12:4. He was of course not exceptional in giving prominence to this verse, but its use in this case seemed particularly apposite since, as previously noted, Twisse reported at the same time that he had recently read a manuscript drawing attention to evidence which appeared to validate Daniel's text. The manuscript pointed out that in accordance with the prophecies of Daniel 'the opening of the world by navigation and commerce, and the increase of knowledge, should meet in one time or age'.[44] Twisse gave no further details concerning his manuscript source,

43. Stoughton (272), p.133.
44. Mede (187), sig. A3r.

but in all probability he was referring to Francis Bacon's fragment 'Valerius Terminus of the Interpretation of Nature', which was not published until 1734. We know that Bacon's followers collected and studied his manuscripts after his death in 1626. Different collections of posthumous writings were produced in 1626-7, 1629 and 1638, and preparations were made for the publication of many others. Nothing is known about the precise history of the manuscript of *Valerius Terminus* before it passed into the hands of the Earl of Oxford later in the century, but even modern commentators have recognised that, although it is one of the most disconnected and fragmentary of Bacon's works, 'it is at the same time full of interest, inasmuch as it is the earliest type of the *Instauratio*'.[45] There is every reason to believe that this work would have had a strong appeal for Bacon's puritan disciples, particularly in view of its opening chapter, 'Of the limits and end of knowledge', one of the four entire sections of the manuscript.[46] This chapter was designed to solve one of the basic dilemmas facing the protestant intellectual. If man originally transgressed and fell owing to his pursuit of knowledge, how could it be possible for him again to seek knowledge, without falling from grace? Bacon reconstructed the story of the Fall of Adam from the points of view of both God and man. He believed 'that knowledge is of the number of those things which are to be accepted of with caution and distinction'. He concluded: *'all knowledge is to be limited by religion, and to be referred to use and action.'*[47] This conclusion was perfectly adapted to the puritan position; investigations conducted into secondary causes, and with utilitarian ends in mind, would incur no risk of transgression, but instead glorify God, and restore man's dominion over nature. Moses and Solomon had successfully followed this course and were regarded by Bacon as an inspiration for later ages. If their example were followed, it would be revealed that 'many and noble are the inferior and secondary operations which are within man's sounding.' This message was of fundamental importance to the seventeenth century; God appeared to have sanctioned the rise of experimental science by a special prophecy. Bacon appreciated that he was making an enormous claim, but his conviction was expressed with firmness, if with humility.

> 'This is a thing which I cannot tell whether I may so plainly speak as truly conceive, that as all knowledge appeareth to be a plant of God's own planting, so it may seem the spreading and flourishing or at least the bearing and fructifying of this plant, by

45. Ellis in Bacon *Works,* iii, p.202.
46. *Ibid.,* pp.217–24.
47. *Ibid.,* p.218. Italics as in the original. See also pp.221–2: 'evermore it must be remembered that the least part of knowledge passed to man by this so large a charter from God must be subjected to that use for which God hath granted it; which is the benefit and relief of the state and society of man.'

a providence of God, nay not only by a general providence but by a special prophecy, was appointed to this autumn of the world: for to my understanding it is not violent to the letter, and safe now after the event, so to interpret that place in the prophecy of Daniel where speaking of the latter times it is said, *Many shall pass to and fro, and science shall be increased;* as if the opening of the world by navigation and commerce and the further discovery of knowledge should meet in one time or age.'[48]

Thus, the prophecy of Daniel was integrated by Bacon into the first draft of his philosophical programme. This religious foundation of his philosophy was not left to one side when he proceeded to the slow task of elaborating the plan for the Instauration and then completing the constituent parts. The very fact that shortly after the composition of *Valerius Terminus* Bacon decided to baptise his system, the *Instauratio Magna,* is probably indicative of a conscious desire to relate his philosophy to the Christian historical framework.

Examination of the first drafts of individual sections of the Instauration confirms the impression given by *Valerius Terminus.* Bacon's approach remained fundamentally historical and eschatological. Man's dominion over nature was sacrificed at the Fall; but the Bible gave many instances of the restoration of knowledge under God's grace. Bacon believed for instance that the philosophy of the Presocratics was basically uncorrupt, but that subsequently the schools of Greek philosophy had brought about total intellectual degradation. Their authority had persisted until Bacon's own day, but he confidently predicted that their tenure of power was almost ended. Already the scholastic edifice was under attack and there were unambiguous signs of regeneration. In *Cogitata et Visa,* Bacon enlarged upon his view of the providential course of history, with particular reference to one of his favourite maxims, 'that truth is the daughter of Time'. He expanded upon the omens described in *Valerius Terminus*: the recent ambitious voyages of discovery (per longinquas illas navigationes et peregrinationes) he argued, had provided a material basis for a new philosophy. Philosophy could also expect to benefit from the rise in the mechanical arts, which seemed to be inspired by a 'vital breath'. Printing had revolutionised communications to permit discoveries and opinions to be disseminated 'like a flash of lightning'. It would be tragic if this expansion of human horizons were not carried over into philosophy, owing to the latter's confinement within the narrow boundaries of scholastic knowledge. Europe seemed to be moving into a new state of political and religious tranquillity, creating conditions which would be favourable for the contemplation of the power, wisdom and goodness of God's works. Time seemed to promise a great instauration.[49]

48. *Ibid.*, pp.220–1.
49. *Cogitata et Visa,* Bacon *Works,* iii, pp.612–13.

Another of Bacon's early writings, a speculative sociology of knowledge, was the rather grandiloquent sketch *Redargutio Philosophiarum.* This also distinguished between the independent-minded Presocratics and their more influential successors. The former adopted a fruitful and pragmatic approach to nature, but their views were readily suppressed by later Greek philosophers who enforced their corrupt opinions by constructing systems and establishing schools. Bacon's caricatures of the ancients ended with an appeal to men to shake off their chains and become masters of themselves. The limits of the intellectual globe had not been defined by the ancients; the voyages of exploration gave insight into the wonderful potentialities offered by God to man. He returned to the comparison between philosophy and cosmography, already mentioned in *Cogitata et Visa* :

> 'It would disgrace us, now that the wide spaces of the material globe, the lands and seas, have been broached and explored, if the limits of the intellectual globe should be set by the narrow discoveries of the ancients. Nor are those two enterprizes, the opening up of the earth and the opening up of the sciences linked and yoked together in any trivial way. . . . Not only reason but prophecy connects the two. What else can the not at all obscure oracle of the prophet mean which, in speaking about the last times says : *Multi pertransibunt et multiplex erit scientia?* Does he not imply that the passing through or perambulation of the globe of the earth and an increase or multiplication of the sciences, were destined to occur in the same age and century? (ac si orbis terrarum pertransitus sive peragratio, et scientiarum augmenta sive multiplicatio, eidem aetati et saeculo destinarentur)'.[50]

Once again key importance was attached to the prophecy of Daniel. Indeed its frequent appearance in Bacon's early writings suggests that it may well have constituted an important element in his personal motivation. Although in his mature works Bacon became preoccupied with detailed philosophical or scientific issues, the historical, providential and millennial themes were never far from sight. Hence in *Novum Organum* he confidently reiterated his interpretation of Daniel's prophecy to mean that 'the passage through the world (which now by so many distant voyages seems to be accomplished, or is in the course of accomplishment) and the advancement of the sciences, are destined by fate, that is by Providence, to meet in the same age.'[51] This millennial passage might be overlooked, but the theme would constantly be brought to mind by Bacon's philosophical terminology, or by the decorative title-pages of *Novum Organum* and *De Augmentis Scientiarum* which gave

50. *Redargutio Philosophiarum,* Bacon *Works,* iii, p.584.
51. *Novum Organum,* I, 93.

emblematic expression to the motto *'Multi pertransibunt et augebitur scientia'*.[52]

When it is appreciated that Bacon's philosophical system evolved in the context of the Calvinist code of ethics as well as of the providential and millenarian view of history, it is not surprising that his works came to be regarded by the Puritans as the philosophical complement to Foxe's *Book of Martyrs*. The one promised a successful conclusion to the religious reformation, the other provided the blueprint for philosophical reform. Hence Bacon's writings, for such divines as Stoughton, Hakewill and Twisse, assumed an almost canonical status. This influence extended, until Bacon became the most important philosophical and scientific authority of the Puritan Revolution. It is therefore only a slight exaggeration to regard Baconianism as the official philosophy of the Revolution. The 'Advancement of Piety and Learning' became inseparably associated aims in the programme of the puritan intelligentsia. And as Beale's letters indicate, descriptions of the millennial revival of knowledge tended to be written in terms of the fulfilment of the Baconian Instauration.

There were of course other philosophical reformers who appealed to the Puritans. It is notable in this context that Comenius, the figure who ranked nearest to Bacon in their estimation, tended to reinforce the religious and millenarian associations of the new philosophy. This bias is not surprising in a figure who had been educated in the Calvinist academy at Herborn and who was an immediate pupil and friend of Alsted. But the millenarian idea was greatly re-emphasised in writings produced in connection with his brief visit to England on the eve of the Civil War. Particularly important in this respect are *Pansophiae prodromus*, 1637 (translated in 1642 as *A Reformation of Schools*) and the manuscript of *Via Lucis*, a work which was composed in 1642, but not published until 1668.

Like Bacon, Comenius conducted the defence of his new pansophic philosophy in historical terms; the scriptural foundation for his position was even more explicit. The causes for the intellectual decline of western society were examined, and avenues proposed for the rescue of civilisation from the darkness of barbarism.[53] Comenius provided a slightly different perspective on the dawning of the promised age of light as indicated by the appearance of printing and the improvement of navigation. By the former, God provided 'A mechanism for communication with all the epochs of the past'; through navigation 'communications have been opened up between men scattered through various continents'. Not unexpectedly these innovations were identified as the fulfilment of the prophecy of Daniel: 'For this end God permits, nay, even compels, so many men to run to and fro, in order

52. This title-page also probably alludes to Isaiah 11:9, 'the earth shall be full of the knowledge of the Lord, as the waters cover the sea.'

53. Comenius, *Via Lucis* (55), especially pp.34–7, 103–11.

that knowledge may be increased.' If these improvements were complemented by 'an easie way of teaching all men all things' there would be nothing to hinder the Golden Age of knowledge which was eagerly awaited.[54]

The new age was described in terms reminiscent of *Felicitas ultimi saeculi.* Drawing on the same scriptural texts as Stoughton, Comenius produced a vivid sketch of the glorious state of the church on earth. This age of light was not yet realised, but its appearance was guaranteed: 'for it is necessary that all that has been pre-determined by the counsel of God and foretold by his word must first be fulfilled and brought to completion.'[55] Positive policies for this situation were explained by Comenius in terms of the imagery of light. This metaphor was of course a Christian commonplace, but the millenarians made it peculiarly their own. Since God reserved his greatest gifts for the last age, this was the age of the greatest light, and most profound enlightenment. The emergence of the age of light out of unsettled conditions was both described and given emblematic expression by Comenius.

> 'But it sometimes happens that rain or mist comes on in the morning, and then the sun dispels the darkness of the clouds with more difficulty and more slowly, and only succeeds at last towards the evening in pushing forth its conquering rays, and rejoicing the inhabitants of the world with its full vision. And it is not otherwise with the intellectual light of the soul, namely, Wisdome.'[56]

This image must have seemed particularly pertinent to conditions in England and Europe at that time, when storm clouds were gathering and when there were few signs of the conquering rays of light.

On intellectual matters Comenius followed Bacon in calling for an emancipation from Greek philosophy, which had 'inflicted so many injuries upon the Christian spirit.' This release would prepare the way for a totally new philosophy which, in Comenius's case, involved a syncritical fusion of elements from rational, empirical and biblical sources. The Comenian philosophical programme for the regenerate age was framed with explicit reference to the millennial goal. The plans for a Universal College, Universal Schools, Universal Knowledge and Universal Language, which were initially outlined in *Via Lucis,* ultimately became the foundation for the exhaustive *Consultatio Catholica,* which may be regarded as the Comenian complement to Bacon's *Instauratio Magna.*[57] Both systems were conceived as a means of completing the restoration of that harmony of nature which was sacrificed at the Fall. Their final aim was no less than 'Light, Peace,

54. *Ibid.*, pp.105–8; *A Reformation of Schooles* (52), pp.3–4.
55. *Via Lucis* (55) p.44.
56. *Ibid.*, pp.101–2.
57. This was largely completed by 1657, but it was not published until 1966.

Health . . . and that golden age which has ever been longed for.'[58]

The work of both Bacon and Comenius was unfinished. Inevitably philosophical programmes which were framed with universalist and millennial aims in mind, and undertaken virtually single-handed, were destined to a fragmentary conclusion. But the edifice was sufficiently complete to serve as an inspiration to puritan intellectuals at a time when the revolutionary ideology was in process of forming.

(vi) The Great Instauration

When reinforced by the philosophical doctrines of Bacon and Comenius, millennial eschatology, already exploited to lend weight to the cause of ecclesiastical and political reform, could emerge as an inducement to total reformation. A new dimension was thereby added to the puritan programme; the Puritans in general became aware of the significance of the new philosophy and the advocates of intellectual reform cemented their attachment to the puritan cause. The revolutionary ideology was thereby strengthened in an important respect.

For puritan intellectuals the millennial context was of vital importance in determining the tone of their scientific effort. In certain connections they investigated subjects which are relevant to the 'enduring scientific debates' of the historians of science. However, this element constitutes an insignificant proportion of puritan science, which was dominated by the millennial and universalist aims of the Great Instauration. Millennial ideas were all-pervasive, causing attention to be directed towards particular fields of research, as well as determining conceptions of ultimate goals. Programmes of a utopian character were elaborated and there was every confidence that these would receive providential sanction.

The Puritan Revolution accordingly appeared to mark the time appointed for the restitution of man's dominion over nature. Nothing should be allowed to distract attention from the ultimate millennial goal. Bacon's frequent reference to the fable of Atalanta was designed to inspire vigilance against the distractions of ephemeral and limited rewards. When planning the work of the reformers, Joachim Hübner declared that 'All must bee done in relation to a perfect reformation'. It was unlikely that Comenius would be able to fulfil all of his promises, but Hübner believed that 'the world will always remaine indebted unto him for setling that notion that wee must know all Things'. Comenian *pansophia* assumed special significance in the providential scheme.

> 'Certainly God hase some special aime in bringing this notion of a pansophical learning into the world, though it bee so imper-

58. *Via Lucis* (55), p.9.

fectly as Comenius does it. It seemes to bee a preparation for that happy promised state of God's church and a forunner to bring men into that blessed and wished for unity and union, by stating of all the universal principles aright.'[59]

On the eve of the Revolution the Puritans became engaged in discussions about the exact course of the intellectual reformation; it was essential that their energies should be used to maximum effect. As Milton had stressed, they might not be given a second opportunity, if their effort were dissipated in the first attempt to frame an 'Idea' of reformation. It was therefore necessary to operate according to an agreed plan: Hübner for instance suggested that 'there should be first an *Idea Reformationis* elaborated and published, then the *Prodromus* with the *didactica,* then the *Pansophia.*'[60]

Although in the everyday scientific work of the Puritans it was not necessary to make explicit reference to the underlying theme of the Great Instauration, this idea was never far below the surface. Thus, Dury's apologetical introduction to Boate's draft of a Baconian natural history of Ireland, drew attention to the 'neer approaches of . . . Liberty, and the advancement of the ways of Learning'. Cromwell, Fleetwood and the army had broken the former tyranny and established a political climate congenial to intellectual change. The day was approaching when the earth would be full of knowledge, as the waters covered the seas.[61]

'*The father hath reserved in his own hand the times and seasons,* [Acts 1:7] wherein these promises are to be fulfilled, yet as by the dawning of the day we can know that the Sun is neer rising, so by the breaking forth of yoakes and the breaking forth of the meanes of more perfect knowledge, both in Natural and Spiritual things, wee may see the drawing neer of the promises, which will in their own times Constitute *the day of Salvation unto all the Earth, wherein all flesh shall see the glory of the Lord together*' [Is. 40:5].[62]

Winstanley expressed his confidence in the dawning of a new age in very similar terms. The persecuted sons and daughters of Zion should gain comfort from the knowledge that the Beast's reign, although 'very hot, yet it will be short'. The Sun of Righteousness was about to disperse the cold, rainy clouds and 'make the earth (mankind) to become like the summer season, full of light, heat, fruitfulness and comfort'. The millennial idea was not confined only to Winstanley's social planning, or to the imperialistic economic designs of

59. Ephemerides 1639.
60. *Ibid.*
61. *Irelands Naturall History* (30), sig. A4r. Isaiah 11:9.
62. *Irelands Naturall History* (30), sig. A4v.

Worsley; it also impinged upon such mundane considerations as the life-span of fruit trees.[63]

Certainly not all puritan intellectuals subscribed to the millennial idea with the enthusiasm shown by Dury, Beale, Worsley, Stoughton or Winstanley. Others remained within the more conservative eschatological tradition expressed by Hakewill. But their idea of the latter-day glory of the church absorbed many elements from the more radical thinkers. Hakewill believed in the great providential design, the restoration of learning, and in the imminent destruction of Babylon. Thus an extremely broad group of Puritans looked forward to the Great Instauration. John Wilkins and John Wallis may be taken as representative major figures who adopted the more conservative position. Before their elevation to the universities, both were closer to the advocates of universal reformation than is customarily acknowledged. Wilkins's early interest in universal language is well-known. His first major writing *The Beauty of Providence* (1645) came near to the millennial writings in its treatment of the doctrine of providence. Recent chaotic changes might have suggested that there was no order or purpose in events; Wilkins appealed to his readers to examine the course of history more carefully. Then they would find that disorder and confusion were not in things themselves, but that all events were divinely ordained and history would resolve itself into 'the greatest serenity'. In many ways *The Beauty of Providence* was an updated, more concise, and popular exposition of the work of Hakewill; it also reflected the general spirit of Ralegh's preface to the *History of the World*. A considerable part of Wilkins's book was designed to dispel apprehensions about the disquieting course of contemporary events. In spite of civil disruption and 'revolutions' of government, the outcome (parliamentary supremacy) was sanctioned by Providence. The better-known sections of Wilkins's work, dealing with the divine plan in nature, were designed to reinforce the more general providential argument.[64]

John Wallis composed his first philosophical tract with the aim of correcting the epistemological ideas of Robert Greville, Lord Brooke. But while repudiating many of Greville's ideas on the unity of knowledge, he fully shared the latter's admiration for the pansophic endeavours of Comenius. Greville, a Platonist and patron of Comenius, was completely convinced of the intrinsic unity of nature. It was therefore with enthusiasm that he greeted the work of Comenius 'that mighty man [who] doth happily and rationally indeavour to reduce *all* into one.' Like the Cambridge Platonists, Greville applauded Comenius's attempt to unify philosophy and theology into a single body of Christian Philosophy.[65]

63. Winstanley, *The Breaking of the Day of God* (London, 1649), Preface; Beale, *Herefordshire Orchards* (23), pp.61–2. Malachi 4:2.

64. Wilkins, *The Beauty of Providence* (332), pp. 63–7.

65. Robert Greville, Lord Brooke, *The Nature of Truth*, 1640 (124), p.124.

Wallis adopted a more empiricist epistemology and was extremely suspicious of premature attempts to establish the unity of phenomena. But, no doubt attracted by the practical aspect of Comenius's philosophy, he advocated public support for the pansophic design.

> 'And indeed I wish as heartily as his Lordship that *Comenius* his designe of *reducing all into one,* might proceed. And great pity it is that so worthy a design is not prosecuted at a public charge, that such a shining light should be extinct for want of Oyl; if there may be hopes of effecting it.'[66]

It is apparent from the above comments that millenarianism played a considerable part in moulding the puritan conception of the Great Instauration. Science was pursued not as an end in itself, but for its value in confirming the power of providence and for its applicability to social amelioration. The puritan reformers diagnosed the deficiencies of current knowledge and sought solutions to all fundamental intellectual and social problems; in order to make headway with this ambitious programme, an essentially new attitude to knowledge was called for. It would be necessary for individuals to dedicate themselves in a totally disinterested manner to a great collaborative enterprise. The philosophies of Bacon and Comenius provided initial guidance on epistemology, methodology and science policy. Through the development of their ideas a new philosophy could be evolved which would be consistent with the spiritual enlightenment of the Puritans. Through universal education the young could be protected from the evils of pagan scholasticism and be exposed to a genuine Christian philosophy. Experimental medicine could solve the problems of disease; agricultural innovation could restore the plenty of a Garden of Eden; general economic reform might bring undreamed-of prosperity and elevate Britain to a position of world supremacy. This programme was an expression of a utopian mentality. Not only was there interest in the utopias of Bacon or Andreae; the new science of the Puritan Revolution was inaugurated by *Macaria* (1641), an ambitious plan cast in the utopian mould, but designed for immediate implementation by the Long Parliament. This idealistic spirit persisted; it was evident in new utopian works, projected utopian societies and the social programmes of authors such as Winstanley or Worsley, who cast aside the literary veneer of the older utopian literature in order not to obscure their essentially practical purposes. As Milton declared, it was not their aim to 'sequester out of the world into *Atlantick* and *Eutopian* polities', but to frame proposals which would bring about a world reformation.[67]

In view of these express priorities it is not appropriate to follow conventional practice in the historiography of science by examining puritan science in terms of contributions to the separate sciences of

66. John Wallis, *Truth Tried,* 1643 (301), p.91; quotation slightly abbreviated.
67. Milton, *Areopagitica, CPW,* ii, p.526.

anatomy, botany, optics or mechanics. Rather the central sections of this book will be concerned with the evolution of puritan opinion on communications, education, medicine, technology, economic planning and agriculture. These subjects represent some of the major categories of scientific effort recognised by the Puritans themselves.

II

The Spiritual Brotherhood

'So that now the question is not whether this Land, and so consequently other Kingdoms may live in worldly happiness and prosperity for ever hereafter, but whether they will do so or not; for if they be willing, they will shew the same by their actions, and then I am sure there is no doubt to be made of the possibility thereof: whereby *Utopia* may be had really, without any fiction at all.'

Gabriel Plattes, in *Samuel Hartlib His Legacy* (1655), p.207.

(i) The Spiritual Brotherhood

A large body of puritan opinion believed that the eagerly awaited reformation of the church would be accompanied by a Great Instauration of learning. Their reflections on the nature of the impending Instauration display a considerable degree of uniformity, both with reference to the interpretation of biblical authorities and in statements about a new philosophy of nature. This unity of outlook may be partly attributed to their common theological or philosophical affiliation, but it is also necessary to take into account the high degree of association between the Puritans themselves. Examination of the interconnections between Mede, Twisse, Goodwin and Stoughton, the major exponents of the millenarian position described in the previous chapter, indicates that they were by no means independent and isolated advocates of a common position. On eschatology as on other matters, a common viewpoint was evolved as a result of active discussion and free communication of ideas within the community of puritan intellectuals.

The substantive basis for the puritan position was provided by *Clavis Apocalyptica;* its author, Joseph Mede, was adopted as a model by the puritan natural scientists—versatile as he was, both as a biblical scholar and as a natural philosopher. Among his pupils at Christ's College Cambridge were John Milton and Henry More, both of whom were important as interpreters of Mede's eschatological position. Mede's work was assisted and promoted by Samuel Hartlib, the foreigner, who would have been able to acquaint the Cambridge scholar with the work of such continental chiliasts as Alsted, Jonston and Comenius, all of whom were among Hartlib's more intimate correspondents. These same associations probably led John Dury towards the millenarian position. Twisse conducted an extensive correspondence with Mede about the millennium, and Hartlib was kept informed on these exchanges. Mede was questioned about some of the issues which Twisse discussed in his introduction to the translation of *Clavis Apocalyptica.* Twisse, in spite of his relative obscurity as rector of Newbury, was no mean scholar.[1] While at Oxford he assisted Savile with a translation of Bradwardine, and he visited Heidelberg as chaplain to Elizabeth, Queen of Bohemia, on the occasion of her marriage. Thereafter Twisse often refused preferment and devoted himself primarily to composing a considerable body of writings defending the puritan theological position against Arminianism. It is possible that his millenarian interests were aroused by his contacts with protestant theologians on the continent. Among the puritan clergy Twisse was obviously an influential figure, as is suggested by his ultimate selection as prolocutor of the Westminster Assembly. Hartlib reported that 'men flocke unto him as unto some Oracle', and noted Twisse's exchanges of ideas with John White (his contemporary at New College Oxford), and with John Stoughton.[2]

Hartlib himself took responsibility for the distribution of Potter's manuscript 'On the Number 666', in the years before its publication. No doubt Hartlib was equally interested in Potter's capacities as a commentator and inventor, talents which might otherwise have gained little recognition, since Potter occupied the remote living of Kilmington in Somerset. By contrast with Hartlib, Hannibal Potter, the influential elder brother of the inventor and Fellow of Trinity College Oxford, regarded his brother's interests with distaste and embarrassment.

Perhaps Hartlib's most direct service to the propagation of puritan millennial ideas was his supervision of the publication of John Stoughton's *Felicitas ultimi saeculi.* This work was composed in about 1638, primarily for the benefit of the Transylvanian protestants. This group was very much influenced by English puritanism and the connection was cemented by the visit of Transylvanian students to England.[3] Stoughton's text was written in the form of a letter to one of the most celebrated Transylvanian visitors, Johann Tolnai, and it was dedicated to Prince Georg Rákóczi I. No doubt appreciating its relevance to the English situation, Hartlib, who was one of the beneficiaries of Stoughton's will, published *Felicitas ultimi saeculi* in 1640, shortly after Stoughton's death.

Stoughton's ideas on the millennium were the result of many years' deliberation about the work of Mede. Gradually he came to differ from the Cambridge scholar on many points. This may have led to direct discussion between them since it was reported that Stoughton 'would

1. *DNB.*

2. Letter from Hartlib to Dury, 30 Sept. 1630, HP VII 30; Ephemerides 1634.

3. Jenö Zoványi, *Puritánus Mozgalmak a Magyar Református Egyházban* (Budapest, 1911); L. Makkai, 'The Hungarian Puritans and the English Revolution', *Acta historica,* 1958, 5: 13–45.

faine communicate divers notions to Mr. Meade. He dislikes that Mead holds afterwards the Church shall come to trouble againe *et* holds Christ will come personally upon earth.'[4]

Stoughton's views on the revival of learning were echoed by John Goodwin. Stoughton and Goodwin were ministers of St. Mary Aldermanbury and St. Stephen's Coleman Street respectively. These parishes were conspicuously and consistently puritan and in both the advowson was under the vestry's control. Stoughton and Goodwin were among the five London lecturers examined for 'inconformity' by Bishop Juxon in 1635.[5] Goodwin, like Stoughton, was associated with Hartlib and Dury; their most important joint work was completed in 1648, when Hartlib published a translation of Acontius's *Satanae Stratagemata* under the combined sponsorship of Dury and Goodwin.[6]

The associations revealed above between the puritan thinkers concerned with eschatology and the revival of learning, are indicative of a wider communion which existed within this group. The authors of theological and philosophical works represent the public face of a structured community which extended from influential patrons, to clergymen, lecturers, academics, schoolmasters and students. Such elder puritan clergymen as John Dod, John White or John Stoughton, owed much of their influence to their intimacy with powerful lay patrons. Although often occupying relatively inauspicious positions, these ministers assumed a much more than parochial function. John White in his Dorchester parish was concerned with the problems of social welfare; his work included the supervision of education and the establishment of a public brewhouse to provide work for the able poor, on the principle of 'knowledge causing piety, piety breeding industry, and industry procuring plenty . . .'.[7] On questions of practical divinity White was described by Hartlib as 'A man of very rare and extraordinarie gifts and endowments.'[8]

It was perhaps this puritan belief in the spiritual value of productive industry which led White in 1623 to play a prominent part in the creation of the Dorchester Company of Adventurers. This Company intended to establish a colony of Westcountrymen in New England, to develop fisheries. This venture, although shortlived, was important in two respects. First, White grafted on to his initial economic proposal the idea of establishing a 'Bible Commonwealth', which could become a refuge for idealistic English Puritans. Secondly, in 1628 many of White's ideas were embodied into the 'New England Company for a

4. Ephemerides 1634.
5. Seaver (258), pp.138, 257; D. A. Williams, 'London Puritanism: The Parish of St. Stephen Coleman Street', *Church Quarterly Review*, 1959, *160*: 462–82.
6. Haller (129), pp.195–9; *Satans Stratagems, or the devils Cabinet-Council Discovered* (London, 1648).
7. S. E. Morison (192), pp.21–50; Frances Rose-Troup, *John White The Founder of Massachusetts* (New York, 1930).
8. Letter from Hartlib to Dury, 30 Sept. 1630, HP VII 30.

Plantation in Massachusetts Bay', which was backed by the powerful interest of the puritan grandees, including the Earl of Warwick, Lord Saye and Sele, and Lord Brooke; John Pym and Richard Knightley were also among the founding members of this Company.[9] In the 1630s the Massachusetts Bay Company became the main avenue for the puritan exodus to New England.

John Dod, by either education, friendship or marriage, was connected with the earlier generation of Cambridge Puritans, Richard Greenham, Richard Sibbes and John Preston.[10] Despite difficulties with the Anglican Bishops, Dod held a succession of livings in Oxfordshire and Northamptonshire controlled by puritan gentry. He also attracted attention as a preacher in London. Finally he settled at Fawsley, Northamptonshire, under the patronage of Richard Knightley; John Preston opted to leave London and spend his last days in Dod's company at Fawsley. From this centre of puritan political manoeuvering Dod played an active part in securing posts for puritan clergymen.[11] Although not directly involved in the migration to New England, Dod was consulted by such ministers as John Cotton and Thomas Hooker about their impending flight. Dod's daughter married Walter Wilkins, an Oxford goldsmith, and their eldest son was John Wilkins, the natural philosopher. After the goldsmith's death in 1625, it is probable that Dod took on the main responsibility for Wilkins's education.[12] Wilkins spent the years 1627-1637 at Magdalen Hall, one of the centres of anti-Laudian influence at Oxford. Thereafter he was ordained and for a brief time assisted his grandfather at Fawsley, before becoming chaplain to Knightley's friend and near neighbour, Lord Saye and Sele of Broughton, near Banbury.[13]

John Stoughton was educated at Emmanuel College Cambridge. After serving for some years as rector of Aller in Somerset, he became in 1632 perpetual curate of St. Mary Aldermanbury, remaining there until his death in 1639.[14] His London parish was one of the main centres of puritan resistance, with the result that Stoughton was in continual conflict with the ecclesiastical authorities. That he remained defiant and unrepentant is illustrated by his arrest in 1635, under suspicion of collecting funds for New England ministers. A sympathiser,

9. Newton (199); Andrews (4), i, pp.344–74.

10. Haller (129), pp.56–63.

11. H. I. Longdon, *Northamptonshire and Rutland Clergy from 1500,* 16 vols. (Northampton, 1938–52), iv, p.107; xv, p.85. Seaver (258), pp.176–8.

12. W. Lloyd, *A Sermon preached at the Funeral of . . . John . . . Bishop of Chester* (London, 1672), p.32.

13. Shapiro (259), pp.12–20; Longdon, *op. cit.,* xv, p.85. According to Woodcock Laud did not think Dod 'worthy of a liveing; but his son [sic] Wilkins was allowed the vaccarige of fawsley and Mr. Dod to be his curate' : *Extracts from the Papers of Thomas Woodcock,* ed. G. C. Moore Smith (Camden Soc. Miscellany, 3rd Series, xi, 1907), p.55.

14. J. C. Whitebrook, 'Dr. John Stoughton the Elder', *Transactions of the Congregational Historical Society,* 1913–15, *6*: 89–107; 177–84.

John Rous, reported with satisfaction that 'within 2 or 3 dayes, *re cognita,* he returned with credite, in the earl of Holland's coach'.[15] An influential figure in the St. Mary Aldermanbury congregation was Sir Robert Harley, who was one of the laymen most active in assisting Stoughton and other leading Puritans to secure livings for their protégés.[16] The Stoughton and Cudworth families were closely associated for the best part of a century. John Stoughton followed the elder Ralph Cudworth as rector of Aller, married his widow and took responsibility for her family. Stoughton was probably particularly conscious of an obligation to the younger Ralph Cudworth who followed his father and stepfather to Emmanuel College, Cambridge. He pursued a successful academic career which began with a fellowship at his own college in 1639.[17] By this time he had probably developed a sympathy for Platonism sufficient to form the foundations for his monumental attempt to integrate protestant theology and Neoplatonic philosophy. Cudworth's Platonism is usually attributed to the influence of Benjamin Whichcote of Emmanuel College, but it is clear that Stoughton's works would have prepared Cudworth to undergo this development.

One of Stoughton's patrons, Henry Rich Earl of Holland, was the first Governor of the Massachusetts Bay Company; Stoughton's stepson James Cudworth, and his two brothers Thomas and Israel Stoughton, became leading Massachusetts settlers and politicians. John Stoughton himself was never obliged to seek refuge in America, but he was clearly interested in colonial policy. For instance, among his papers unearthed by the High Commission was a proposal for 'erecting a place where some may be maintained for learning the language and instructing heathen and our owne and breeding up as many Indian children as providence shall bring into our hands'.[18] This fragmentary document is regarded as the first positive proposal for the establishment of a collegiate educational institution in Massachusetts. The most serious accusation of the High Commission related to the joint activities of Stoughton and White as trustees of a fund designed to 'administer to the necessity of the afflicted brethren at home or abroad'. Operating like the Feoffees for Impropriations, the Trustees had begun to purchase advowsons and provide financial assistance wherever appropriate, either in England or in the New England colonies. One beneficiary was Stoughton's adopted daughter's husband; another was John Dury.[19]

The careers of Dod and Stoughton illustrate the kind of pressures applied against the Puritans. Theologians and philosophers were subjected to the same treatment as politicians. Stoughton, Goodwin, Dury,

15. *Diary of John Rous* (Camden Soc., lxvi, 1856), pp.79–80.
16. Seaver (258), pp.50–2.
17. Whitebrook, *op. cit.*
18. S. E. Morison, *The Founding of Harvard College* (Cambridge, Mass., 1936), pp.161–2, 415–16.
19. *CSPD 1635,* pp.104–5, 377–8, 435–6, 459, 500; Whitebrook, *op. cit.,* pp.97–107; Rous, *Diary,* p.80.

Hartlib and their associates were obstructed, criticised, intimidated, or imprisoned. Their letters were intercepted, their private papers confiscated. However, while they were often disconsolate, and while occasionally there were acts of disloyalty, the puritan movement as a whole suffered no diminution in effectiveness, even on its most exposed flanks.

Puritan influence in the universities was diminished, but the Laudian reconstruction could proceed only slowly. Accordingly pockets of puritan influence were still active in 1640. Christ's College, St. John's College and above all Emmanuel College, at Cambridge, as well as Magdalen Hall at Oxford, continued to harbour substantial numbers of puritan academics and students. Among the figures discussed in this book who were associated with Emmanuel College are John Bainbridge, William Bedell, Benjamin Whichcote, Richard Holdsworth, John Stoughton, Ralph Cudworth, William Croune, Samuel Foster, Walter Foster, Jeremiah Horrox, John Wallis, John Sadler, John Smith, Samuel Cradock, John Worthington, Peter Chamberlen and possibly Samuel Hartlib. Nevertheless, certain prominent puritan academics, including William Ames and Thomas Goodwin, were driven into exile. But even during the Laudian supremacy, foreign protestants like Theodore Haak, Joachim Hübner and Johann Tolnai were able to find congenial companions at Oxford. Otherwise, puritan integrity was maintained by resorting to Trinity College Dublin (e.g. John Winthrop junior, Benjamin Worsley, Miles Symner and Sir Robert King), or to centres in the low countries (e.g. Robert Greville, William Brereton, William Rand, Robert Child and William Petty). There are even signs that the Puritans would have considered establishing alternatives to the English university colleges if the uncongenial religious code were enforced too rigorously. Hartlib's short-lived academy designed 'for the education of the Gentrie of this Nation, to advance Piety, Learning, Moralitie and other Exercises of Industrie', which was established at Chichester in 1630, may have represented a move in this direction. Certainly Hartlib's academy adopted ambitious educational standards. At Chichester, Hartlib was assisted by John Pell, who joined the academy immediately after completing his studies at Trinity College Cambridge. After the failure of Hartlib's academy he set up his own school in Sussex.[20] Perhaps the demise of Hartlib's academy reflects the undiminishing vigour of the puritan party in the universities. After returning from Chichester, Hartlib spent a short time at the London house of Lord Brooke, attempting to gather support for a new academy.

The Puritans continued to exercise considerable influence at the more elementary level of education, often out of necessity while awaiting substantial preferment, or while in retreat from the Laudian authori-

20. *HDC*, pp.16–20, 36–8. For Pell see Aubrey, ii, pp.121–31; Wood *Fasti*, i, pp.461–4; Venn, iii, p.337. Aubrey described Pell's father as 'a kind of Nonconformist'.

ties. For instance, Hugh Peter after graduating at Cambridge taught at Langdon in Essex for two years before seeking ordination. Thereupon the Earl of Warwick granted him the living of Rayleigh, Essex in 1623 and supervised his brief but meteoric career as a London Lecturer in 1626 and 1627.[21] Because Hartlib and Pell were unordained, the assistance they received from patrons tended to be inadequate and more sporadic; Pell positively refused ordination when offered a benefice by Bishop John Williams, although this was the only means of release from schoolteaching. When Hooker was forced out of his lectureship at Chelmsford by Laud, he set up a school at nearby Little Baddow with John Eliot as his usher. In some cases teaching was a chosen vocation and certain well-remunerated posts were available to Puritans. This point is well-illustrated by Felsted School, which was controlled by the Earl of Warwick. In 1628, on the advice of John Preston, Warwick appointed the Cambridge graduate Martin Holbeach as the master of this school. Holbeach was the conspicuously successful teacher of Richard and Henry Cromwell, Henry Mildmay and the mathematicians John Wallis and Isaac Barrow. Sir John Bramston commented that Holbeach 'scarce bred any man that was loyall to his prince.'[22]

A determined attempt was made to regulate the lectureships which, especially in urban areas, had become one of the most active agencies for the extension of puritan influence. The preaching ministry was fundamental to puritanism and the regulation and restriction of preaching was of fundamental concern to Laud's bishops. As indicated above, Thomas Hooker and Hugh Peter were suspended from their lectureships. In 1630 John Humphry, John White's collaborator and Deputy Governor of the Massachusetts Bay Company, reported that Laud had 'silenced many godly men recently', among whom was John Archer, the lecturer at Allhallows Lombard Street and St. Antholin's, who has already been mentioned as the author of the well-known millenarian work, *The Personal Reign of Christ on Earth*.[23] In spite of Anglican anxieties about lectureships and Laud's instinct to embark on a policy of suppression, little reduction in their numerical strength occurred, even in London, where it has been estimated that there were more puritan lecturers in the city in 1640 than in any year before 1626.[24]

The failure of the campaign to discipline the lecturers merely underlines the buoyancy of the mechanism of puritan patronage. Thus when Archer was prevented from lecturing, the Feoffees for Impropriations secured the vicarage of All Saints Huntingdon for him. When Obadiah Sedgwick was suspended, he was presented by the Earl of Warwick

21. Seaver (258), pp.234–7; R. P. Stearns, *Hugh Peter Strenuous Puritan* (270), pp.15–52.

22. *VCH Essex,* ii, pp.531–8; *Autobiography of Sir John Bramston* (Camden Soc., xxxii, 1845), p.124.

23. I. M. Calder, 'The St. Antholin lectures', *Church Quarterly Review,* 1959, *160*: 49–70; *Winthrop Papers,* ii, p.340.

24. Seaver (258), p.226.

with the living of Coggeshall in Essex.[25] This benefice was used to house a whole succession of non-conforming clergymen including the fathers of both John Stoughton and Ralph Cudworth the philosopher. Whether in the form of vestries, corporations or as individuals, the puritan patrons controlled a considerable network of livings, as well as offering posts as secretaries, legal advisers, tutors, chaplains and schoolmasters. This system was maintained by virtue of the close inter-relationships between patrons on one level, and between their protégés at another. It was not possible to control this informal but brilliantly effective mechanism without undermining the entire system of lay patronage. Accordingly, even the suppression of the more formalised Feoffees for Impropriations proved to be only a minor setback to the puritan movement.[26]

Because of the effectiveness of puritan patronage, the church retained its attraction as a principal means of professional advancement. Hence we find that science was dominated by men in holy orders (academics, chaplains, or beneficed); they covered the entire religious and political spectrum, from Beale, Wilkins, Wallis, Cudworth and More, to the radicals Dell, Webster and Pinnel. It is also noticeable that a substantial proportion of the natural philosophers active during the Puritan Revolution were the sons of clergymen. These sociological factors in themselves are sufficient to guarantee the existence of a basically religious spirit in mid-century English science.

Given the above situation it is tempting to conclude that many of those Puritans who went into exile did so as much out of choice as out of necessity. But from whatever cause, even the instances cited above make it clear that migration to the New England colonies became, in the 1630s, a most attractive alternative for the Puritans. The well-worn pattern of exile to the continent was followed by the older generation. When Ames gave up his fellowship at Christ's College Cambridge he settled in the low countries, where he pursued a successful academic and clerical career. However, towards the end of his life Ames felt the lure of the colonies; and after his death in 1633, his wife (a relative of John Winthrop) and family settled in New England. Ames was joined in the Netherlands by many young puritan exiles; some waited for more favourable times before returning to England, but most came to regard the low countries as a staging post in the journey to America. Thomas Hooker and his assistant John Eliot left their school in Essex for the Netherlands; Hugh Peter arrived there after losing his London lectureship. Between 1630 and 1635 these three, as well as James Cudworth, Thomas and Israel Stoughton, Thomas Pell (brother of John Pell), joined John Winthrop father and son, and Sir Henry Vane, in the search for better things in Massachusetts. The

25. Seaver (258), pp.250–1, 260.

26. I. M. Calder, *The Activities of the Puritan Faction of the Church of England 1625–1633* (New York, 1957).

Company which superintended this exodus represented a fusion of interests. Its religious complexion was determined by the puritanism of John White, its prestige by such experienced colonial adventurers as the Earl of Warwick with his allies Brooke, Holland and Saye. Then behind this façade operated political activists like Pym, St. John and Sir Nathaniel Rich. Given this effective initiation, the Massachusetts Bay Company was able very quickly to attract a complete microcosm of the puritan community and to launch its first godly colonial settlements.

Before the Civil War the fortunes of the aspiring generation of Puritans were irrevocably bound up with the affairs of their patrons. Through the constant reiteration of their names in connection with the above puritan biographies, it is clear that a formidable group comprising the peers Warwick, Lord Brooke, Lord Robartes, Viscount Mandeville and Lord Saye and Sele, and the gentlemen Sir Thomas Barrington, Sir Benjamin Rudyerd, Sir Nathaniel Rich, Sir Robert Harley, Sir Henry Vane junior, Sir William Waller, Richard Knightley, John Pym, Francis Rous and Oliver St. John, was involved in deploying the labours and skills of the educated Puritans. In certain cases women were extremely active in matters of patronage. Mary, Lady Vere, Margaret, Lady Clotworthy and slightly later Katherine, Lady Ranelagh were important, either directly as patrons, or indirectly as sources of money and goodwill. Puritan social organisation was comprehensive. The family and the church, the patron and the protégé were welded together as an integrated structure.

The smooth operation of this network of influence has already been illustrated with respect to figures who came to play an important part in science during the Puritan Revolution. A characteristic pattern emerges. John Wilkins and Ralph Cudworth were both left fatherless; both had the advantage of an early upbringing under prominent puritan clergymen; both studied at predominantly puritan colleges and both were ordained. Wilkins's professional career began when he became chaplain to a puritan aristocrat at the height of his political influence. Thenceforth the way was clear for a sequence of moves which culminated in a successful academic career. Cudworth remained at Emmanuel College until the parliamentarian authorities offered him substantial academic preferments. John Wallis constitutes an example of a comprehensively puritan upbringing—son of a puritan clergyman, education at puritan Felsted School and Emmanuel College, and chaplain to the puritan widow, Lady Vere.[27] Through Lady Vere, Wallis became involved in political affairs; of particular importance was his chance introduction to ciphers by the chaplain of Sir William Waller. Wallis found that he had a natural aptitude for deciphering royalist despatches and was rewarded with the benefice first of St. Gabriel

27. Lady Vere's husband, Sir Horace Vere, had employed William Ames as his chaplain.

Fenchurch Street and then of St. Martin Ironmonger Lane.[28] As noted in the previous chapter, he entered into philosophical debate with Lord Brooke, and became assistant to the Clerks of the Westminster Assembly. The ground was by then well prepared for his academic preferment.

Natural philosophy was exploited partly for personal gratification, but it was also a means of enhancing personal reputation by displays of intellectual virtuosity. The early writings of Wilkins and Wallis were designed as much to attract the admiration of the educated public as to make contributions to natural philosophy. Preferment was the appropriate reward; this in turn brought increased leisure and access to like-minded associates, so creating suitable conditions for even more active promotion of the sciences. For Wallis the mathematician, Cudworth the philosopher and Wilkins the virtuoso, the foundation of a career was firmly laid before 1640. For laymen without access to an obvious ladder of preferment in the church or universities, such as John Pell, Samuel Hartlib, Gabriel Plattes or Theodore Haak, the path was more hazardous. This was especially so for those outside the relatively well-remunerated medical profession. Things were perhaps hardest of all for the foreign refugees. In certain cases they had no particular reason for selecting England as their place of exile. On the other hand, many were clearly optimistic about prospects in a nation which was seemingly insulated from the devastation of the Thirty Years War. But upon arrival they found that England was neither prosperous, nor congenial from a political or religious point of view. Hartlib, Hübner and Haak spent some time at the English universities, but refugees were often not formally admitted, and they usually left without taking degrees. Hence no firm basis was established for a professional career, with the result in Hartlib's case that, although a figure of increasing public prominence he experienced more difficulties in obtaining a secure post than his English friends in the puritan ministry.

Hartlib may have been attached to Emmanuel College Cambridge; he was certainly associated with John Preston, the head of that college.[29] After his first professional venture—the academy at Chichester—Hartlib was encouraged, especially by William Speed, the puritan minister of St. Pancras Chichester, to settle in London. But Hartlib never established an adequate basis of support for his operations. Dury attributed his initial difficulties to 'being too charitable to poor scholars, and for undertaking too freely the work of schooling and education of children'.[30] In the 1630s he came to rely on innumerable small contributions from a varied group which included Lord Brooke, Sir Thomas

28. A previous incumbent of this parish was the Puritan, Joseph Simonds, who was ejected by Laud in 1639: Seaver (258), pp.325–6.

29. *HDC*, p.14. For Hartlib see G. H. Turnbull, *A Sketch of his Life and Relations to J. A. Comenius* (284); Webster (320), Introduction.

30. Letter from Dury to Sir Thomas Roe, 7/17 December 1635, *CSPD 1635*, pp.538–9.

Barrington, Sir Nathaniel Rich, John Pym, Richard Knightley, Oliver St. John, John Stoughton, Sir William Waller, Benjamin Whichcote, Archbishop Ussher and Sir Thomas Roe. Although without adequate means himself, Hartlib attempted to assist others, so complementing among laymen the activities of Stoughton and White among the clergy. Hartlib's association with John Pym, one of his most important allies, was probably typical. The politician employed Hartlib's talents for various purposes including the supply of foreign intelligence and assistance in finding a technician to solve the problem of flooding in coalmines at Coventry. Pym corresponded from Fawsley and no doubt Hartlib's news was distributed to other puritan politicians from there. In return Pym made small payments to Hartlib, expected to be asked to assist his public-spirited protégés, and took an active interest in promoting the visit of Comenius to England. From the tone of this correspondence it is clear that a warm relationship existed between Pym and Hartlib. Dury was therefore probably correct in describing Hartlib as 'Mr. Pym's intimate and familiar acquaintance'.[31]

Despite the extremely limited success of his efforts, Hartlib was sufficiently optimistic about the turn of events to encourage other scholars to contemplate settling in England.[32] With the recall of parliament, Hartlib believed that a watershed had been reached; the puritan party had established such a supremacy that the grand schemes outlined by Bacon might be set on foot. All the indications suggested that the advancement of learning would be incorporated into the puritan reform programme. At this time Hartlib strongly recommended his patrons to read the new translation of *De Augmentis Scientiarum*, adding, 'mee thinkes the tyme drawes neare that this Great desideratum [the advancement of learning] all soe shall bee fulfilled for some noble ende which God's providence aymes at.'[33] In response to Hartlib's urgent and dramatic appeals, Comenius decided to visit England, convinced that his visit was sanctioned by parliament itself.[34] This misapprehension was partly induced by the sermon preached before parliament by John Gauden, chaplain to the Earl of Warwick, which in its printed form, included a digression recommending the work of Comenius and Dury.[35] It was unusual for parliamentary sermons to make such specific recommendations. In this case not parliament, but

31. Letters from Pym to Hartlib, 1636–1642, HP XXXI 3: *HDC*, p.270.

32. Young (348), p.44.

33. Letter from Hartlib to Robartes and Sir William Waller, 20 Feb. 1640/1, HP VII 43.

34. Young (348), pp.39–41; H. R. Trevor-Roper, 'Three Foreigners' (283), pp.260–72; G. H. Turnbull, 'The Summoning of Comenius to England by parliament', *Central European Observer*, 1 April 1927, pp.219–20. The suggestion that Comenius was invited by Parliament was first made by Jeremy Collier in the dedicatory letter to Hartlib in *A Patterne of Universal Knowledge*, 1651 (trans. of Comensius's *Pansophiae Diatyposis*, 1643).

35. John Gauden, *The Love of Truth and Peace* (London, 1641). The sermon was preached on 29 November 1640; the invitation to publish it was delivered by Sir Thomas Barrington.

a group of influential parliamentarians were willing to identify themselves with Comenius. Among leading supporters mentioned by Comenius were such powerful figures as John Williams the friend of Bacon and newly appointed archbishop of York, Lord Brooke and John Pym. Comenius described his patrons as 'some good men, theologians and bishops, [who] had in consideration a plan for the propagation of the Gospel among the heathen'. This comment suggests that Comenius was supported by a group which aimed to further the work of Stoughton and White.[36] Hartlib's papers prove that Comenius's presence was valuable in attracting other, more minor figures, such as the Kentish gentlemen Sir Cheney Culpeper and Nicholas Stoughton, into the ranks of the movement for social and intellectual reform.[37] Although individually many were neither particularly prosperous nor well-known, these adherents were active and well-connected. They became the backbone of the movement to promote Hartlib's designs. Hence in spite of the eruption of the Civil War and the decision of Comenius to return to the continent in 1642, an extremely substantial foundation was laid for future attempts to pursue the aims of the Great Instauration.

It is evident that puritan attitudes to natural philosophy or to any other sphere of intellectual enquiry were formed in the context of a well-defined social group. This community appears to have become even more united and resilient under the oppression of the 1630s. The disfavour of the monarch, the increasing dominance of Archbishop Laud, the emergence of a powerful Arminian party in the Church of England, the tendency to appease the continental catholic states, the imposition of unconstitutional taxes and the adoption of non-parliamentary government, only served to invigorate, and expand the appeal of the puritan opposition. Accordingly, even in their embattled position, the English Puritans gave every appearance of power and influence to foreign protestants locked in the devastating conflict of the Thirty Years War.

From the point of view of intellectual history, the experiences of the 1630s were an important inducement to the Puritans to evolve a compelling, coherent and comprehensive system of beliefs. The increasingly close association between Puritans in the decade before 1640 was born out of necessity; reconciliation of conflicting interests, and emphasis on points of common belief were essential for the survival as an opposition party of a group having disparate social, political and religious ends. For the intelligentsia, this powerful association of

36. Young (348), p.44.

37. Stoughton (1592–1648) was from Stoughton, Kent; he was educated at New College Oxford (contemporary with White and Twisse); from 1645 until 1648 he was MP for Guildford, Surrey. Culpeper (1601–1663) was born at Hollingbourne, Kent; his education was at Hart Hall, Oxford; he resided at Leeds Castle and served as secretary to the Kent Committee. His friends included Pym, Vane and Westrowe.

magnates and clergymen was of the greatest importance. In the first place, it offered avenues for preferment and employment shielded from the sanctions of the establishment. Then, it provided a stimulating environment for the debate of intellectual problems. The social ethic of puritanism proved to be thoroughly consistent with the spirit of the new philosophy evolved by Bacon and his followers. Accordingly the puritan movement provided an ideal environment for the cultivation of the ideals of the Great Instauration; and the puritan habits of mutual assistance, free communication and covenant responsibility became important factors in determining the structure of the emergent scientific movement.

(ii) Wunschräume

It is not possible to trace back to any particular point either the desire to construct a utopian commonwealth, or, attempts to further this aim by means of organised groups of activists whether concerned with all aspects of social planning, or with more specific problems such as science, medicine and technology. But from our point of view it is notable that in the first decades of the seventeenth century, figures as different as Campanella, Andreae and Bacon were involved in utopian planning in some sense or other. Bacon's *Instauratio Magna* was a utopian system of philosophy, which was designed to expose the potentialities of science as a means to attain mastery over the environment and a solution to the problem of disease. Within this context, he advocated the establishment of state-patronised brotherhoods of learned men who would supervise the planned exploitation of nature.

England during the 1630s was scarcely the most fruitful territory on which to promote schemes of this kind. Nevertheless it was possible to think in these terms with respect to the colonial ventures, which increasingly absorbed the puritan imagination. Indeed, the 'running to and fro' and the 'increase of knowledge' of Daniel, were thought by the Puritans to relate to the opening up and exploitation of the New World. Even the American Indians had a part to play in this story; John Eliot regarded them as heathens ripe for conversion in the final days, while Mede identified the Indians as the inhabitants of the land of Gog and Magog, who were destined to resist conversion and vex the godly inhabitants of the American plantations. Mede first adopted this pessimistic forecast in correspondence with Twisse, who had been wondering about 'the providence of God concerning that world, not discovered till this old world of ours is almost at an end'. Twisse had hoped that the English plantations might be the seat of the New Jerusalem, a conclusion which was widely shared by his fellow Puritans.[38] The lecturer William Symonds echoed the general puritan atti-

38. Correspondence between Mede and Twisse 1634–5); Mede *Works*, pp.978–96. J. Bowman, 'Is America the New Jerusalem or Gog and Magog?',

tude to North America; it was 'a Land more like the Garden of Eden: which the Lord planted, then any part else of all the earth.'[39]

New Atlantis, the utopian fragment published shortly after the death of Bacon in 1626, was ultimately known for its description of the ideal scientific institution, Solomon's House, but for the Puritans *New Atlantis* would have had further relevance as an account of the harmonious and devout society of the island of Bensalem—'a Christian people, full of piety and humanity.'[40] This island was situated off the coast of America and Bacon's vision of a perfect society was undoubtedly influenced by the imaginative and optimistic accounts of America and the Islands of the West Indies, published by Hakluyt, Ralegh and Harriot, or even by the stream of propaganda on the wonders of the New World issued by the promoters of the Virginia Company between 1606 and 1624. Bacon himself devoted one of his *Essays* to the subject 'Of Plantations' and took an active interest in schemes for the plantation of Ireland, Virginia and Newfoundland.[41]

The puritan aristocracy and gentry invested considerable resources in colonial adventures, which were at first regarded primarily as speculative business undertakings. In the 1630s the colonial ventures took on a more positive significance, as the pressures on the Puritans increased until, for many, normal vocational and spiritual life became impossible in England. Colonisation ultimately emerged as a means to preserve the spirit of the reformation among the English people.

John White was the leading apologist on behalf of the Massachusetts colony. In his view 'God especially directs this worke of creating Colonies unto the planting and propagating of Religion'. Furthermore God had ordained that this work would be undertaken in the 'Western parts of the World' during the last age of history.[42] As well as emphasising the fundamentally religious constitution of the new colony, White was aware of the need to create an harmonious and well-balanced community, which would be free from the social evils and poverty of England. John Winthrop shared White's feeling that the faithful in England were about to experience the most severe trials and calamities. It was in this spirit that in 1630 he accepted the invitation to become Governor of Massachusetts, believing that 'God had chosen this country to plant his people in'.[43]

Proceedings of the Leeds Philosophical and Literary Society, 1950, *6*: 445-52. For other biblical texts relating to America, see Bridenbaugh (34), pp.401–2.

39. William Symonds, *Virginia. A Sermon Preached at White Chapel* (London, 1609), p.26.

40. Bacon, *New Atlantis, Works,* iii, p.134.

41. Bacon's essay on plantations was composed c. 1620; Andrews (4), i, pp.72, 85, 303–4. Bridenbaugh (34), pp.400–10 for a summary of popular writings.

42. John White, *The Planters Plea* (London, 1630), pp.11–12. Andrews (4), i, pp.385–7.

43. Letter from John Winthrop to Lord Saye and Sele, 1640, Winthrop *Journal,* i, p.234.

In the small American colonies, religious and political conflicts proved no easier to escape than in England; intimidated minorities were guided by such religious leaders as Roger Williams to establish separate utopias elsewhere in New England.

Among the primitive institutions of the new colonies there was no place for a sophisticated establishment like Solomon's House, but the effective exploitation of resources assumed high priority with some of the Massachusetts settlers, as illustrated by the partnership between Robert Child and John Winthrop Jr.[44] The latter left England in 1635 after studying at Trinity College Dublin, to establish a settlement at Saybrook on behalf of Saye and Brooke. Child came from a prosperous Kent family; after graduating at Cambridge, he followed the not uncommon practice of studying medicine at Leyden and Padua.[45] Upon his first visit to New England, sometime between 1638 and 1641, Child discovered a close identity of outlook with Winthrop. Each studied his environment closely, prospected for profitable minerals or other useful raw materials, and investigated a variety of innovations in agriculture. They both built up extensive libraries, dominated by works on chemistry, the subject which they saw as the key to the understanding of agriculture, medicine and industry.[46] Many of their pilot schemes failed, but their ironworks were extremely successful. In their scientific and industrial work they were joined by such figures as the technician Richard Leader, or the physician and alchemist George Starkey. Thus Winthrop and Child gained experience in New England which proved invaluable to the English Baconians. Indeed, it may be claimed that they were well ahead of their English contemporaries in pursuing the ideals of Solomon's House.

North America was also considered for a brief time as a suitable location for settlement by Hartlib and his continental associates, whose proposed colony was styled *Antilia*. This was partly an imitation of the German utopian societies founded by Andreae and partly an agency for establishing a settlement for a group which was anxious to escape from the unsettled conditions of Europe. Hartlib received correspondence relating to Antilia between 1628 and 1635; he attempted to interest his continental colleagues in settlement in Virginia, but they favoured the nearer and better known north-eastern states of Europe. As late as 1639

44. The standard biographical sources are G. L. Kittredge, 'Dr Robert Child the Remonstrant', Colonial Society of Massachusetts *Transactions,* 1919, *21*: 1–146; G. H. Turnbull, 'Robert Child' (290); Robert C. Black, *The Younger John Winthrop* (New York and London, 1966). R. S. Wilkinson of Washington is preparing a study of the life and scientific labours of Winthrop. R. P. Stearns's monumental *Science in the British Colonies of America* (271) is surprisingly deficient in the treatment of this seminal phase in American science.

45. Child obtained his MD at Padua in 1638.

46. R. S. Wilkinson, 'The Alchemical Library of John Winthrop Jr. and his Descendants', *Ambix,* 1963, *11*: 33–51; 1966, *13*: 139–86. W. J. Wilson, 'Robert Child's Chemical Booklist of 1641', *Journal of Chemical Education,* 1943, *20*: 123–9.

Hartlib was recording the views of Hübner, St. Amand and Waller on the advantages of establishing 'universal colonies'.[47] Unfortunately no writings survive which definitely relate to plans for Antilia, but it may be assumed that its *Confessio* and *Leges* were based on equivalent texts drafted by Andreae for his Societas Christiana. However, one manifesto may relate to the formative phase of Antilia. This firstly suggested the establishment of an international fraternity of scholars, along the lines laid down in Bacon's introduction to Book II of *De Augmentis Scientiarum*. Secondly, it outlined plans for the creation of a network of colleges, many of which would have been concerned with aspects of science and technology.[48] This latter project belongs more to the world of utopian phantasy than to the practical scheme for an Antilian colony in Virginia.

(iii) Macaria and the Universal College

The Antilian manifesto was not practical and it was probably, like *Christianopolis,* framed primarily for the pious edification of German protestant scholars at a time when the calamities of the Thirty Years War precluded any chance of utopian social reconstruction. In England, during 1640 and 1641, the clouds lifted and it became possible to take advantage of the groundswell of sentiment in favour of reform and to place before parliament schemes for intellectual organisation which would revive the projects that had lain dormant since the death of Bacon.

Macaria may have owed its general inspiration to Hartlib, but its immediate author was Gabriel Plattes.[49] Virtually nothing is known of Plattes's biography, except that his patron was the inventor and drainage engineer William Engelbert; he may well have worked with Engelbert. Plattes's first two publications were issued in 1639, when their author was probably in his forties; the first dealt with husbandry and the second with mining. They were unorthodox, provocative and were obviously the fruit of considerable first-hand experience. Plattes was an experimental philosopher by instinct rather than by conscious imitation of the maxims of Verulam. In his agricultural work, *A Discovery of Infinite Treasure,* Plattes advocated the creation of a 'Colledge for Inventions in Husbandrie'.[50] This idea was consistent with the principle which he often reiterated, that practitioners were morally obliged to utilise their skills to the maximum public good. Plattes's tracts immediately attracted the attention of Hartlib, who drew Plattes into his orbit and encouraged

47. *HDC,* pp.69–76; Ephemerides 1639.

48. This document is headed, 'In nomine Dei Omnipotentis!'; it is given in full by Turnbull (289), pp.166–70. For discussion see *HDC*, pp.75–6 and Webster, 'Samuel Hartlib and the Great Reformation' (321).

49. Webster, 'The Authorship and Significance of Macaria', *Past and Present,* 1972, no. 56: 34–48.

50. Plattes (217), p.72.

the preparation of 'other tracts which will more particularly instruct all sorts of people how to procure their own and the public good'.[51]

The first fruit of this new phase of Plattes's activity was *Macaria,* a brief utopian dialogue dedicated to Parliament and issued to coincide with the opening of the second session of the Long Parliament. Notwithstanding its use of the utopian genre, *Macaria* is quite evidently intended as a straightforward set of proposals on economic and social reform which were designed to complement the suggestions made in various petitions for the redress of grievances, which emanated from many sources at this time. The utopian framework permitted the author to illustrate the advantages of economic planning and state patronage of scientific research and development. In *Macaria* each aspect of the economy was regulated by a Council, which had the authority to introduce appropriate laws.[52] Then, like Bacon's Island of Bensalem, 'a Colledge of experience' was responsible for preparing new medicines and rewarding innovators who could contribute to 'the health or wealth of men'. Plattes used *Macaria* to reinforce his previous scheme for the state to endow and administer a college for research into technology, agriculture and medicine. Like Winthrop and Child he believed that chemistry was the science which would reveal the mechanisms of nature.[53] Accordingly the college would be dominated by its laboratory. While Plattes made no specific proposals, he probably conceived the college primarily as a loose association of expert practitioners, who would meet periodically to pool their knowledge. No prospective members of the college were mentioned, but Plattes probably had in mind, as well as himself, such figures as the mathematician Pell, the inventors Caspar Kalthoff and Johann Christoph de Berg, and the chemist Johannes Hunniades, all of whom were already associated with Hartlib in some capacity. Plattes was insistent that state supervision was essential, not only for verification of results, but also to ensure the dissemination of useful information to the widest public. In both *Macaria* and *The Profitable Intelligencer* (1644) Plattes insisted that his major work 'The Treasure House of Nature Unlocked' could not be published until it had been granted the imprimatur of a parliamentary committee. Only by such a mechanism could the fruits of scientific research 'be made common to all'. Then it would be appreciated that 'as God is infinite, and men are infinite by propagation, so the fruits of the Earth for their food and cloathing are infinite, if men will consent to put their helping hand to this commendable Design'.[54]

Macaria was published shortly after Comenius's arrival in London. Comenius like Plattes was hoping that England's rulers would take up

51. Letter from Hartlib to Roe, 10 August 1640, *CSPD 1640,* p.568.

52. Plattes, *Macaria* (219), pp.3–5.

53. Letter from Winthrop to Hartlib, 16 December 1659, in Turnbull (292), p.39, which demonstrates that Winthrop had actually met Plattes.

54. *Macaria* (219), pp.11–12; *Mercurius Laetificans,* quoted from *Hartlib his Legacy* (142), p.174.

the ideas of Bacon about the Universal College expressed at the opening of Book II of *De Augmentis Scientiarum.* The appearance of a new translation of this work by Gilbert Watts of Lincoln College, a friend of Hübner at Oxford, was regarded by the Czech prophet as auspicious.[55] Comenius hoped that this translation would prepare the ground for universal restoration (universalia universalis restaurationibus) by promoting the compilation of 'Universal Books' and the organisation of a system of 'Universal Schools'. Initially he proposed that a college should be founded in London, with six or seven members, who would divide responsibilities and correspond with learned men throughout the world about discoveries and inventions.[56] Already in 1638, Dury, Hartlib and Comenius had decided upon a convenient distribution of labour. Dury was to continue to 'promote the councells of peace ecclesiasticall'; Hartlib was 'the sollicitor of humane learning for the reformation of schooles', with Comenius as his 'coadiutor' producing works on 'schooling and pansophicall learning'.[57] In the following year Hartlib described a slightly different arrangement: Pell was suited to produce 'a perfect enumeration of all things', Hübner 'for that which hase an evident use in *vita humana'*, and Comenius 'for methodizing and contracting, cutting of all verbosities and impertinencies whatsoever'.[58] Comenius attributed this scheme for collaboration to a friend (almost certainly Hartlib), who by 'a certaine, fervent and extraordinary desire of promoting the publick good . . . drew us forth with our endeavours into the publick'. Afterwards, various 'choyser wits' were persuaded to co-operate in the matter, and it was agreed that they should all meet 'to distribute the tasks amongst us'.[59] Among other prospective participants in this Universal College, would have been Joachim Hübner, Theodore Haak, and John Pell; at one stage the orientalist Johann S. Rittangel was courted.

According to Comenius, Culpeper and Stoughton, parliament considered assigning to them either the Savoy Hospital, Chelsea College or the hospital of St. Cross Winchester, 'whereby a certain number of learned and hard-working men, called from all nations, might be honourably maintained either for a term of years or permanently'.[60]

Pansophiae prodromus, a translation of which was issued in 1642, provided a general indication of the pansophic aim of Comenius. But his more specific recommendations concerning the Universal College

55. Young, pp.54–5, 65; *MGP* II, pp.100–2, where Hübner describes meetings with Watts to discuss Bacon and Comenius.

56. Letter from Comenius to Hartlib, 7/17 February 1641, HP VII 84; *HDC,* p.350; D. Čapková, *Acta Comeniana,* 1970, *26*: 286–9. The term *Collegium Lucis* was used interchangeably for *Collegium universale.*

57. Letter from Dury to Edward Montague Viscount Mandeville, Trinity College Dublin MS C. 2.10, fol. 7; reproduced by O. Odložilík, *The Slavonic Review,* 1930–1, *9,* No. 25: p.86.

58. Ephemerides 1639.

59. Comenius, *Patterne of Universal Knowledge* (53), pp.172–3.

60. Young (348), p.54; *HDC,* pp.361–2; letter from Culpeper to Hartlib [c. April, 1642], HP XIII.

were contained in *Via Lucis,* the main work composed during his English visit.[61] Like Plattes, Comenius insisted that the members of this college should be dedicated to public service :

> 'For this task fit men will be chosen from the whole world, men of quick and industrious temper, of piety, warmly devoted to the welfare of the people, taken indifferently from laymen engaged in public affairs and of ecclesiastics; these must be set, as it were, in a watch-tower to look out for the well-being of mankind, and to see every possible way, means, or occasion of seeking whatever will be beneficial to all men.'[62]

Again like Plattes, Comenius was concerned, not merely to advance knowledge, but to ensure that the gifts of God were 'enjoyed in widest commonalty'. The prophets of the college should be on constant guard against any tendency to benefit the few without attention to the common good, to pursue one study without reference to other disciplines, or to favour one sectarian opinion at the expense of the universal church. They were to be guided by the principle of universality.

Following Bacon, Comenius encouraged the college to communicate with colleagues throughout the world. Hence the society might become an 'Invisible College', its members being bound together by 'ties of sacred laws'. In the tradition of the German fraternities, Comenius drafted a brief set of rules to guide the members of this Universal College.[63] The focus of activity would be England, in view of its suitability as a centre of international communications. In line with the general millenarian spirit of *Via Lucis,* Comenius pointed out that Drake's voyages 'gave us a prelude of this universal concert of the nations' based on England.[64]

In view of his emphasis on universality, it would have been inappropriate for Comenius to outline limited functions for his college. He contended that what was essentially new about his project was 'its universal range, nothing in fact less than the improvement of all human affairs, in all persons and everywhere'.[65] Nevertheless, *Via Lucis* suggested certain basic areas of action—the promotion of universal education, a critical synthesis of knowledge into a pansophic system, the production of a series of graded textbooks which would make this knowledge available to all age groups and all social classes, and finally the elaboration of a universal language.

Plattes and Comenius placed their colleges in a utopian context, because utopian solutions seemed appropriate to the conditions in which they were writing. They themselves believed that influential promoters would support institutions conceived in these terms and that the state

61. *HDC,* pp.362, 367.
62. Comenius, *Via Lucis* (55), p.167.
63. *Ibid.,* pp.173–6.
64. *Ibid.,* p.172.
65. *Ibid.,* p.6.

would ultimately come to superintend ambitious schemes of social reconstruction. Their schemes were therefore strictly practical in intention and they were conceived with reference to a widely supported social programme. However, the Civil War rapidly extinguished any possibility of parliament's establishing a national institution for the advancement of learning. In 1642 Comenius and Dury left for the continent disillusioned about the possibility of fulfilling their mission in England; Hübner saw no point in remaining at Oxford and he too left in 1642; Pell had taken up an academic appointment in Amsterdam by 1643; Plattes became destitute and one day fell dead in the street on his way to visit Hartlib. So ended the Universal College and temporarily Hartlib moved from the centre of the stage. However, *Macaria* and the Universal College are valuable in indicating the extent of puritan commitment to the organisation of intellectual effort and for highlighting the central place of science and medicine in their schemes. Indeed the scientific problems discussed at this time remained central to the concerns of puritan intellectuals during the Commonwealth and Protectorate.

(iv) The 'New Philosophy' in London

After the initial traumas of the Civil War there was an immediate renewal of initiative on intellectual and social reform. There assembled in the capital both aspiring puritan intellectuals, and discredited royalists in search of rehabilitation. Science and medicine offered useful gambits for both parties, with the result that from 1645 onwards London witnessed an impressive variety of plans for intellectual organisation, introduced by such activists as Hartlib, Haak and Worsley.

There were many dimensions to London science. The College of Physicians, the Barber-Surgeons Company and the Worshipful Society of Apothecaries, while primarily concerned with professional matters, inevitably took on educational and scientific functions. These organisations will be considered in detail in Chapter IV of this book. Each of these professional groups was extremely diverse from the point of view of political and religious outlook; it would not have been in the interests of any of them for one section of their membership to attempt to force the whole society into a partisan attitude. In view of their specific vocational function, none of these bodies was equipped to become the major centre for lay participation in science. Gresham College on the other hand was by its constitution and traditions better adapted to serve this purpose.[66] Much has been written about the merits of Gresham, but it must be remembered that of the seven chairs, only in Geometry and Astronomy was a conspicuously successful tradition established. It has been demonstrated that Gresham assumed importance as a meeting

66. John Ward, *Lives of the Gresham Professors* (305); F. R. Johnson (159); Hill, *Intellectual Origins* (149), pp.37–61.

place for mathematicians and as a centre for the dissemination of innovations in practical mathematics to an audience of London merchants and seamen. But it is also clear that even in mathematical subjects the college was extremely variable in its effectiveness, in both its research and teaching capacities. Henry Briggs was the supremely successful teacher, and his work was continued by Edmund Gunter, Henry Gellibrand and Samuel Foster. Each of these figures had fairly pronounced puritan associations, although the professors as a whole were not obviously puritan. Henry Gellibrand was brought before the High Commission, Foster had been described as a 'zealous nonconformist'; his brother, also a mathematician, occupied the Emmanuel living of Aller in Somerset which has already been mentioned in connection with Stoughton and Cudworth.[67]

By the late 1630s all was not well at Gresham. A hint of the unsatisfactory state of affairs there was given by Hartlib: 'The Professors therof . . . who excepting few have beene very idle, should bee made at least to publish all their lectures.' Boswell, Hartlib's informant, excepted only Briggs and Gellibrand from this criticism.[68] Hartlib's impressions are confirmed by a brief inspection of the Gresham professoriate in 1640. In 1636 Samuel Foster took over from Gellibrand the prestigious chair of astronomy, but after a year he was obliged to vacate the position, being replaced by the king's nominee, Mungo Murray. Murray held the post in conjunction with a benefice in Norfolk, until he resigned in 1641, to allow Foster to reoccupy the chair. Richard Holdsworth, the capable Cambridge scholar held the chair of divinity, but university politics, and his duties as Master of Emmanuel College, would have prevented him from attending to duties at Gresham. John Greaves the professor of astronomy since 1630, undertook an expedition to the Middle East in 1633 and did not return until 1640. Eventually he was 'removed from his Gresham professorship, on account of his long absence, and the neglect of his lecture'. Similarly Thomas Eden the professor of law was an active politician having 'several other imployments, which interfering with his attendance at Gresham, he resigned that professorship upon the 27 July 1640'. Richard Knight professor of music, Thomas Winston professor of physic and John Goodridge professor of rhetoric were nonentities, who made virtually no impression on Gresham College or on their subject.[69] One restriction operative at Gresham, which is invariably overlooked, is the confinement of appointments to unmarried scholars, who were expected to reside in the college and live communally in a manner very reminiscent of the university colleges. Thus there was a severe danger that an institution designed to give versatile young scholars the opportunity to energise the intellectual life

67. For Gellibrand, see *DNB* and Ward (305), pp.81–5; for the Fosters, *DNB* and Ward (305), pp.85–8. Walter Foster was ejected from his living in about 1652, which suggests Presbyterian affiliation: *Walker Revised*, p.313.

68. Ephemerides 1639.

69. Ward (305), pp.56–65; 88–90; 135–53, 217, 240–4, 266–8, 314–17.

of London, would lapse into an almshouse for eccentric old bachelors.[70]

One is left with the impression that the most important scientific activities in London were taking place outside the above institutions, at private discussions in the shops and houses of mathematical practitioners, physicians, surgeons, apothecaries, or laymen with no professional stake in science. The Gresham mathematical professors had risen into celebrity through their work on magnetism and the application of logarithms to navigational tables and instrument making.

These were basically indigenous developments. On the continent other aspects of the physical sciences were being studied with equal success by groups of experimenters whose discoveries were rapidly disseminated throughout Europe by such active correspondents as Marin Mersenne. In Italy the experimenters were beginning to institute formal academies.[71] It was inevitable that the English intellectuals should wish to be drawn into this international network.

Cosmopolitan figures like Sir Charles Cavendish made frequent reports from the continent about topical scientific developments. Among the regular correspondents of Cavendish was John Pell, who was no doubt active in promoting the new science in England, until his own departure in 1643. Pell's patron Samuel Hartlib was by this time absorbed with Comenian pansophy and with the work of various inventors. He was aware of the Italian and French scientific work, but it interested him only to a limited degree, and while he was in favour of initiating a correspondence with such figures as Mersenne, Hartlib himself was happy to remain a bystander. He consequently delegated this specialised aspect of the pansophic undertaking to his friends Pell, and Theodore Haak, the Palatinate exile. Pell had attained the reputation of being a mathematical prodigy, while Haak was well-qualified to undertake the mission in view of his longstanding interest in mathematics, dating back to his studies at Oxford under Thomas Allen and Henry Briggs.[72]

Haak was also fully acquainted with the revival of Bacon's ideas about a universal college. He was on good terms with Hartlib, Dury, Pell and Hübner; all five were included on Comenius's list of particular friends who met him upon his arrival in England.[73] Haak initiated a correspondence with Mersenne by sending Pell's *Idea Matheseos* and Comenius's *Conatuum Comeniorum Praeludia*, works published by Hartlib to stimulate interest in the pansophic system.[74] The correspondence with Mersenne was not entirely satisfying to either party. Mer-

70. Ward (305), p.23: 'none shall be chossen to reade any of the said lectures, so longe as he shall be married, nor be suffered to reade any of the said lectures after that he shalbe married.'

71. Harcourt Brown (36); W. E. Knowles Middleton (177).

72. For an excellent biography of Haak, see Pamela R. Barnett, *Theodore Haak* (20). For the letters between Mersenne, Pell and Haak, see vols. 7–10 of C. de Waard *et al.* (eds.), *Correspondance du M. Mersenne.*

73. Young (348), p.64.

74. Barnett (20), p.38; *idem,* 'Theodore Haak and the early years of the Royal Society' (19), pp.207–9.

senne solicited information on various technical subjects under discussion in France and he wanted allies in his conflict with Robert Fludd; Haak would have preferred to discuss the ideas of Comenius and he felt no sympathy with Mersenne's attempt to discredit Fludd. Accordingly it is not surprising that Haak became increasingly more unresponsive to Mersenne's requests, until in 1640 he brought the correspondence to a close. Nevertheless the experience had been valuable in providing an up-to-date impression of scientific work in France.

According to John Wallis, Haak was the figure who in about 1645 'gave the first occasion, and first suggested' the regular scientific meetings which are generally regarded as the source of the Royal Society.[75] Although Wallis wrote his account of the history of the Royal Society as late as 1697, there is no reason to doubt the basic accuracy of his record. The absence of reference to the 1645 meetings by Sprat in his *History of the Royal Society* (1667) can be explained by his lack of concern with the early history, his ignorance of the events, or his positive desire to suppress an account of events which might attract attention to the puritan and pansophic associations of the early Society. There is one other point of difficulty—Wallis made no reference to Haak in his *Defence of the Royal Society* (1678).[76] However, he was not at that date concerned with the question of the origins of the 1645 meetings. In this more polemical discourse he wished primarily to shed light on the career of John Wilkins. Despite this difference in bias, what is notable is not the discrepancies, but rather the basic similarities between the 1678 and 1697 accounts of the 1645 meetings. It is impossible to sustain the view that his detailed impressions of the 1645 meetings were a figment of Wallis's imagination—or a product of his disingenuity. It is therefore permissible to adopt the long-established view that Wallis provides a basically accurate account of the origins and nature of the 1645 meetings of the originators of the Royal Society.[77] As far as we can detect, Wallis had no ulterior motive for singling out Haak for special mention. Haak was therefore likely to have initiated the 1645 meetings, and as Syfret and Barnett suggest, Haak's involvement with Comenius and the Universal College must be of considerable significance in explaining the origins of his enthusiasm for organised scientific activity.[78]

Besides Wallis and Haak, the other members of the 1645 group

75. Wallis, 'Account of Some Passages of his own Life' (257), p.39.

76. Wallis, *A Defence of the Royal Society* (302).

77. Purver (230), pp.161–82 is the only author seriously to question the accuracy of Wallis's account. For the alternative position, see D. Stimson, 'Dr. Wilkins and the Royal Society', *Journal of Modern History,* 1931, *3* : 539–64, and the contributions by Hill, and A. R. Hall and M. B. Hall in *Notes and Records of the Royal Society,* 1968, *23*, no. 2.

78. Syfret, 'The Origins of the Royal Society' (276); Barnett, *Theodore Haak* (20), pp.75–83; *idem,* 'Theodore Haak and the early years' (19), pp.209–12.

Turnbull, 'Samuel Hartlib's influence on the early Royal Society' (287), pp.104–6, without any sound basis attempts to dissociate Haak from the pansophic activities of Comenius.

mentioned by name in 1697 were John Wilkins, Jonathan Goddard, George Ent, Francis Glisson, Christopher Merrett and Samuel Foster; the 1678 description included Charles Scarburgh, but omitted Haak.[79] This group represents a fusion between two equal elements. The first consists of Glisson, Ent, Scarburgh, Goddard and Merrett, who were academically qualified physicians (the first three being already associated with the College of Physicians in 1645 and the other two becoming so shortly afterwards) all of whom displayed fairly catholic interests in experimental philosophy. All except Goddard were protégés of Harvey. The other members (Wallis, Wilkins, Foster and Haak) were primarily involved with the mathematical sciences; with the possible exception of Wilkins they were in some way connected with the celebrated mathematics teacher William Oughtred, as was the physician Scarburgh. This division correlates to a certain extent with those in religious and political outlook. All of the mathematicians were parliamentarians and Puritans. Of the physicians only Goddard was an active parliamentarian, although Glisson (brother of Henry Glisson, Physician-General in the parliamentary army) was likely to favour parliament. Ent and Scarburgh were particularly committed royalists. In view of this division of allegiance, it is understandable that 'matters of Theology and State Affairs' were excluded from consideration.[80]

There is no direct evidence to indicate how the above group came together. Any reconstruction must be purely conjectural. Haak may have met Wilkins and just possibly Christopher Merrett at Oxford in 1631. More likely his acquaintance with them began much later. His friendship with Oughtred and Pell would probably have led to association with Wallis, Foster and Scarburgh.[81] If they had not met earlier, Wilkins and Haak would have met through Karl Ludwig, the Prince Elector Palatine, whom Wilkins served as chaplain in 1644. Wallis may have been the link with the medical men, in view of his acquaintance with Francis Glisson, the Regius professor of physic, before whom he conducted a defence of Harvey's theory of circulation while a student at Cambridge. Circumstantial evidence of this kind renders it entirely feasible that the group described by Wallis should have come together at the suggestion of Haak; there is nothing in the biographies of the eight figures to preclude Haak from having played this role. Because of his aptitude for mathematics, Haak was encouraged by Hartlib to take up work which led him first to Mersenne and then inexorably into association with Wallis, who was also interested in Comenius but whose main work was drifting towards pure mathematics. This in turn would have led Haak into participation with figures who were primarily

79. Wallis, *Defence* (302), p.8.

80. Wallis, Autobiography (257), p.40; *idem, Defence* (302), p.8.

81. Wallis in his capacity as assistant to the Clerks of the Westminster Assembly may have had dealings with Haak, who knew various members and obtained authorisation from the Assembly for his *Dutch Annotated Bible*: Barnett (20), pp.114–19.

interested in classic experimental and mathematical problems. Hartlib's experiences led in an altogether different direction and it is apparent that he knew virtually nothing about the important association forming around Haak.

The history of the '1645' Group is relatively straightforward. There is no reason to doubt that the meetings began in 1645, although the group could have been formed by the end of the previous year, since Haak returned from his diplomatic mission to Denmark in May 1644. The leading participants were named by Wallis, but he also noted that 'many others' attended, or that 'our numbers encreased'. In 1697 he mentioned weekly meetings, but in 1678 he had been more expansive; they 'met weekly . . . at a certain day and hour, under a certain Penalty, and a weekly Contribution for the Charge of Experiments, with certain Rules agreed upon amongst us'—suggesting a degree of formalisation similar to that adopted at the Oxford meetings of the 1650s.[82] In both accounts Wallis listed various meeting-places adopted by the experimental philosophers, placing slightly more emphasis on Gresham College in 1678 than in 1697. In both accounts the first locations mentioned were Goddard's lodging in Wood Street and the Mitre nearby; they also used the Bull-head in Cheapside. During term-time they gathered at Foster's lecture at Gresham and afterwards repaired either to his lodgings or to some other convenient place nearby.[83] In view of the above evidence about membership and meeting-places the common practice of characterising Wallis's 1645 associates as the 'Gresham Group' gives a rather misleading impression. Gresham and its professors were probably not dominant factors, although Foster's lecture perhaps increasingly proved to be a convenient meeting-point for their group during term-time. Goddard's lodgings were an alternative centre of operations. Goddard was an extremely active and ambitious young physician who would have been eager to establish himself as one of the leading experimental philosophers in London. As Wallis noted, he performed a valuable service by maintaining an operator at his house, who was employed in grinding lenses for microscopes and telescopes.

The primary interests of the London meetings were defined by Wallis as 'the New Philosophy or Experimental Philosophy' after the manner of Galileo and Bacon.[84] It was hoped that this embryonic scientific society would enable England to equal Italy, France and Germany in the cultivation of the new philosophy. The range of their investigations was extremely wide—'Physick, Anatomy, Geometry, Astronomy, Navigation, Staticks, Magneticks, Chymicks, Mechanicks and Natural Experiments.'[85] Wallis was quite specific; the discoveries investigated were (as he rightly claimed) either entirely new or not generally known at that

82. Wallis, *Defence* (302), p.8.
83. Wallis, Autobiography (257), p.39; *Defence* (302), p.8.
84. Wallis (257), p.39.
85. *Ibid.*, p.40.

time. The circulation of blood and the lymphatics were discoveries of the 1620s, but they were still under debate in 1645. Topics discussed also included the latest work on the weight of air and the vacuum, or the Torricellian experiment (1644). It is known that work began in earnest in England at this time on the improvement of telescopes. Both this and the astronomical problems mentioned by Wallis were soon taken up at Oxford.

The London group remained intact until parliament set in motion the first major wave of ejections at Oxford in 1648. This severely depleted the academic ranks and it is not surprising that in view of their commendable intellectual initiative, the politically reliable members of the London group were selected for preferment. Glisson was already established at Cambridge; Wilkins, Wallis and Goddard moved into prestigious posts at Oxford. Once established in the university they resumed their regular scientific meetings. This offshoot of the London Group will be considered in Chapter III. The royalists Scarburgh and Ent were left in London, as was the Gresham professor Foster, who died in 1652. Wallis emphasised in both his accounts that the London meetings continued 'as before', but in view of the predominance of physicians in the 'rump' it is probable that for some time the College of Physicians became the centre for this activity.

(v) The Invisible College

When considering this much-discussed fraternity, it is essential to remember that the term 'Invisible College' was only referred to directly in three letters written by Robert Boyle during 1646 and 1647. In addition there are two other references which seem to relate to the Invisible College.[86] Boyle himself offered few hints about the positive identification of this short-lived and obscure society. However, the Invisible College is important, since it provided the occasion for Boyle's first serious excursion into science. Accordingly, the College is relevant to our understanding of Boyle's intellectual development, and it may throw light on the wider problem of intellectual organisation among the Puritans.

Considerable confusion has been generated on this issue because none of the commonly held identifications of the Invisible College is compatible with the basic facts of Boyle's biography. The first hypothesis derives from Thomas Birch in the eighteenth century; he was peculiarly well-qualified to pronounce on this subject since he was editor of both Boyle's works and the early records of the Royal Society. In view of this background it is not at all surprising that Birch identified the Invisible College with the group of experimental philosophers

86. In basic interpretation this section repeats my 'New Light on the Invisible College: The Social Relations of English Science in the Mid-Seventeenth Century', *Trans. R. Hist Soc.*, 1974, *24*: 19–42, which cites in full the evidence relating to the Invisible College.

whose meetings in 1645 were recorded by Wallis.[87] This solution, which conveniently connects Boyle with the origins of the Royal Society, has had widespread subsequent appeal.[88] However, it is open to two basic objections. First, Boyle's description of the utopian and utilitarian outlook of the Invisible College is difficult to reconcile with the disinterested experimental case-history approach of Wallis's associates. Secondly, Boyle was not acquainted with the members of the 1645 Group until a much later date. Accordingly, any hypothesis identifying the Invisible College with any group including the originators of the Royal Society must be ruled out. If as some recommend Birch's 'Invisible College' is expanded to include members of the Hartlib circle, the first objection is answered in part, but the second is strengthened, since neither Boyle, *nor* Hartlib and his closer associates were familiar with the activities of the group described by Wallis, or involved with any of its members except Haak.[89] Hence it is not helpful to suggest that the Invisible College consisted of a loose federation of two quite distinctive groups—one of which was completely forgotten when Wallis wrote his account of the origins of the Royal Society.

An obvious escape from this dilemma is to equate the Invisible College with the Office of Address, a project which was evolved by the Hartlib circle during 1646 and 1647.[90] However, once again a seemingly productive line of investigation is ruled out by the facts of Boyle's life. During 1646, when the Invisible College was formed, Boyle was not acquainted with Hartlib. His contact with Hartlib was not made until about March 1647 and he was not introduced to the Office of Address proposals until then. Equally, Hartlib knew nothing about the Invisible College until he was informed about it by Boyle in May 1647. No amount of evidence illustrating the deep sympathy between Boyle and Hartlib after that date is sufficient to implicate Hartlib or the Office of Address in anything but the later stages of the Invisible College. This does not quite exhaust the range of attempted solutions, but all tend to founder, either because they are incompatible with Boyle's biography, or because they are irreconcilable with his comments about the aims and activities of his associates. Ideally, the members of the College should rank among Boyle's known asso-

87. Boyle *Works,* i, p.xlii; Birch (26), i, p.2.

88. See C. R. Weld, *History of the Royal Society,* 2 vols. (London, 1848), i, pp.39–40; R. F. Young, *Comenius in England* (348), pp.17, 77; D. Stimson, 'Comenius and the Invisible College', *Isis,* 1935, *23*: 373–88; G. H. Turnbull, 'Samuel Hartlib's influence on the early Royal Society' (287); P. R. Barnett, 'Theodore Haak' (19): *idem, Theodore Haak* (20), p.81; R. F. Jones, *Ancients and Moderns* (163), pp.177–8.

89. Proponents of this point of view include D. Masson, *The Life of John Milton,* 7 vols. (London, 1859–94), iii, pp.662–6; Margaret L. Bailey, *Milton and Jakob Boehme* (16); R. H. Syfret, 'The Origins of the Royal Society' (276); F. A. Yates, *The Rosicrucian Enlightenment* (346), pp.182–4.

90. See M. Boas, *Robert Boyle and Seventeenth Century Chemistry* (Cambridge, 1958), pp.5–32; M. Purver, *The Royal Society* (230), pp.206–34; B. J. Shapiro, *John Wilkins* (259), pp.26–7.

ciates in 1646 and their scientific outlook must accord with the direct references made to the Invisible College in his letters.

The Birch edition of Boyle's letters gives the impression that the only scientific correspondence of Boyle in 1646 and early 1647 is that in which he transmitted information about the Invisible College to Marcombes in October 1646 and to Tallents in February 1647. However, closer examination of the letters printed by Birch reveals that Boyle also wrote two letters to Benjamin Worsley during this period, in November 1646 and February 1647.[91] These letters were obviously written to an intimate scientific companion.[92] Although no direct reference to the Invisible College was made, the tone of these letters is so consistent with Boyle's description of the College that Maddison has quite justifiably suggested that Worsley was involved with this venture.[93] In private correspondence between initiates there would have been no need to mention the College by name. If this view is accepted, these letters may be used to provide further insight into the mechanism of the Invisible College.

The first letter was written just after Boyle, at Stalbridge in Dorset, had received the news that Worsley's project to manufacture saltpetre had received parliamentary approval. This venture, which will be considered more fully in Chapter V, illustrates the faith of Worsley and Boyle in the potentialities of chemical technology in both peace and war. Boyle's other 'grand employment' at this time was 'to catechise my gardener and our ploughmen concerning the fundamentals of their profession'. He hoped soon to convey information which would further Worsley's 'great design' to publish a discourse *de usu partium* for the 'great world'.[94] In the second letter Boyle developed a theme mentioned in the first, that active correspondence could partly compensate for separation. In extravagant terms Boyle begged Worsley to continue the correspondence in order 'to sweeten my unwelcome separation from you'. His immediate quest was for information about practical chemistry from Worsley's laboratory, pending the arrival of a wagon containing chemical apparatus which would form the nucleus of his own laboratory. He was clearly excited by the prospect of establishing a laboratory and frustrated by delays in the transport of his apparatus. But in spite of these initial difficulties chemistry was praised for having cemented their friendship. Intense admiration was expressed

91. R. E. W. Maddison, *The Life of the Honourable Robert Boyle* (185), p.70. Neither letter is dated, and the recipient of the second is wrongly given by Birch as Oldenburg.

92. Boyle *Works,* vi, pp.39–41.

93. However, Maddison has made his position slightly less tenable by suggesting that Dury, Hartlib's closest associate in the Office of Address, was associated with the Invisible College: 'Studies in the Life of Robert Boyle FRS. Part VI, the Stalbridge Period, 1645–1655', *Notes & Records,* 1963, *18*: 104–24; *Life of Boyle* (185), pp.67–70.

94. Letter from Boyle to Worsley [c. 21 November 1646], Boyle *Works,* vi, pp.40–1.

for Worsley, whose letters were described, using one of Boyle's characteristically cumbersome metaphors, as being 'more fertile in philosophy, than news, as oysters are in pearls, than in rattles.' Boyle recognised that he would be the main beneficiary from the correspondence, but he believed that Worsley would gain in stature, just as the brightness of planets reflected the virtues of the sun. In addition, Worsley's free communication of knowledge was morally edifying.[95] In view of the extremely close relationship between Boyle and Worsley exposed by the above letters, it is reasonable to suppose that they were jointly involved in the formation of the Invisible College, some time late in the summer of 1646. From the tone of the letters it is clear that Worsley, who was eight years older than Boyle, would have been the senior partner in this enterprise and perhaps its originator. Worsley may well have been the figure who was described by Lady Ranelagh to Boyle in June 1647 as 'one of your own fraternity, who thinks himself in the highest class of your philosophical Society'.[96]

The explicit references made by Boyle to the Invisible College expand upon themes introduced in the letters to Worsley. Boyle's primary aim was to follow Worsley's example by establishing a chemical laboratory. However, upon the arrival of his apparatus, he was disconsolate to find that the furnace, the centre-piece of his laboratory, had 'crumbled into as many pieces, as we into sects'.[97] In his letter to Marcombes about the Invisible College, Boyle solicited information about continental husbandry, presumably to assist his improvements at Stalbridge, but also to supply the useful information promised to Worsley.[98]

The aims of Boyle's fraternity were stated with varying emphasis in his letters to Marcombes, Tallents and Hartlib. To the Cambridge tutor Francis Tallents he underlined their emancipation from scholasticism —'school-philosophy is but the lowest region of their knowledge'. Following Bacon's maxim, they would learn from 'the meanest, so he can but plead reason for his opinion'. 'Narrow-mindedness' (probably the idle curiosity and avarice criticised in the first letter to Worsley) was not tolerated; instead they were guided by 'charity', or 'universal good-will', and so took 'the whole body of mankind for their care'. This latter maxim was also applied in the first letter to Worsley which expressed similar universalist aims and defended economic enterprise providing that it was conditioned by 'the good they may do with it'.[99] Boyle employed the continental scholar Isaac Marcombes as an agent for procuring useful 'receipts' (chemical experiments, or medicines) or choice books; for his benefit Boyle identified the fraternity's interests

95. Letter from Boyle to Worsley [February 1647], Boyle *Works*, vi, pp.39–40.

96. Letter from Lady Ranelagh to Boyle, 3 June [1647], Boyle *Works*, vi, p.522. For the dating of this letter see Webster (*op. cit.* n.86), p.21.

97. Letter from Boyle to Lady Ranelagh, 6 March 1646/7, Boyle *Works*, i, pp.xxxvi–xxxvii.

98. *Ibid.*, i, p.xxxiv.

99. Letter from Boyle to Tallents, 20 Feb. 1647, Boyle *Works*, i, pp.xxxiv–xxxv.

as 'natural philosophy, the mathematics, and husbandry, according to the principles of our new philosophical college, that values no knowledge, but as it hath a tendency to use'.[100]

It may be presumed that Boyle would have wished to expand the scope of the Invisible College. In March 1647 he was introduced to Hartlib, to whom he acknowledged the 'Utopian' character of the Invisible College in a letter written in May of that year.[101] He realised that his correspondent would be sympathetic, since it was well-known that Hartlib had been involved in similar utilitarian and utopian ventures. There are no indications that Boyle solicited support from members of the 1645 Group. He may perhaps have known about their weekly meetings, but the subjects described by Wallis were not of primary interest to Boyle at this time. Both the Invisible College and the 1645 Group were ostensibly concerned with such subjects as mechanics, natural philosophy and chemistry, but the 1645 Group was fascinated by a miscellaneous collection of 'New Discoveries' which were under discussion throughout Europe, whereas Boyle was only concerned with knowledge which 'hath a tendency to use'. Hence, at least for a time, the scientific work of the two groups of experimental philosophers diverged in accordance with their different premises and priorities. The experimental work of the 1645 Group was suited to a membership which was politically heterogeneous: unity could best be preserved if topics having social relevance were avoided. The Invisible College on the other hand was pledged to social action. It was therefore difficult for its members to avoid partisan political involvement, as illustrated by the saltpetre project: this was intended to supply many economic benefits and also to alleviate a public grievance, but it was also directly designed to facilitate the supply of gunpowder to the parliamentary army.

It is unlikely that the Invisible College ever aspired to more than an informal existence. The College was 'Invisible', not out of a desire for secrecy of the Rosicrucian type, but because its members were likely to be geographically separated. Andreae's Societas Christiana in Germany was maintained on an exactly similar basis of correspondence between widely separated members. Secrecy would have been incompatible with Boyle's public aims. Worsley in London and Boyle in Stalbridge provided the basic axis of the fraternity, and they no doubt expected to be able to sustain its character. The letters cited above suggest that the Invisible College maintained its identity from the late summer of 1646 at least until June 1647. Boyle's College was still described as 'new' in the letter to Tallents, written in October 1646. There is no indication of when its identity was finally lost, but the Office of Address discussed below perhaps provides the answer to this question.

100. Letter from Boyle to Marcombes, 22 October 1646, Boyle *Works*, i, pp.xxx–xxxiv.
101. Letter from Boyle to Hartlib, 8 May 1647, Boyle *Works*, i, pp.xl–xli.

Apart from Worsley and Boyle, who were the members of the Invisible College? Isaac Marcombes and Francis Tallents were canvassed for support, but it is unlikely that they were more than peripheral adherents. Hartlib would certainly have given his unqualified approval, but he was approached too late. Hartlib's most intimate correspondents, Culpeper and Dury, seem to have known nothing about the Invisible College.

Boyle kept his sister Lady Ranelagh fully informed about his philosophical and scientific work. She also knew Worsley well. Her familiarity with the affairs of the Invisible College is shown by the letter of June 1647 which transmitted correspondence from Worsley to Boyle. While as a woman she may have been reticent about formal membership, there are numerous testimonies of her forceful participation in religious, political and philosophical debates among puritan intellectuals. Even as a young woman, she was venerated by her family and acquaintances alike. In time her reputation became inseparably linked with that of her brother. Hence in his funeral eulogy of Boyle Burnet also commemorated Katherine, as the woman who had 'made the greatest figure in all the revolutions of these Kingdomes for above fifty years'.[102] Accordingly her role was much more than that of a patroness and clearing house for correspondence. She would certainly have exerted as much influence as a full member and her numerous associates would have provided a clientele for recruitment. The meetings of the enthusiasts of the Invisible College probably centred around Worsley's laboratory, and Lady Ranelagh's London home in Pall Mall.

The close relationship between Boyle, Worsley and Lady Ranelagh once established, it is possible to consider whether the social group in which they operated provides a plausible base for the wider Invisible College. The obvious common denominator between Worsley, Boyle and Lady Ranelagh was their Irish connection, a factor which probably explains, among other things, Worsley's early acquaintance with the Boyle family. Katherine, the seventh child of the first Earl of Cork, married Arthur Jones, second Viscount Ranelagh, whose family had allied with Cork against Strafford before 1640. Through Jones, Katherine became the sister-in-law of Sir John Clotworthy and the niece of Dorothy Moore (the future wife of John Dury), who was the sister of the planter Sir Robert King. At the outset of the Irish Rebellion Katherine was besieged in Athlone Castle for nearly two years, before being allowed safe conduct to England. Once established in London, her home became a focal point for meetings of Irish protestants in exile or on political missions to parliament.

When Robert Boyle returned from his European tour with Isaac Marcombes, he gravitated immediately to Katherine's home where

102. Gilbert Burnet, *A Sermon Preached at the Funeral of the Honourable Robert Boyle* (London, 1692), p.33.

'with thankfulness to God, acknowledg'd as a seasonable Providence . . . since first in the heat of his youth, it kept him constantly in a Religious family, where he heard many pious discourses, & saw great store [of] pious examples, . . . Besides by this means grew acquainted with several Persons of power & interest in ye Parliament and their party, which being then very great, & afterwards the prevailing one, prov'd of good use, & advantage to him . . .'[103]

Katherine undertook responsibility for the education of members of her family, entrusting Richard Barry second Earl of Barrimore, and her own son Richard Jones, to John Milton. Another tutor involved with the Boyle family was Francis Tallents of Magdalene College, whom Robert Boyle introduced to the Invisible College.[104] Boyle having completed his formal education was introduced to parliamentarians and puritan intellectuals. In Katherine's immediate household, Boyle would have encountered her sister-in-law, Margaret, Lady Clotworthy, wife of the prominent Presbyterian parliamentarian.

By 1646 Robert Boyle's elder brother, Roger, Lord Broghill, had come to assume a leading role in Irish political and military affairs. In parliament, he became identified with the party of Philip Sydney, Lord Lisle, who became Lord Lieutenant in April 1646. This alignment involved Broghill in political manoeuvres in both London and Dublin.[105] Lisle's party included Sir William Parsons, Sir John Temple and Arthur Annesley, all of whom were accused of 'Independency' by their major opponent the Lord President. Parsons and Temple were long-standing associates of the Earl of Cork, while at this time Arthur Annesley was entrusted by Robert Boyle with the management of his estates in Connaught.

By 1646 Broghill and most members of his family were advocates of a vigorous war policy in Ireland, with the result that they were thrown into alliance with the Independent party, and against royalist advocates of compromise, as well as the more obvious catholic enemy. The war policy was seen as the most effective means of protecting the planting interest and of preventing the suppression of protestantism. The alignments involving Broghill in 1646 were very largely a continuation of associations which had been formed during opposition to Strafford.[106]

103. Robert Boyle, Autobiographical fragment, British Museum Sloane MS 4229, fol. 68; Maddison, *Life of Boyle* (185), pp.53–4.

104. Maddison, *Life of Boyle* (185), p.65; Historical Manuscripts Commission Report, *Egmont,* i, pp.474–5, 491–2.

105. K. S. Bottigheimer, *English Money and Irish Land: The Adventurers in the Cromwellian Settlement of Ireland* (Oxford, 1971), pp.91–108.

106. Historical Manuscripts Commission Report, *Egmont,* i, pp.367–74. In March 1647 Inchiquin pleaded with Lady Ranelagh to intercede with her brother on his behalf: *ibid.,* i, pp.374–5. H. F. Kearney, *Strafford in Ireland 1633–41* (Manchester, 1959), pp.10–11. Maddison, *Life of Boyle* (185), p.65. Kathleen Lynch, *Roger Boyle* (Knoxville, Tenn., 1965), pp.38–69.

Worsley was involved with Irish affairs in a modest capacity. His career began in the service of Strafford, and then, at the outbreak of the rebellion, he became an army physician. But he soon left the army service and entered Trinity College Dublin. After obtaining a degree he returned to England, settling in London under the patronage of Sir John Temple, whose propagandist history of the Irish Rebellion was published in 1646. Subsequently Temple probably played an important part in securing Worsley's preferment in the Irish civil service. Temple's growing participation in Anglo-Irish politics was signified by his election to the House of Commons and his membership of the Committee for Ireland formed in August 1646. Broghill was also actively involved with this committee, which was effectively dominated by the Lisle interest.[107]

Worsley first received official recognition in 1647, when the House of Commons decreed that 'Dr. Gerard Boate, Mr. Benjamin Worsley, and Mr. Marmaduke Lynne, be appointed physician, Surgeon-General and Apothecary of the Army in Ireland, and sent to Dublyn.'[108] This may have been the topic under consideration in the letter from Lady Ranelagh to Boyle already mentioned. Worsley and Boate were not able to take up their appointments in Ireland immediately, probably because internal dissension in the parliamentarian party reduced the level of military assistance given to Dublin until 1649.

The date of Worsley's earliest acquaintance with Boyle is not known precisely, but it probably occurred at the end of 1645 or the beginning of 1646. Worsley knew Hartlib, but he would have found Boyle a more congenial choice for participation in the Invisible College. Thereafter the Invisible College was revealed to dependants of the Boyle family such as Marcombes and Tallents, or to other members of Lady Ranelagh's circle, and Lisle's party. There is much circumstantial evidence to suggest interaction between the scientific and political groups which crystallised around Lady Ranelagh during 1646.

Two obvious candidates for the Invisible College within the Ranelagh circle are the brothers Gerard and Arnold Boate, both physicians of Dutch origin whose London careers had been punctuated in the previous decade by conflicts with the College of Physicians.[109] Sub-

107. For Worsley see Bodleian, Clarendon MS 75, fols. 300–1: autobiographical letter from Worsley to Lady Clarendon. J. B. Whitmore, *Notes and Queries* (1943), *185*: 123–8; Maddison, *Robert Boyle* (185), pp.63, 136. Historical Manuscripts Commission Report, *Ormonde,* n.s. ii, pp.256–7, 284–5. Temple and Sir William Parsons were signatories of letters on behalf of 'Chyrurgian-General' Worsley in 1643. For a recent excellent summary, see Aylmer (12), pp.270–2, 416–17. For Temple see Bottigheimer, *op. cit.,* pp.101–8; also D. Underdown, *Pride's Purge* (Oxford, 1971), pp.43, 82; *DNB.*

108. *CJ,* v, p.247, 17 July 1647.

109. For Gerard (1604–1650) and Arnold Boate (1606–1653), see *Nieuw Nederlandsch Biografisch Woordenboek,* iv, pp.211–12; Sir George Clark, *History of the Royal College of Physicians* (50), i, pp.262–3, 297. Historical Manuscripts Commission Report, *Ormonde*, n.s. ii, pp.155–6. *CSPD 1649–1650*, pp.66, 588; Samuel Hartlib (ed.), *Irelands Naturall History* (30), sig. A6r–8r; Bottigheimer,

sequently they became involved with the Boyle family, Worsley and various Anglo-Irish politicians. Arnold settled in Dublin in 1636, where his patients included both Ussher and Strafford. Thereafter for some years his career resembled that of Worsley. He joined the army medical corps, as physician-general to the army in Leinster; he then returned to England at about the same time as Worsley, joining his brother in London from May to October 1645, before leaving for Paris. Gerard Boate remained in London and his patients included Robert Boyle and Lady Ranelagh, as well as other members of the Boyle family. One of Robert Boyle's early medical notebooks has entries derived from Worsley and Gerard Boate.[110] Just before the establishment of the Invisible College Gerard Boate began work on a comprehensive natural history of Ireland, based on information collected by Arnold Boate, Sir William Parsons and his son Richard Parsons. The involvement of Gerard Boate and Worsley in the Ranelagh circle may have facilitated their joint appointment to the Irish army medical service in 1647. Gerard Boate arrived in Dublin in late 1649, only a few months before his death. The Boates display the characteristic attributes of the Invisible College, enthusiasm for Baconian natural history, and anti-authoritarianism both in natural philosophy and in medicine. Their first publication, less radical philosophically than its title suggests — *Philosophia naturalis reformata id est philosophiae Aristotelicae accurata examinatio ac solida confutatio* — was dedicated to Robert Sidney, Earl of Leicester and published in Dublin in 1641. Similar antiperipateticism may have been inherited by Worsley's patron Sir John Temple from his father, the celebrated Ramist Sir William Temple, Provost of Trinity College Dublin.

In view of the pronounced antiperipateticism of Boyle, Worsley and the Boates, their Invisible College would have undoubtedly attracted the sympathy of Miles Symner, a little-known figure, who was prebendary of Kilmacallan in Connaught from 1634, under the patronage of Sir John King. In 1648 we find Symner writing to his patron's son Sir Robert King, declaring his enthusiasm for 'reall & experimental Learning' and inveighing against the 'ventosities, froth & idle speculations of the Schooles' which were fatal to university education.[111] There

---

op. cit., p.177: Boate invested £180, in expectation of a reward of 847 acres; see below, p.435. T. C. Barnard, 'The Social Policy of the Commonwealth and Protectorate in Ireland' (18), pp.332–5.

110. 'Memorials Philosophical', Royal Society, Boyle Papers XXVIII.

111. Letter from Symner to King, 24 October 1648; copies in British Museum Sloane MS 427, fol. 85 and HP XLVII 6. For Sir William Temple (1555–1627), see W. S. Howell, *Logic & Rhetoric In England 1500–1700* (Princeton, 1956), pp.194–6, 205–6. Temple's main antiperipatetic work was *A Dissertation concerning the Unipartik Method . . . an Explanation of Some Questions in Physics and Ethics* (London, 1581). T. C. Barnard has kindly reminded me that Sir Robert King's brother, Edward King, was the friend of Milton whose name is mentioned in connection with *Lycidas*.

is no direct evidence to connect Symner with the Invisible College in 1646, but it is quite possible that he had been in contact with Boate and Worsley in Ireland before that date. Subsequently Symner became chief engineer to the Irish Army, professor of mathematics at Trinity College Dublin, and an active participant in the Irish Survey.[112] Symner reflects Boyle's description of the Invisible College as consisting of 'men of so capacious and searching spirits that school-philosophy is but the lowest region of their knowledge'.

The Anglo-Irish intellectuals associated with the Boyle family provide a much better potential basis for the Invisible College than alternative groups previously put forward. There is nothing in Boyle's early biography to preclude this Irish connection and it is supported by much circumstantial evidence. Hence the Invisible College may have been initiated in the late summer of 1646 by Worsley and Boyle, as a means to propagate their conception of experimental philosophy among their immediate associates. Initially, active participation came from Lady Ranelagh, Gerard and Arnold Boate, and possibly also from such figures as Miles Symner or John Sadler.[113] This fraternity was well-prepared to receive the ideas developed by Worsley and Boyle. Within the Anglo-Irish group, the Invisible College would have found many patrons, who were not intimately involved with philosophical, scientific or economic affairs, but who were in a position to provide encouragement and information. This class includes Broghill, Temple, Sir Robert King, Sir William and Richard Parsons, Sir Charles Coote and Sir John Clotworthy. If the above identification is correct, 'Invisibility' would have been forced on the group by virtue of their unsettled fortunes and obligations outside London. While London provided a focus, it was necessary to maintain communications with Stalbridge, Ireland, Paris and various other locations on the continent and perhaps even New England. Although there is no positive evidence to support their association, Robert Child and John Winthrop Jr. were so close in outlook to Worsley and Boyle, that they would have made invaluable members of the Invisible College. It is interesting in this context that Winthrop was educated at Trinity College Dublin, and that his father had been concerned with Irish plantations. Child arrived in England in 1647 for his second visit; he soon made preparations to visit Ireland. He landed in Ireland in 1651 and remained there until

112. Symner was the brother-in-law of Henry Jones, Bishop of Clogher. H. Cotton, *Fasti Ecclesiae Hibernicae*, iv (Dublin, 1850), pp.149–50. Barnard (18), pp.399–441; *idem*, 'Miles Symner . . .', *Jnl. Roy. Soc. Antiquaries of Ireland*, 1972, *102*: 129–42. John Sadler and King were appointed members of the 1653 Committee for the Advancement of Learning: *CJ*, vii, p.287; Firth & Rait, ii, pp.355–7.

113. John Sadler (1615–1674), the London lawyer who became Master of Magdalene College Cambridge in 1650, was often mentioned in conjunction with Worsley in letters received by Hartlib in 1647. See below, n. 162. In 1648 Hartlib recorded that Sir William Parsons, 'a very rational gentleman', was passing medical information to Lady Ranelagh: Ephemerides 1648.

his death in 1654.[114] Once established in England Child became acquainted with Boyle and Worsley, but unfortunately there is no evidence that he corresponded with them from America.

Although small in membership and short-lived as a formal association, the Invisible College was by no means unproductive. Through this agency Robert Boyle was launched into his scientific career inspired with missionary zeal and single-minded dedication. He believed that Histories of Trade and Nature of the kind undertaken by his friends were as much a fertile basis for scientific enquiry as a means to promote economic innovation. The ideas announced in letters about the Invisible College received definitive expression in his *Usefulness of Experimental Natural Philosophy.* A characteristic manifestation of the work of the Invisible College was Boate's *Irelands Natural History,* the first stage of a comprehensive regional economic survey—perhaps a contribution to Worsley's *de usu partium* of the 'great world'. From the saltpetre project Worsley moved quickly into the area of general economic theory, proposing measures designed to create a favourable atmosphere for the exploitation of innovations. Support from politically active patrons of the Invisible College was probably important in securing Worsley's appointment to civil service positions from which he could further promote his utopian schemes. The activities of the Invisible College clearly illustrate the manner in which the direction of scientific research is determined by social factors. The investigations into chemistry, metallurgy, agriculture and surveying were to a large degree a reflection of the aspirations of a social group whose primary ambition was to re-establish profitable Irish plantations.

(vi) The Office of Address

While separate groups of experimental philosophers were crystallising around Wallis and Boyle, Hartlib was attempting to resuscitate the ashes of the Universal College. After 1641 there was no possibility of establishing Comenius's College on an institutional basis, but the more modest idea of an international correspondency among scholars was not entirely lost from view. Dury in particular hoped that a correspondency of this kind—sometimes called the College of Reformation—might assist with negotiations between the protestant churches of Europe.[115] His attendance at the Westminster Assembly doubtless gave him an opportunity to gather support for this protestant correspondency.

This religious correspondency was never finally relinquished, but Hartlib applied himself primarily to furthering the economic reform

114. G H. Turnbull, 'Robert Child' (290).

115. [John Dury], *A faithfull and seasonable Advice, or, the necessity of a Correspondencie for the advancement of the Protestant Cause* (London, 1643). The background to this tract is given in a letter from Dury to Hartlib, 9/29 September 1642, HP II 42. See also Dury, *The Reformed Spiritual Husbandman* (London, 1652).

proposals announced in *Macaria.* He no doubt increasingly believed that any scheme involving ecclesiastical negotiations would soon be undermined by sectarian squabbles. Accordingly, the model on which Hartlib decided to operate was the Parisian *Bureau d'adresse* of Théophraste Renaudot. This pioneering French agency for intellectual communication and the exchange of information on trade, manufacture and employment attracted widespread attention.[116] Hartlib first commented on the Bureau in 1639, but his correspondence suggests that he did not receive copies of French tracts describing the Office, or a detailed first-hand report of Renaudot's work, until much later. There was considerable interest in the Parisian Bureau when the practical details of the Office of Address were being worked out.[117] The Office of Address proposal also absorbed elements from Bacon, Comenius and Plattes.

The first references to an 'Office of Address' are found among Hartlib's papers dating from the beginning of 1646. It is therefore reasonable to suppose that the scheme was evolved in the latter part of the previous year. As with the Universal College of Comenius, the Office of Address was conceived as a state-regulated institution. In this respect it was different from both Wallis's group and the Invisible College. Ideas about the Office were never entirely fixed, but in the preliminary discussion two basic aims predominated. First, it was hoped that the office would serve as an international correspondency for the advancement of learning. Secondly, it would direct the efforts of inventors, presumably along lines described by Plattes and amplified in the correspondence of Culpeper. Although Gabriel Plattes had died, there appeared to be no deficiency of inventors equipped to continue his work. Hartlib and his collaborators believed that such innovators as Hugh l'Amy, Peter le Pruvost, William Wheeler, William Petty, Benjamin Worsley and others even less well-known (Harrison, Barton, Joiner, Duckett, etc.) might be persuaded to remain in England and serve the public interest, if only the state would take on the responsibility of patronage.

The Office of Address was discussed throughout 1646 by Hartlib, Dury and Culpeper. At first Culpeper was pessimistic about the possibilities of obtaining state support. He advised Dury that he should settle for a London lectureship, which might then become 'a braine center for all kindes of correspondency'. To Hartlib, Culpeper remarked: 'your resolution to persist in your office of addresse showes me your life of faythe, & how in this (as in the rest of your life) you wrastle not onely without but againste hope'. The 'monopolising Corporations'

116. Harcourt Brown (36), pp.18–31; Gilles de la Tourette, *La Vie et les Oeuvres de Théophraste Renaudot* (Paris, 1892); I. Rosenthal & F. Hartmann, *Théophraste Renaudot: Idee und Form seiner Tätigkeit als Polikliniker* (Hanover, 1967); H. M. Solomon, *Public Welfare, Science and Propaganda in Seventeenth Century France: The Innovation of Théophraste Renaudot* (Princeton, 1972).

117. Ephemerides 1639; *HDC*, pp.80–1, 123–4; letters from Culpeper to Hartlib, 29 October 1646 and 9 April 1647, HP XIII.

were blamed for the opposition to Hartlib's philanthropic schemes.[118]

The Office of Address was first announced to the public by Dury in 1647.[119] By this stage the Office was conceived in extremely elaborate and ambitious terms. Its aim was no less than to ensure that 'all that which is good and desirable in a whole Kingdome may be by this means Communicated unto any one that stands in need thereof'. The Office would function in two quite separate sections. One part, the Office of Address for Accommodations, would follow the pattern of Renaudot's Bureau and serve as a comprehensive labour exchange. This proposal was further elaborated by Hartlib, who passed on responsibility for establishing this Office to an 'Agent', the capable merchant and economic reformer, Henry Robinson. Once Robinson's Office was underway, it inspired a whole series of complements, rivals and imitations, produced by members of the Hartlib circle, or by unwelcome interlopers.[120]

Dury and Hartlib expected to be much more directly involved with the second part of the institution, the Office of Address for Communications. This was designed to maintain registers of information on 'matters of Religion, of Learning, and of all Ingenuities, which are Objects of Contemplation and delight unto the Mind, for their strangenesse and usefulnesse unto the life of Man'.[121] There were thus three main divisions of information, Religion, Learning and Ingenuities. Dury's religious correspondency was the first division. The second was designed to further the philosophies of Bacon and Comenius, while the third would fulfil the aims of the College of Experience outlined by Plattes. The Agent for Communications was expected to undertake a predominantly secular programme:

> 'Secondly, in Matters of Humane sciences, the End of his Negotiation should be, 1. To put in Practice the Lord Verulam's Designations, *De Augmentis Scientiarum*, amongst the Learned. 2. To help to perfit Mr. *Comenius* Undertakings, chiefly in the Method of Teaching, Languages, Sciences, and of Ordering Schooles for all Ages and Qualities of Scholars.
>
> Thirdly, in the Matters of Ingenuity his End should be to offer the most profitable Inventions which he should gaine, unto the benefit of the State, that they might be Publikely made use of, as the State should think most expedient.'[122]

118. Letters from Culpeper to Hartlib, 24 February and 4 March 1645/6, HP XIII.

119. John Dury, *Considerations tending to the Happy Accomplishment of Englands Reformation in Church and State* (86).

120. *Englands Reformation* (86), pp.20–58; Samuel Hartlib, *A Further Discoverie of the Office of Publick Addresse for Accommodations*, 1648 (136); *HDC*, pp.85–7. For further discussion, see below, Chapter V. Many of the Office proposals were collected by Hartlib: HP LVII 3, LXIII 7. For Robinson, see *DNB;* W. K. Jordan, *Men of Substance* (Chicago, 1942); Aylmer (12), pp.225–6, 403.

121. *Englands Reformation* (86), pp.45–6.

122. *Ibid.*, p.47.

This brief shows that the Office of Communications was designed to be at least as comprehensive in its scope as the Universal College of Comenius. The Agent for Communications was enjoined to make his office a 'Center and Meeting-place of Advices, of Proposalls, of Treaties and of all Manner of Intellectual Rarities'. He was to encourage English scholars, entertain visitors and keep up an international correspondence. It was particularly important for him to employ the librarians of major libraries to supply useful information from their collections of books and manuscripts.[123] Therefore, from even this first brief exposition of its aims it is apparent that the Office of Address for Communications was designed to embrace a national agency for research and development in science and technology.

The utopian associations of the Office of Address for Communications are emphasised by Hartlib's employment in 1647 of John Hall to translate two documents relating to Andreae's Societas Christiana, and his subsequent use of these tracts to publicise the Office.[124] The Hartlib circle realised that such a major institution would not be easy to establish. Further publicity was given the Office of Communications at the beginning of Petty's *Advice of W.P. to Samuel Hartlib* (1648), in a memorial preceding Hartlib's *Further Discovery of the Office of Public Address* (1648) and in Dury's *Seasonable Discourse* (1649). Although these documents were similar in all major respects, certain trends are apparent. First, the Office of Address increasingly became known as the 'Correspondencie and Agencie for the Advancement of Universal Learning' or the 'Agencie for Universal Learning'.[125] It was also common for the Office or Agency to be called a 'College'.[126] This was partly a reference back to Bacon and Comenius, but this usage also helped to prevent confusion with the Office for Accommodations. Secondly, Dury had originally proposed Oxford as the most appropriate location for the Agent for Communications, undoubtedly because of the importance of the Bodleian Library.[127] But after discussion with other members of the Hartlib circle it was decided that London would be the best location for both offices.[128] It was still hoped that the Agent for Communications would receive an income from a 'place of profit' at Oxford, but this idea was soon discarded.[129] Thirdly, the specifically theological

123. *Ibid.*, pp.48–9.

124. J. V. Andreae, *A Modell of a Christian Society* (Cambridge, 1647). The letters from the translator, John Hall, to Hartlib make frequent references to the Office of Address: HP LX 14. A letter from Joshua Rawlin, 11 May 1648, makes it clear that Hartlib was circulating the Andreae text as a means of promoting the Office of Address: HP X 11.

125. Hartlib, *Further Discoverie* (136), p. (i); Dury, *Seasonable Discourse* (87), pp. 21–6.

126. Letter from Boyle to Hartlib, 8 May 1647, Boyle *Works,* i, p. xl. Letter from Dury to Hartlib, 26 March 1649, HP IV.

127. *Englands Reformation* (86), p.53. See Appendix I below for a plan to integrate the Office of Address into an academic institution.

128. Letter from Culpeper to Hartlib, 22 July 1649, HP XIII.

129. *Further Discoverie,* p.(ii).

responsibilities of the Communications Office were gradually abandoned, although this whole venture remained completely religious in spirit and motivation. Dury's *Reformed Spiritual Husbandman* (1652) showed that he hoped to establish a completely independent protestant correspondency at Chelsea College. Fourthly, the decision of the Council of State on 8 June 1649 to make an annual payment of £100 to Samuel Hartlib was taken as tacit recognition of his position as 'Agent for the Advancement of Universal Learning'. Thereafter Hartlib himself used this title, and others addressed him as the State Agent for Universal Learning.[130] Finally, there was a tendency to distil the original discursive account of the Office for Communications into a set of specific proposals. Thus in 1649 the following plan was put forward by Dury:

1. The Agent already designated by parliament should be given an adequate subsistence.
2. The Agency should be governed by a Board of Trustees for the Advancement of Learning. They would administer funds—a £500 or £1,000 'yearly allowance from the State'—and receive additional legacies. Among their duties were international correspondence, and the administration of all schools and schoolmasters.
3. Two secretaries should be appointed, one for Latin and one for the 'Vulgar' tongues.
4. A hospital should be established for the entertainment of visitors. (Dury had Charterhouse in mind for this purpose.)
5. The Agency should have permission to establish a printing press.[131]

When translated into a set of proposals of this kind, the Office for Communications could be presented as a more practicable objective by its advocates. A similar list of suggestions headed 'A Memoriall for the Advancement of Universal Learning' was used as a basis for discussion, and for distribution to potential supporters.[132] It is noticeable that the *Memorial* abandoned both the specifically religious, and educational clauses of Dury's proposal, concentrating almost entirely on the 'Advancement of Learning and Ingenuities'. This *Memorial* was anonymous, and it is probably best to regard it as a product of joint discussions within Hartlib's circle. However, Dury hinted that Hartlib was its author, whereas Petty seems to claim that it was his work—a possibility which certainly cannot be ruled out, in view of Petty's known support for the Office of Address from an early stage.[133]

Who were the members of this 'College'? Hartlib's state pension immediately established him as the Agent, and he attempted to pro-

130. *CSPD 1649/50*, p.177. For the details of the state pension paid to Hartlib before 1660, see Turnbull, *Samuel Hartlib* (284), pp. 48–51.

131. Dury, *Seasonable Discourse* (87), p.24.

132. The Memorial is given in full in Appendix VIII.

133. Letter from Dury to Hartlib, 26 March 1649, HP IV. Letter from Petty to Boyle, 17 Feb. 1657/8, Boyle *Works*, vi, pp.139–40.

mote the activities outlined in the *Memorial* regardless of the chances of further state patronage. Most members would have served as 'trustees' or 'feoffees'. These trustees were in a sense the secular counterpart of the former Feoffees for Impropriations. Among the original advocates of the Office of Address, John Sadler, Dury and Culpeper would rank as trustees; William Petty might have expected to serve in some more specific capacity, but his name is not included in any of the lists of members yet examined. In looking for further support, Hartlib naturally turned to the members of the Invisible College, Worsley, Boyle and Gerard Boate. They would certainly have realised that the Office of Address was an ideal vehicle for promoting their own utopian and philanthropic aims. Hence by the summer of 1647 the Invisible College, having served its purposes, was allowed to lose its identity. Documents relating to the Office were despatched to Boyle immediately after his introduction to Hartlib. Boyle was quickly converted and soon he was expressing hopes of contributing towards the building of 'that *college*, whereof God has made you hitherto the midwife and nurse'.[134] Thereafter Boyle became one of the most influential and committed supporters of the Agency. Dury described the venture to Boate, who immediately declared 'his willingnes, to be a reader, in the Colledge, eyther of Philosophie or phisiques, or both, and that at present hee would take little or be content with nothing; untill a settlement for the provision of the professors heer after.'[135]

Perhaps because of the possibility of establishing his Office at Oxford, Hartlib adopted a collegiate pattern of organisation for his associates. His plans were headed 'Foundation of a New College' or 'Oxford. To Raise et Correspondency', and contained general lists of names—presumably of the trustees. In this category were Dury, Sadler, Pell, Worsley, Boyle, Culpeper and the physician Thomas Coxe. Also included were the Dutchman Adam Boreel and the inventor Harrison, both of whom were recommended to Hartlib as men of ability. The Agency was to be divided into sections or 'Offices', each being headed by a professor. Various methods of distributing labour were proposed; the following list is a representative reconstruction, derived from the various drafts:

Office of Divinity—Dury
Office of Mechanics—Boyle
Office of Agriculture and Traffic—Worsley and Culpeper
Office of Experimental Philosophy—Worsley, Coxe and Boyle
Chamber of Rarities—Caspar Godeman
Medicine—Gerard Boate, Worsley and Justin van Ascher.[136]

134. Letters from Boyle to Hartlib, 8 May 1647, 16 November 1647, n.d. [1647], Boyle *Works,* i, pp.xli, xlvi–xlvii; vi, p.76. In the first of these letters Boyle divulged the existence of the Invisible College to Hartlib.

135. Letter from Dury to Hartlib, 31 August [1647], HP IV.

136. HP XLVII, 1, 9, 20. For Thomas Coxe, physician to Boyle and one of the

The Office of Address provided an extremely effective test of parliament's long-standing, but rather vague promise to assist the Advancement of Learning. Culpeper and Sadler were Hartlib's main contacts with the increasingly dominant Independent party in the Commons. In March 1646 Culpeper offered to become 'bothe an example & a sollicitor in the behalfe of the Office of Addresse & I make noe question but Mr. Westroe will be (by me) drawne into become a merchant venturer'.[137] Besides Thomas Westrowe, MP for Hythe, Culpeper reported that Andrews was likely to join them. Westrowe informed Culpeper of his approaches to various officers; of these Oliver Cromwell was found to be greatly in favour of a foreign correspondency.[138] Later Culpeper reported that Francis Rous had undertaken 'to propose somethinge on your behalfe & [I] am confidente . . . your office of addresse would not stay longe after'.[139] Sadler was able to exert parliamentary influence through his Dorset relatives John Trenchard and William Sydenham, both of whom entered the Commons in 1645.[140] Negotiations of this kind provided the background to the parliamentary sermon delivered on 31 March 1647 by Stoughton's stepson, Ralph Cudworth, who had by this stage risen to become Master of Clare College Cambridge. This was the only occasion on which Cudworth was selected to speak before parliament and his sermon was a characteristic statement of Christian Platonism of the kind also espoused by Francis Rous. Cudworth prefaced his sermon with an appeal for parliament to promote 'Ingenious Learning'.[141] This move was reminiscent of Gauden's appeal on behalf of the Universal College. Immediately after Cudworth's sermon parliament recommended the payment of £300 to Hartlib, and the newly formed Committee for Oxford was ordered to take account of the deserts of Hartlib and other well-wishers of the

---

closest medical associates of Hartlib, see Munk (195), i, p.247; Maddison (185), p.219; F. H. Ellis, in *Notes & Records,* 1963, *18*: 36–8. See also below, n. 140. For Boreel, see W. Schneider, *Adam Boreel, Sein Leben und Sein Schriften* (Giessen, 1911); Oldenburg *Correspondence,* i, *passim.* Godeman was steward to Philip Herbert, Earl of Pembroke, and a friend of Kynaston.

137. Letter from Culpeper to Hartlib, 1 March 1647, HP XIII.

138. Letter from Westrowe to Culpeper, 20 February 1647, HP XIII. Westrowe served with Culpeper on the Kent Committee. He had the reputation of being a Fifth Monarchist. Yule (349), p.124; Brunton & Pennington (38), pp.41, 51; A. Everitt, *The Community of Kent and the Great Rebellion* (Leicester, 1966), pp.137, 151. The other supporter may have been Thomas Andrews, the London merchant who was Lord Mayor in 1650: Pearl (206), pp.309–11.

139. Letter from Culpeper to Hartlib, 15 March 1647/8, HP XIII.

140. John Sadler married Trenchard's daughter; Trenchard's other daughter married William Sydenham. It is perhaps not entirely coincidental that Thomas Sydenham (younger brother of William) was introduced to medicine by Thomas Coxe, one of the collaborators in the Office of Address project. Hutchins, *Dorset,* i, pp.426–35; ii, pp.546–58; iii, pp.325–31. Brunton & Pennington (38), pp.160, 172; Yule (349), p.121; Keeler (171), p.364; K. Dewhurst, *Dr. Thomas Sydenham* (London, 1966), pp.15, 43, 63.

141. Cudworth (64), sig. A1r–2r.

'Advancement of Learning; and to recommend him to some Place of Benefit in the University of Oxon.'[142] The Hartlib circle saw this recommendation as a spontaneous and prompt response to the Office of Address proposal announced in *Englands Reformation*. In May Boyle expressed his delight over the news from parliament that further developments were expected. However, despite active canvassing the momentum was not maintained. In 1649 Dury wrote to Oliver St. John mentioning that Trenchard and Sadler had notified him of their intention to press on with the Office of Address 'which is lookt upon by many as very useful'. On this occasion Hartlib's supporters probably made use of a brief petition on Hartlib's behalf outlining the advantages of an Office of Address and arguing for state regulation on the grounds that its usefulness would otherwise be impaired by rivalry between competing offices.[143] Once again no action was taken but this was not quite the end of hopes for the establishment of the Office of Address. The reconquest of Ireland, followed by the successful surveys which involved Symner, Worsley, and above all Petty, made it possible to assess the value of confiscated estates. Most of this property was of course earmarked for the repayment of parliamentary debts. Hartlib's supporters detected that this mechanism of settling debts with Irish land could be turned to the advantage of the Agency for Universal Learning. In 1655 Richard Eccleston and James Rand presented a petition asking permission to buy up debentures for arrears due to officers and soldiers in Ireland, and certificates for supplies to the army in Ireland. These debentures and certificates, to the value of £10,000 or £12,000, would then be satisfied with forfeited houses and the profits deployed for the support of Hartlib's schemes as outlined in the *Memorial for the Advancement of Universal Learning*.[144] The *Memorial* and associated documents show that by 1655 Hartlib's Agency was almost exclusively designed to promote the advancement of secular learning, and particularly Baconian science and technology. The aims expressed in 1655 were:

> 'For the cherrishing & incouraging of Persons that are singular for any Faculty or Art. For the holding & maintaining a Correspondency, as well within this Nation, as in forreigne parts with Persons excelling in one & the same faculty or Art. For the makeing some further progresse & Advancement in a usefull improvement of Experiments, to the more cleare elucidation as well of things Naturall as Artificiall. For the raising a Stocke towards the pur-

142. *CJ*, v, pp.131–3.

143. Letter from Dury to St. John, 26 February 1648/9, HP IV 1. 'The humble petition of Sam. Hartlib Esqr . . . for the erection of an Office of Addresse and entries': *HDC*, pp.83–4. This was associated with a draft Act to make Robinson the superintendent of the Office for Accommodations, and Hartlib and Dury the joint superintendents of the other office: HP LXIII 7.

144. For James Rand the prominent London apothecary and his son William Rand, see below, Chapter IV. Richard Eccleston was an Excise Office official.

chasing or towards the printing or translating out of any of the Moderne Tongues or other Tongues, such choice pieces, as are now perhaps not commonly knowne. Towards the purchasing & collecting alsoe of such other things as are or may prove to bee much desired by Learned Men. All which as it is the Intent of the Petitioners they should bee soe farr communicate & made publick, as may bee of use to this Nation.'[145]

John Beale's plan, produced shortly afterwards at Hartlib's request, further shifted the Office of Address in the direction of science and technology. Beale proposed that the first aim of the Office should be that of supplying 'intelligence of all necessary, convenient, pleasant & allowable accommodations, Noveltyes, Rarityes, advertisements & instructions to all parts of this Nation, & to all considerable places abroade'. Beale believed that the Office should be established at public expense, and furnished with a staff of professors. Its central feature would be a 'Colledge of Noble Mechaniques & Ingenious Artificers', which would concentrate on mathematics and inventions. This 'College' was designed to be 'the emulator of all Universityes', which would 'in due season bring forth the fruits perfect of happy industry'.[146]

Hartlib and the other trustees hoped to take advantage of the Protector's 'great Care for the preservation of Learning in this Nation', as well as his 'extraordinary Endeavour for the mainteyning a Unity & Correspondency with Persons eminent for Abilityes, Learning & Piety beyond the Seas.' They judged the mood of Cromwell correctly: the sentiments expressed to Westrowe in 1647 had not changed. In December 1656 the Eccleston-Rand petition was referred by the Council of State to a committee which included Hartlib and was dominated by his supporters.[147] In August the committee reported favourably and the Council of State issued an order to Lord Deputy Henry Cromwell and the Council of Ireland to implement the Rand-Eccleston proposals. The Hartlib circle were jubilant over this outcome and Benjamin Worsley was prepared to facilitate the work in Ireland. At last Hartlib seemed to be guaranteed a secure income for his agency. Henry Oldenburg, the tutor to Lady Ranelagh's son wrote to congratulate Boyle on this achievement: he was 'hugely pleased, that the councill hath granted your desires for the promotion of knowledge'.[148]

This optimism proved to be premature. Very considerable sums were invested in debentures, but no property was acquired. Petty, out of envy and animosity for Worsley, used his position as secretary to the Council in Ireland to obstruct the implementation of the order relating

145. HP XLVII 4, slightly abbreviated.

146. Letter from Beale to Hartlib, 10 January 1656, HP XXX 1.

147. For state response to this petition, see *HDC*, pp.54–6; O'Brien (202), pp.36–9.

148. Letter from Oldenburg to Boyle, 22 September 1657, Boyle *Works*, vi, p.142; Oldenburg *Correspondence*, i, pp.136–8.

to the Agency. Worsley claimed that Petty was determined to deflect the revenues for his own ends; he was amazed that any individual dared to usurp funds designated by the state for use by its appointed trustees. According to Wood, Petty (perhaps in order to justify his action) was encouraging the establishment of a separate Office of Address in Dublin; he might have wished to deflect the Rand-Eccleston revenues for this purpose. Petty would undoubtedly have exercised considerable influence in an Irish Office, whereas he realised that a London agency was likely to be dominated by his bitter rival, Worsley, rather than by Hartlib.[149] Worsley contrasted the rapacious self-interest of Petty, with the 'piety, integrity, and worth' of the most recently nominated trustees.[150] Faced with Petty's intransigence, the trustees (Boyle, Hartlib, Dury, Sadler, Worsley and Beale) spent nearly two years writing countless letters and conducting endless negotiations in order either to pacify Petty, or to countermine his actions. However, particularly after the death of Cromwell, their efforts were counterproductive.[151]

By 1659, a state-endowed institution having ambitious and long-term goals for the advancement of learning and its application to the public good was entirely out of place. Nevertheless, the Office of Address was not entirely a wasted exercise. The Office for Accommodations publicised Renaudot's *Bureau,* and as a scheme it was both useful and popular; it was also a valuable stimulus to economic planning. The Office for Communications became the foundation for Hartlib's attempt to improve the efficiency of puritan intellectual organisation. It also furnished a convenient platform for use in the recruiting of new associates and political allies. Once formed, the group of scholars could collaborate fruitfully regardless of the existence of a formal agency, and the nucleus of political patrons could be persuaded to support other humanitarian ventures. As the revolutionary decades wore on, Hartlib recognised that it would not be possible to implement his ambitious social and religious programme. The Agency accordingly took on a different character. Ultimately Hartlib and the other trustees came to regard the Agency primarily as an association for the promotion of the sciences and technology; it was possible to pursue this objective without state involvement. It was hoped that through private initiative, the Agency would still be able to contribute to the public good. This was a vestigial manifestation of the original Office of Address proposals, but the utopian ideal still provided the basic motivation for the maintenance

149. Letters from Robert Wood to Hartlib, 1657, HP XXXIII 1. Worsley commented sourly that the obstruction was owing to the 'intention & aime that some others have for the disposing & encouraging of [the Office]': Letter to Dury, 26 May 1658, HP XXXIII 2.

150. Worsley as cited in letter from Hartlib to Boyle, June 1658, Boyle *Works,* vi, p.110.

151. See particularly the numerous extracts from letters by Worsley, HP XLVII 3; and the Boyle-Hartlib correspondence, Boyle *Works,* vi, pp.94–116.

of this organisational effort. Finally, the constant preoccupation with revising and perfecting the Office of Address proposals stimulated more general interest in scientific organisation. By the end of the Protectorate the Office of Address had passed through a complex evolutionary process and documents relating to it were universally known. Perhaps more than any other factor it was responsible for publicising among scientific intellectuals, the merits of a national scientific institution.

(vii) The Servants of God

The foregoing examples of scientific organisation indicate how quickly the social position of puritan intellectuals was transformed after 1641. Before that date they operated from the entrenched position of the puritan ministry, or as laymen they were supported on an inadequate and piecemeal basis by wealthy sympathisers. Given the intellectual restrictions and economic lethargy at home, many ambitious young men were tempted to seek their fortunes abroad. The Universal College of Comenius illustrates how quickly the mood changed. In July 1641 Hartlib addressed three separate letters to Comenius making a dramatic appeal for him to visit England immediately—'Come, come, come; it is for the glory of God: deliberate no longer with flesh and blood!'[152] It was time for the servants of God to gather in one place and prepare the table for the coming of the Lord's annointed. During the prelude to the millennium every turn in events was significant; men began to live their lives with a new sense of urgency, feeling that they were witnessing the passing of the last phase of the degenerate condition of fallen man. The saints could not choose but to return from the wilderness and rededicate themselves to their mission. It was a time for activism, ambitious goals, and renewed aggression. As Culpeper exclaimed: when one evil was destroyed, then 'many more wee shall have in chase & what one hownde misses, another will happen in the sente of & thus will Babilon tumble, tumble, tumble, tumble . . .'[153]

Millennial propaganda was important in cementing loyalty to parliament at home and it significantly affected the image of Britain abroad. As England came to assume a more active role in world reformation, its attractiveness to exiles and foreigners increased. In 1641 the preachers Thomas Goodwin and John Archer returned from Arnhem. Soon Massachusetts Puritans like Hugh Peter and Israel Stoughton returned home to stiffen the parliamentary party. England was soon more tolerant of and congenial to Puritans than Massachusetts. The physicians Robert Child and George Starkey visited England, and never returned to America. The immigrant community of continental scholars and arti-

152. Young (348), p.39.
153. Letter from Culpeper to Hartlib, 4 March 1645/6, HP XIII.

sans greatly increased. The Huguenots Hugh l'Amy and Peter le Pruvost hoped that parliament would support their schemes for utopian plantations. Comenius's assistant Georg Ritschel was maintained by Culpeper and Stoughton while working at the Bodleian Library on his textbook on metaphysics.[154] Johann Brun (alias Unmussig) the Paracelsian physician, after travelling as far as Transylvania and Constantinople, arrived in England to take advantage both of the unrestricted practice of medicine and of the fresh enthusiasm for medical innovation.[155] Other foreign adepts who sought their fortune in England at this time include Joachim Polemann, Johann Hartprecht and Peter Staehl. Balthazar Gerbier, after making cautious enquiries, decided that England was preferable to France as a base for his entrepreneurial activities. The diplomat from Brandenburg, Johann Friedrich Schlezer joined in the medical and alchemical work of the Hartlib circle. In 1653 Henry Oldenburg arrived as an envoy from Bremen. He soon became an active participant in English intellectual affairs.[156] The Küffelers returned to England to carry on the dye-works begun by Drebbel; Johann Sibertus Küffeler shared his father-in-law's gifts for ingenuity and self-advertisement. Even during the final years of the Puritan Revolution the crocodile of utopian planners continued. Peter Cornelius Plockhoy appealed to Cromwell in 1658 for support for his utopian settlement.[157] In 1659 Bengt Skytte visited England to seek patronage for his grandiose scientific academy and was still there at the restoration; he then readjusted his sights and attempted to capture the king's support for the scheme.[158]

Most of the foreign visitors established only a tenuous foothold and soon left in search of greater rewards elsewhere. The more modest and industrious remained; Georg Ritschel became first a successful schoolmaster, then a parish priest. Henry Oldenburg became tutor to Lady Ranelagh's son, and entrenched himself as an invaluable adjunct to Hartlib as an informant on continental affairs.

For the well-established English or foreign allies of the parliamentarian regime attractive vocational prospects opened up. Instead of dependence on private patronage they could expect to move into positions of security and prestige, either through being employed by the state directly, or by intrusion into situations made vacant by state interference with the church or universities. There were inevitably more candidates than vacancies, but the scientific intellectuals were extremely well-placed to capture attention and esteem. The new philosophy was com-

154. For the numerous petitions relating to the Huguenots (1645–7), see especially HP LIII 14. R. F. Young, *A Bohemian Philosopher at Oxford* (347).

155. Ephemerides 1648–1650; Boyle *Works*, vi, pp.81ff.

156. Ephemerides 1654–7; Oldenburg *Correspondence*, i, Introduction.

157. L. & M. Harder, *Plockhoy from Zurik-zee. The Study of a Dutch Reformer in Puritan England and Colonial America* (Newton, Kansas, 1952); Schenk (255), pp.144–8.

158. Purver (230), pp.220–33.

pletely compatible with the ideology of the parliamentarians, and the Baconians discovered that the advancement of learning provided an infallible mechanism for advancing themselves.

There were many routes forward. The puritan members of the 1645 Group (Wilkins, Wallis and Goddard) were advocates of the new philosophy, but they were also tolerant of traditional forms of higher education. Accordingly they were acceptable for university preferment, from the point of view of both parliament and the academic bodies. John Wilkins was spectacularly successful. He rose from the position of a private chaplain to become Warden of Wadham College; he then married the sister of Oliver Cromwell; in 1655 he was described as 'the rising sun' of Oxford. His influence was certainly considerable; in 1658 Hartlib expected him to succeed Francis Rous as Provost of Eton College, but a year later he transferred instead to the lucrative Mastership of Trinity College Cambridge. By this stage, according to one source, Wilkins, Philip Jones and Roger Boyle were the three cabinet councillors to Richard Cromwell.[159] Jonathan Goddard was only slightly less successful. He was as resourceful in the vocational context as he had been in that of the 1645 Group. He volunteered to serve as a physician in the army and rose to be physician to and 'a great confidant' of Oliver Cromwell. His services during Cromwell's illness in Scotland were rewarded with the post of physician-general to the army in Ireland and then the Wardenship of Merton College, a post which had been granted by Charles I to William Harvey only a few years previously. He was also appointed professor of physic at Gresham College, probably owing to the intervention of Cromwell. These preferments were not undeserved if we are to believe the laudatory address to Goddard composed by the royalist Seth Ward in 1653. According to Ward, Goddard was as skilled in the physical sciences and mathematics as in the art of medicine. His collection of mathematical and astronomical instruments was praised, and he was even credited with constructing the first telescope ever made in England. Goddard was obviously a valued servant of Cromwell and he rose to become a member of the Council of State, an MP for Oxfordshire in the Saints Parliament and a member of various committees. In 1658, according to Haak, he was considering leaving Oxford to become Master of the Savoy Hospital.[160] John Wallis earned his preferment by service to the Westminster Assembly and as a cipher expert. He was selected as Savilian professor of geometry at Oxford in 1649 and he aroused con-

159. Wood *Athenae*, iii, pp.967–71; *Biographia Britannica;* Aubrey, ii, pp.299–302; *DNB;* Shapiro, *John Wilkins* (259). Letter from Timothy Halton to Joseph Williamson, 1 August 1656, *CSPD 1656–7*, p.51. Edmund Ludlow, *Memoirs*, 3 vols. (London, 1688–99), ii, p.632. Letter from Hartlib to Boyle, 16 December 1658, Boyle *Works*, vi, pp.115–16.

160. Wood *Athenae*, iii, pp.1029–30; *Biographia Britannica;* Munk (195), i, p.240; *DNB;* M. B. Rex, *University Representation* (240), pp.185–6; Barnett, *Theodore Haak* (20), p.120.

siderable animosity by securing in addition the post of Custos Archivorum. These gains were modest, but secure, since unlike the more active public figures Goddard and Wilkins, Wallis was spared ejection in 1660.[161]

For the most part the associates of the Office of Address and of the erstwhile Invisible College were not attracted by academic careers. This group had no affection for the universities; their ideal was radical reform, but in the absence of any real reform they tended to treat the universities with contempt, or as a source of revenue for use elsewhere. None of these attitudes appealed to academics and in spite of tentative moves on behalf of Hartlib and various of his associates, the only member of this group to take up a university position was John Sadler. His appointment as Master of Magdalene College Cambridge in 1650 was a reward for his services as a lawyer and constitutional theorist. His position was analogous to that of Goddard : he was a friend of Cromwell, MP for Cambridgeshire in 1653 and a member of the Council of State. He served with Goddard on the Committee for the Advancement of Learning in 1653. Sadler refused Cromwell's offer of lucrative legal preferment in Ireland.[162]

Most of the work of the 1645 Group related to the aspects of natural philosophy and medicine treated in the academic curriculum. It was therefore entirely logical that they should gravitate towards the universities. The Invisible College and the Hartlib circle on the other hand were concerned with subjects which had no place in academic studies. In view of their concern for social and economic problems they tended to favour a public service career. This path was somewhat uncertain, but it could be extremely lucrative and might lead to positions of considerable public influence.

Hartlib's appointment as Agent for Universal Learning has already been described. This position nominally gave him about £100 per annum, about half the salary of a head of college, but with assistance from other sources Hartlib expected to secure a salary of £200 or more. This was the amount which Dury also received for his services to the state.[163] In order to avoid his having to rely on this rather insecure state pension, Dury and Henry Langley unsuccessfully proposed Hartlib for the post of Bodley's Librarian, with a salary of £200 per annum.[164] Hartlib's determination to concentrate on the work of his Agency con-

161. Wood *Athenae,* iii, pp.1073–6; Aubrey, ii, pp.280–3; *Biographia Britannica; DNB;* Scriba (257).

162. *DNB;* Worthington *Diary,* ii, part 2, pp.252–5; M. B. Rex (240), pp. 212–28; A. Fraser, *Oliver Cromwell* (107), p.350 and *passim.* Veall (296), p.81.

163. *CSPD 1654,* p.280; *HDC,* pp.27–34. For general biographical details of Dury, see *HDC,* part 2; J. M. Batten, *John Dury Advocate of Christian Reunion* (Chicago, 1944).

164. Dury served as Library Keeper at St. James's Palace, 1650–52; see *HDC,* pp. 268–70. For general biographical details of Hartlib, see G. H. Turnbull, *Samuel Hartlib* (284); *HDC,* part 1; C. Webster, *Samuel Hartlib* (320), Introduction.

demned him to insecurity. He was often able to assist others, but was rarely able to assist himself.

Other members of Hartlib's circle followed more customary vocational pathways. Worsley and Gerard Boate entered the army medical service in Ireland at the outset of the rebellion and during their Invisible College period they were reappointed. Boate in the meantime built up a successful medical practice in London, whereas Worsley through his saltpetre project was initiated into general economic planning. In 1650 powerful political allies were able to secure for Worsley the post of Secretary to the newly formed Council of Trade, which included Sir Cheney Culpeper among its members. Worsley's salary was £200. Thereafter he was attracted into the Irish civil service, serving first as Secretary to the Irish Commissioners and later as Surveyor-General.[165]

Ireland assumed considerable importance for the puritan intellectuals. Once pacified, this territory needed capable administrators and surveyors, who could prepare the way for its plantation and profitable exploitation. The country possessed many of the attractions of New England, but it was geographically more conveniently situated. Gerard Boate, Worsley, Symner, Child and Wood, as well as many minor figures were lured to Ireland in the 1650s, but there were many difficulties; the Irish civil service constituted a severe test of administrative abilities.[166] Worsley proved to have little aptitude for the survey, whereas Petty, who arrived in Ireland in 1652 as physician-general to the army, was able to take up this work and complete it in an exemplary manner. Petty's Down Survey was a remarkable achievement by the standards of any age.[167] Although completely lacking the advantages of noble birth or wealth, Petty obtained a cosmopolitan and sophisticated education on the continent before returning to England in 1646 at the age of twenty-three. Once established in London, he applied his energies in various directions. Hartlib knew him first as an inventor of technical instruments and agricultural machinery. But Petty had also studied medicine at Leyden and he probably resumed his medical studies in London. For Hartlib he composed a brilliant essay on technical and medical education, which was published in 1648.[168] This tract probably assisted the London parliamentarians Edmund Wylde and John

165. For sources on Worsley, see note 107 above.

166. For a general survey of social policy in Ireland, see Barnard (18). Dr. Barnard informs me that Johann Brun was appointed as a physician in Cork.

167. Wood *Athenae*, iv, pp.214–20; *Biographia Britannica; DNB;* Lord Fitzmaurice, *Life of Sir William Petty* (London, 1895); E. Strauss, *Sir William Petty* (London, 1954); Innes Smith (157), p.181; Munk (195), i, pp.270–2. Mr. L. G. Sharp of The Queen's College Oxford is engaged in a detailed study of the life and work of Petty. I am grateful for his comments on sections of this book relating to Petty.

168. *Advice of W. P. to Samuel Hartlib* (210); Petty first wrote to Pell on 8 Nov. 1645 (BM Sloane MS 4279, fol. 183); he is first mentioned in Hartlib's correspondence 25 Jan. 1647, by Sir Cheney Culpeper (HP XIII); on 16 Nov. 1647 Hartlib described Petty to Boyle (Boyle *Works*, vi, p.76).

Graunt to secure for Petty the modest post of assistant to the Tomlins Reader in Anatomy at Oxford. This paved the way for an Oxford MD and a fellowship at Brasenose College. Petty also proved his abilities as a natural philosopher when in 1648, at the invitation of Hartlib, he conducted a spirited defence of Baconianism and an assault on Descartes against a formidable opponent, the Platonist Henry More of Christ's College Cambridge. Hartlib hoped that Petty's talents would be efficiently employed in a new College of Mechanics or at Gresham College. In this context Petty probably drew up a scheme which Hartlib possessed for the reorganisation of Gresham. Although undated, it probably antedates Petty's appointment as Gresham professor of music in 1651, which again was facilitated by John Graunt.[169] At Oxford he immediately became one of the leading members of the scientific group. The impression made in London and Oxford quickly recommended him to a position of responsibility in the Irish civil service, his first post being physician-general to the army in succession to Jonathan Goddard.

Others followed the pattern set by Worsley and Petty. Robert Wood was intruded into a fellowship at Lincoln College by the authority of the parliamentary Commissioners, and once there, he joined in the work of the Experimental Philosophy Club. As a mathematician he turned to speculations about monetary theory and currency decimalisation; these brought him outside recognition and promotion to Ireland, where he worked as an assistant to Henry Cromwell. His service in Ireland probably helped him to secure appointment as professor of mathematics at the new College at Durham. Miles Symner served in the Irish Army as an engineer. After the pacification he assisted with the survey and distribution of lands, as well as being the first incumbent of the chair of mathematics at Trinity College Dublin.[170]

The careers of Goddard, Worsley, Petty and Symner illustrate the value of the army as an avenue of preferment. Daniel Whistler also followed this course. After obtaining an MD at Leyden, he returned to practise medicine in London. He then achieved considerable success in the administration of the naval medical services and was rewarded with a fellowship at Merton College and the chair of geometry at Gresham College.[171] Another successful army physician was Thomas Coxe, the friend of Hartlib, Sydenham and Petty. Both Coxe and Whistler built up large London practices, but both ultimately died in poverty. Thomas Sydenham and Joshua Sprigg owed their election to

169. 'Mr. Petty's letter in answer to Mr. More', HP VII 123; quoted in full in Webster (319), pp.367–8. For Petty's proposals for Gresham, see Appendix VII below; Ward, *Lives of the Gresham Professors* (305), pp.217–27.

170. For sources on Symner and Wood, see above, n.112 and below, pp.416, 532.

171. Wood, *Athenae*, iv, pp.167–8; Munk (195), i, pp.249–51; Ward (305), pp.155–6; A. M. Cooke, 'Daniel Whistler', *Journal of the Royal College of Physicians of London*, 1967, *1*: 221–30; J. J. Keevil, *Medicine and the Navy* (172), ii, pp.13–55.

All Souls fellowships to their service in the army. Sydenham, like his influential brother William, had been a combatant and he returned to Oxford to follow Coxe's advice that he should study medicine. Sprigg had been an army chaplain.

The chaplains varied greatly in their fate. As a group they tended increasingly to religious and political radicalism. Accordingly such figures as Dell, Webster, Saltmarsh and Pinnel were regarded with suspicion by the universities and the more orthodox religious groups. These fears were confirmed by the behaviour of William Dell, who used his position as Master of Caius College Cambridge as a platform from which to attack the learned clergy. John Webster was left to fulminate against the universities at lectures delivered at Allhallows Lombard Street, before retiring to a living in his native Yorkshire. Henry Pinnel abandoned the army to become a separatist preacher at Brinkworth in Wiltshire. During 1647 John Saltmarsh became acutely depressed and declared to Fairfax that the 'army had departed from God'; two days after making this statement he died.[172] All of these chaplains made substantial contributions to the literature of spiritual religion, and some were important exponents of the hermetic philosophy.

Foreign service was another area in which the puritan intellectuals could seek advancement. Work of this kind was Dury's whole life. Hartlib, assisted by his son Samuel junior, a secretary to the Council of State, relayed a constant stream of foreign intelligence to the Council. Haak undertook similar work and had the same difficulty as Hartlib in securing his stipend. Georg Rudolph Weckherlin and from 1649 onwards John Milton, were the official Secretaries for Foreign Tongues. Haak was one of the two persons chosen in 1643 to represent the British interest in Denmark. Although this was a modest venture it was the first diplomatic mission sent by parliament to the continent, with the exception of Walter Strickland's Residency in the Hague. Haak later refused to serve as British Resident in Zürich, but he successfully recommended John Pell for this post. This represented a rather belated recognition of Pell's abilities. At the beginning of the Civil War Pell was persuaded by Boswell and Haak to take up an academic career in the low countries, pending the return of settled conditions in England; he was then overlooked in the race for preferment at Oxford and Cambridge. Wallis occupied the only public lectureship in mathematics at the universities and Whistler was installed as professor of geometry at Gresham. When war with the Dutch seemed imminent in 1652, Pell returned to England and petitioned the Council of State for assistance. He was granted £200 per annum and a house for use with respect to an as yet unspecified mathematics lectureship. But before this scheme materialised, he was offered the post in Zürich. When God-

172. Apart from Leo Solt's slight *Saints in Arms,* there is no adequate study of the chaplaincy of the parliamentary army. Anne Lawrence of Linacre College Oxford is currently investigating this topic.

dard was considering moving to the Savoy, Haak hoped that the Wardenship of Merton College could be obtained for Pell. The letter which Cromwell wrote to the Gresham Committee in 1656 may represent a rather belated attempt to assist Pell.[173]

It was suggested that John Dury should accompany Bulstrode Whitelocke on his embassy to Sweden in 1653, but Dury remained in England and Whitelocke was attended by Daniel Whistler. At one stage Sir Cheney Culpeper and Whitelocke were being considered as candidates for the post of 'Ambassador Extraordinary from England to Germany to unite the Protestant Princes'.[174]

From the examples cited above it is apparent that the advocates of the new philosophy were extremely successful in recommending themselves to the new men who assumed power during the Puritan Revolution. They came to occupy important niches in the administrative and educational structure of the Republic, and their initiative and efficiency encouraged the authorities towards further recruitment from the ranks of the experimental philosophers. Consequently there was a marked elevation of science and medicine in the public esteem and an acceleration in the pace of scientific development. The settled academic climate at Oxford was conducive to the reconstruction of the regular scientific meetings begun in London; the civil service provided convenient vantage points for promoting the social and economic ideas of the group associated with Hartlib.

Under the Commonwealth and Protectorate, a natural philosopher who was willing to conform could look forward to a successful career in academic and public life. There was considerable flexibility and he was encouraged to combine academic with political, diplomatic or administrative work. A versatile young physician like Whistler could establish a medical practice in London, serve as medical adviser to important military and political figures, become a leading power in the College of Physicians, secure a chair at Gresham College, be rewarded with a fellowship at a university, and travel abroad as an envoy. Whistler was successful, but he was not exceptional. Wilkins, Goddard, Sadler, Wallis, Worthington, Cudworth, Ray, Wood, Petty, Worsley, Symner, Haak, Pell, Hartlib and Dury, to mention only the figures with specifically scientific interests, illustrate the degree to which the energetic intellectual could succeed in achieving a position of advantage during the Puritan Revolution. A regular salary of £200 could be anticipated, and initiative could secure considerably more, and perhaps lay the foundation for considerable wealth as in the case of William Petty. Preferment was the reward for loyalty to parliament in the case of the more mature figures, and an inducement to conformity in the rising generation.

It is not possible to regard every academic or civil service appoint-

173. Barnett (20), Chapters V & VIII. Abbott, iv, pp.160–1, 9 May 1656.
174. *HDC*, pp.272, 280–1; Aylmer (12), p.271.

ment as a reward for political loyalty. However, the close associations between puritan patrons, politicians and intellectuals developed during the 1630s and cemented during the Civil War, proved to be an important factor in the careers of the figures listed above. Without the support of influential figures, brought about through adherence to common religious, political and social beliefs, it would not have been possible for the puritan intellectuals to rise to positions of security and esteem, and in turn it would have been difficult for them to realise their potentialities or exercise their full influence in science or medicine. This affiliation with the parliamentary party conveyed more than marginal advantages. In the interests of its protégés the parliamentary authorities were willing to break precedents and circumvent rules. This is aptly illustrated by the celibacy rule in academic institutions, a minor point which was nevertheless of key importance for many natural philosophers. This rule was modified at Wadham, and Wilkins became the first married head of this college—in his case the marriage being one of considerable importance for his immediate career. Thomas Horton, the teacher of John Wallis, was Gresham professor of divinity. He rose to become Vice-Chancellor of Cambridge, and married in 1651. An order was obtained from the parliamentary committee permitting him to retain his Gresham chair despite his marriage and this order was renewed in 1656 and 1660. This action constituted an important precedent and could have paved the way to an entirely different pattern of social composition in the Gresham professoriate.

It is notable that during the final years of the Protectorate even staunch royalists of the older generation were coming to accept the new settlement. Seth Ward had left Cambridge for conscientious reasons, but he took up a Savilian chair at Oxford. Royalists entrusted their sons to John Wilkins at Wadham; Digby, Evelyn and Aubrey began correspondence with Hartlib. Two typical opportunists, Abraham Cowley and Thomas Sprat, began to court the dominant party. By this stage the puritan movement was so fragmented and diluted that it is possible to detect only traces of the coherent intellectual programmes of the previous decade.

(viii) Lux in Tenebris

The process of petitioning and promotion continued even up to the last moments of the Republic, but there was an increasing sense of insecurity and most action was defensive and dispirited. Wood and Petty oscillated between England and Ireland, being unsure where their energies were best applied. Gradually during 1659 Hartlib relinquished his plan to establish the Office of Address; Worsley attempted unsuccessfully to succeed Thurloe in the management of the Post Office. Tong sought to restore state support for Durham College. The future appeared totally uncertain. Prognostications varied greatly and only a few weeks before the dissolution of the Republic Oldenburg confidentially reported that affairs were moving towards a republican settlement.[175]

The work of Hartlib's group was seriously undermined by the ending of the Protectorate, since so much importance was attached to state assistance of humanitarian goals. State intervention for the public good was confidently anticipated right until the end of the Protectorate. But with the gradual extinction of hope for general reformation, it was necessary for Hartlib and his associates to attempt a radical readjustment of perspective. This situation was not entirely new. Hartlib had experienced similar disappointments during the Laudian oppression of the 1630s, or before that during the Thirty Years War in Germany. During the earlier crisis he had followed the example of Andreae and taken part in the formation of fraternities dedicated to the preservation of the spirit of reformation. In 1659 he responded in a precisely similar manner and even called the new fraternity by the name of the old—Antilia, or sometimes Macaria after the utopian work by Plattes with which he had been so closely involved. It is possible that the new Antilia had no more than a notional existence, but it was nevertheless important psychologically in maintaining the morale of Hartlib and his friends. Antilia also buttressed their faith in an ultimate, millenarian utopia.

Prophecy again became a subject of discussion, especially after the distribution of Comenius's *Lux in tenebris* (1657). In June 1657 the author sent twelve copies of this work to Hartlib, specifically for the benefit of the Council of State, and with one bound in skin especially for Cromwell, which Hartlib was asked to deliver personally. Hartlib was known to be cautious about the prophecies of Drabicus, Poniatovia and Kotter, but Beale found that Comenius's interpretations agreed precisely with his own.[176] Beale increasingly believed in his own prophetic abilities and he wrote for the benefit of Lady Ranelagh a tract showing that 'scripture, reason & experience sheweth How wee may bee restored to paradyse on Earth'. Recent developments in experimental philosophy were regarded as millennial omens by Beale; Daniel and the Apocalypse showed that still more 'powerful mysteries' could be revealed, perhaps by reviving astrology. If only men would allow themselves to be infused by the light of God, they might be given complete mastery over nature.[177] This enlightenment was promised, and it was necessary for the spiritual virtuosi to cherish the ideal as best they could. Those who had seen a glimpse of paradise, could not

175. Letter from Oldenburg to Becher, 2 March 1660, Oldenburg *Correspondence*, i, p.359.

176. *HDC*, pp.336–8; letter from Beale to Hartlib, 18 January 1658/9, HP LI.

177. Letters from Beale to Hartlib, 15 Sept. 1657, 12 June 1658, 26 March 1659, HP XXXI. Letter from Beale to William Brereton, 18 January 1658/9, HP LI

easily abandon their transcendental goals. As Hartlib commented, he had 'grown too old to lay aside the thoughts of promoting learning, philosophy and the tongues, for all the vulgar pretences.'[178]

A brief but intensive discussion about Antilia occurred at the end of 1659. From the enquiries which were being made about the organisation of Moravian communities in Transylvania, it is apparent that Antilians were once again thinking in terms of a discrete settlement gathering together a body of religious idealists who would eventually become the spearhead of a movement for world reformation. Beale exclaimed: 'O for a Paradyse in which wee might retreate from the noyse of Trumpet & drum.' He had composed a work which has not survived entitled, *A free discovery of the true, lawful, holy, and divine expedient for the propagation of the gospel, and establishment of an universal peace all over the world,* which Hartlib felt deserved to be published at the expense of Macaria, since its 'scope it is most professedly to propagate religion and to endeavour the reformation of the whole world'.[179] By January 1660, Beale, Boyle, Worthington, Hartlib and Joachim Polemann were involved in the Antilian correspondence and Worthington at least was anticipating the imminent establishment of Macaria.[180] After a sudden burst of interest, Macaria and Antilia are not mentioned for some time in the correspondence; then in October 1660 Hartlib announced that he had been misled, there had been no serious intention to establish an Antilian colony and 'the name & thing is as good as vanished'. Nevertheless, he had interested Pell in the scheme and his acquaintances had decided that the Bermudas would be an ideal location for their colony. Thereafter Hartlib wrote many letters apologising for the vanity of his hopes of Antilia. No doubt he initially thought that it was conceived as seriously as the earlier Antilian project, and that it represented the adaptation of this to more recent use.[181] The name Antilia possessed such sentimental appeal that Hartlib had abandoned caution and seen this fraternity as a projection of his own utopian aspirations. Even when the fictional nature of Antilia was generally appreciated, Hartlib continued to believe that, though 'the smoke is over, but the fire is not altogether extinct. It may be it will flame in due time, though not in Europe.'[182]

178. Letter from Hartlib to Worthington, 20 July 1659, Worthington *Diary*, i, pp.144–5

179. Letter from Beale to Hartlib, 4 Nov. 1659, BM Additional MS 15948, fol. 82r–v; letter from Hartlib to Boyle, 15 Nov. 1659, Boyle *Works*, vi, p.132.

180. Letter from Worthington to Hartlib, 30 January 1659/60, Worthington *Diary*, i, pp.162–77; see also letter from Worthington to Hartlib, 8 July 1660, BM Additional MS 6268, fol. 21r.

181. Letter from Hartlib to Worthington, 15 October 1660, Worthington *Diary*, i, pp.210–15; see also pp.227–30, 233–9, 239–41, 253–6, 338–41.

182. Letter from Hartlib to Worthington, 26 June 1661, Worthington *Diary*, i, pp.341-3.

(ix) The Royal Society

The Royal Society of London for Improving of Natural Knowledge (Regalis Societatis Londini pro scientia naturali promovenda) received its second charter on 22 April 1663. This invalidated the previous charter and established the rules by which the Society felt able to operate. On this date the Society received the name by which it has since been known. The Royal Charter containing this name was mainly concerned with constitutional and legal points, but it also briefly defined the aims of the Society, as the advancement of the knowledge of natural things and useful arts by experiments, to the glory of God the creator and for application to the good of mankind.[183] The Society was administered by a president, and a council of twenty-one, one member of which served as treasurer and two as secretaries. The list of Fellows compiled after the granting of this charter totalled one hundred and fifteen. The imposing roll of founder Fellows shows that the Society had made a considerable impression; it attracted able and influential members who rapidly steered it towards permanent organisation. After only a short time it joined the ranks of the chartered corporations of London. All of this occurred within the first three years of the reign of Charles II.

The extremely rapid consolidation of the Royal Society suggests that a sound basis must have been developed for scientific organisation in London before the formal charters were granted. It is this question of origins, rather than the functioning of the Royal Society which is relevant to the present study. In particular it is important to establish the degree to which the Royal Society was influenced by the puritan experiments in intellectual organisation already described.

The restoration history of the Royal Society is well documented. In July 1662, when the first charter was granted, the title 'Royal Society' was first legitimately adopted. But this charter was granted after regular weekly meetings had been in progress for a year and a half. The event which inaugurated the Society as a regularly constituted body occurred on 28 November 1660, when a group of friends meeting at Gresham College decided to initiate formal meetings to be held on Wednesday afternoons in Laurence Rooke's chambers at Gresham College during term-time, and at William Balle's rooms in the Temple during the vacation. An admission fee and a weekly fee were to be charged. In the first instance John Wilkins was appointed Chairman, William Balle as Treasurer and the physician William Croune as Registrar. There were twelve at this meeting and these drew up a list of forty others who might be expected to support the Society. At

183. Birch (26), i, pp.221–30: 'studia ad rerum naturalium artiumque utilium scientias experimentorum fide ulterius promovendas in Dei Creatoris gloriam & generis humani commodum applicanda sunt.'

a second preliminary meeting a week later, a brief set of rules was drawn up and a form of subscription adopted. The rules described the group's aims simply as 'the promotion of experimental learning'. On 19 December the first specifically scientific question was raised and the scientific meetings began in earnest.[184] At this point the society was constituted in the same way as the Oxford Experimental Philosophy Club or the even earlier 1645 Group.

There has been much disagreement about the origins of the Royal Society. To a large extent the conclusions reached have been determined by the procedures adopted, which in most cases have yielded relatively little insight into the Royal Society as it really existed. Most studies of the origins have rested on prosopographical methods. Attracted by the size of the sample, one author has undertaken a painstaking statistical analysis of the Fellows of the Royal Society enlisted during the first decades of its operation. Another convenient starting-point is the list of 191 Fellows included in Sprat's *History of the Royal Society* in 1667. Another basis for estimates about the early years is provided by the definitive list of 115 Fellows which was compiled in May 1663, shortly after the grant of the second charter. However, any analysis conducted on the basis of these large samples is seriously deficient, in view of the fact that the majority of Fellows subscribed their names out of idle curiosity and never played more than a nominal part in the activities of the Society. It is therefore necessary to establish a basis for procedure which enables us to determine exactly who the founders were, before going on to ask questions about the background of these founders. Some method of selection must be adopted which gives a reasonably accurate impression of the *active membership* of the Society during its first phase. One valuable list is provided by the twelve names in attendance at the foundation meeting in November 1660, but certain founders might have been absent from this meeting for accidental reasons. Their names would have been included in the list of forty prospective members, but this list would also have contained many names included for politeness' sake only.[185] Fortunately the Journal Book of the Society, which was edited by Birch, provides an approximate basis for estimating degrees of participation, since it includes a record of the day-to-day experimental work of the Society. This method has certain drawbacks; for instance, it is likely to give more prominence to members of higher social rank; but it is unlikely to record the active participation of Fellows who were completely absent. If this procedure does not give a completely accurate, positive picture, it does provide a useful basis for the exclusion of nominal members. Accordingly, accepting that this technique is approximate only, the first part of Birch's

184. Birch (26), i, pp.3–7.

185. For some unaccountable reason Boyle and Wren were on both lists. See L. Mulligan in *Past and Present*, 1973, No. 59: 92–116, as part of an ongoing debate involving other contributions to this journal.

History, covering the period from December 1660 to 24 June 1663, has been divided into five equal temporal divisions; the number of references to each Fellow has been noted for each division. Any Fellow has been deemed to be an 'active member' if he is either mentioned on five or more occasions in each of any two divisions, *or* if he is mentioned on three or more occasions in each of any three divisions. This is an extremely low requirement for 'active membership', but it is a satisfactory basis for preliminary sorting.

A preliminary conclusion is that the great majority of names are mentioned on five or fewer occasions over the *whole* two-and-a-half-year period. The complete membership lists are therefore totally unreliable guides to participation in the work of the Society. Equally, of the list of forty prospective members, only ten became active members. But of the twelve attending the inaugural meeting, only two (Bruce and Hill) were not active members. Therefore the official lists in the records of the Royal Society provide us with a list of twenty active members. But there were also a few scientists who became active participants, but were neither at the original meeting, nor included on the list of prospective members. They were elected at a later date. However, this category is small (ten Fellows), and most are either marginal cases, or alternatively became active towards the end of the period. This increases the list of initial active members to thirty. Their names are given in Table 1 (p.92), which illustrates the perfectly symmetrical construction of the early Society, with three sets of ten members drawn from respectively, the attendance at the original meeting, the list of prospective members, and among the ranks of subsequent recruits.

It is not difficult to reduce this list still further. Graunt, Hoskins, Hooke, Merrett and Winthrop were not much involved during the first eighteen months; Hooke then became a key figure owing to his employment as curator of experiments, but it is unlikely that he was able to exert much influence until his reputation was more established. Balle, Clarke, Colwall, Digby, Ent, Henshaw, Neile, Palmer, Pope, Power, Tuke, Wallis and Whistler were continually involved with the Society, but their attendance was numerically not very considerable. Therefore the first two-and-a-half-years' life of the Society was sustained by a nucleus of twelve members, consisting of Boyle, Brouncker, Charleton, Croune, Evelyn, Goddard, Moray, Oldenburg, Petty, Rooke, Wilkins, and Wren—precisely the number which attended the inaugural meeting. This corrected list of the founding 'active nucleus' of the Royal Society consists of eight of those who attended the November meeting, three from the list of prospective members (Croune, Evelyn and Oldenburg), and only one subsequent recruit, Walter Charleton. If it is remembered that Croune had expected to attend the November meeting, the list of those at this meeting is found to correlate extremely closely with the statistics of attendance. Evelyn was not at the November meeting because an illness contracted on a visit to Sayes Court kept him away from London from 27 November until 5 December. Upon his return to London he immediately began attending meetings of the 'Philosophical Society now meeting at Gresham'. The young immigrant Oldenburg was perhaps diffident about assuming a leading part, until invited by more influential figures. Charleton may have been omitted from the original list by an oversight, but as an opportunist and populariser he was not particularly well-liked, and his recent experiences with the College of Physicians showed that he had enemies. However, this is not an important issue since Charleton was one of the first elected members of the Society.[186] Evidence from other sources tends to confirm the view that the figures mentioned above dominated the work of the early Royal Society.

Questions about the more distant background of the Royal Society should be examined in terms of the intellectual biographies of the active nucleus of twelve, rather than with reference to larger groups which had only a nebulous connection with the Society. To what extent did the active group exist in a coherent form before 1660 and extend back into the previous decade to interlock with the organisations generated under puritan auspices? Sprat, a not altogether reliable source, suggested that the regular meetings at Gresham began in 1658, when the greater part of the Oxford Experimental Philosophy Club transferred to London. However, as Birch has pointed out, the events which Sprat mentioned in connection with these meetings occurred in 1659, not 1658. Accordingly the meetings either began in 1658 without the 'greatest number' of the Oxford group (an interpretation not congenial to the Oxonian Sprat), or alternatively the meetings began in 1659 not 1658.[187]

There is one excellent piece of evidence to suggest that Sprat's date was right, but his construction wrong. In November 1658 the mathematical practitioner Anthony Thompson passed via Hartlib a message to Pell inviting him to a meeting 'in the moorefields of some Mathematicall freinds (as you know the costam hath beene); there will be Mr. Rook and Mr. Wrenn, my Lord Brunkerd, Sir Pauel Neile, Dr. Goddard, Dr. Scarburow etc.' Thompson hinted that the number invited to the meeting—twelve—was smaller than Pell would normally expect.[188] This number happens to be precisely the same as the total of the active nucleus of the Royal Society as here defined. Of the six names mentioned by Thompson, four were from this nucleus, while Neile became an active member. Of the other mathematicians mentioned in this letter, Pell and Scarburgh were less active Fellows, while Thompson was perhaps excluded on social grounds. Wren, Rooke and Goddard were

186. Evelyn (97), iii, pp.261–2, 266–7. For Charleton see Clark (50), i, pp.281–2; Birch (26), i, pp.13, 19, 23. A forthcoming paper by Mr. L. G. Sharp will deal with Charleton's difficulties with the College of Physicians; see also his 'Walter Charleton's Early Life . . .', *Annals of Science,* 1973, *30*: 311–40.

187. Sprat (266), pp.57–8; Birch (26), i, p.3.

188. BM Birch MS 4279, fol. 273. Punctuation inserted.

TABLE I

THE ACTIVE MEMBERS OF THE ROYAL SOCIETY 1660–1663

	Names	Divisions of the period December 1660–June 1663					
		1	2	3	4	5	TOTAL
A	William Balle	3	3	9	3	20	38
A	Robert Boyle	23	16	31	20	26	116
A	Lord William Brouncker	18	12	11	15	26	82
C	Walter Charleton	5	7	2	25	12	51
B	Timothy Clarke	5	8	2	1	18	34
C	Daniel Colwall	7	—	4	5	3	19
B	William Croune	4	21	10	21	24	80
B	Sir Kenelm Digby	6	6	—	1	4	17
B	George Ent	2	4	3	6	7	22
B	John Evelyn	15	7	6	12	18	58
A	Jonathan Goddard	15	23	15	39	47	139
C	John Graunt	—	—	3	5	8	16
B	Thomas Henshaw	4	6	3	6	16	35
C	Robert Hooke	1	—	—	15	79	95
C	John Hoskins	—	—	—	5	10	15
B	Christopher Merrett	8	2	—	23	16	49
A	Sir Robert Moray	17	19	19	59	58	172
A	Sir Paul Neile	7	5	—	1	7	20
B	Henry Oldenburg	3	7	5	11	24	50
C	Dudley Palmer	2	2	3	3	14	24
A	William Petty	15	7	13	11	16	62
C	Walter Pope	2	6	2	5	11	26
C	Henry Power	2	2	5	8	6	23
A	Laurence Rooke	8	9	12	7	2	38
C	Samuel Tuke	6	8	—	3	7	24
B	John Wallis	5	—	2	6	6	19
B	Daniel Whistler	4	4	4	4	4	20
A	John Wilkins	7	20	20	19	27	93
C	John Winthrop	—	1	6	9	9	25
A	Christopher Wren	10	7	13	11	13	54
	Period	5 Dec. 1660– 28 May 1661	5 June 1661– 18 Dec. 1661	1 Jan. 1662– 2 July 1662	9 July 1662– 31 Dec. 1662	3 Jan. 1663– 24 June 1663	Number of references in Birch (26)

A = Attendance at Meeting on 28 November 1660: Birch, i, p. 3.

B = Inclusion on tentative list of members, 5 December 1660: Birch, i, p.4.

C = Active membership, but not on list A or B.

by this time professors at Gresham. It is clear from Thompson's letter that the meetings were a well-established phenomenon by the end of 1658. There is no evidence about the origination of these meetings, but a hint is perhaps contained in Wallis's quite unambiguous claim that the London meetings initiated by Haak 'continued, and . . . were increased . . . and were afterwards incorporated by the name of the Royal Society'.[189] It may therefore be taken as a working hypothesis that the 1645 liaison between mathematicians and physicians was maintained by Samuel Foster until his death in 1652 and after that date by his successor at Gresham College, Laurence Rooke. As in 1645, the later meetings would have been held at various locations. Continuity with the earlier work was probably maintained by Goddard, Scarburgh and perhaps Ent. The group would have expanded with the arrival of Rooke and Wren from Oxford to take up chairs at Gresham in 1652 and 1657 respectively. Brouncker and Neile would have been able to attend the meetings throughout this decade. Because of the growing dominance of Gresham professors, this group would increasingly have tended to revolve around Gresham College. Sprat was probably correct in suggesting that in addition to the figures listed by Thompson, the nascent society was joined by William Brereton, John Evelyn, Thomas Henshaw, Henry Slingsby, Timothy Clarke, George Ent, William Balle, Abraham Hill and William Croune—perhaps some in 1658, and others in 1659. Most of these names occupied a small, but regular part in the records of the Royal Society; Croune and Evelyn became extremely active. Thus a substantial basis of scientific meetings in London had been established even by the time of the death of Oliver Cromwell. New recruits continued to filter into the meetings until the time of the dissolution of the Republic in the spring of 1660.

Sprat's description of the origins of the Royal Society in terms of the establishment of the Oxford Experimental Philosophy Club at Wadham by his patron John Wilkins, and its transference to London shortly before the restoration, is a severe distortion. The Club at Oxford was itself an offshoot of the London group, and it followed the same pattern of organisation. The two groups maintained a close association, until first Rooke and later Wren migrated to London. Wilkins, Petty, Boyle, Oldenburg and Goddard had also taken part in the Oxford meetings at some stage, but they were not affiliated with the Oxford Club to the exclusion of all other scientific associations. Indeed, diversity of outlook and experience was one of the most considerable advantages of the active nucleus of the Royal Society. This is illustrated by the details of association given in Table 2 (p.94).

It is almost superfluous to ask whether the active nucleus of the Society was mainly puritan and parliamentarian, or Anglican and royalist. The Society gradually evolved over a period of nearly twenty years, during which there were constant shifts in membership and

189. Scriba (257), p.40.

TABLE 2

THE SCIENTIFIC ASSOCIATIONS OF THE ACTIVE NUCLEUS OF THE ROYAL SOCIETY

Association / Names	College of Physicians: Candidate or Fellow	Gresham College: Professor	1645 Group	Oxford Club	Hartlib's Agency	Visitor to Continental Academies	Gresham Meetings: 1657–
Robert Boyle				1654–	1647–		1660–
Lord William Brouncker							1658–
Walter Charleton	1650–					c. 1648	1661–
William Croune	1663–	1659–					1659–
John Evelyn					1659–		1659–
Jonathan Goddard	1643–	1655–	1645–	1651–5			1657–
Sir Robert Moray						1655–60	1660–
Henry Oldenburg				1656–7	1655–	1657–60	1660–
William Petty	1655–	1651–		1650–1	1647–	–1646	1660–
Laurence Rooke		1652–		1650–2			1657–
John Wilkins			1645–8	1648–59	1658–		1660–
Christopher Wren		1657–		1650–7			1657–

scientific interest. Consequently the question of religious and political bias can be addressed to many different situations. It is therefore not surprising that no simple solution is forthcoming; no factor is supremely important and none irrelevant. It is also necessary to bear in mind that religious belief and political persuasion were themselves subject to fluctuation during the formative period.

However, religious and political factors are most relevant to our understanding of the natural philosophy of the individual founders of the Royal Society. Indeed, it was more likely the depth of disagreement on these issues, rather than adherence to some kind of latitudinarianism, which led to the 1645 Group to organise its activities in such a way as to circumvent ideological conflict. They avoided religion and politics and concentrated on experimental and mathematical problems which were free from obvious political or religious connotation. Accordingly this group was from its outset and by intention, of extremely mixed religious and political constitution and this tradition persisted into the

Royal Society. The active nucleus of the Society exhibited the same balanced structure as the original 1645 Group. Half of its members (Boyle, Goddard, Oldenburg, Petty and Wilkins) had actively collaborated with the parliamentarian regime, while the other half (Brouncker, Charleton, Evelyn, Moray and Wren) had been its intransigent opponents.[190] As one would expect the first group tended towards puritanism whereas the second were mostly orthodox Anglicans. Of the Gresham professors Whistler, Goddard and Petty were active parliamentarians, whereas Rooke and Wren were not.

The conscious decision of the originators of the Royal Society to avoid contentious issues was important for the survival of their group. Whereas the fate of Hartlib's Agency was completely bound up with political developments, the activities at Gresham were unaffected by the disintegration of the Republic and the re-institution of monarchy. Before 1660 the parliamentarian members tolerated their erstwhile royalist opponents, and after 1660 the dominant royalist element assisted with the rehabilitation of their parliamentarian colleagues. Their scientific work was insulated from ideological friction.

It remains to consider to what degree the evolution of the Royal Society was influenced by specifically puritan ideas on intellectual organisation. It has already been demonstrated that the involvement of Haak (and to a lesser extent Wallis) with the Comenian pansophic enterprise was relevant to the genesis of the 1645 Group. Accordingly puritan idealism played a part at this crucial first stage. Thereafter the meetings persisted primarily because of a momentum deriving from the intrinsic interest of the subjects under investigation. The period between 1645 and 1660 was enormously productive, both in mathematics and experimental science. Such novelties as the improved telescopes and microscopes of the London group were responsible for increasing the popular appeal of the new science, so laying the foundations for a viable scientific society. Puritan utilitarianism was probably incidental to this phase of growth and consolidation.

The regular meetings at Gresham College were not impaired by the absence of formal organisation, partly because of the degree of continuity and leadership provided by the Gresham professors. There appears to have been no pressure for a change in status of the meetings before 1660. But in that year there was an influx of new members, owing to the arrival in London of such figures as the prominent Scottish politician and royalist, Sir Robert Moray, from the continent, Wilkins from Cambridge after his ejection from Trinity College, Petty from Ireland after the lapse of his office, Boyle from Oxford, and Oldenburg from his visit to the continent with Richard Jones. It is probably members of this incoming group who initiated moves, first towards more

190. The position of Croune and Rooke is not clear. The former, as a product of Emmanuel College and friend of Abraham Hill and Hartlib, was probably a parliamentarian, whereas Rooke may have been a royalist.

formal organisation, and then to the attainment of status as a national institution and to a definition of aims which accorded with Bacon's *Instauratio Magna*. Very quickly the intimate and informal assembly of enthusiasts at Gresham metamorphosed into a large corporation, having a President, Council, two Secretaries, two or more Curators of Experiments, the rights to appoint one or more official printers and engravers, to print matters relating to the Society, to obtain the cadavers of criminals for the purpose of anatomical demonstration, and to build in London or its environs one or more colleges to house the assemblies of the Society.[191] Once this framework was established, the able apologists Sprat, Glanvill and Cowley could claim that the heterogeneous group of experimental philosophers at Gresham were the legitimate heirs of Bacon's *Instauratio Magna,* and the Royal Society was eulogised as the embodiment of Solomon's House.

The character of the expanded Society was moulded by various interests. The politicians Moray and Brouncker would have been able to ensure good relations with the court. A particularly important part was played by the members who were committed to transforming the Gresham club into a Baconian institution. This ideological reorientation was probably supervised by such figures as Evelyn, Boyle, Petty, Wilkins and Oldenburg, all of whom had developed a very definite, broader conception of the social role of natural science, as well as appreciating its intrinsic interest as a problem-solving mechanism.

At this stage puritanism again becomes relevant. With the exception of Evelyn this group had been conspicuously implicated with the parliamentary party. They had also been involved with the puritan experiments in intellectual organisation. Each in his separate way had become an advocate of Baconian scientific organisation.

Wilkins had followed the progress of the Gresham meetings since their inception; he was the teacher or friend of a majority of the members who met in November 1660 and he became the first chairman of their meetings. At an extremely early stage Evelyn addressed Wilkins as 'President of our Society at Gresham College'. It may have been his long-cherished scheme for a 'Mathematico-Chymico-Mechanical School', which was under discussion at Gresham on 28 November, that was meant when it was reported that 'something was offered about a design of founding a college for the promoting of physico-mathematical experimental learning'.[192] This item was directly followed by the proposal to establish the formal society. Wilkins's project was reported by Hartlib, Boyle and Evelyn, and it was presumably known to many members of the Oxford Club. There can be no doubt that Wilkins would have favoured the expansion of work at Gresham to include reference to both 'luciferous' and 'fructiferous' experimental knowledge, in accordance

191. Birch (26), i, pp.228–30.

192. For Wilkins's scheme, see below, pp.171–2. Letter from Evelyn to Wilkins, 17 Feb. 1659/60 [sic?], Evelyn (96), iii, p.129–31.

with the dictates of Bacon. It will be recalled that an essentially similar plan was advocated by Beale in 1656. His 'College of Noble Mechaniques & Ingenious Artificers' was designed to be constructed at public expense, and to emulate the universities in its fruitful research.[193]

Boyle's dedication to the 'Usefulness of Experimental Natural Philosophy' began with the Invisible College in 1646 and continued owing to his position as a trustee of Hartlib's Agency for the Advancement of Universal Learning. In its mature form, as described in 1655, this Agency was primarily designed 'for the makeing some further progresse & Advancement in a usefull improvement of Experiments, to the more cleare elucidation as well of things Naturall as Artificiall'. As already indicated, the Agency was conceived as a national institution headed by an Agent and a council of trustees, with two permanent secretaries employed on foreign and internal correspondence as its principal officers. It was expected to employ inventors, experimenters and artists on an *ad hoc* basis, to build up a museum and establish a laboratory; it would employ draftsmen and undertake the printing of important books and useful information. Hartlib's Agency was thus extremely close to the Royal Society in general structure and purpose, but its income would have been derived from the state, rather than from the subscriptions of a large body of Fellows. This dissimilarity entailed a very great difference in the social roles of the two bodies and there is every indication that the Royal Society purposely avoided entanglement with national policy. Accordingly the Royal Society was freed from state regulation, but it was also divested of a large element of the humanitarianism and utopianism of the Agency for Universal Learning. Independence of operation was assured, but the absence of direct public responsibility may have reduced commitment to the systematic Baconian programme, thus impairing the effectiveness of committees established to investigate particular problems of economic relevance.

The Agency for Universal Learning was extremely well-known. It was publicised continually from 1647 and it had stimulated much comment in correspondence. This Agency was particularly familiar to the Baconian architects of the Royal Society. Boyle and Petty were completely familiar with the Agency in every stage of its evolution; it was also revealed to Wilkins, whom Hartlib expected to be appointed 'president of the . . . standing council of universal learning' at the beginning of their difficulties with Petty. It is interesting that Hartlib at this stage should accord the names 'President' and 'Council' to the Agency's chairman and its board of trustees.[194] The documents relating to the Agency and to Beale's College were probably sent to Evelyn, who first entered into correspondence with both Beale and Hartlib at this time.

193. Letter from Beale to Hartlib, 10 January 1656/7, HP XXXI 1. Beale became one of the most active provincial Fellows of the Royal Society.

194. Letter from Hartlib to Boyle, 16 December 1658, Boyle *Works*, vi, pp.115–16.

Certainly Hartlib supplied Evelyn with Andreae's *Model of a Christian Society*. This entire group became preoccupied with discussions about the most effective 'Model' for a society of natural philosophers. Having noted the failure of Hartlib and Wilkins to establish a Solomon's House, Evelyn outlined his own scheme for a residential college, which he hoped would be established on a thirty or forty-acre site outside London. This would support a society of gentlemen involved in the study of experimental science. While generally favourable to this idea, Hartlib believed that Evelyn's model was not 'comprehensive' enough.[195] He no doubt realised that Evelyn's college was conceived completely without reference to the public-spirited goals of the Agency for Universal Learning.

Evelyn's monastic society is typical of the schemes for colleges and settlements which were introduced around the time of the restoration by idealists from the left and the right of the protestant church. Plockhoy, Hartlib, Worthington and Beale planned their utopian colonies as a means of salvaging the work of the Reformation. Evelyn, Cowley and Skytte designed colleges to appeal to the tastes of the élite in the individualistic atmosphere of the restoration. The most ambitious plan of this kind emanated from the Swedish visitor Skytte, who attended the meetings at Gresham while visiting London in 1659. Skytte wished to obtain a Royal Charter for the establishment of a utopian community, which would be organised on a luxurious scale, and contribute to the advancement of useful arts and sciences. This scheme, called by Hartlib 'the other Antilia', was totally impracticable, and opportunistic. Hartlib was probably correct in believing that 'the other virtuosi will not have it that it should go forward'.[196] The Gresham group were much more satisfied with Abraham Cowley's scheme for a 'Philosophical Colledge' which it was hoped to establish outside London. Cowley may well have been influenced by Evelyn; his published description was dedicated to the 'Honourable Society for the Advancement of Experimental Philosophy'.[197] Although Hartlib believed that Cowley's 'Pansophical College' had not materialised, schemes of this kind undoubtedly exerted a strong influence on the leading members of the embryonic Royal Society. During 1660 the Gresham enthusiasts would have been exposed to a whole array of schemes for scientific organisation, ranging from Hartlib's Agency to Skytte's Royal College. They realised that if they as a group failed to take advantage of this opportunity to establish a national scientific society, an organisation of this kind might be established under the aegis of a less responsible agent, who would

195. Letter from Evelyn to Boyle, 3 September 1659, Evelyn (96), iii, pp.116–20. Letter from Hartlib to Worthington, 20 July 1659, Worthington *Diary*, i, pp.140–58.

196. Letter from Hartlib to Worthington, 2 April 1661, Worthington *Diary*, i, pp.295–6. For a useful discussion of Skytte's project, see Purver (230), pp.220–34.

197. Cowley, *A Proposition For the Advancement of Experimental Philosophy*, 1661 (63). Letter from Hartlib to Worthington, 22 August 1661, Worthington *Diary*, i, pp.353–6.

employ the new science for entrepreneurial ends. The rapid evolution of the Royal Society during 1661 and 1662 was accordingly prompted partly by commitment and partly by expediency.

A Baconian ideology was adopted at an early stage. Long before the Society's records made reference to Baconian aspirations, Evelyn announced to the public that the society at Gresham College aimed to 'improve practical and Experimental knowledg, beyond all that has been hitherto attempted, for the Augmentation of Science and universal good of Mankind'.[198] This grand conception was successfully imposed upon the Royal Society; it was incorporated into its charters, promulgated by Oldenburg's *Philosophical Transactions,* epitomised in Sprat's *History of the Royal Society,* and reinforced by the writings of Boyle, Evelyn and many minor apologists. Thus the Royal Society contrasts with the 1645 Group, the Oxford Experimental Philosophy Club and the 1658-1660 Gresham meetings, none of which was self-consciously organised according to Baconian principles. The Baconian inspiration was provided mainly by the newcomers Boyle, Petty, Oldenburg, Wilkins and Evelyn, who had not been intimately involved in the routine scientific activities at Gresham. These new recruits became 'active members' and they qualify to be included in the all-important 'active nucleus' of the Royal Society. They had one other important experience in common. All had in some way been involved with Hartlib's Agency for the Advancement of Universal Learning—Boyle and Petty from its inception as the Office of Address, and the whole group in the period immediately before the formation of the Royal Society. It is therefore quite possible that the Agency provided the model which guided the architects of the Royal Society on certain important matters of organisation and philosophical orientation. Hence the specifically puritan ideal of intellectual organisation is relevant, both to our understanding of the initiation of the 1645 meetings and to the process of institutionalisation which occurred between 1660 and 1663. The Royal Society was by no means the complete realisation of the puritan ideal of a Universal College for the advancement of piety and learning; but its similarity was sufficiently close to merit Comenius's dedicating *Via lucis* to the Society in 1668, in the hope of encouraging the Fellows to direct their energies towards the ultimate goal of world reformation.

198. Evelyn, *A Panegyric to Charles the II* (London, 1661), p.14.

III

The Advancement of Learning

'The end then of learning is to repair the ruins of our first parents by regaining to know God aright, and out of that knowledge to love him, to imitate him, to be like him, as we may the neerest by possessing our souls of true vertue, which being united to the heavenly grace of faith makes up the highest perfection.'

Milton, *Of Education* (1644), p.1.

'Illius scopus est reparari ad imaginem Dei amissam, sive ad amissam liberi arbitrii perfectionem, quae consistit in electione boni et reprobatione mali, ut nempe Homines discunt.'

Comenius, *Pampaedia,* VII 7.

'It were some extenuation of the Curse, if *in sudore vultus tui* were confinable unto corporal exercitations, and there still remained a Paradise, or unthorny place of knowledge. But now our understandings being eclipsed, as well as our tempers infirmed, we must betake our selves to wayes of reparation, and depend upon the illumination of our endeavours. For, thus we may repair our primary ruines, and build our selves Men again.'

Browne, *Pseudodoxia Epidemica* (1646), I, 5.

(i) The New Pedagogy

Assertion of the primarily religious aim of education linked Milton and Browne with a wide range of humanist scholars. In the *pietas litterata* advocated by Tudor humanists, all learning was judged by its relevance to the service of God. Such a duty, belonging to both secular and religious life, was owed to a beneficent Creator.[1] An additional dimension to this theme was provided by the puritan insistence on the catastrophic ruin of human abilities after the Fall. Pre-occupation with the deficiencies of the senses and reason, awareness of the inherent defects of the cultural inheritance, and appreciation of the degree of labour required for correction, induced a sharpened awareness of the difficulties of education. At the same time it was realised that childhood and youth were God's gift to each generation, constituting a perpetual challenge to man to redeem his state of corruption. Each new mind was a *tabula rasa;* every child was as impressionable as wax. The inherited

1. Vives, *De tradendis disciplinis libri quinque* (Antwerp, 1531), quoted from Foster Watson, *Vives on Education* (Cambridge, 1913), pp.28–30. Ascham, *The Scholemaster* (London, 1570), p.46.

seed of evil was therefore more readily contained at this stage than in later life. In accordance with this view of education, protestants gave priority to the virtuous upbringing of youth through family discipline and the catechism of the church. Education was seen as a battle-ground, on which society's educational mechanisms were tested against the impinging forces of evil. Through education, the Kingdom of God came within the reach of each generation, but failure to exploit its potentialities had perpetuated man's ruinous condition. Education was accordingly both a source of hope and a reminder of human inadequacy. The Puritans were accustomed to speak of the cultivation of 'those plants of Paradise, Christian children', whose nature was constantly threatened and too often overcome by a tangled undergrowth of thorns and brambles.[2]

Belief in the impending millennium prompted the Puritans to redouble their educational efforts, so that the ground might be prepared for the Great Instauration. In the final age the barriers to knowledge would be removed, but only after dedicated individual effort, and the total utilisation of human resources, would God grant his full Light of Wisdom. It was therefore necessary to contemplate education on a scale even more ambitious than that envisaged by the educational pioneers of the Reformation. Puritan educational reformers encouraged higher standards of individual attainment, but also the extension of education to a broader spectrum of society. The latter principle was taken to its logical extreme by Comenius, who called for 'Universal Schools' which would provide education 'not only for all nations and tongues and orders of men, but for every single individual to rise out of the darkness of ignorance and barbarism'.[3]

John Dury emphasised that education was performed under the dispensation of God's grace; like all things it was practised entirely at his pleasure. Therefore the teacher was involved in a divine rather than secular mission. 'Celestial agriculture' provided an ideal opportunity to work with God and to abide by the apostle's admonition to take the fullest advantage of the power of grace (2 Cor. 6 : 1). God reserved the power to multiply the fruits, requiring only man's co-operation in planting and irrigation. Under this superintendency the infernal tares would be extirpated, enabling the teacher to reap the mature fruits of the human mind and to lay the foundation for the celestial state. For success it was imperative to realise that the active principles of growth flowed from heaven and would only be forthcoming if teachers practised the virtues of zeal, diligence, labour and sweat, in daily cultivation. For those undertaking this labour rewards were guaranteed—'in due season we shall reap, if we faint not.'[4] Accordingly the Puritans believed in the

2. Comenius, *Didactica Magna* (56), p.61; *ODO,* i, p.39.
3. Comenius, *Via Lucis* (55), p.164.
4. Dury, 'De summa curae paedagogicae seu spirituali agricultura exercitatio' [1628], HP I 27.

sanctity of the educational mission; schoolmasters were as necessary as ministers in guiding society towards New Jerusalem. Educational activists pressed for the creation of a body of godly teachers to complement the comprehensive preaching ministry.

This appreciation of the value of education prompted a considerable investment in schools and colleges in England which resulted in an expansion of educational opportunities for many sections of the community. In the period 1560-1640, this movement was sufficiently dramatic to be described as an 'educational revolution'.[5] It is difficult to quantify the impact of this development on basic literacy and elementary education, but in 1640, university expansion had made higher education available to 2.5 per cent of all males of appropriate age, a figure not exceeded until the 1930s.[6] The English population as a whole at this time may well have reached an educational level which was not exceeded until the late nineteenth century. None the less, however impressive this expansion may seem to the modern observer, it was no source of complacency to the puritan reformers, who in 1640 began in earnest their campaign for universal education.

Under Laudian supervision every attempt had been made to contain education within a restricted religious framework. But, as indicated in the previous chapter, the Puritans were successful in cultivating education for their own purposes at all levels. Even stringent regulation of the universities was not able to loosen the puritan hold on many colleges and halls. Recruitment to the puritan cause was accelerated by the growing number of 'alienated intellectuals', whose aspirations were frustrated by the restrictions imposed under the Laudian regime.[7] Each new group of grammar-school-leavers or university graduates gave added strength to the opposition party. This phenomenon attracted considerable comment; Hobbes came to regard the universities as the 'core of rebellion', while William Cavendish included the 'abundance of grammar schools and Inns of Court' among the root causes of disaffection. James Howell seriously regretted that among the English people there was 'such a general itching after Book-Learning, and I believe so many Free-Schools do rather hurt than good'.[8]

All parties knew that it was necessary to control education. Accordingly the Puritans, when in power, submitted the teachers and academics as well as the ministry to religious and political tests; but the degree of positive guidance which the administration exercised was never sufficient to satisfy the educational reformers. Lady Ranelagh

5. L. Stone, 'The Educational Revolution in England, 1560–1640', *Past and Present,* 1964, No. 28: 41–80.

6. *Ibid.,* pp.68–9.

7. M. H. Curtis, 'The Alienated Intellectuals of Early Stuart England', *Past and Present,* 1962, No. 23: 25–43.

8. Memoirs of Cavendish, quoted by Stone, *Past and Present,* 1963, No. 24: 101–2. James Howell, *Familiar Letters* (156), pp.525–6; See also Bacon's essay, 'Of Seditions and Troubles', Bacon *Works,* vi, p.410.

regretted that the Puritans had neglected the training of schoolmasters owing to their preoccupation with short-term military objectives. The only way to lay 'the foundation of the Kingdom of Christ' was by 'timely and good instruction', leading to piety and virtue among all social classes.[9] Lady Ranelagh shared Dury's view that authority was not aware, and indeed happy to remain unaware of the significance of the educator's task (nescit enim aetas nostra, neque scire satagit, quantum Paedagogis incumbant). Teachers had the capacity to promote or to destroy human happiness. They were doctors of minds (Medicos animarum), capable of curing the desperate ailments of the church and state. The puritan preacher Thomas Gataker declared that 'nearest to God are ministers, and next to them schoolmasters'.[10] The reformers believed that until parliament could be persuaded to adopt a broader definition of its educational role, it would not be able to consolidate its military victories or establish a stable puritan state.

Education became a common denominator in the programmes for social reform which matured during the Laudian oppression and proliferated in print under parliament. Practical proposals, petitions, comprehensive schemes and utopian models, emanating from a wide range of authors, demonstrate the existence of a strong educational imperative among puritan reformers.

In an attempt to expand the horizons of education, theorists explored the neglected regions of early childhood and adult life. For total intellectual regeneration it was necessary for the community to evolve a comprehensive programme of training for all its members, from earliest childhood to full maturity. Thus writers on education no longer concentrated on defining the duties of the grammar school master, but instead paid attention to the widest range of pedagogical problems.

Great originality was displayed in devising schemes for educational expansion. Winstanley believed that the phases of formal education, 'childhood' and 'youth', should extend from early childhood to the age of forty. The whole community was expected to participate in educational lectures on the sabbath. Efficient education for all sections of the community was a necessary condition for achieving mastery over nature and subsequent social amelioration.[11] Comenius also believed that the social and religious significance of education was such that it was to be extended into adult life. He advocated *Scholae Virilitati,* which were designed to combine vocational training with spiritual

9. Letter from Lady Ranelagh to Hartlib, January 1660, Worthington *Diary,* i, p.166.

10. Dury, 'De summa . . .'; Gataker, *Davids Instructor* (London, 1620), p.16.

11. Winstanley, *Law of Freedom* (336), pp.56–8, 68–76. R. L. Greaves, 'Gerard Winstanley and Educational Reform in Puritan England', *British Journal of Educational Studies,* 1969, *17*: 166–76.

guidance.[12] By this means adults would be better equipped to educate their children. But Comenius's main originality lay in his insistence on the great educational potentialities of early childhood. Parents were urged to become aware of the significance of this stage, and to take the maximum advantage of its opportunities.

Theologians stressed the severe harm which would result from carelessness about wet-nursing, which might lead to the imbibition of a sinful disposition from an ungodly nurse. Furthermore it was realised that a harmonious relationship between mother and child was essential for temperamental stability in later life.[13] Humanists such as Ascham, Brinsley, and Burton pressed for the humane treatment of young children during their grammatical studies. It required the intuition of Comenius to develop the full pedagogical implications of this principle. Throughout his writings, beginning with the *Informatorium školy mateřské* (pre-1632), considerable prominence was given to early childhood. The significance of this stage was stressed by constant reference to his favourite metaphor of the cultivation of saplings or the planting and tending of seeds.[14] Enlightened parents were enjoined to nurture children in such a way as to implant desirable attitudes to social life, a fruitful understanding of nature, and sympathy for religious goals. Comenius's preoccupation with early education, his search for an educational programme suited to immature minds and his appreciation that this was to be adapted to rapid psychological and physical development, precipitated his emancipation from conventional practices. He was obliged to conclude that the universal education designed for the new age could make only the most limited use of the pious edifice of humanistic pedagogy.[15]

In England the ground was well-prepared for a favourable reception of the ideas of Comenius. There was increasing disillusionment with humanistic education. John Beale was not exceptional in emerging from his studies with a deep feeling of insecurity about spiritual election. Only when his energies were diverted to the study of experimental philosophy was he sufficiently confident to launch into full and enthusiastic participation in the intellectual community.[16] Beale's intellectual salvation owed much to his teacher and patron Sir Henry Wotton, through whom he imbibed an enthusiasm for the philosophy of Francis Bacon. The

12. Comenius, *Pampaedia,* Chapter 13.

13. 'Matrem ipsam lactare infantem' had become a medical commonplace: for a representative discussion, see Burton, *Anatomy of Melancholy* (Everyman edn.), i, pp.331–3. One of Robert Boyle's first writings was 'The Duty of Mothers being a Nurse asserted' (15 August 1647), two copies of which are preserved in BP XXXVII.

14. Comenius, *Didactica Magna* (56), Chapter XXVIII.

15. Comenius, *Informatorium školy mateřské* (Leszno, pre-1632); German edition, 1633; Latin variant, *ODC*, i, pp.198–250. Dagmar Čapková, *Předškolní výchova v díle J. A. Komenského* (Prague, 1968). *Idem*, 'The Significance of Comenius' ideas on the theory and practice of pre-school education', *Durham Research Review,* 1969, no.22: 333–45.

16. Beale, autobiographical letter, 28 November 1659, HP LX 1.

Advancement of Learning had dwelt prophetically on the weaknesses of humanism. Excessive admiration for classical authors, reaction against the barbarism of the schoolmen, concentration on the study of languages and a taste for elaborate preaching had resulted in 'an affectionate study of eloquence and copie of speech'. As this grew to excess, 'men began to hunt more after words than matter.' Thus the great humanist educational theorists, such as Sturm and Ascham, were accounted responsible for enticing intellectuals into an idolatrous worship of the linguistic arts (grammar, rhetoric and logic), and away from the more profitable sciences, which represented the true springs of human knowledge. In order to restore a balanced education, combining contemplation with action, Bacon advocated the first-hand study of Nature, which was 'a rich storehouse for the glory of the Creator and the relief of man's estate'. Recoiling even further from humanistic standards, Winstanley demanded a more radical revision of education. Languages were seen as a total encumbrance, leading men 'to know nothing'. By contrast 'the young people may learn the inward knowledg of things which are, and find out the secrets of Nature'; Winstanley adopted the common maxim that 'to know the secrets of nature, is to know the works of God'. Comenius believed that while the dictatorship of grammar continued, learning could not become a 'delightful pleasure'. A radical reorientation was needed, which would inevitably deepen the gulf between the new pedagogy and humanism. Languages would only be acquired with ease if taught naturally, 'in attaining knowledge in things themselves, which yet hath not hitherto beene put in practise'.[17]

A similar view was emerging in the debates on language teaching among the schoolmasters in Hartlib's circle. In the search for means of deposing the 'Grammatical Tyranny of teaching Tongues' Hartlib was first attracted to William Webbe, the impecunious and eccentric catholic polymath, whose patent for teaching languages 'after a new method without Rules' had been granted in 1626.[18] Webbe may have been inspired by another catholic, William Bathe, whose *Janua linguarum* (1611) eased the path to classical authors by assembling a large collection of simple Latin sentences, with parallel vernacular translations. This would have provided a convenient introduction to Webbe's projected parallel Latin-English editions of such authors as Terence. Both Latin and English texts were to be divided into numbered equivalent clauses. The complexity and expense of this method rendered it impracticable; furthermore it perpetuated dependence upon classical authors at early stages in language learning. Thus in spite of his hermeticist outlook Webbe was firmly within the tradition of humanist language teachers, relying on an early introduction to classical texts to instil idiomatic

17. Bacon, *Advancement of Learning* (1605), Book I, sections iv 2, vii. *Idem, De Augmentis* (13), pp.17, 25. Winstanley, *Law of Freedom* (336), pp.43, 58. Comenius, *Reformation of Schools* (52), p.7.

18. Vivian Salmon, 'An Ambitious Printing Project of the Early Seventeenth Century', *The Library*, 5th Series, 1961, *16*: 190–6.

fluency. The radicalism of his method consisted in its total renunciation of grammar. This provoked objections from other schoolmasters, notably John Brooke. Brooke's method admitted grammar at later stages, but discarded classical authors in early language learning in favour of a 'sensual' approach, beginning with the names of simple objects. Hartlib ensured that this debate was widely publicised; the respective merits of Webbe and Brooke were debated by his correspondents throughout Europe. These exchanges suggest that English schoolmasters were locked in lively discussion; whether favourable to reform or not, they were obliged to adopt precise attitudes to language, psychology and epistemology. New perspectives were introduced and a considerable body of opinion became receptive to reform. The rapid evolution of sympathy for the new pedagogy is indicated by the writings of the London puritan teacher, Hezekiah Woodward. His *A Light to Grammar and all other Arts and Sciences* (1641), exhibited complete familiarity with the debates of the previous decade, and receptivity to the ideas of Comenius and Bacon. He shared the antigrammatical inclinations of Webbe, but was more directly aligned with Brooke on method. However Woodward advocated an extension of the sensual method, to provide a graduated introduction to the 'book of Nature'; style, idiom, imitation and grammar were to be relegated to a subordinate role. Like Bacon and Comenius he adopted the metaphor of the parrot for contemporary linguists, whose eloquence concealed ignorance of all significant knowledge.[19]

Further emancipation from tradition was gained by increasing the use of the vernacular. Brooke's method put a value on the vernacular in early exercises, whereas Woodward wished to see English used as the general medium for education. *A Light to Grammar* represented the characteristic puritan reaction against the prevailing humanistic standards of Elizabethan and Stuart courtesy literature. Woodward was committed to universal education, and convinced that a child could 'doe his worke playing, and play working'. He no longer accepted the grammar school model which had seemed natural to his fellow Puritan Brinsley a few decades earlier. Classical authors and Renaissance commentators tended to fade into the background. Woodward felt an instinctive sympathy for any pedagogical principle emphasising the superiority of individual judgement and personal experience. In the manner of the Platonists in religion he felt that his method of 'precognition' was superior since it 'conveys a light unto the understanding, which the child hath lighted at his own candle.' Although developed in a loose and aphoristic form, and expressed in terms of facultative psychology, Woodward's ideas were based on an empiricist epistemology. Through the gradual exploration of nature, reinforced by experiment and artistic representation, the child would naturally cultivate the faculty of under-

19. Woodward, *A Light to Grammar* (341), sig. a4r; Comenius, Preface to *Janua linguarum reserata*. Woodward was quoted in Charles Hoole's preface to his translation of Comenius's *Orbis sensualium pictus* (1659).

standing; thereafter the faculty of memory would develop without effort. As the analogue of religious experience, God would be revealed through 'the Vestigia of His power, and wisdome, of all His attributes in the glorious Workmanship of the world'.[20]

Discussion among the language teachers increasingly led to an appreciation of the educational value of the empirical sciences, and sympathy for the philosophy of Francis Bacon. Bacon had recognised the weakness of humanistic philosophy and education. His system embraced an epistemology consonant with new ideas on child psychology, a methodology suited to the theory of precognition, and a view of the social role of knowledge consistent with the puritan advocation of an active life. Bacon's experimental philosophy accordingly provided an ideal context for the puritan view of childhood.

The new pedagogy favoured by the Puritans was sufficiently comprehensive to embrace the needs of early childhood, adolescence and maturity. In its first application it would direct the natural exploratory behaviour of childhood, when 'All is newes to him, and thereof our nature is greedy. It is as a little Ape taken up by imitation.' Schools would become 'Scholas, & ludos literarios, meaning, that the study of learning was but a pleasant paines-taking or serious recreation'.[21] By a reversal of the priorities of traditional education, languages would be acquired only where relevant to an increased understanding of the natural world. The foundation of knowledge would be the solid learning of science and mathematics, conducted in the vernacular:

> 'Children also must be framed to be men by handling humane things; and by having all manner of occurences of this life represented both to their notice, and practice while they are in Schooles. Yea, all Philosophy in generall must be so ordered, that it may be a lively image of things, a secret fitting and dressing of mens minds for the businesses of this life.'[22]

Thus the process of education would lead naturally into vocational life, each member of the community being equipped for public service conducted out of a sense of religious obligation.

In order to prevent the degeneration of the new pedagogy into pious slogans and utopian dreams, it was essential for it to acquire a more definite expression. Francis Bacon provided inspiration and a philosophical framework, but his writings lacked detailed and specific comment on educational questions. What was needed was a comprehensive range of writings exhibiting the merits of the new pedagogy to the heads of families, schoolmasters and social administrators. As with all idealistic movements, the central problem was one of translating general policies

20. Woodward (341), pp.14–19, 24.
21. Woodward (341), p.27; Comenius, *A Reformation* (52), p.7.
22. Comenius (52), pp.20–1.

into concrete terms: in this case, textbooks or practicable schemes for school organisation. The continental Cartesians effectively transposed Descartes's writings into a series of textbooks covering the same ground as the established scholastic works. By contrast Bacon's writings generally stopped short of the systematic exposition of metaphysical and scientific issues. The *Novum Organum* might supplant traditional logic, but its methods precluded structured natural philosophy of the type elaborated by Descartes. Thus Bacon's works lacked any obvious basis for reformulation as a system of textbooks. Nevertheless Bacon unambiguously demanded both the reform of early education and greater cultivation of the sciences in higher education. His *Instauratio Magna* provided guidelines for this reorientation, but the specific educational application of his ideas was devised by Comenius. The Czech took the lead in the attempt to evolve a comprehensive new pedagogy.

The 'Christian philosophy' or *pansophia* of Comenius infused into Bacon's empiricism a strong religious element.[23] Harmony between the senses, reason and the scriptures was the essential foundation for pansophia. Accordingly Comenius incorporated the inductive philosophy into a more explicitly religious framework, embracing the ideal of man's intellectual and social regeneration, but within the strictly protestant view of world reformation. Pansophism, with its ambitious philosophical pretensions and encyclopaedic scope became, in the hands of the majority of its advocates, an esoteric and inaccessible system of knowledge. Comenius gained greater authority among the English Baconians perhaps because he avoided this introspective tendency; although his pansophia involved a mystical dimension, it was primarily conceived as a body of knowledge to be attained by the combined, empirical labours of all classes. Comenius's success in rendering pansophia intelligible to a wide public was assisted by his composition of a system of textbooks suitable for all stages of intellectual development. By constant reference to the pansophic idea he was able to use even language textbooks as an introduction to an encyclopaedic investigation of nature and as a vehicle for his enlightened pedagogy.

Comenius first attracted attention through his involvement in the reform of language teaching. His *Janua linguarum reserata* (1631) was a sensational success as a language primer, being adapted for numerous vernaculars as well as classical languages. Combining the antigrammatical method of Webbe, with the approach to early studies through 'sensuals' of Brooke, the *Janua* achieved immediate popularity among the English language reformers and occasioned a lasting friendship between Comenius and Hartlib. Two separate editions were promptly published in England by John Anchoran and Thomas Horne, the latter being a participant in the language discussions of the 1630s. Anchoran's English-Latin-French *Porta linguarum trilinguis reserata* (1633)

23. For the sources of Comenius's pansophia, see Schaller (254).

was reprinted four times, while the more popular edition by Horne, *Janua linguarum reserata* (1636), was constantly revised and augmented, nine editions appearing before 1660.[24] Together with the appended and even more elementary 'Vestibulum', the *Janua* was intended as a first reader, appropriate for teaching either the vernacular or Latin, or both together. The author acknowledged a debt to the Jesuit *Janua*, but the resemblances between the two primers are largely superficial. Bathe was primarily concerned with moral precepts and the cultivation of style, and with paving the way to an acquaintance with the moral philosophy of classical authors and catholic theologians.[25] Comenius, on the other hand, preferred a progressive organisation, beginning with very simple phrases and avoiding difficult abstract concepts throughout. The soundest subject matter for such a primer was in his opinion the systematic description of the natural world. In a hundred brief chapters the *Janua* sought to provide a synopsis of things themselves (*res ipsae,* or *rerum ipsa universitas*).[26] It opened by surveying the macrocosm and microcosm, beginning with a description of the universe, the earth and living organisms, and passing on to human anatomy and physiology. The central and longest parts of the book were concerned with domestic and social life. Finally, a few chapters dealt directly with religious practices, eschatology and the final heavenly order. The book consequently embraced the entire *scala natura,* starting with the physical universe and ending with the spiritual realm. Throughout the emphasis was on language and idiom suitable for everyday communication. An axiom of this method was the necessity of parallel development of the intellect and language. This combination of the practical with the linguistic was guaranteed to have great appeal among puritan educators. The Latin language was only taught in its relationship to the vernacular; it was only used where necessary as a vehicle for useful communication; pagan writings were brought into a new perspective, being no longer regarded as idols for imitation, but as sources of information having no assumed superiority over other literature. The English editors of the *Janua* fully exploited its practical aspect, even to the extent of overburdening the vocabulary and obscuring the linguistic aims of the original. In the 1631 *Janua,* sentence 134 listed twenty grassland plants whereas Thomas Horne's 1650 edition gave thirty-nine. The next two sentences in Horne's edition gave twenty-eight species of culinary herbs and nearly one hundred medicinal plants, the latter being classified according to use. Thus the *Janua* evolved into a thesaurus, its sentences bulging with useful

24. For a list of editions, see Webster (320), p.208.

25. Corcoran (59), compares Bathe and Comenius in a manner strongly biased in favour of the former.

26. Comenius, *Janua linguarum reserata,* Preface. The full title of this primer reveals its aims: *Janua linguarum reserata, sive seminarium linguarum et scientiarum omnium, hoc est compendiosa Latinam (et quamlibet aliam) linguam una cum scientiarum artiumque fundamentis per discendi methodus.*

information on all aspects of daily life, from the moral responsibilities of each member of the family to techniques of ploughing.[27]

This stress on the active life, involvement in economic affairs, and exploration of the natural world, was quickly imitated by Woodward and other educational writers. Indirectly, Comenius influenced the outlook of a much wider range of reformers. Detecting the sympathy for Comenius in England, Hartlib and Hübner assiduously furthered his interests among the Puritans. Their major *coup* was the publication at Oxford of the first edition of *Pansophiae prodromus,* the preliminary exposition of Comenius's pansophic philosophy. This work was issued without the author's permission and its publication involved adroit manipulation of the censor. After Comenius's objections had been overcome, the work was reissued in London, and then translated as *A Reformation of Schools* (1642), a title chosen to underline the educational relevance of pansophia.[28] Comenius defined the educationalist's duties in the broadest pansophic terms, as 'the art of readily and solidly teaching all men all things'.[29] Hartlib distributed this book widely, with the intention of establishing England as the focus for debate on educational and philosophical matters.

The educational aspect of pansophia was foremost in the discussions preparatory to Comenius's visit to England in the winter of 1641/2. The Czech detected sympathy for his objectives, noting that proposals were under discussion for the reform of schools throughout the kingdom so that 'all young people should be instructed, none neglected'.[30] By this time Comenius had completed major unpublished writings such as *Didactica Magna* and *Via Lucis,* containing his detailed views on education. Education held a high place among the duties of the projected Universal College described in *Via Lucis.* Comenius envisaged that the members of the college would supervise the establishment of a national system of schools, and draft a series of books which would determine the course of educational reform. The impressive series of handbooks envisaged consisted of:

1. *Excitatorium universale;* a plea to magistrates and rulers stressing the urgency and necessity of reforming schools for all sections of the community.

27. *ODO,* i, pp.259–60; *Janua linguarum reserata* (London, 1650), sentences 134–6. An example of a typical information-packed sentence is 391, which deals with ploughing—'He who laieth it upon rigs, with one hand he holds the plough handle, for fear of running beside the furrow, with the other the plough staff & the coulter with the plough share, fastened into the plough beam, breaking up the furrows until the task be completed.'

28. *Conatuum Comenianorum praeludia* (Oxford, 1637); *Pansophiae Prodromus* (London, 1639). Hartlib composed different prefaces to the two editions.

29. Comenius, *A Reformation* (52), p.47; original—'omnes omnia prompte et solide docendi artificium exhibens.' For Dury's definition of pansophia, see below, p.113.

30. Letter from Comenius to his associates in Leszno, 8/18 October 1641, quoted from R. F. Young (348), p.65.

2. *Informatorium ad Parentes;* advice to parents on pre-school education, based on his *Informatorium scholae maternae.*
3. *Tirocinium Literarum;* a new alphabet for children aged five or six.
4. *Encyclopaedia sensualium;* a work perhaps inspired by the English reformers who used this term to describe an elementary introduction to natural objects. They also conceived that this might be illustrated, a point only developed later by Comenius, in his *Orbis pictus* (1658).
5. *Bibliorum Epitome Historica;* a digest introducing students to the use of the scriptures.
6. *Praxis Biblica;* a guide to Christian ethics.
7. *Medulla Biblica;* a summary of Christian faith, based on the catechism.
8. *Priscianus Vernaculus;* a grammar to be applied to both the vernacular and Latin tongues.
9. *Informatorium ad Scholarum Vernacularum Moderatores;* a guide to those organising vernacular education, whether in the family or school. This would outline the aims of elementary education and provide details of the regimen.
10. *Latinitatis Vestibulum;* the elementary Latin primer.
11. *Janua Latinitatis;* the expanded form of the *Janua linguarum reserata,* with dictionary and grammar.
12. *Palatium Latinitatis;* a more advanced Latin textbook, giving an introduction to classical authors.
13. *Informatorium ad Latini studii Magistros;* advice on the organisation of the more advanced Latin school.
14. *Panhistoria: sive Singularium historia Scientialis;* a survey of empirical knowledge covering each branch of natural philosophy, crafts and trades, approximating to Bacon's natural histories or histories of trades.
15. *Pandogmatia;* a survey of the range of human opinion on philosophical questions, analogous to Bacon's *De Augmentis Scientiarum,* Book III, Chapter 4.
16. *Pansophiae opus;* the culmination of these endeavours would be a digest of human wisdom, which would then be disseminated for the benefit of mankind.[31]

Because of the Civil War Comenius was obliged to accept Swedish patronage for his ambitious schoolbook programme. Nevertheless his brief visit to England served an important function. Comenius's great prestige further enhanced Hartlib's position among the parliamentarian leaders. The Long Parliament was receptive to positive social policies, and Comenius's ideas on schools, schoolbooks and a system of know-

31. Comenius, 'Ad excitanda publice veritatis et pacis (hoc est communis salutis) ope Dei studia. Elaborandorum Operum Catalogus', HP VII 90. Edited by G. H. Turnbull (289), pp.17–26.

ledge related to social needs, were congenial to the puritan intelligentsia. If *Ad excitanda publice* was more conventional in its attitude to classical studies than his initial pansophic writings, this only served to restore confidence among more cautious members of the puritan party. Thus a party within parliament, prompted from outside by an active group of educational enthusiasts, became favourable to the advancement of learning.[32]

In June 1641 parliament resolved that all Deans and Chapters should be completely abolished and their lands employed 'to the Advancement of Learning and Piety'.[33] This was accompanied by the appointment of committees to examine the state of free schools and universities.[34] The Anglican spokesman John Hacket expressed alarm that these measures would only serve to destroy the nation's principal grammar schools, placing education at the mercy of fanciful schoolmasters 'introducing new Methods and Compendiums of teaching, which tend to nothing but loss of time and ignorance'.[35] It is easy to detect in this sentiment a fear that education would be unduly influenced by Comenian schoolmasters, whose ideas were at that time being voiced in Woodward's writings.

The textbooks of Comenius and the organisational skills of Hartlib were sufficient to prevent the complete collapse of this educational endeavour during the Civil War. Woodward expressed the widely-felt debt to the foreigners:

> 'But (I thanke you againe) since you came into these parts, those discouragements about our Schoole points began to weare out; such hath beene your activenesse therein. And which is the greatest meanes to make our way clearer, you have beene a meanes to make Comenius knowne amongst us, the greatest light to this Kinde of Learning, that was ever set up in the World.'[36]

In the absence of the greatest light, it rested on Hartlib to promote reformed pedagogy, develop a practical programme for universal education and ensure that parliament was reminded of its obligations to apply ecclesiastical revenues to the advancement of learning. Largely owing to Hartlib's initiative authors were found to write tracts on all aspects of education. Often their work was influenced by Comenius, but increasingly the English puritan educational writings took on a separate identity. Hartlib and his associates completely dominated the educational literature of the Puritan Revolution, being responsible for at least fifty educational works between 1640 and 1660.[37] About half

32. Webster (320), pp.22–38.
33. *CJ*, ii, pp.159, 176, 204.
34. For schools, 16 April 1641, *CJ*, ii, pp.121–2, 126; for universities, 22 April 1641, *CJ*, ii, pp.126, 167, 233.
35. Hacket, *A Century of Sermons*, ed. Thomas Plume (London, 1675), p.xx.
36. Woodward, *A Light to Grammar* (341), sig. a5v.
37. For a complete list of these writings, see Webster (320), pp.208–11.

these works were produced between 1647 and 1651, when Hartlib was most active as the parliamentary 'Agent for the advancement of learning'. This association with parliament was an added incentive for authors to frame their proposals in practicable terms. The educational literature of this period represents an almost complete break with tradition, bearing only a remote resemblance to the grammars, texts, courtesy books and advices to the schoolmaster composed during the previous decades. Milton is perhaps the only leading writer to embody a compromise between the new and old pedagogies.

In 1642 Hartlib claimed that educational reform and the Baconian advancement of learning were absolutely necessary for the 'true and fundamentall Reformation' of the state.[38] Dury revised the list of educational writings projected for the Universal College, but without acknowledgment to Comenius.[39] Apart from directions to teachers and administrators about the ordering of schools, Dury advocated three sets of books, designed to deal with religion, languages and the sciences. The surveys of the sciences would contribute towards pansophia, 'shewing the universall method of ordering the thoughts, to finde out by our owne industry any truth as yet unknown, and resolve any question which may be proposed in nature, as the object of rationall meditation'.[40]

It was of course impossible to follow Comenius's programme exactly. Indeed Comenius himself was overwhelmed by the scope of his project and the masterwork of his scheme, *Consultatio Catholica,* although completed, was not published until recently. His revised and augmented Latin primers lacked the qualities of simplicity and appeal to practical experience of the earlier versions; they also tended to revert to the traditional humanist pattern. On the whole Comenius's English adherents found greater appeal in his pansophic sketches and simpler textbooks; their approach to education remained more uncompromisingly antihumanistic. *Janua linguarum reserata* (1631) was subjected to continual editorial attention, the editors ignoring many of his later, less inspired, and laborious grammatical works. The pansophic sketch of 1637, it will be recalled, was published by Hartlib as *A Reformation of Schools* (1642). In 1651 an anonymous translator produced *Natural Philosophy reformed by Divine Light,* while at Hartlib's request Jeremy Collier translated *A Pattern of Universal Knowledge*.[41] Comenian pansophia provided an explicit biblical sanction for Baconian empiricism, so cementing the integration of Bacon's philosophy into the puritan

38. Hartlib, *Englands Thankfulnesse* (134), p.9; Webster (320), p.74.

39. Dury, *A Motion Tending* (84), pp.23–4; Webster (320), pp.104–6. For general discussions of Dury's educational writings, see H. J. Scougal, *Die pädagogischen Schriften John Durys* (Jena, 1905); T. H. H. Rae, *John Dury: Reformer of Education* (Marburg/Lahn, 1970).

40. Dury, *A Motion Tending* (84), p.24; Webster (320), p.105.

41. *Physicae ad lumen divinum reformatae* (Leipzig, 1633); *Pansophiae diatyposis* (Danzig, 1643).

worldview and underlining the relevance of that philosophy to educational reform. Furthermore, Comenius's work demonstrated that educational reform was an integral element in the eschatological scheme. The universal provision of schools was a necessary precondition for the 'extension of light over all men universally', which would ensure that all men, from the greatest to the least, would honour God (Jer. 31 :34). With the extension of pansophic education man would achieve full faith, unity and knowledge, approaching the stature of Christ, and be a child no longer (Isa. 65 :20).[42] Such biblical pronouncements inspired puritan intellectuals with a passion for intellectual exploration; they now demanded of educational institutions that 'they should be able to teach all things to all men'.[43]

The call for universal education begun in the writings of Comenius was quickly taken up by the puritan social reformers and it was incorporated as an axiom into the reform literature of the Puritan Revolution. Criticisms of scholastic education began cautiously, but soon achieved full expression with Hartlib and his associates Dury, Milton and Hall, while even more radical criticisms came from the army chaplains Dell, Webster and Pinnel. Having cleared the ground, Hartlib's protégés rushed forward with plans for workhouses, elementary schools, agricultural colleges, and academies, designed for both sexes and for all social classes. These were an open demonstration of the means by which the precepts of Bacon and Comenius could be translated into social action. Political supporters were pressed to reinforce the influence of pamphleteers; parliament and the Council of State were never allowed to forget their acknowledged obligation to advance learning. Educational reconstruction during the Puritan Revolution was only possible if the reformers could operate successfully on the conscience of the legislators. Tentative exercises in state investment in education, discussed below, indicate some cautious sympathy for the aims of the reformers. The necessity of intervention in education was accepted in principle; but complete reorganisation of education, the destruction of scholasticism and the introduction of universal education, implied social experiments too ambitious for the taste of the new rulers. Accordingly the state fell back on the traditional form of participation in education, regulating practitioners and institutions according to political and religious tests. It was hoped by this means to protect the social fabric against aberrant intellectual fashions. As the reformers predicted, failure to implement more positive educational reforms undoubtedly contributed towards weakening the foundations of the puritan state.

This situation exposed deep rifts among the puritan educators. The reformers regarded educational reconstruction as a necessary prerequisite for the creation of the millennial state. Others were driven

42. Comenius, *Via Lucis* (55), pp.196–7.
43. Hall, *An Humble Motion* (127), p.27.

to defend scholastic education out of fear of the social consequences of unbridled reform. Conflict developed on a whole range of educational issues, but the debate was fiercest over the universities, which, to the reformers, were symbols of an alien intellectual and religious order.

The foundations for conflict over education were laid at an early stage. In the *Grand Remonstrance* of 1641, parliament expressed an intention to 'purge the fountains of learning, the two Universities, that the streams flowing from thence may be clear and pure'. The reform of scholastic education and overthrow of the authority of the Anglican church within the universities was a clearly defined goal which was within the reach of parliament. Without purification of the universities the people would lack sound spiritual guidance and teachers would continue to mislead the young. This issue thus provided a symbolic test of parliament's intention to pursue the advancement of learning. Since the innovators increasingly regarded experimental science as an integral part of puritan education, the introduction of the sciences into the universities became a central issue in the fierce debates on educational reform which accompanied the Puritan Revolution.

(ii) Science and Medicine in Academic Studies before 1640

In an assessment which must be allowed to have considerable authority, Oxford's restoration chancellor Lord Clarendon admitted that, notwithstanding the general barbarism of the interregnum, Oxford had during that period 'yielded a harvest of extra-ordinary good and sound knowledge in all parts of learning'.[44] This was an opinion shared by all but the severest high-church critics of the parliamentarian regime, who, once reinstalled in the universities, embarked upon a course of retribution which precluded acknowledging any grain of merit in the offending Presbyterian and Independent parties. Clarendon's estimate is confirmed by the well-informed Anglican and royalist physician Walter Charleton, an eye-witness who extolled 'The noble successes of those Heroicall Wits among our Country-men, who have addicted themselves to the Reformation and Augmentation of Arts and Sciences, and made a greater Progresse in that glorious design, than many ages before them could aspire to.'[45] Oxford and the London College of Physicians were singled out for special mention in Charleton's eulogy of his countrymen's contribution to the various facets of experimental science. This rise of experimental natural philosophy at the universities impressed many other observers, eliciting comment in orations delivered during the interregnum by academics of many persuasions. Claren-

44. *History of the Rebellion,* ed. W. D. Macray (Oxford, 1847), iv, p.284. For a similar estimate in an oration delivered in 1654 by Vice-Chancellor Owen, see *The Oxford Orations of Dr. John Owen,* ed. P. Toon (Linkinhorne, 1971), p.15.
45. Charleton (46), p.33.

don was probably impressed by the increasing reputation of the scientific virtuosi, but intellectual vitality was not the only reason for the debt of the restoration to the natural philosophers who rose to prominence during the interregnum. They had proved to be exemplary guardians of the academic institutions moulded by Archbishop Laud.

In order to arrive at a balanced view of the role of science and medicine in the universities during the Puritan Revolution it is necessary to draw attention to the conditions prevailing in the earlier part of the century. There is considerable divergence of opinion on this subject. At one extreme it is felt that the period of Laudian dominance was characterised by intellectual stagnation, which was effectively counteracted by parliamentarians, to allow free flowering of the new philosophy.[46] Others would claim that the new science became firmly rooted in the Laudian universities and that this tradition was merely maintained during the subsequent upheavals.[47] Both points of view rely on substantially the same sources of evidence: the autobiographical and apologetic writings of Ward, Wilkins and Wallis, and the 'Directions for a Student' attributed to Richard Holdsworth. All of these documents were composed after 1640, but they have been cited as guides to earlier educational attitudes, a purpose for which they must clearly be used with the greatest caution.

Whatever view is taken about the rise of science in the universities, it must be appreciated that the 'sciences' which captured the imagination of Brian Twyne at the beginning of the seventeenth century had little in common with those pursued by the students of John Wilkins fifty years later. In the course of that time each facet of science developed and metamorphosed. The new systems of Telesio, Campanella, Descartes and Gassendi greatly diversified the conceptual approach to natural philosophy. Most of the experimental activities, mathematical problems and philosophical debates recorded by Wallis for the originators of the Royal Society would have been foreign to the experience of natural philosophers at the beginning of the century. Developments of this kind cannot be ignored when assessing the intellectual atmosphere in the English universities. Accordingly it is as frivolous to deny that there were any substantially new developments after 1640 as it is to assert that puritanism provides a sufficient explanation for the change.

It is not possible to enter into a discussion of academic response to the sciences without some reference to the problems of definition.

46. 'A Note on the Universities', Hill (149), pp.301–14.

47. Curtis (69), pp.227–60; P. Allen, 'Scientific Studies in the English Universities of the Seventeenth Century', *JHI*, 1949, *10*: 219–53; also B. J. Shapiro, 'The Universities and Science in Seventeenth Century England', *Journal of British Studies,* 1971, 10: 47–82. Shapiro suggests that 'Universities had shown continuous interest in science, that Puritan intervention did not significantly alter the pattern of scientific concerns . . .'. For a valuable review of sources, see Frank (106).

It is for example important to bear in mind that the term 'university' is customarily used for an institution and the statutory activities of its members, but that it may also be legitimately applied to cover the wider, informal activities of the community of scholars associated with the institution. In the seventeenth century at least it was possible for individuals to play an institutional role little related to their private intellectual life. The universities may therefore be assessed according to various standards. The institutional structure, statutory teaching regulations, and examination mechanisms seem the most obvious basis on which to make a judgement. But this evidence usually provides only limited and superficial indications about the scope of formal education. At the other extreme, we possess considerable information about the informal intellectual activities of the university in the wider sense. Between these two extremes of university life lies the *terra incognita* of tutorial studies and independent student enterprise. Some tutors would have taken the fullest advantage of any opportunity of introducing their students to the latest intellectual developments; ambitious students took the initiative themselves, sometimes even against their tutors' advice. In view of the fragmentary preservation of student records, our estimation of general tutorial response to the growth of the sciences must be largely speculative.

The scientific disciplines which could be most readily assimilated into university studies were medicine and mathematics. The former had a venerable history as a postgraduate discipline, while the latter was a potentially important constituent of the liberal arts curriculum. In addition, natural philosophy received some attention during the later stages of the arts course. The exact role intended for these subjects is not easy to determine. The statutes were specific and detailed, but these complex documents are extremely difficult to interpret. In some cases, later statutes were intended to complement the earlier, while in others they were to supplant them. The two universities differed slightly in their requirements, but some tuition was offered in arithmetic, geometry, music, cosmography, and astronomy.[48] Under the Laudian code at Oxford, arithmetic, geometry and music were stipulated for undergraduates, while at Cambridge only natural philosophy was authorised. Thus during the four-years preparation for a BA, little attention to mathematics and natural philosophy was required, particularly at Cambridge. During the subsequent three years of study for an MA, these subjects assumed greater importance. Both universities required some reading in astronomy, geometry and natural philosophy.[49] The stipulated texts for these studies were predominantly classical, or later didactic works based on obvious classical sources. The texts of Euclid, Galen, Ptolemy, or Aristotle were often an excellent starting-point for wider investigations, but there is little indication that the average stu-

48. Curtis (69), pp.86–90.
49. Gibson (116), pp.xcii–xcvi, 378.

dent was made aware of the changing horizons of scientific knowledge. Pedagogical routine increasingly stood in the way of a flexible and creative approach to the sciences in both English and continental universities.

Student notebooks probably give a reliable impression about the general tone of formal studies.[50] They confirm the dominance of standard classical texts and exhibit a degree of formalisation and didactic simplification characteristic of the systematic but desiccated textbooks of the protestant scholastics. By their capacity to administer precisely to the statutory requirements of undergraduates, rather than by genuine intellectual appeal, the scholastic textbooks of the seventeenth century gained a tenacious hold which was only slowly overcome by textbooks representative of the new philosophy. Even in the eighteenth century, Tristram Shandy could be made to remark with simulated astonishment that his father 'had never in his whole life [had] the least light or spark struck into his mind, by one single lecture upon Crakenthorp or Burgersdicius, or any Dutch logician or commentator'.[51] But virtue was not entirely absent from these writings. Besides their sharp disputes on logical and ethical questions, such authors as Alsted and Ramus made distinct moves away from Aristotelianism, preparing the ground for more eclectic approaches to education and philosophy. Both Alsted and Ramus were successful textbook writers in natural philosophy and mathematics, but they were inclined to overreach themselves in their enthusiasm for comprehensiveness.[52] The restlessness of a young intellectual with a desire to escape from scholastic values, but without clear insight into a means of emancipation, is instanced by Nathaniel Carpenter. His *Philosophia Libera* was a work on natural philosophy explicitly intended to undermine Aristotelian orthodoxy, but whose author was totally imprisoned by scholastic concepts and terminology.[53]

Those who were tempted to explore neglected areas of knowledge found little encouragement, incentive or guidance. Brian Twyne's father warned him against premature reading of medical works.[54] None the less, Twyne accumulated medical books and quickly moved into even more disputed territory, studying mathematics and astrology under

50. W. J. Costello (61); H. Kearney (170), pp.77–90, 102–9.

51. Laurence Sterne, *The Life and Opinions of Tristram Shandy,* Chapter XIX. For an earlier remark of a similar satirical nature, see Joseph Glanvill, *Plus Ultra* (London, 1668), p.118. For the neo-scholastics, see P. Miller (189), pp. 102–4, 510–12; N. W. Gilbert, *Renaissance Concepts of Method* (New York, 1960); P. Dibon, *La philosophie néerlandaise au siècle d'or: Tome I* (Paris, 1954). For a review of recent research, see C. B. Schmitt (256). For textbooks, Patricia Reif, 'The Textbook Tradition in Natural Philosophy 1600–1650', *JHI*, 1969, *30*: 17–32.

52. W. J. Ong, *Ramus: Method and the Decay of Dialogue* (Cambridge, Mass., 1958).

53. Madan (184), iii, p.312.

54. Letter from Brian Twyne to Thomas Twyne, 6 July 1601, Bodleian MS, Gr. Misc. d. 2, fols. 40r–41v; quoted from *Bodleian Quarterly Record,* 1926/9, *5*: 217.

Thomas Allen of Gloucester Hall, at a time when 'astrologer, mathematician and conjurer were accounted the same things'.[55] With this danger in mind Ascham had warned against too great an interest in mathematics, while the most active exponents of this subject, Dee, Allen and the Harriot circle, earned notoriety as 'juglers'.

Under these circumstances the serious student of mathematics was an isolated figure, often displaying an almost religious devotion and enthusiasm for his new-found interest. The most influential mathematics teacher of this period, William Oughtred, described his mathematical apprenticeship in fervent terms:

> 'I redeemed night by night from my naturall sleep, defrauding my body, and inuring it to watching, cold, and labour, while most others tooke their rest. Neither did I therein seek only my private content, but the benefit of many: and by inciting, assisting, and instructing others, brought many in to the love and study of those Arts, not only in our own, but in some other Colledges also.'[56]

Oughtred's new obsession gave him intense satisfaction, which he transmitted to younger disciples. Through such ardent advocates as Oughtred, mathematics became available to a small but active 'sect' of academics. It reached a wider audience through Oughtred's textbook, *Clavis mathematica* (1631), which greatly enhanced the status of the subject. The astronomer William Gascoigne reported that he turned to Oughtred's book after he had failed to obtain guidance in mathematics at Oxford.[57] Many other provincial gentlemen shared Gascoigne's experience. Even those who spent many years at university were likely to find that mathematics was a neglected subject, its appearance in the notebooks of Twyne being an exception.[58] John Wallis was exceptionally fortunate in attending Felsted School, where the rudiments of arithmetic were taught. He regretted that 'this was my first insight into Mathematicks, and all the teaching I had'. At Cambridge he found that mathematics was thought appropriate to seamen and artisans, no assistance being available in 'what books to read, or what to seek, or in which method to proceed'. Of the two hundred students at his college Wallis knew only two who possessed reasonable skill in mathematics. He knew that mathematics was thriving in London among the mathematical practitioners, with whom he was soon able to asso-

55. Aubrey, i, pp.26–9.

56. Oughtred, *The Circles of Proportion* (London, 1633), appendix, 'The Just Apologie', sig. A4v–B1r. A. J. Turner (293), draws attention to the importance of instruments in seventeenth-century mathematical education. Aubrey noted that 'countrey people did beleeve that he [Oughtred] could conjure' and that 'He was an astrologer and very lucky in giving his judgements on nativities': Aubrey, ii, pp.108–9. For further consideration of this subject, see Thomas (281), pp.349–54.

57. Gascoigne 'Left both Oxford and London before [he] knew what a proposition in geometry meant': Letter to Oughtred [1640], Rigaud (245), i, p.35.

58. W. J. Costello (61), pp.102, 149.

ciate, owing to his decision to leave university and enter the ministry.[59] Seth Ward at Sidney Sussex College had similar experiences; upon finding mathematical books in the college library, he was unable to find any Fellow able to help him. This position was only remedied when his ejection in 1644 led to his association with the London mathematicians and with William Oughtred.[60]

Such biographies suggest that before 1640 colleges at Oxford and Cambridge placed very little emphasis on mathematics and virtually none on experimental science. As Costello concludes, the neatness and convenience of their existing arrangements insulated them 'from any obligation to rethink the old curriculum in terms of the busy findings of the new mathematics and the New Science'.[61] There appears to have been a willingness to surrender these subjects to the London mathematical practitioners, or to the professors of Gresham College. The close interrelationship between scholars and practitioners in London may have convinced most academics that mathematics was irrelevant to liberal education in the universities. This attitude continued to prevail until the middle of the nineteenth century.

The medical faculties offered an alternative basis for the assimilation of science into higher education. If natural philosophy had been neglected in arts studies, there were no counter-attractions to deflect the student from its study during the long period of preparation for an MD.[62] The capacity of medical studies to lead to productive research in a wide range of scientific problems is illustrated by the careers of Gilbert and Harvey. However, their personal success was not due to the vitality of English medical schools. The medical schools at Padua, Bologna, Leyden and Montpellier had become centres of humanistic learning, anatomy, natural history and clinical training. Their counterparts at Oxford and Cambridge were not active in these directions, although Thomas Linacre and John Caius attempted to bridge the gulf between English, and continental medical education. Each university had been furnished with a Regius professor in medicine since the reign of Henry VIII. Linacre endowed medical lectureships at both Oxford and Cambridge, but these never became properly functional. A few colleges had medical fellowships; Caius was exceptional in establishing two at his college.[63]

Before 1640 the English medical faculties appear to have adopted an extremely traditional approach to medical education. The pro-

59. Scriba (257), pp.26–7, 29–30. See above, pp.40–1.
60. Walter Pope (223), pp.9–10, 16.
61. Costello (61), p.148.
62. The precise length of time spent in preparation for an MD is difficult to estimate. According to the statutes, after obtaining an MA in seven years, an MD was confirmed after a further four to seven years. However, in almost all cases, graces were obtained to reduce this period of study. For a brief survey of this topic, see P. Allen, 'Medical Education in Seventeenth-Century England', *J. Hist. Med.,* 1946, *1*: 115–43.
63. Curtis (69), pp.152–5; Costello (61), pp.128–35; Macalister (182).

fessors were orthodox and almost uniformly undistinguished. Considering the extreme length envisaged for medical studies, the statutory provisions were vague and fragmentary. Nothing like a comprehensive medical curriculum emerged. Thus when as regularly happened a dispensation was granted so that requirements might be reduced, no dilution of standards was involved. The essential ingredients were lectures and the study of small sections of the Galenic and Hippocratic corpus. The occasional revisions of the statutes betrayed no significant response to developments in humanistic medicine.[64]

There was no move towards the kind of clinical teaching adopted in certain Italian medical schools. More surprisingly, dissection appears not to have been practised more than sporadically although the Edwardian statutes prescribed two anatomies for each incepting MD. Various graces were passed to prompt more active attention to dissection, but to little avail.[65] The disputation subjects for this period reflect the intellectual tone of the medical faculty. Most disputations related to elementary Galenic and Hippocratic tenets. Diet, alcoholic drinks and exercise were discussed in the frequent questions on regimen. There was also considerable discussion about the correct practice of phlebotomy and purgation. In one exceptional instance Robert Fludd debated the virtues of chemical therapy (1605). Discussion of points of anatomy was almost unknown, while physiological questions were general and elementary. Edmund Deane was asked whether respiration was necessary to sustain life; others were asked about the nutritive functions of blood. Humoral pathology and the doctrine of temperaments were the basic components of these disputes.[66] Medicine was evidently a literary study, but its practical aims should not be overlooked. The knowledge acquired from the texts studied at university was intended as a substantial foundation for medical practice.[67]

The numbers graduating in the medical faculties fluctuated widely before 1640. Occasionally the faculties must have hovered on the edge of extinction, since in some years no MB or MD was granted. For the period 1620-1640 Oxford produced an average of 2.5 MBs and one MD each year, while the equivalent figures for Cambridge were 1 and 1.5. The medical faculties of both universities were important as licensing agencies, granting incorporations to physicians with foreign MDs, and dispensing licences for practice 'pro regnum Angliae'. Incorporation was uncontroversial, since it was primarily intended to supply a qualification for membership of the College of Physicians. However,

64. Gibson (116), pp.ciii, 346, 379; Clark (48), ii, part 1, pp.123–9.

65. Macalister (182), pp. 10–11.

66. Clark (48), ii, part 1, pp.189–94; Univ. Oxon. Arch., Congregation Registers 1623–1640.

67. This contradicts the opinion of the editor of the Oxford registers: 'The faculty of Medicine . . . had already lost touch with the requirements of professional study, and presented very much the features which it has at the present day [1885]'. Clark (48), ii, part 1, p.123.

the College asserted that its position was being undermined by physicians who were using the university licence as an excuse to practise in London.[68] Furthermore, the College believed that the universities were unduly generous in granting medical licences. Soon after his appointment as Regius professor at Cambridge, Ralph Winterton 'observed and grieved to see sometimes a Minister, sometimes a serving man, sometimes an Apothecary admitted to a licence to practice in Physick'.[69] Both he and his predecessor were anxious to confine the grants of licences to those possessing a classical education but, according to the College of Physicians, arbitrary licensing continued.[70] Licences for the practice of medicine may have been given indiscriminately in a few cases, but at least as far as the Oxford records show, licences were almost invariably given to physicians having an MB or MD qualification.

For a more substantial medical training it was customary for medical students to visit one of the major continental universities. This expedient offered an insight into the full complexities of humanistic medicine. Foreign travel also served to familiarise English scholars with continental developments in mathematics and natural philosophy. Strong links were often forged between English and foreign physicians, which were maintained after the English scholars returned home, thus ensuring that they continued to be exposed to the most recent debates and advances in their specialities. The taste for continental medical education had been firmly established by the humanists in the first part of the sixteenth century. Linacre returned from Italy with a considerable reputation as a translator of Galen. His example was followed by Caius, who even incorporated a provision for such peregrinations in the statutes of his college. Caius had known Vesalius at Padua and later he collaborated with Conrad Gesner in compiling his *Historia animalium*. When faced with Vesalius's revisions of Galen however he reacted in favour of tradition. By contrast, Thomas Mouffet, who also visited Gesner in Switzerland, became an advocate of Paracelsus. Exposure to continental influences led to diversification of outlook within the medical profession, but it was an extremely long time before the new ideas became reflected in educational practice.

(iii) New Trends

From the point of view of the sciences an important watershed occurred around 1620, when the institutional status of science was greatly improved at Oxford, and means were sought to promote similar developments in Cambridge. The foundation of the Savilian chairs of astronomy

68. For the sources of the statistics quoted, see below, note 153. Averages are given to the nearest 0.25 per cent. G. Clark (50), i, pp.112–13; 209–10.
69. C. Goodall (119), p.443. Letter to the College of Physicians, 25 August 1635.
70. Clark (50), i, pp.260–1.

and geometry in 1619 provided the incentive for this transformation.[71] The immediate repercussions of Savile's carefully conceived benefaction are apparent from the letter written by Henry Briggs, the first Savilian professor of geometry, to his friend Samuel Ward, Master of Sidney Sussex College Cambridge. A copy of the Savilian statutes was enclosed, with the suggestion that the time was opportune for endowing similar posts at Cambridge. Out of respect for his 'mother Cambridge', Briggs expressed willingness to assist any benefactor in arranging an endowment. He reported that Sir William Sedley, Savile's son-in-law, had donated £2,000 for a lectureship in natural philosophy at Oxford, and that Henry Danvers, Earl of Danby, had made generous provision for a botanical garden, which was ultimately to have both a keeper and a professor of botany. An impressive foundation ceremony at the garden had taken place only a few days before. Briggs optimistically concluded 'I would very gladly have as great hope that Cambridge would follow a pace, as I have that Oxford will go further'.[72]

Oxford indeed went a little further. The Westminster merchant Richard Tomlins made a modest bequest for an anatomy lecture which was to be conducted annually by the Regius professor or his deputy.[73] But at Cambridge, while there was undoubtedly a nucleus of support for the sciences, no institutional expression was immediately forthcoming. Great expectations were aroused by Francis Bacon's somewhat belated expressions of respect for his *alma mater*. Bacon's will designated that two lectureships should be established at each university; of these at least one was to be devoted to the promotion of natural philosophy and related sciences. His executors were ordered to follow the Savilian statutes in framing these lectureships. Bishop Williams had hinted to Bacon that it was desirable to establish the endowment primarily at Cambridge in order to counterbalance the recent developments at Oxford.[74] Further consideration of these lectureships proved to be superfluous owing to Bacon's insolvency. In fact there were no further permanent scientific foundations at Cambridge, until the endow-

71. 'Statuta Saviliana', 19 August 1619: Gibson (116), pp.528–40; Griffiths (125), pp.244–53.

72. Letter from Briggs to Ward, 6 August 1621, Bodleian, Tanner MS 73, fol. 68. Briggs was a graduate of St. John's College Cambridge. Sedley's lectureship was founded under his will dated 29 October 1618: Wood *Hist. & Antiq.*, ii, pp.869–71; Griffiths (125), pp.36–7, 254. For the botanical garden, see R. W. T. Gunther, *Oxford Gardens* (Oxford, 1912); S. H. Vines & C. G. Druce, *An Account of the Morisonian Herbarium* (Oxford, 1914); C. G. Druce, in *Botanical Exchange Club Supplement*, 1925, *7*: 335–66.

73. 'De lectura anatomatica', Gibson (116), pp.550–5. Entered into the statutes 14 December 1624. This statute was exceptional in being framed in English. For a draft variant see Bodleian MS Wood F27, fol. 135r; Latin form, Griffiths (125), pp.258–61.

74. J. Spedding, *Letters & Life of Bacon* (263), vii, pp.544, 546, 547–8. Will dated 19 December 1625. There is some ambiguity whether one or both lectureships were intended for natural philosophy; see Mullinger (194), iii, pp.65–7; *idem*, 'The Relations of Francis Bacon Lord Verulam with the University of Cambridge', *Proc. Camb. Antiq. Soc.*, 1896/8, *9*: 227–37.

ment of the Lucasian chair in mathematics in 1663.[75] Its founder, Henry Lucas, had been secretary to the Laudian chancellor of Cambridge; hence he may have been indirectly influenced by the proposals of Briggs and Ward.

If the above institutional developments lacked the capacity to prompt an educational revolution, they at least provided Oxford with an agency for the dissemination of interest in science. Enthusiasts were given an institutional base which was not available at Cambridge. This factor probably affected scientific development at the two universities during the interregnum. Analogous intellectual movements are detectable at both, but from 1620 onwards science tended to be conducted on a more organised basis at Oxford.

The Savilian statutes made explicit reference to both practical and textual studies. The comprehensive and precise rubric of these statutes would have given new stimulus to the younger generation of mathematicians and astronomers, and there are many indications that the Savilian professors operated according to the spirit of Savile's maxims. They were authorised to use standard classical or Renaissance works as a starting-point, with the provision that they should make reference to any source necessary for the complete coverage of the subject, in both its theoretical and practical aspects. The technical subjects navigation and geodesy were encouraged, while astrology was strenuously prohibited. For the purposes of practical instruction, regular astronomical observation and the use of instruments in the field (in agris universitati vicinis) were recommended. It was envisaged that the endowments would support scientific expeditions, or the purchase of instruments and books. The professors were ordered to give informal instruction in the vernacular whenever appropriate, in order to propagate their subject.[76]

Briggs and his Cambridge friend John Bainbridge, both of whom had been associated with Gresham College, were the first holders of the Savilian chairs. The Gresham spirit was thereby effectively transferred to Oxford and quite soon Briggs and Bainbridge were framing ambitious proposals for a collection of instruments and a mathematical library.[77]

Less is known about the other benefactions but they served to reinforce the spirit of the Savilian statutes. Since Sedley was not specific about the functions of his lecturer, the university stipulated a range of Aristotle's texts, designed to cover major aspects of natural philosophy. It is not known how the first two lecturers[78] interpreted these statutes, but the parliamentarian nominee Joshua Crosse and

75. See below, p.136 for a lectureship in mathematics temporarily established in 1647.

76. Gibson (116), pp.528–35.

77. Draft letter from Bainbridge, 30 March 1629, headed 'Instrumentorum Mathematicorum Catalogus', Bainbridge MS, Tritinty College Dublin.

78. Edward Lapworth; John Edwards (ejected 1648).

his successor Thomas Willis were prominent advocates of experimental natural philosophy.

An inducement to a more adventurous approach to medical studies was created by the foundation of the Tomlins lectureship and the botanical garden. Tomlins gave instructions for there to be two series of lectures and practical demonstrations each year, the first illustrated by a dissection and the second by a skeleton. This was the first occasion on which explicit provision for anatomical lectures was made at an English university, whereas anatomy had been an established part of Italian medical education for almost a century. Tomlins may have been prompted to endow his anatomical lectureship by the success of the anatomical lectures delivered since 1616 at the London College of Physicians by William Harvey. These must have drawn attention to the intrinsic value and interest of anatomical demonstrations. Although it was many years before anatomical lectures became well established in the universities, there are increasing signs of attention to dissection after 1620. Positive statements in favour of dissection were made by the medical lecturers; Joseph Mede recorded attendance at a dissection and the grisly experience of a surprise encounter with a drying skeleton in a college garden.[79] Cambridge appointed Francis Glisson, Harvey's most distinguished English disciple, as Regius professor. Under Glisson physiology flourished; John Wallis claimed to have been the first of his pupils to defend the theory of circulation in a public disputation.[80] At Oxford there was an even earlier defence of circulation. Edward Dawson, a former member of Samuel Ward's college, transferred to Oxford and in 1633 defended the thesis 'An circulatio sanguinis sit probabilis?'[81] Particularly among younger scholars there is ample evidence of a spontaneous interest in anatomy, regardless of statutory provisions.

The humanistic botanists of the sixteenth century exercised perceptible influence in the continental medical schools; hence botanical gardens had been established at universities throughout Europe by the end of the sixteenth century. In England botany became the passion of apothecaries and of gentlemen. It was therefore appropriate for Henry Danvers, Earl of Danby, to endow a botanical garden at Oxford.[82] At the opening ceremony orations were given by the Regius professor, Thomas Clayton, and the young medical student Edward Dawson. The garden developed slowly and at great expense, but under its German curator, Jacob Bobart, it grew into an important botanical collection. In letters of commendation for Parkinson's herbal, Clayton and Bainbridge took the opportunity to advertise the Oxford garden

79. Macalister (182), pp.10–11; Costello (61), pp.130–1.

80. Scriba (257), p.29.

81. For Dawson's disputation see C. Hill, 'William Harvey and the Idea of Monarchy', *Past and Present*, 1964, No. 27, p.59. For Dawson, see Munk (195), i, p.218.

82. Gunther, *Oxford Gardens*, p.2.

as 'compleately beautifully walled, and gated, now in levelling, and planting, with the charges and expences of thousands by the many wayes Honourable Earle of Danby'.[83] For fifty years this was the only botanical garden in Britain.

The above trends suggest that within the English universities of the period before 1640 there was active interest in natural philosophy and growing receptivity to recent developments in experimental science. If the advocates of new subjects were not able or inclined to transform undergraduate studies, a sound basis was provided for the further cultivation of science, mathematics and medicine. Vitality in this area was matched by similar initiatives in the classical languages, oriental studies and history.[84]

Although the innovators were able to achieve some institutional recognition, the centre of gravity of these operations remained informal. There is evidence that around particular tutors and at certain colleges, groups of enthusiasts equalled their better-known interregnum successors in their enthusiasm for natural philosophy. Thomas Allen of Gloucester Hall Oxford, and William Oughtred of King's College Cambridge, pioneered the teaching of mathematics. Another prominent teacher was Joseph Mede, who, as described by his pupil Worthington, was an 'acute Logician, an accurate Philosopher, a skilfull Mathematician, an excellent Anatomist (being usually sent for when they had any Anatomy at Caius College)', as well as a botanist, linguist, historian and chronologist.[85]

William Watts of Caius College, Cambridge, is primarily known as a collaborator in Sir Henry Spelman's linguistic studies, but he also composed 'To the venerable Artists and younger Students in Divinity, in the famous University of Cambridge', in which he attacked Aristotelianism and appealed for closer attention to practical mathematics and geography in university studies.[86] This combination of traditional erudition and new learning characterised many of the advocates of science during this period. Indeed few would have countenanced single-minded investigation of a single subject.

It is difficult to generalise about the distribution of interest in science in the universities before the civil wars, but its strongest advocates were often found in the areas in closest contact with London and where there was greater sympathy for puritanism. Christopher Hill has already underlined the role of London as a pacemaker; mathematics flourished at Gresham College and medicine at the College of Physi-

83. John Parkinson, *Theatrum botanicum* (London, 1640), sig.(a)1r.

84. For differing points of view on the history chairs, see C. Hill (149), pp.173–80; H. R. Trevor-Roper, *History and Theory,* 1966, 5: 61–82; Rebholz (237), pp.293–302. J. Fück, 'Die arabischen Studien in Europa vom 12. bis in den Anfang des 19. Jahrhunderts', in *Beiträge zur Arabistik, Semitistik und Islamwissenschaft,* ed. R. Hartmann & H. Scheel (Leipzig, 1944), pp.85–253.

85. John Worthington, Introduction to Mede's *Works,* pp.iv–viii.

86. Published as an appendix to Henry Gellibrand's *Appendix concerning Longitude* (London, 1633).

cians, the Barber Surgeons' Company, and the Apothecaries' Society. These agencies constituted a reserve of talent, and new ideas, which gradually penetrated into the universities.[87] Constant movements of personnel and active correspondence consolidated this effect and provided avenues for reciprocal influence between London and the universities. A generation of intellectuals developed owing allegiance to both metropolitan and academic life. Glisson and Harvey were influential both at the universities and in the College of Physicians; Briggs and Bainbridge were drawn from London to initiate the Savilian chairs at Oxford; Comenius installed his agent Joachim Hübner at Oxford and Hartlib was in close touch with Mede at Cambridge. For information about mathematics in the universities, Hartlib relied on Henry Gellibrand of Gresham College.

Support for a more liberal approach was not confined to one religious party within the universities, but from our point of view it is important to note that academics who were opposed to the prevailing ritualism of the Anglican church, and in sympathy with the Calvinist position inherited from Elizabethan puritanism, were among the most conspicuous advocates of innovation. Particular attention has already had to be given in this study to students of Emmanuel College Cambridge. Outside Emmanuel College, Samuel Ward and Joseph Mede were particularly influential. The former was a close friend of Henry Briggs formerly of St. John's College Cambridge, who gained Hartlib's approval as 'a judicious godly man'.[88] Many of Ward's pupils exhibited scientific interests; they included Edward Dawson, Seth Ward, William Dugard, George Ent, John Stearne, Gilbert Clark and Richard Holdsworth. Some of these students were puritan, others were not. Oliver Cromwell also experienced his brief taste of university life at Ward's college. Samuel Ward considerably revived the fortunes of Sidney Sussex College, increasing its membership to a level not again achieved until recent times. He became one of the most influential Cambridge opponents of Laud, unfashionably supporting the first Brooke history lecturer, Isaac Dorislaus.[89] Towards the end of Ward's career Hartlib reported of him that he was engaged in the unusual religious exercise of 'meditating upon the spiritual uses of the loadstone in Latin'.[90] Common puritan sympathies may have led the Emmanuel College students John Wallis and John Worthington to associate with Ward.

At Oxford, Lincoln College was a centre of puritan influence. One of its Fellows, Gilbert Watts, took an ardent interest in Bacon and

87. Hill (149), pp.14–84.

88. Ephemerides 1635. In a letter to Ward, Briggs wrote of the desirability of appointing the puritan Robert Johnson as the first White's reader in moral philosophy (Bodleian, Tanner MS 73, fol. 68). Merton College may have been inclined to puritanism during Briggs's tenure, as witnessed by the small number of ejections in 1648. For Emmanuel College, see above, p.37.

89. Curtis (69), pp.207–11; *DNB*.

90. Ephemerides 1635. Ward's last published work was *Magnetis redactorium theologicum* (London, 1637).

Comenius, producing in 1640 the celebrated Oxford edition of the *Advancement of Learning*. The halls are generally thought to have ceased to play a significant role at Oxford by the beginning of the seventeenth century, but this is certainly not true. They continued to attract students and were particularly important for medical studies. Broadgates Hall was transformed into Pembroke College under the direction of Thomas Clayton, the Regius professor of physic, who was probably responsible for the concentration of medical students in his college. Gloucester Hall had gradually declined but then begun to enjoy new vigour under its Principal Degory Whear, first Camden professor of history. Like his counterpart Dorislaus at Cambridge, Whear gravitated to the Calvinist camp. Thomas Allen 'the Atlantes of the mathematic world' had made Gloucester Hall the centre of mathematical studies for a long period before his death in 1632.[91] Another resident of this hall was William Gilbert, a graduate of Lincoln College, described by Hartlib as 'wholly spending himself in a Verulamian Philosophi for the Natural part'.[92] Gilbert was also a mathematician, in correspondence with Henry Gellibrand in London. The reputation of Whear and Allen led Theodore Haak to settle at Gloucester Hall during his studies at Oxford between 1628 and 1631.[93] Other foreign visitors of Hartlib's acquaintance may have been attached to Gloucester Hall. This type of association may be the explanation of how Joachim Hübner could be so closely involved in Oxford affairs without leaving traces in the university records.[94] Christopher Merrett and Ralph Bathurst, both prominent physicians and participants in scientific meetings, were educated wholly or partly at Gloucester Hall.

New Inn Hall had a puritan Principal, Christopher Rogers (a Lincoln College MA), from 1626 until 1660. John French and Tobias Garbrand, two physicians who later promoted the study of practical chemistry, were educated there. Both were parliamentarians, Garbrand being rewarded with the headship of Gloucester Hall following the death of Whear. The army chaplain Henry Pinnel, who graduated from St. Mary Hall, shared in the growing enthusiasm for chemistry.

Magdalen Hall, under its puritan head, John Wilkinson, expanded to become one of the largest teaching societies in Oxford.[95] The little direct evidence available about teaching at this hall indicates that a liberal approach to the curriculum was adopted. Ralph Verney's tutor John Crowther sent him astronomy notes and offered to visit his home during the vacation to provide instruction in geography.[96] These subjects

91. Wood *Athenae*, ii, pp.542–3. For Whear, see sources cited in note 84.

92. Ephemerides 1634. Wood *Fasti*, i, p.411.

93. Barnett (20), pp.19–20.

94. *MGP* II, p.95; Hübner on Whear's historical writings, 1637.

95. Wood *Hist. & Antiq.*, ii, p.686; this hall had 300 members in 1624, 40 of whom were MAs, 'mostly inclined to Calvinism'.

96. F. P. Verney, *Memoirs of the Verney Family*, 2 vols. (London, 1892), i, pp.118–20.

were probably conceived in a predominantly scholastic manner, if we are to accept the impression given by the autobiographical comments of Thomas Hobbes, a student of Magdalen Hall, and the scientific writings of William Pemble, the hall's versatile reader in divinity. However, there was obviously a high level of intellectual activity and a freedom from religious and scholastic restriction sufficient to engender a sympathetic response to new ideas in Hobbes, John Wilkins, Thomas Sydenham, Jonathan Goddard, Walter Charleton, John Chandler the translator of van Helmont, and Theophilus Gale the pioneer of nonconformist academies.

After 1635 the universities were increasingly disrupted by plague, religious strife and eventually civil disturbances. The effect of these traumatic experiences was to dislocate formal academic activity. Oxford was firmly in royalist hands until 1646, while Cambridge was controlled by parliament from the outset of the Civil War. The additional problem of political allegiance was superimposed on long-standing religious divisions. Puritan academics generally supported parliament and vacated their posts at Oxford, while Anglicans gradually drifted away from Cambridge. However the correlation was by no means perfect. In certain cases, the threat of civil strife was sufficient to precipitate Puritans back into the Anglican fold, as witnessed by Samuel Ward's loyalty to Charles I and subsequent imprisonment at Cambridge.

(iv) The Purification of the Academies

Normal academic functions were almost completely undermined during the initial disruptive phases of the civil wars, but informal intellectual activities were less affected. Indeed the very circumstances of the war brought about new associations and influences which served to stimulate philosophical and scientific inquiry.

Under royalist control, Oxford enjoyed an artificial extension of Laudian dominance until 1646. Intellectual affairs were secondary to defending the city against the parliamentarian army, but there is firm evidence that scientific pursuits were not completely submerged. Indeed such subjects as astrology and the military sciences were highly relevant to the new situation. The vacuum left at Oxford by the flight of parliamentarians was more than filled by the royalist court, administration and army. Elias Ashmole settled in Oxford after a period of restlessness and he developed a taste for studying in the libraries. Quickly he made acquaintance with Captain George Wharton the leading royalist astrologer, and Sir John Heydon, Lieutenant General of the Ordnance, who was an alchemist and astrologer. Astrology, a common vehicle of scientific interest in the universities, became a consuming passion with Ashmole.[97] This aroused his interest in more orthodox scientific subjects such as botany, perhaps in association with his

97. C. H. Josten, *Elias Ashmole,* 6 vols. (Oxford, 1966), i, pp.20–30; ii, pp.350–70.

fellow royalist William How of St John's College, whose *Phytologia Britannica* (1650) was annotated by Ashmole.[98] Each served for a short time in the royalist army.

Virtuosi like Ashmole were joined by scholars with more substantial scientific reputations. Upon the death of the first Savilian professor of astronomy in 1643, this post was granted to John Greaves, the negligent Gresham professor of astronomy.[99] Greaves's interest in oriental astronomy had prompted him to undertake a scientific expedition to the Middle East before the Civil War. This excursion led to his gaining the patronage of Anglican orientalists, and paved the way to preferment at Oxford. He, in turn, was able to secure the appointment of William Harvey as Warden of Merton College. A little earlier, after the battle of Edgehill, the elderly physician had been granted an Oxford MD. Harvey established himself at the head of a small but distinguished scientific circle in Oxford.[100] In this company he resumed his researches on embryology; John Aubrey recorded Harvey's visits to George Bathurst's rooms at Trinity College to inspect incubating eggs.[101] Greaves may also have shared this interest, since he brought back from Egypt details of a technique for artificial incubation. Harvey considerably influenced the attitude to science of a number of young royalist scholars at Oxford. These younger men vindicated Harvey's methods and constructed a new system of physiology based on circulation. Harvey's brief digression into academic life was consequently of the greatest importance for the development of physiology.[102] His closest disciple at this time was Charles Scarburgh, who abandoned Cambridge to join Harvey's company at Oxford. Harvey's group probably also included Ralph Bathurst, Thomas Willis, and Walter Charleton. Even Aubrey and Abraham Cowley may have been peripherally involved with the group.

This interlude during the Civil War is a valuable indicator of the changing tone of English natural philosophy. The work of such figures as Harvey and Galileo generated considerable interest in experimental science. The success of Harvey at Oxford proves that certain aspects of the new science were congenial to the Anglican mentality. The emergence of Harvey's group also indicates how close experimental science had come to the threshold of scientific organisation. The crucial condition for further development was social stability, a requirement spectacularly absent from Oxford under military siege. The restoration of

98. *Ibid.*, ii, pp.478–9. In the preface to the 1647 edition of *Clavis mathematica*, Oughtred thanked How for assistance and commended his abilities in alchemy.

99. Taylor (278), p.209; T. Birch, *Miscellaneous Works of Mr. John Greaves*, 2 vols. (London, 1737).

100. G. Keynes, *Life of William Harvey* (Oxford, 1966), pp.299–300.

101. Aubrey, i, p.300.

102. For Harvey at Oxford, see Keynes, *op. cit.*, pp.284–314. The present estimate revises Keynes's view that Harvey's Oxford career was 'well-known, though relatively unimportant' (p.298).

normal academic life by the parliamentarian regime provided the necessary social stability for the further maturation of science in the universities. Would the Puritans and their allies prove as capable of accommodating themselves to the new science as their Anglican predecessors?

Once parliament gained control of the universities, the normalisation of academic life was encouraged. However, the new authorities were not able to permit the training ground for the professions to remain in the hands of disaffected academics. Hence it was necessary to replace delinquents with scholars who sympathised with the religious and political settlement. 'Whilst the Universities continued unreform'd their Work was but half done' was Walker's assessment of the situation.[103] The wholesale ejections which followed the covenant test at Cambridge in 1644, and the Oxford visitation of 1648, fulfilled immediate objectives, but dissension within the parliamentarian party precluded any uniform attitude to intrusions, or a positive approach to reform. University affairs during the period of parliamentary rule became punctuated by sporadic ejections, with appointments and policy a matter of dispute between the parliamentary committee for universities, the vice-chancellors, the boards of visitors, and various committees representing the college interest. Of these bodies, only the colleges maintained a degree of continuity and consistency, while the rest fluctuated according to the mood of the central authority.

This situation would scarcely be expected to favour the smooth running of the universities. Indeed royalist preachers, on the eve of the Civil War, forecast their decline under an anti-episcopal parliament.[104] Pamphleteers gave lurid descriptions of the desecration of colleges during military occupation and these stories were embellished into martyrologies by Walker after the restoration. Indisputably there was some disruption of academic activities and considerable changes in personnel, but equilibrium was restored at both universities with remarkable speed under the new regime. The royalist academics were at all levels replaced by men of comparable abilities and backgrounds. There was no difficulty in recruiting a complement of MAs from the puritan ministry to replace the expelled royalist tutors. Parliament's concern to guarantee the status of the most senior academics is indicated by the decision to supplement the salaries of heads of colleges and halls.

Cambridge achieved its 'settlement' first.[105] Cromwell garrisoned the town during the early stages of the war, effectively stifling attempts by the university to assist Charles I. In 1644 an ordinance was passed appointing a committee of sequestrators to remove scandalous members from the university.[106] All heads of colleges and Fellows were called

103. Walker (300), p.108.

104. Mullinger (194), iii, pp.212–26; see especially the sermons of Holdsworth and Thomas Stephens.

105. G. B. Tatham (277), pp.93–151.

106. Firth & Rait, i, pp.371–2; 'Ordinance for Regulating the University of Cambridge etc', 22 January 1643/4.

to Cambridge in order to subscribe to the oath and covenant. As with all such tests, there was wide divergence of opinion about the severity of the requirement and the manner of its enforcement. Some known objectors were allowed to escape penalty, but ten heads were finally ejected, while only six conformed.[107] The colleges varied greatly; Sidney Sussex and Emmanuel Colleges had relatively few expulsions, while only one Fellow was undisturbed at Peterhouse and most of the members of Trinity College were ejected. It is difficult to give a precise total to the ejections, but Matthews records 254, a figure comprising mainly heads and Fellows.[108] These were rarely replaced in the traditional manner, all appointments coming under the scrutiny of the parliamentary commissioners. Because officials had no criteria to guide them, a wide range of puritan divines found themselves in academic positions, the Westminster Assembly providing a particularly fertile ground from which to recruit clergymen with avowed reservations about episcopacy.

Academic discipline was not long disrupted; the war had been longer-lasting than the plagues and more severe than the Laudian interference of the previous decade, but its effects were not catastrophic. For instance, student admissions at St. John's College Cambridge, which fell off sharply between 1642 and 1644, quickly rose above the pre-war level and maintained this position throughout the period of parliamentary rule. Similarly university matriculations rapidly regained the pre-war level.[109]

At Oxford the situation was confused and disruption more persistent.[110] The royalist occupation brought with it the retirement of puritan academics and a concentration on politics and war; disputations were not held and degrees were granted by special dispensation.

Oxford surrendered to parliament on 24 June 1646. Harvey was exceptional in resigning his post immediately. The major part of the university elected to await the pleasure of parliament. The first major change was the appearance of an antagonistic army, containing lay enthusiasts and chaplains who proceeded to harangue their abject opponents. Boyle remarked that the non-submitting academics were ranked 'with the greatest enemies of the state'.[111] But the new Board of Visitors was not able to exercise its authority until 1648. As at Cambridge six heads of colleges submitted and ten were ejected.[112] At Corpus Christi College virtually the whole college was expelled, while Lincoln and Merton were exceptional in the extent of their submission. Oxford had a total of 370 ejections from senior positions, which created considerable preferment opportunities for ambitious young Puritans from Cambridge.[113] As at Cambridge, recruits were drawn from a variety of parties; some

107. Tatham (277), pp.119–20.
108. Tatham (277), pp.121–3; *Walker Revised*, p.xiii.
109. J. B. Mullinger, *St. John's College Cambridge* (London, 1901), pp.84, 126, 147; see Mullinger (194), iii, Appendix E, for university matriculations.
110. Burrows (42), pp.lxxvii–cxxxiii; Tatham (277), pp.152–97.
111. Letter from Robert to Richard Boyle, 14 July 1646, Boyle *Works*, vi, p.44.
112. Burrows (42), p.lxxxii.
113. *Walker Revised*, p.xiii.

colleges were even allowed to retain non-submitters providing no disturbance was made. The university was functioning normally by 1649.[114]

At both Oxford and Cambridge university officials and heads of colleges gave academic discipline high priority. In view of the dilatoriness of parliament over reforming the university statutes, the puritan academics were obliged to fall back on the Laudian regulations. Hence, paradoxically, the parliamentarians became guardians of the system of higher education framed by their religious adversaries. Changes in the formal life of the university centred on the chapel and theological disputation subjects. In this area the 'novelties' of the Laudian regime were ruthlessly erased in accordance with the stricter spirit of the English reformation. By contrast, there was a striking continuity between academic studies of the earlier and later periods.

The liberal arts curriculum, a common denominator of all university studies and the only aspect of higher education experienced by the majority, exhibited the greatest conservatism. The popular neo-scholastic texts continued in vogue, extant student notebooks being indistinguishable from those of earlier decades.[115] Even at Wadham College, the centre of scientific studies, the surviving notebook of Nicholas Floyd is of an entirely scholastic nature.[116] The continuing conservative pattern of scholastic education was the chief ground of Milton's discontent with the universities. He believed that the 'scholastic bur in their throat . . . both stopped and hindered all true and generous philosophy from entering'.[117] But the gentry at large had little apprehension of Milton's intellectual goals, and they were quite satisfied that the modest rhetorical equipment provided by the colleges was adequate and appropriate for their sons. This general satisfaction with traditional studies was used by Floyd's teachers at Wadham College as a key argument against innovation.[118] Complacency over the current situation was also expressed in a dialogue by the Anglican clergyman Clement Barksdale, formerly of Gloucester Hall. He defended the secular and religious aspects of Oxford life against those who desired to see the eradication of the ministry and universities. A balanced diet of ancient and reformation Latin authors was recommended. Such a course was intellectually invigorating and pleasant. He advised his readers that he would 'let Logick alone, and employ my time in Classical Authors, Greek & Latine, with a little mixture of Arithmetic and Geometry, and the use of the Globe, and a little of Musick'.[119] It is illuminating to note that Barks-

114. Burrows (42), p. cxxi. L. Stone, 'The Size and Composition of the Oxford Student Body', in Stone (ed.), *The University in Society* (Princeton, 1974), pp.3–110; esp. Tables 1 and 18, pp.91 and 110.

115. Kearney (170), pp.112–28.

116. *Ibid.*, p.124.

117. Milton, *The Reason of Church Government urged against Prelacy* (London, 1641); *CPW*, i, pp.854–6.

118. See below, pp.204–5.

119. C. Barksdale, *An Oxford Conference of Philomathes and Polymathes* (London, 1660). For Barksdale, see Wood *Athenae*, iv, pp.221–5.

dale was not entirely conservative; he looked forward to some modest acquaintance with the mathematical aspects of the quadrivium, and he was quite content to abandon traditional logic completely.

Barksdale's comments suggest that, as in previous decades, there was room for flexibility of approach within the framework of the original statutes. This conclusion is supported by both circumstantial and direct evidence. The college libraries received donations of representative collections of contemporary books on science and philosophy. The 'advices' to studlents composed during this period made increasing reference to this recent literature. Holdsworth's directory, drawn up as the result of teaching experience acquired before 1640, made only limited reference to new works. Bacon's *History Natural and Experimental of Life & Death* and Browne's *Pseudodoxia Epidemica* were recommended, but only for subsidiary purposes.[120] A younger writer of similar social and religious outlook, Thomas Barlow of Queen's College Oxford, was slightly more adventurous, recommending principally scholastic authors for natural philosophy but adding as an afterthought Magnan, Gassendi, Descartes, Digby, White and Bacon's *Sylva Sylvarum.* This list of the major exponents of the new philosophy reflects library acquisitions made at this time.[121]

Many teachers took up the new doctrines. Seth Ward was reported as bringing 'the Astronomy Lectures into Reputation, which had been for a considerable time disused and wholly left off', as well as providing teaching in mathematics *gratis* to any pupils desiring it.[122] This probably represented a conscientious attempt to realise the intentions of the Savilian statutes. At Cambridge Henry More of Christ's College introduced his pupils to Descartes's *Principia*, and established his university as a notorious centre of Cartesian influence. Such was More's reputation that Joseph Glanvill regretted he had first studied at Oxford, since the 'new philosophy and art of philosophising' was better developed at Cambridge.[123] At Trinity College Cambridge, the young tutors John Ray and Isaac Barrow pressed for increased attention to experimental philosophy and mathematics. In an oration delivered in 1651, Barrow argued eloquently for the educational virtues of mathematics, geometry, geography, astronomy, optics and Arabic. He asserted that the distinction between ancient and modern learning should be disregarded in the disinterested search for truth.[124]

120. H. F. Fletcher, *Intellectual Development of Milton* (Urbana, 1961), ii, Appendix.

121. De Jordy & Fletcher (74), pp.3–4. St. John's College Oxford Library is probably representative. Immediately after the Civil War, acquisitions included works by Descartes, Gassendi, Mersenne, Torricelli and Digby. See also Curtis (69), pp.108–13, 131–4, 289–90; Kearney (170), pp.103–4; Hill (149), pp.207–9.

122. Pope (223), pp.23–4.

123. Webster (319), pp.360–1; Wood *Athenae,* iii, p.1244.

124. Barrow, *Theological Works* (22), ix, pp.19–34; 'Oratio Moderatoria', 1651. For Ray, see below, pp.150–3.

Increasingly students displayed signs of acquaintance with the new philosophy and, simultaneously, an increasing dissatisfaction with scholastic authorities. This trend was, if anything, accentuated by the vigorous condemnation of Descartes by a broad spectrum of churchmen. Robert Baillie, the influential Scottish academic, was so disturbed about the spread of Cartesianism and Jesuit textbooks that he warned his colleagues in England and the Netherlands that the misguided heretic Descartes (*fatuus haereticus Cartesius*) could only be undermined by an orthodox, sound and clear body of philosophy which could be used in all protestant academies.[125] But no such effective rival emerged and the Cartesian vogue continued. Thus, when John North was at Cambridge after the restoration, Cartesianism was still unstemmed. He found

> 'such a stir, about Descartes, some railing at him and forbidding the reading him, as if he had impugned the very Gospel, and yet there was a general inclination, especially of the brisk part of the university, to use him, which made me conclude, there was somewhat extraordinary in him.'[126]

Oliver Heywood recorded his tutor's exemplary attention to practical divinity and religious exercise; the same tutor, Alexander Akehurst, was known to Hartlib as 'chymically given', employing the alchemist Hartprecht to construct a furnace at Cambridge. Heywood regretted that he had not taken advantage of the opportunity to study natural philosophy under Akehurst.[127] The Cambridge religious controversialist, Charles Hotham, was known to have constructed a laboratory in his rooms at Peterhouse; he also projected an edition of the mathematical works of Horrox.[128]

Novel philosophical attitudes began to appear in philosophical disputations. At Oxford, in 1651, to the sceptical proposition 'An nihil sciatur' Edmund Dickinson was expected to answer in the affirmative, while previously the opposite reply had been given. In the following year a question about animals having the power of reasoning was certainly inspired by the Cartesian theory of the beast-machine. In 1654, a commonplace of earlier views was reversed, when it was accepted

125. Baillie (15), iii, p.268, see also p.274. Letter to G. Voetius, September 1654.

126. Roger North, *The Lives of the Norths,* 3 vols. (London, 1826), iii, pp.335–6. For a typical adverse comment on Descartes composed in 1667, the year of North's entry to Jesus College Cambridge, see the letter by John Worthington, formerly head of the college—'they are enravish't with it, and derive from thence notions of ill consequence to religion': Worthington *Diary*, ii, p.254. James Duport, teacher of Ray and Barrow, spoke of Descartes with scorn in *Musae Subsecivae* (Cambridge, 1676).

127. Joseph Hunter, *The Life of Oliver Heywood* (London, 1842), p.46; Ephemerides 1653. For Akehurst, see Venn, i, p.11.

128. A. M. W. Stirling, *The Hothams,* 2 vols. (London, 1918), i, pp.116–24; Ephemerides 1652, 1653; Venn, ii, p.412.

that 'Novitas sit Antiquitati praeferenda'. The exact nature of the achievement of the moderns was probably the response required to two questions of topical relevance, the first being concerned with the ability of arts to flourish in times of war, the second claiming that 'Institutio academiarum sit utilis in republica'. Significantly this latter subject was raised in 1653, the crisis year for the universities.[129]

It is noticeable that the universities took no steps to systematise the teaching of mathematics, chemistry or botany by establishing new teaching posts. State interference was generally not welcome, while private patrons were generally too poor, or politically disaffected. The Council of State wished to establish Pell in a mathematical lectureship at Cambridge, presumably to fulfil a function equivalent to that of the Savilian professors at Oxford, but this proposal was not effected. Private initiative was equally unsuccessful, although Thomas Smith reported that 'The Mathematical Lecture is begun, hath been read 2 or 3 times, & I hear from divers that Sir John Wollaston gives 20 lb. a yeere to it, promising that if the University shall like it he will make it up hereafter 60 lb. per annum'.[130]

The medical faculty was one of the sections of the university most exposed to new ideas. Galen and Hippocrates continued to dominate general teaching, but once anatomy and physiology were given serious consideration, they became an obvious avenue for the dissemination of new doctrines about vital processes. Francis Glisson at Cambridge was particularly resourceful in fostering experimental physiology. He may have become an absentee after the restoration, but his notebooks from the parliamentarian period describe practical investigations and discussions involving Cambridge medical students. Like Petty at Oxford he also took dissection more seriously, but it is doubtful whether practical anatomical teaching ever became systematic or even persistent at either university in the seventeenth century.

An indication of the new spirit of enquiry among medical students is provided by two of Glisson's Yorkshire pupils, Matthew Robinson and Henry Power. They followed the basic arts curriculum during their first years at university, but soon became attracted by new ideas and convinced of the sterility of scholasticism. This impatience with scholasticism is apparent from Robinson's verdict on his early studies:

> 'As to ethics . . . and physics (abstracted from anatomy, astronomy, meteorology, and the natural history at large) he thought these jejune studies not exceeding one month's enquiry: and for the new philosophy he was *inter primos*.'[131]

129. Univ. Oxon. Arch., 2 a 17, 1648–1659.

130. Letter from Smith to Hartlib, 20 November 1648, HP xv vii. There is no evidence as to the identity of this lecturer.

131. *Autobiography of Matthew Robinson,* ed. J. E. B. Mayor (Cambridge, 1856), p.21. Robinson entered St. John's College in 1645; Fellow 1650–54: Venn, iii, p.472.

Both young scholars were attracted to medicine. Significantly, neither visited foreign medical schools, although Robinson gave this course of action some consideration. Quite possibly the level of activity in medicine at Cambridge had reached a threshold sufficient to satisfy the requirements of conscientious students, since neither Power nor Robinson detected any disadvantages in their English medical education.

The changing attitude in England to medical studies is indicated by the celebrated letter of advice sent to Power at Christ's College by Sir Thomas Browne. Galen and Hippocrates were still regarded as the basic authors, but Browne went far beyond the popular textbooks to recommend a wide range of medical works composed by humanistic and modern authors. This example indicates the ease with which the inquisitive humanist could assimilate experimental natural philosophy. A recurrent theme in Browne's letter is the importance of 'observation and experience'. Hence Power was referred immediately to Harvey's work and Bartholin's up-to-date anatomy; he was advised to undertake practical investigations of plants, animals and minerals, pharmacology, and 'the useful part of chymistry'. Power followed this advice conscientiously, his correspondence enabling us to trace the progress of his medical studies under the influence of Browne and Glisson. An early progress report described simpling expeditions in the Cambridge region and the study of recent anatomical works. Power was especially attracted to 'Harvey's circulation, and the two incomparable authors Des-Cartes and Regius, which, indeed were the only two that answered my doubts and quaeries in that art'.[132] Power went beyond Browne in his appreciation of Cartesianism, as might be anticipated from the prevailing philosophical climate at Christ's College. But Power's attraction to Regius also points to the effectiveness of the Cartesians as compilers of textbooks designed to rival their scholastic counterparts. For the medical student, this would represent an advantage not apparent to the erudite Browne.

Power and Robinson became particularly enthusiastic students of botany, chemistry and physiology.[133] Power became one of the most able of Harvey's disciples, extending the techniques and ideas developed during work on the circulation of blood, to other physiological systems.[134] Harvey's *De Generatione* (1651) had an equally pervasive influence. Browne, who was familiar with this work before its publication, had displayed an interest in embryology in *Pseudodoxia Epidemica* (1646). Power corresponded with Browne about plant morphogenesis

132. Letter from Browne to Power [1646], G. Keynes (ed.), *The Works of Sir Thomas Browne*, 4 vols. (London, 1968), iv, pp.255–6. Mayor, *Autobiography of Robinson*, p.32, suggests that similar advice was given by Browne to Robinson, but these letters were to Reuben Robinson of Maldon, Essex, another friend of Power: Venn, i, p.473.

133. Letter from Power to Browne, 15 September 1648, Browne, *Works*, iv, pp.259–60. Power was a student in Christ's College Cambridge from 1642 to 1655: Webster (318), pp.150–78.

134. Mayor, *Autobiography of Robinson*, pp.30–2.

and embryology.[135] Embryology attracted the attention of Walter Needham of Trinity College Cambridge, who also conducted anatomical investigations during his medical studies, in 1654, publishing this work at Boyle's request many years later.[136]

Our evidence about these Cambridge scholars gives an impression of a spontaneous vitality in medical studies, more attributable to the assimilation of recent ideas than to active direction from the university. Glisson was as much a collaborator in this movement as its architect and leader. The university provided the formal framework of discipline and residence, and looked with passive acquiescence on the changing spirit within the medical faculty.

A similar impression is given by the situation at Oxford. There the leadership was even weaker. The Regius professor, Thomas Clayton Jr., was an ambitious university politician and an intellectual nonentity; from 1649 his assistant as Tomlins Reader was the prodigious William Petty, but Petty was active in Oxford for only a brief period. By contrast the Botanic Garden, although not supplied with its professor, prospered under the capable management of Jacob Bobart. When Evelyn visited the garden in 1654 his attention was absorbed by the behaviour of the sensitive plant.[137] More important were the expanding collections of indigenous and alien plants, brought together by a number of little-known botanists at Oxford. In 1648 they produced their first catalogue, of about 1,600 plants; ten years later this was augmented by Philip Stephens and William Browne.[138] Once again the initiative in medical studies was taken by the students themselves, in conjunction with such lay enthusiasts as Robert Boyle, or the local royalist physician Thomas Willis. The Experimental Natural Philosophy Club, discussed below, also helped to generate a momentum within the medical faculty.

Disputations delivered in the Oxford medical faculty between 1651 and 1660 reveal the deep and swift permeation of new ideas. The new spirit of enquiry developed during informal medical studies was not reserved for private colloquia, but was given ample opportunity for expression in the schools. Although the university was not the instigator of this trend, official consent was required for the disputation topics. Owing to the Civil War, no disputation topics are recorded for the period 1640-1650. On a direct comparison then between the periods of Laudian and parliamentarian control, there was no gentle assimilation of new ideas; the difference between the two periods is striking and absolute, representing two contrasting medical ideologies. Dispu-

135. Webster (318), pp.154–67.

136. Walter Needham, *Disquisitio anatomica de formato foetu* (London, 1667); J. Needham (197), pp.131–3, 158–62. Walter Needham was a Fellow of Queen's College Cambridge, 1655–60: Venn, iii, p.239.

137. Evelyn, *Diary* (97), iii, pp. 109–10.

138. *Catalogus plantarum horti medici Oxoniensis* (Oxford, 1648); anon. but generally attributed to Bobart. *Catalogus horti botanici Oxoniensis* (Oxford, 1658). Madan (184), ii, p.475; iii, p.77.

tations before 1640 were, as already indicated, elementary, uniform, practical and usually related to the more popular prescribed texts. Simple questions on therapeutics and humoral theory were dominant, while anatomy and biological theory were almost entirely ignored. Dawson's discussion of circulation stands out as an exceptional concession to contemporary issues, in a period of Galenic supremacy.[139]

The first recorded medical disputation of the parliamentarian period occurred in 1651.[140] Of the three *quaestiones* disputed *in vesperiis,* one was a conventional point relating to diet, while the other two considered the problem of the relationship between spirits and blood, and whether the blood was composed of the four humours.[141] These two latter questions had been of central concern to Harvey; the final chapters of *De Generatione* (1651) were critical of the established view, that blood was constituted from humours, atoms or elements and that 'spirits' were super-added to provide its vital faculty.[142] Two of the three questions *in comitiis* reflect similar sources. One related to the nourishment of the foetus by maternal blood. In the same year, Harvey concluded that the foetal circulation was not continuous with the maternal.[143] A further question asked whether concoction in the stomach was caused by an acid ferment or by heat. This is indisputably a reference to the theory of digestion by chemical fermentation recently announced by van Helmont.[144] The respondent on this occasion was Ralph Bathurst of Trinity College, whose notes on disputation subjects allow us to confirm that these exercises were used as a vehicle for the discussion of recent ideas.[145] Bathurst was familiar with ancient authors, but the medical classics were treated with no more respect than were contemporary works. His disputation on foetal nutrition began with an acknowledgment of Harvey's work. The complex debate on this subject was surveyed, before he reached the independent conclu-

139. See above, pp.121–5.

140. The *quaestiones* for this period are preserved in Univ. Oxon. Arch. 2 a 17, 1648–1659. The *quaestiones* were for many years printed as broadsides, many of which are listed in E. N. Cordeaux & D. H. Merry, *A Bibliography of Printed Works Relating to the University of Oxford* (Oxford, 1968), pp.191–4.

141. For the latter a positive answer was anticipated in 1651, whereas in 1657 the same question assumed a negative reply, in accordance with Harvey's views.

142. Harvey, *De Generatione* (London, 1651), Exercitationes LII, LXXI & LXXII, 'De sanguine, prout est pars principalis', 'De calido innato', & 'De humido primogenio'. W. Pagel, *William Harvey's Biological Ideas* (Basel, 1967), pp.252–65.

143. Harvey, *De motu cordis* (1628), Chapter VI; *De Generatione*, Ex. LXIX & LXX. The continuing dominance of Harvey is evidenced by later *quaestiones.* For example, all three topics disputed by William Page in 1653 were derived from Harvey: 'An dentur spiritus a sanguine distincti? An omnia animalia oriantur ex ovo? An embryo sugat in utero materno?'

144. J. B. van Helmont, *Ortus medicinae* (Amsterdam, 1648), Chapters XIX, XXVIII & XXX. Further influence of Helmont (and Glisson) is illustrated by the 1654 set of disputation subjects of Robert Fielding: 'An detur catarrhus e cerebro in pulmones defluus? An lien sit fermentationis organum? An rachitis proveniat a debita sanguinis fermentatione et circulatione impedita?'

145. T. Warton (309), pp.211–38. The date is 1651, not 1654 as stated by Warton.

sion that the foetus was nourished partly by a liquor passing through the umbilical vessels, partly by oral ingestion of a different nutritive liquor. Bathurst's disputation on digestion explored a wide range of experimental evidence. He criticised the traditional view that digestion was caused by heat, citing a variety of evidence to support Helmont's theory that an acid ferment was produced by the stomach.

From many points of view, Bathurst's 'Praelectiones tres de Respiratione' (1654), the three stipulatory lectures delivered by him as an incepting MD, are even more interesting.[146] They were composed in a form suitable for publication, but although this was periodically considered, the lectures were not printed until after Bathurst's death. However the text was widely circulated in manuscript form before publication, and probably had a considerable influence on the physiological outlook of such authors as Boyle and Mayow. Hence Bathurst may have felt that his ends had been achieved without publication. In the lectures he provided a comprehensive survey of the physiology of respiration, establishing the role and mode of operation of the various organs involved for man and other vertebrates. Arguing from a wide range of authorities to support his own explanation of respiration, he concluded that: 'Dicimus itaque inspirationem praecipue inservire ad pabulum nitrosum animali subministrandum, quo sanguis ita contemperetur, ut, spiritibus, ad obeunda vitae munia generandis, idoneus fiat.'[147] The Galenic theory of the cooling function of air in respiration, which was supported even by Harvey, was opposed in favour of a chemical theory which postulated that a nitrous component in air was absorbed into the blood to support basic vital functions. Tradition was again assailed, when it was claimed that respiration was common to all animals and plants. Bathurst's lectures show a wide command of ancient and modern opinions and an independence of judgement which can rarely have been matched by his contemporaries. He had taken a very long step away from scholastic medicine, and had come within reach of the celebrated physiological researches of John Mayow.

The medical disputations submitted after 1651 continued to reflect interest in the new physiology. The ideas of van Helmont and Harvey were predominant, but other new theories were discussed soon after they were announced. In 1652 no less than six candidates offered medical disputations. Their topics involved discussion of Pecquet's recent theories about the movement and concoction of chyle, and Glisson's explanation of rickets.[148] Helmontian influence was reflected in a question about the possibility of producing a 'universal medicine'. In 1657 all the questions discussed by Edward Stubbe related to Glisson's

146. *Ibid.*, pp.127–210.

147. *Ibid.*, p.184. Note the similarity with the disputation subject for 1654, 'An suffocatis fiat ob defectum pabuli spiritualis nitrosi omnium animatorum spiritus perpetuo reparantis?'

148. Jean Pecquet, *Experimenta nova anatomica* (Paris, 1651); Eng. trans., 1653. Francis Glisson, *Tractatus de rachitide* (London, 1650); Eng. trans., 1651.

view that a nutritive fluid passed through the nerves rather than through the lymph ducts.[149] Opposition to Glisson's theory was anticipated by Stubbe's examiners, possibly out of deference to the ideas of George Joyliffe, an Oxford graduate, who claimed the independent discovery of the lymphatics. Another of Glisson's favourite themes discussed in 1657 questioned the dominant role of the liver in sanguinification, and considered whether this function occurred instead in the heart.[150] These and other disputation subjects advanced at Oxford were listed among the 'New Tenents' described by Charleton as subjects under discussion at the College of Physicians.[151]

Whatever the quality of formal medical education at the universities, the disputation topics indicate that the students incepting for MDs were not bound by the texts prescribed in the statutes. The medical faculties during the interregnum adopted an interpretation of their function flexible enough to allow a generation of ambitious medical students unrestricted licence to transform their education and develop a medical outlook sympathetic to the new doctrines of Harvey, van Helmont and Descartes. The gulf between advanced research or the colloquia at the College of Physicians, and the university medical faculty considered as a whole, had been closed. This provides a complete contrast with the Laudian period, when even Harvey's theory produced a scarcely perceptible reaction in the universities. During the interregnum new ideas were rapidly assimilated; occasionally they were even current in academic discussion before being announced in print. There is consequently every indication that, instead of performing a purely formal and ceremonial function, the medical disputations became a forum for the debate of new theories. Traditional topics were not entirely absent, but they were subordinated to subjects derived from the new physiology; Galenic pathology and therapeutics retreated into the background. This change in mental attitude to medicine brought no necessary improvement to practice, but the more vigorous intellectual atmosphere would have encouraged initiative and provoked a generally critical approach to professional work.

This vitality within the medical school was founded on the achievement of major innovators, but the actual dissemination of new doctrines was primarily the achievement of informal associations of minor medical enthusiasts. Most were students in the higher faculties, but some were laymen. Through their efforts, and in the absence of any strong official doctrine or active teaching of statutory texts, it was possible to induce a revolutionary change of attitude to medicine within the university medical faculties. The high standard of English medical publications between 1650 and 1680 bears witness to the fertility of this movement within the universities, which gave stimulus to numerous minor re-

149. Glisson, *Anatomica Hepatis* (London, 1654), Chapter XLV.
150. *Ibid.*, pp.299–327.
151. Charleton (46), pp.38–40.

searchers like Henry Power, Timothy Clarke, William Croune, George Joyliffe, Thomas Millington and Ralph Bathurst, as well as to such celebrated figures as Richard Lower, John Mayow and Thomas Willis. Thomas Sydenham's association with Oxford, although subject to much comment, must remain conjectural.

This renaissance of medicine in the universities is also reflected by quantitative factors. Before 1640, as already suggested, the medical faculties were relatively small; the incorporation of medical graduates from foreign universities was a major function. After the civil wars this situation quickly changed. Financial pressures, political circumstances and intellectual fashions led increasing numbers of students to undertake the relatively long course of study for an English MD. During the 1650s an important factor directing such figures as Ralph Bathurst into medicine was distaste for the theological faculty as controlled by the puritan faction. This must have driven into medicine many young Anglicans who might otherwise have entered the church. Clinically, continental medical schools were superior, but they could no longer outshine English anatomy and physiology. The production of advanced textbooks and the rise of English medical publishing also reduced the advantages of continental travel. For the first time English textbooks were being produced which were capable of competing with their continental counterparts. For instance, the Oxford physician Nathaniel Highmore composed a systematic text which effectively combined new theories of physiology with current anatomical knowledge, and Walter Charleton's popular physiological handbook was even more influential.[152]

With the recruitment of increasing numbers of students the medical faculties for the first time became fully viable units. Licensing was no longer a major function; the numbers of students taking English medical degrees soon equalled and then out-stripped the number of incorporations. There was a considerable increase in the numbers of medical degrees granted. Between 1649 and 1660, an average of four MDs per annum were granted at both universities. For the same period 0.75 and 4.25 MBs were granted per annum at Oxford and Cambridge respectively. The decline in MBs granted at Oxford does not mask the general overall growth trend.[153] The increased level was sustained until the end of the century.[154] Although the numbers graduating in medicine were never large, they represented a considerable percentage increase, bringing the faculty of medicine for the first time into parity with

152. Highmore, *Corporis humani disquisitio anatomica in qua sanguinis circulationem prosecutus est* (The Hague, 1651). Charleton, *Oeconomia animalis* (London & Amsterdam, 1659).

153. These figures are derived from the Oxford University Congregation registers; those for Cambridge were kindly supplied by Dr. A. Rook of Cambridge. Averages are given to the nearest 0.25 per cent. See also A. Rook, 'Medical Education at Cambridge 1600–1800', in A. Rook (ed.), *Cambridge and its Contribution to Medicine* (London, 1971), pp.49–64. See also above, p. 121 and note 68.

154. A. Rook, 'Medicine at Cambridge 1660–1760', *Medical History*, 1969, *13*: 107–21; pp.111–14.

those of law and theology. It should also be noted that the long period of residence increased the numerical strength of the medical schools. At any one time during this period, there would have been at each university twenty or more students preparing for a degree in medicine. Given this numerical strength, under the conditions already described, the medical faculties could be expected to develop a corporate spirit, a lively habit of debate, and continuity of research interests. Hence during the interregnum the English universities could for the first time have claimed to possess fully effective medical schools. In structure they were less formal than their continental counterparts; accordingly they were less durable, but in the short term they worked exceptionally efficiently as promoters of medical education and research. Inevitably this more dynamic structure soon had repercussions on the College of Physicians and on provincial medicine; and the English-trained physicians provided, among other things, a reservoir of talent which was later tapped by the Royal Society.

The above survey of the role of science and medicine in university studies during the period of parliamentary dominance indicates the fulfilment of many of the aspirations of such pioneers as Thomas Linacre, John Caius or Sir Henry Savile. The medical faculties exhibited the most obvious transformation. Although the arts curriculum retained its scholastic bias, many tutors and students explored new pathways of knowledge. Where the tutor's influence was a negative one, the student could, at Oxford, receive assistance from the Savilian professors or study at the flourishing botanical garden. Even more important, both universities had small groups of academics who, in an informal capacity, propagated interest in a wide variety of scientific subjects. Speaking from long experience of Oxford, Wallis claimed that the '*privata collegia*', which he instanced, could provide instruction in 'any part of usefull knowledge proper for scholars to learn'. Any defect was caused by 'want of learners not teachers'.[155]

Our evidence points to the steady infiltration of new ideas into higher education. This was accompanied by little of the antagonism which similar developments aroused in the Dutch universities. In some subjects there was a sharp confrontation between the new and the old; in others, innovation could occur by gradual assimilation into established disciplines. Thus the introduction of Cartesianism created tension, whereas the growth of mathematics and anatomy did not. More subtly, new subjects competed for attention with the old. Thus, when Sancroft returned to Emmanuel College Cambridge, he reported that there was evidence of serious scholarship, but that Hebrew and Greek were out of fashion; while 'the rational learning they pretend to [is] neither the old philosophy, nor steadily any one of the new'. The 'old genius' of the college was gone.[156] This is reminiscent of Tuckney's assertion twenty years before, that

155. Wallis (303).
156. G. D'Oyly, *The Life of William Sancroft*, 2 vols. (London, 1821), i, p.128;

Whichcote's entanglement with philosophy had caused a decline in his abilities as a teacher and disputant.[157]

Whether intentionally or not, parliament created conditions favourable to intellectual experiment in the universities. Thus by 1660 the change in atmosphere was sufficient for Laudian academics to feel a sense of discomfort upon their reinstatement. However, consolation could be drawn from the survival of statutes and of academic discipline. This provided a sufficient basis for the preservation of tradition against further encroachment. Those academics opposed to innovation correctly recognised that the strength of the new science and philosophy lay outside formal studies, in the scientific clubs which had sprung up in both universities during the interregnum. Hence Clarendon's praise of the puritan academics had a double significance. He was probably genuinely impressed by their spirit of enterprise and innovation, but his gratitude was the greater because the virtuosi had refrained from interfering with the basic structure of higher education.

(v) Academies within the Academies

Because of its alleged connection with the Royal Society, the Oxford Experimental Philosophy Club has overshadowed analogous development at Cambridge during the period of parliamentary rule. In recent writings, only C. E. Raven's exhaustive biographical study of John Ray has drawn sufficient attention to the growth of informal scientific activity at Cambridge. Even Mullinger's impressive history of Cambridge during this period barely touched upon this issue, although paradoxically the author fully appreciated the importance of Oxford as a focal point of scientific activity.

Even before the Civil War experimental science was cultivated on an informal basis at Cambridge. Samuel Ward and Joseph Mede gave prestige to this movement. Hence it is not surprising that Milton (and other young puritan scholars) took up the Baconian philosophy, the ideals of the Great Instauration being reflected in the academic prolusion 'Beatiores reddit Homines Ars quam Ignorantia'.[158]

Mede and Ward died before they could play any part in the scientific movement of the Puritan Revolution. Their pupils not only took an interest in this new philosophy; they also rose to occupy positions of great influence, under the aegis of the parliamentarian authorities. A propitious omen for this group was given in 1642 when the future editor of Mede's works, John Worthington, was proposed for a fellowship at Emmanuel College.[159] His supporters were in a minority but four of

---

letter from Sancroft to Ezekiel Wright. For a similar 'Lamentation' on the 'Decay of Learning' by Anthony Wood, see Wood *Hist. & Antiq.*, i, pp.422–3.

157. Whichcote (328), pp.36–7.

158. *CPW*, i, pp.288–306.

159. Worthington *Diary,* i, pp.12–17.

them successfully called for parliamentary intervention to secure his election. Of these, three (Whichcote, Sadler and Cudworth) were appointed as heads of colleges under parliament, Worthington himself securing the mastership of Jesus College. Together with Henry More, Mede's pupil at Christ's College, this group constituted a substantial section of the Cambridge Platonist movement which exhibited its greatest vitality and influence during the interregnum. Its members were united by strong bonds of friendship and marriage, as well as by philosophical affinities.[160] Our particular concern with the Platonists is occasioned by their increasing involvement with natural philosophy. Of the father-figures of this group, Benjamin Whichcote was not intimately involved with the problems of natural philosophy. On the other hand, Cudworth's stepfather, John Stoughton, was a keen advocate of the *Instauratio Magna* of Bacon and the 'Christian philosophy' of Comenius. Of the next generation, More and Cudworth became deeply concerned with natural philosophy; Worthington and Sadler displayed superficial curiosity about a variety of scientific questions. Because of their great personal reputations, important academic positions, and the long-lasting influence of their writings, the Platonists were one of the most important formative influences on English natural philosophy in the second half of the seventeenth century. Cambridge graduates ranging in stature from Newton and Ray to Power and Hall, were noticeably susceptible to Platonic philosophy.

More's sympathy for Platonism was evident as early as the publication of his first poems (1642). Whichcote and More led a reaction against protestant scholasticism, and in favour of Platonic authors, who were designated guides to a truly Christian philosophy. This route had already been well-surveyed by the Renaissance Platonists and their followers who had, like the Cambridge scholars, plunged into a wide range of ancient writings in the search for a *prisca theologia,* a sacred genealogy tracing the sources of wisdom to:

> 'Egyptian Trismegist, and th'antique roll
> Of Chaldee wisdome, all which time hath tore
> But Plato and deep Plotin do restore.'[161]

The Platonists believed that through all ages a continuous succession of spiritually enlightened thinkers had acted as guardians of a truly religious philosophy, against the recurrent tendency to atheism. The revival of these ancient doctrines was thought particularly desirable in a period which appeared to be witnessing a revival of interest in ancient

160. General works on the Cambridge Platonists include J. Tulloch, *Rational Theology and Christian Philosophy in England in the Seventeenth Century,* 2 vols. (London, 1872); E. Cassirer, *The Platonic Renaissance in England* (New York, 1953); Rosalie L. Colie, *Light and Enlightenment. A Study of the Cambridge Platonists and the Dutch Arminians* (Cambridge, 1957); J. D. Roberts, *From Puritanism to Platonism in Seventeenth Century England* (The Hague, 1968).

161. 'Psychozoia' (1642), in More, *Philosophical Poems* (40), p.12.

atomism and materialism. The Neoplatonic authors were largely inaccessible without a wide armoury of knowledge, which included mathematics and natural philosophy. Worthington reported John Smith's attainments in Egyptian learning as including: 'the mysterious hieroglyphical learning, natural philosophy, music, physic and mathematics.'[162] This description, written shortly after Smith's premature death, could equally have been applied to the other Platonists, who emphasised that their pointedly mystical and cabbalistic leanings prevented their being satisfied with scholastic digests, or the 'outward shell of words and phrases' of a topic.[163]

Canon Raven has perhaps over-stressed the sympathy of the Cambridge Platonists for the empirical study of the 'Book of Nature'.[164] Platonism certainly could lead in this direction, as is manifest in the example of Sir Thomas Browne who exploited his enjoyment of the minutiae of the natural world to the advantage of his metaphysical ideas. Hence the empirical perspective was certainly not precluded, but the initial bias of the Cambridge scholars was in an altogether different direction. On the whole they felt no call to experimental studies and they developed only the remotest contacts with the Baconian Royal Society. Any familiarity they might have had with developments in experimental philosophy tended to be secondhand. There was a deep conviction that the external senses, and over-involvement with the material world constituted a barrier against the mystical and rational appreciation of the deepest truths of religion and philosophy. Henry More contrasted the 'blundring Naturalist' with the 'deep-searching soul' who would 'thy God seek out, and leave Nature behind'.[165] John Smith quoted the precedent of the ancient sects of philosophers who prepared their disciples for the contemplation of the truly intelligible, by purging their minds of 'early dregs of sense and passion'. One means to this purgation was the study of mathematics, which represented knowledge completely divorced from sensual experience.[166] Thus, in spite of outpourings about the beauty of nature, the Cambridge Platonists felt deeper concern for the metaphysical problems of science. In their assault upon materialism they strove to explain new ideas about matter and causation, cosmology and cosmogony in terms of ancient theological doctrines.

The Platonists even suspected that experimental philosophy deflected attention away from issues of fundamental importance, or worse still led to the pernicious error of enthusiasm. The Paracelsians in particular were regarded by More as liable to these transgressions. More epitomised

162. Smith (261), pp.xvi–xix.
163. *Ibid.*, p.7.
164. Raven (236), i, pp.110–11.
165. 'Psychozoia' (40), pp.37–8; see also N. Culverwell, *Discourse of the Light of Nature* (68), pp.176–7.
166. 'The True Way or Method of Attaining Divine Knowledge', *Select Discourses* (261), pp.10–22.

the chemist, as opposed to the 'finer spirits' who had a true regard for reason, as 'that more Mechanical kind of Genius that loves to be tumbling of and trying tricks with the Matter (which they call making Experiments) when desire of knowledge has so heated it that it takes upon it to become Archetectonical and flie above its sphere. . . . This is that that commonly makes the Chymist so pitiful a Philosopher.'[167] This criticism was probably directed particularly at Hermeticists like Thomas Vaughan, who had recently engaged in an heated exchange of pamphlets with More. Vaughan, as well as his twin brother Henry, was a Paracelsian. Had he heeded More's warnings he might have escaped death in a laboratory explosion![168] More's opinion of chemists is symptomatic of his reservations about the value of empirical investigations in general. He felt that, if not positively harmful, experimentalism represented a dissipation of energies. Accordingly he was unsympathetic to much of the scientific activity of the English Baconians. He expressed this in extremely strong terms in a letter to Hartlib: he admits the humanitarian value of Hartlib's labours, but Baconians are warned that 'without the superintendency and assistancy of these more raysed faculties aforementioned . . . men dig and droyle like blinde molewarpes in the earth, and yet never be able to emerge *in dies luminis orae,* but ly dead and buryed in a heap and rabble of slibber sauce experimentes'.[169] More continued with further highly uncomplimentary remarks about 'low Spiritts' who adopted the practices of artisans, under the illusion that they were assembling a body of profound knowledge. These sentiments must have caused considerable concern to Hartlib, who solicited an opinion about More's remarks from his young protégé William Petty. Petty had just published his first work, *The Advice of W. P. to Samuel Hartlib* (1648), in which he advocated precisely the kind of experimental science censured by More. In response to Hartlib's appeal, Petty provided a brief but most effective statement of the Baconian position; he regarded philosophical systems as premature and vacuous, and metaphysical speculation as unproductive. The useful activity of the inventor, Cornelius Drebbel, was contrasted with the worthless endeavour of the speculative philosophers. Petty accepted that Descartes was the most proficient exponent of the new philosophy, but any person equipped with sound empirical knowledge would be able to detect gross defects in even his system. Many oblique criticisms were aimed at philosophers like More who disputed about phenomena without taking the trouble to familiarise themselves directly with the evidence. This basic defect was attributed to the weakness of university education. Academic

167. *Enthusiasmus Triumphatus: A Brief Discourse of Enthusiasm* (1656), quoted from More (191), p.36.

168. Vaughan was known to have spent years trying 'chymical or physical conclusions', joining forces eventually with Thomas Henshaw at the latter's laboratory in Kensington: Ephemerides 1650.

169. Letter from More to Hartlib, 11 December 1648, HP XVII, quoted from Webster (319), p.365.

authors were equipped to write elegant and compendious works, but they could not effectively disguise their lack of acquaintance with 'things themselves'.[170] One of the main aims of Petty's *Advice* had been to restore a more balanced approach by proposing a Baconian reform of education.

Two other Cambridge correspondents of Hartlib supported Petty's ideas about experimental philosophy and scholastic education. Thomas Smith, a member of More's college, complained that his colleagues had 'their thoughts so taken up with Platonisme, or other high and aery speculations of Divinity or Philosophy, that they will scarce vouchsafe to cast a glance on such a new invention, or anything which is not in their way or in their aime'.[171] Thus, no cultivation of natural philosophy by academics in the universities would satisfy the Baconians unless it was accompanied by a more empirical outlook. This view was elegantly formulated by John Hall of St. John's College in his pamphlet on university reform addressed to parliament in 1649.[172]

The Platonist aspiration to establish a system of theologically orientated philosophy having the facility to undermine both sceptics and materialists led promptly to an extremely strong interest in the writings of Descartes. Few of the Platonists were untouched by this influence, and Henry More was affected to an extreme degree. Its basis in introspection, explicitly theological foundations, comprehensive ramifications, and the certitude of its rational operations, were some of the obvious attractions which Cartesianism had for the Platonist. Initially it was hoped that Cartesianism, more than any other new philosophy, could be adapted to religious purposes, although it was felt necessary to expunge certain latent materialistic tendencies. In 1648 More was persuaded by Cudworth and Hartlib to begin his famous correspondence with Descartes.[173] His initial expectations were high: 'I never found any account of Nature so sound and consistent as this of his is, nor ever hoped to meet with anything this way of that perfection, whereof having no controversy with anything in his writings, that is essential to it . . .'[174] Such expressions typify the spirit of the letters to Descartes, Hartlib and Petty written by More during the winter of 1648/9. Although these first hopes were quickly blighted More had already infected his Cambridge pupils with enthusiasm for the 'new philosophy'. As previously indicated this trend, once initiated, was not readily contained, and Cartesianism came to assume an important role in philosophical discussions at Cambridge in the pre-Newtonian period. Even after his disillusionment with

170. Letter from Petty to More (n.d.), HP VII 123; printed in full in Webster (319), pp.367–8.

171. Letter from Smith to Hartlib, 20 November 1648, HP XV vi.

172. *Humble Representation Concerning the Advancement of Learning: and Reformation of the Universities* (London, 1649).

173. Webster (319), p.364. *Epistolae quatuor ad Renatum Des Cartes* (London, 1662); included in More (191).

174. Letter from More to Hartlib, 11 December 1648, HP XVII, quoted from Webster (319), pp.365–6.

Descartes, More continued to use the *Principia* and *Discours* for the introductory philosophical studies of his college and private pupils, translating part of the *Principia* for their benefit.[175] More's views are probably echoed in Isaac Barrow's philosophical disputation 'Cartesiana Hypothesis de materia et motu haud satisfacit praecipuis naturae phaenomenis' (1652). Barrow's view was that even if the mechanical hypothesis was not acceptable as a comprehensive explanation of natural phenomena, it remained the most original and convincing theory to emerge during the recent revival of natural philosophy, providing the most convenient and best-informed source for the further consideration of scientific problems.[176] From the major figures such as Cudworth, More and Barrow, to their minor disciples, Power, Glanvill and Finch, Cartesianism became the common framework for the discussion of problems in natural philosophy.[177] However, the religious premises of the Platonists necessitated a constant vigilance against materialism which led inevitably to a reaction against many basic tenets of Cartesianism. Hence, paradoxically, Platonism created a fertile ground for the reception of Cartesianism but firmly denied it the opportunity to develop into a consistent philosophical movement.

The basic tensions between More and Descartes were apparent in their very first letters. More's introductory felicitations contrast sharply with the severe reservations about many aspects of the Cartesian theory of matter which immediately follow. Gradually, More was drawn into disputes over technical points and was obliged to move beyond criticism of Descartes's handling of classic scientific problems, to search for counter-instances to support his own anti-materialist position. Inevitably this involved a reliance on experimental investigations and natural history, with the result that he found common cause with the Baconians (and even Paracelsians) whom he had previously so contemptuously dismissed. More realised that the most effective means of undermining the mechanical hypothesis was to collect examples of phenomena which could only be explained by reference to divine agency. Hence he was obliged to fall back on the form of Platonism expressed in Browne's *Religio Medici*. Book II of More's *Antidote against Atheism* (1653) recited a comprehensive series of examples proving the active participation of God in nature.[178] The doctrine of the Spirit of Nature

175. M. Nicolson, 'The Early Stage of Cartesianism in England', *Studies in Philology*, 1929, *26*: 356–74; *idem, Conway Letters: The Correspondence of Anne, Viscountess Conway, Henry More and their Friends, 1647–1684* (New Haven, 1930). Raven (235), notes that the *Discours* and *Principia* of Descartes were among Ray's early reading.

176. Barrow, *Theological Works* (22), ix, pp.79–104.

177. J. A. Passmore, *Ralph Cudworth: An Interpretation* (Cambridge, 1951); Lydia Gysi, *Platonism and Cartesianism in the Philosophy of Ralph Cudworth* (Berne, 1962); Webster (319).

178. Richard Baxter was involved in a similar enterprise: see G. F. Nuttall, 'The Correspondence of John Lewis, Glasrug, with Richard Baxter and with Dr. John Ellis, Dolgelly', *Journal of the Merioneth Historical & Record Society,*

was gradually elaborated by More and Cudworth in order to explain the exact means by which God mediated with His creation. Barrow came to similar conclusions; he argued against the mechanical philosophy, believing that 'experimentis fructiferis ac Naturali Historiae' exposed numerous examples of phenomena which could only be explained by recourse to spiritual agencies.[179]

In their reaction against Cartesianism the Platonists at once appreciated the value of natural theology. The growing body of evidence accumulated by naturalists provided a substantial basis for the 'Universal Principle of Wisdom and Counsel.'[180] Hence More paid increasing attention to natural history, and this was the science which most flourished at Cambridge during these years. Cudworth had been sympathetic at an earlier stage; in 1647 he had appealed for the general encouragement of learning, defending natural history as 'the true Contemplation of the Wisdome, Goodnesse, and other Attributes of God, in this great Fabrick of the Universe [which] cannot easily be disparaged without a Blemish upon the maker of it'.[181]

This religious sanction would have strengthened interest in the biological studies which were already much in evidence in the Cambridge medical faculty. Medical students and pious naturalists were drawn into close association. John Ray exemplifies the Platonist scholar's conviction that 'the study of nature is essentially a religious duty'.[182] Ray came into prominence at Trinity College during the Republic and was ejected in 1662. At his college, he lectured in Greek, mathematics and humanities. To private classes he taught natural theology, compiling notes which were published much later as *The Wisdom of God Manifested in the Works of the Creation* (1691), the most popular of his writings and one of the best informed and most influential works in this genre.[183] He also became the centre of an active group of naturalists. Ray expressed considerable dissatisfaction with a scholastic curriculum which took such little account of 'real Experimental Philosophy in this University, and . . . those ingenious Sciences of the Mathematicks [which] are so much neglected by us'.[184] If divinity was a basic study, natural history was basic to divinity, since it was the most effective means of displaying the workings of providence. Of the authors who determined Ray's theological standpoint, More and Cudworth were pre-eminent.

1953–6, 2: 120–34; published as *The Certainty of the World of Spirits* (London, 1961).

179. 'Cartesiana hypothesis . . .', Barrow (22), ix, pp.86–7, 103–4.

180. More, *Antidote against Atheism,* quoted from More (191), p.40.

181. Cudworth (64), sig. A1v.

182. Raven (235), p.49.

183. Raven (235), Chapter XVII. Ray's work was based on discourses delivered in 1659 and 1660.

184. *Wisdom of God,* 2nd edn. (London, 1692), pp.162–8.

But *The Wisdom of God* was a far more effective vehicle for natural theology than the writings of the Platonists. It converted the dry and superficial instances of More's *Antidote* into a vivid and well-authenticated survey of the Divine plan.

Natural theology provided Ray and his friends, as it had done Sir Thomas Browne, with a direct incentive to the study of natural history; no phenomenon was too small or obscure to merit detailed scrutiny. Ray's first botanical work began as a diversion in the spring meadows while he was recuperating from an illness, and quickly grew into an intensive study of the flora of the Cambridge region. His was one of the first local surveys to be completed.[185] This flora represented a dramatic break with the traditional 'herbals', which consisted primarily of compilations from earlier sources and contained mixed botanical, medical and even astrological information. Henry Power recorded similar simpling journeys in the locality; within a short time he, like Ray, had detected the deficiencies of existing herbals and had begun assembling a herbarium collection.[186] He may have joined Ray's small group of naturalists while at Cambridge. Another member of this circle, Francis Willughby, became Ray's patron and main collaborator after the restoration.[187]

It is possible to provide a reasonably detailed impression of the informal scientific activities at Cambridge during the 1650s. Botany was a main concern, but there are also records of dissections, vivisection experiments and the use of Glauber's distillation apparatus. After leaving Cambridge, Power wrote to one of Ray's friends mentioning the 'excellent & noble discourses Physicall, mathematicall & Anatomicall' of the group.[188] Worthington also drew attention to the liberal scientific activities at Cambridge:

> 'Glisson is writing *De Ostreis* [sic]. Botanical Garden is already in such request that Lord Lambert sent for some plants out of it. Also a Graecian [Ray] is there to teach the Greek tongue and to erect a Laboratory.'[189]

185. *Catalogus plantarum circa Cantabrigiam* (Cambridge, 1660); Raven (235), Chapter IV. The proposal of Cambridge botanists to publish a 'Phytologia of such herbs as are within 10 miles of Cambridge' was known to Hartlib in 1658: letter from Hartlib to Boyle, 2 February 1657/8, Boyle *Works,* vi, p.101. Ray's work was published anonymously, probably in order to emphasise the collaborative aspect of its compilation.

186. Letter from Power to Browne, 15 September 1648, Browne, *Works,* iv, pp.259–60.

187. Barrow dedicated to Willughby his *Euclidis elementorum libri XV* (Cambridge, 1655).

188. Letter from Power to Thomas Pockley, 30 August 1654, BM Sloane MS 1342, fol. 3. Power's scientific associates included Ralph Widdrington who ousted Barrow for the Greek chair, and John Tillotson, the future archbishop of Canterbury. For Pockley, see Raven (235), p.45.

189. Ephemerides 1657. Glisson was studying muscles, not mussels! Ray was Greek lecturer at Trinity College in 1656.

Besides collecting chemical apparatus, Ray was establishing a botanical garden at Trinity College.[190] This may have been the garden which captured Lambert's interest. Perhaps the first proposal for such a garden was made by Robert Child, who suggested that parliament should purchase the garden and collections of Tradescant, to provide Cambridge with a rival to the university garden at Oxford.[191] This provision would have supplemented the substantial parliamentary grants made for the extension of the University Library and for promoting oriental studies.[192] Although no university garden was established, private collections of 'many hundreds' of plants prospered. According to Worthington's reports these gardens, and studies in comparative anatomy were the work of 'divers fellows' involved with preparing the Cambridge Catalogue of plants.

In an oration given just before he left Cambridge in 1654 Barrow commented on the improvement which had taken place in the status of science in the university since his oration of 1651. He noted the general revival of learning since the late troubles; many subjects had prospered, and he could mention achievements in both ancient and modern languages. However his most extensive comments were reserved for the sciences. Scholastic philosophy was severely censured and his colleagues were applauded for following the narrow path of certain knowledge. Then, of his own speciality, he reported with pride that mathematics and allied subjects previously regarded as too formidable to be undertaken, were now pursued with enthusiasm. His admiration was also aroused by the 'innocent cruelty' of vivisection experiments and by the serious botanical work undertaken even by freshmen (*neophytis*), who kept gardens and were able to identify plants unknown to Dioscorides. Finally, even the arcane science of chemistry was studied, and the university possessed scholars capable of understanding even the most obscure writings of Paracelsus.[193]

Although the evidence about the 'divers fellows' who had made such progress in anatomy and botany is fragmentary, Barrow's 1654 oration suggests that Ray's circle was not appreciably inferior to the more

190. Raven (235), pp. 108–10; letter from Hartlib to Boyle, 2 February 1657/8, Boyle *Works*, vi, p.101; letter from Worthington to Hartlib, 13 July 1661, Worthington *Diary*, p.345.

191. Ephemerides 1649.

192. On 24 March 1648 parliament voted £2,000 for extending the Cambridge Library, and £500 to purchase Thomason's collection of oriental books. On 10 October 1648, £40 or £50 was granted for printing Arabic books. *CJ*, v, pp.512, 560. Extracts of letters from Abraham Wheelock (HP XXXIII 4, 1647) indicate that Hartlib was attempting to obtain Arabic and Syriac type-faces for Cambridge, as well as seeking a Maronite to read difficult oriental manuscripts. Thomas Smith commented, 'not myselfe only but the whole Commonwealth of learning are eternally obliged to you for your earnest & happy endeavours for the promotion of all kind of learning especially Oriental'. Letter to Hartlib, 11 Oct. [1648], HP XV vii.

193. Barrow, 'Oratio ad Academicos in Comitiis', *Theological Works* (22), ix, pp.34–47.

celebrated Experimental Philosophy Club at Oxford. There were differences in emphasis; for instance the Platonist and Cartesian bias was almost exclusive to Cambridge. In Ray's circle there was a stronger interest in biological subjects, while at Oxford the physical sciences were dominant. None of the Cambridge scholars was active in the formation of the Royal Society, although many were associated with it at some stage. All of these factors have tended to focus the attention of historians of science on Oxford rather than on Cambridge. Only recently, with the recognition of Newton's debt to the Platonists, has the natural philosophy of Cudworth and More come to be regarded as of more than antiquarian interest. The terminology, concepts, literary sources, theological orientation, biblicism and even the critique of Cartesianism of the Platonists, provided a starting-point for Newton's studies in natural philosophy. The Platonists were also a force which was fully appreciated by Leibniz. At the more conventional level of estimation in terms of relevance to modern science, Barrow, Ray, Glisson and Power are certainly in the same class as their Oxford counterparts. There was a difference in the scale of operation; owing to institutional circumstances and the personalities of certain dominant figures, experimental science developed on a slightly more ambitious scale at Oxford.

One immediate effect of the parliamentarian settlement at Oxford was to sweep away the informal circle of natural philosophers surrounding Harvey. Their leader went into retirement; George Bathurst was killed; others continued military careers for a brief period; many settled in London, and their scientific meetings were partially reconstituted around Charles Scarburgh, who established a successful London medical practice. However in spite of the upheavals between 1640 and 1650, the development of informal scientific activity was only temporarily interrupted. Once stability returned, the pace accelerated, leading among other things to the formation of the Oxford Experimental Philosophy Club.[194] As indicated above, these developments had repercussions for formal academic studies, particularly in the medical faculty.

As at Cambridge, parliamentary interference with the university operated greatly to the advantage of natural philosophy. Involvement in experimental philosophy was probably regarded with favour, since its practitioners generally seemed moderate and politically reliable. The confidence of the authorities in this respect was largely rewarded, since the natural philosophers in academic posts tended to avoid highly

194. This term will be generally used to describe the Oxford group of natural philosophers. The earliest references spoke of 'the club' or 'philosophical club' or 'experimental philosophy club'. The latter term (derived from Aubrey, ii, p.301) aptly characterises the prevailing tone of their natural philosophy. Recent discussions of this group include Purver (230), Chapters IV–V; Shapiro (259), Chapter IV; especially informative is R. G. Frank, Jr. (105).

partisan religious alignments, a characteristic which they shared with their Platonist counterparts at Cambridge.

The natural philosophers recruited to Oxford were drawn from various backgrounds and many had the particular advantage of involvement in practical scientific work at the scientific meetings which had been held in London since 1645. One of the first and most significant acts of the Visitors was to nominate John Wilkins as Warden of Wadham College.[195] No single factor accounts for the appointment of Wilkins. He was not as senior as most of the divines appointed to headships, but he possessed sound credentials as a Puritan and had made a small but favourable impression as a chaplain and scholar. Jonathan Goddard owed his appointment as Warden of Merton College to services as physician to Cromwell. John Wallis's background was similar to that of Wilkins, but he was more obviously in the parliamentarian orbit, through his association with the Westminster Assembly. Wallis replaced the little-known Peter Turner as Savilian professor of geometry. By a complicated manoeuvre, the ejected professor of astronomy, John Greaves, was able to secure the appointment of a fellow royalist, Seth Ward, arguing that the parliamentarians would otherwise 'give it to some Cobler of their Party, who never heard the name of Euclid, or the Mathematics'.[196] As Ward's biographer fairly admits, parliamentarian action over the geometry chair had given no grounds for these suspicions. Although the two divines occupying the Savilian chairs under parliament had very different political and religious allegiances, they developed an amicable association and became distinguished exponents of their subjects. At a more junior level, Joshua Crosse was appointed Sedleian lecturer while William Petty became assistant to the Professor of Physic in the latter's capacity as Tomlins anatomical lecturer. Both were politically conformist and Petty in particular was ambitious for further preferment.

Once these leading figures were established in Oxford, they resumed scientific meetings of the kind previously held in London and found numerous scholars receptive to their ideas. In the stable and sheltered atmosphere of the university, the small informal gatherings prospered. As with the 1645 Group, in the interests of productive scientific enquiry harmonious relations were maintained between scholars of very different religious and political persuasions. Such tolerance was encouraged by Wilkins, who rapidly emerged as both the natural leader of the Oxford scientific community and as a dominant figure in university administration. Scholars from a wide religious and political spectrum were attracted to Wadham, with the result that Wilkins became unpopular with certain of his puritan colleagues; but this proved no disadvantage

195. Shapiro (259), pp.80–3; R. B. Gardiner (112), pp.170–1; Wilkins's name was registered at Wadham, 7 April 1648.

196. Pope (223), pp.18–24. Ward had been ejected from Sidney Sussex College Cambridge.

to his career. Like Goddard and Petty, Wilkins came to wield an influence outside Oxford which elevated him beyond the reach of critical academics.

From the time of Wilkins's appointment, his lodgings became a centre for Oxford science. Aubrey was probably correct in describing him as the 'principal reviver of experimental philosophy . . . at Oxford, where he had a weekeley experimentall philosophicall clubbe, which began 1649'.[197] But the society had other roots in Oxford. A few members had been associated with William Harvey's group. Wallis drew attention to the meetings held at the lodgings of William Petty at Buckley Hall; these probably began soon after Petty's arrival in Oxford in 1650. Petty would certainly have embarked on this programme with great zeal, in order to secure preferment and gain influence at Oxford. His first post as anatomy lecturer paid only £15 per annum, but he looked forward to benefiting from the 'new evacuation of the University about the Engagement'.[198] His appeals for assistance from Dury, Hartlib and Rous were fruitful; he was installed in a fellowship at Brasenose College. Once established in Oxford, Petty perhaps aimed to complement the Wadham interest in the physical sciences, by specialising more in the medical sciences and in chemistry. His lodgings were conveniently situated for this purpose, above the shop of the apothecary John Clarke who, according to Graunt, was an expert chemist and bee-keeper, formerly apothecary to William Harvey.[199] The gatherings at Petty's lodgings may have continued until his appointment as Physician-General to the army in Ireland in 1652, but it is more likely that Petty had left Oxford by April 1651. During his stay in Oxford, Petty made a considerable impression with such feats as the resuscitation of the hanged body of Ann Green and participation in the experiment of 'blowing a boy [buoy] or boat over London bridge'. He was soon attempting to assist Oxford friends, as witnessed by his letter soliciting Hartlib's help in securing the Gresham chair of astronomy for Richard Rawlinson.[200]

During the final year of the interregnum, upon Wilkins's removal to Cambridge, scientific meetings were held in Boyle's rooms at Deep Hall, the house of the apothecary John Crosse. Near neighbours were Jacob Bobart the botanical garden keeper and William Day the surgeon. This location may well have encouraged the interchange of ideas between gentlemen, academics and practitioners. Boyle's patronage had considerable significance. Since Boyle avoided taking up any official university appointment, he was well placed to superintend Oxford science

197. Aubrey, ii, p.301.

198. Letter from Petty to Dury, 26 August 1650, Yale University Library, Osborn Collection, 64/3.

199. Purver (230), pp.118–20, for an identification of Petty's lodgings. Ephemerides 1653.

200. Letters from Petty to Hartlib, 16 December 1650 and 17 May 1652, Yale, Osborn, 64/3.

during the upheavals of the restoration, which entailed the ejection of many of his colleagues from their academic positions. Boyle may also have played an important part in revitalising the Oxford club. In February 1658 Petty reported that 'the club is restored at Oxford', and Hartlib sent Boyle a narrative of the life of Joachim Jungius for the benefit of 'your whole philosophical club'.[201] As described below, the impression formed by Hartlib and Petty, that Boyle had come to dominate organised science at Oxford, was shared at a later date by Evelyn. The potential importance of Boyle had soon been recognised by Wilkins, who solicited him to settle in Oxford 'where you will be a means to quicken and direct us in our enquiries.'[202] Boyle's reputation at Oxford was greatly enhanced by the work of his assistant, Robert Hooke.

A set of eight rules framed in 1651 for an unnamed group of experimenters almost certainly relates to the Oxford Experimental Philosophy Club.[203] The first three rules give the terms of admission; the fourth deals with subscriptions, a proportion of which was to be used for the purchase of instruments. The fifth relates to the removal of persistent absentees from 'the catalogue'. The sixth and seventh provide instructions for the ordering of exercises or experiments. The society expected to commission experiments from its members, a fine being due if the task was not performed within a reasonable period. A final rule establishes that the meetings were to be held weekly, before 2.00 p.m. on Thursdays. There is no evidence that these rules were formally adopted or enforced. More probably the club operated in a less formal manner, groups of specialists meeting according to their particular requirements. However the formulation of rules is significant in indicating a sense of unity of purpose and a desire to extend the regular scientific meetings which had so fruitfully begun in London. It was therefore appropriate to follow the precedent of the 1645 Group and elaborate rules to guide their proceedings. As in the case of many academic statutes, the rules themselves were most explicit on incidental or routine points, and silent on intellectual aims. But the members were united in their enthusiasm for the 'new philosophy' and they would have accepted a common approach to the solution of scientific problems. Among other things, they appreciated the value of a pool of instruments, which would be accessible to the whole group. As shown below, there quickly emerged a plan to establish 'a Magneticall, Mechanicall, and Optick Schoole, furnished with the best instruments, and Adapted for the most usefull experiments in all those faculties'.[204] Thus, once the embryonic scientific society was estab-

201. Letter of Hartlib to Boyle, 2 Feb. 1658; Petty to Boyle, 17 Feb. 1658; Boyle *Works*, vi, pp.101, 139.

202. Letter of Wilkins to Boyle, 6 Sept. 1653, Boyle *Works*, vi, p.634.

203. Bodleian, Ashmole MS 1810, 23 October 1651; dated exactly two years after the appointment of Ward and Wallis—perhaps a coincidence. Purver suggests that the rules are in Gerard Langbaine's hand. The rules are given in full by McKie (183), pp.25–6.

204. Ward (307), p.36.

lished, its work led naturally to a desire for further institutionalisation; laboratories, an observatory, technicians, even a collegiate form of organisation were soon regarded as desirable. Such precocious ambitions were certain to arouse the hostility of the university's scholastic party.

Soon after the above rules were framed, Ward confirmed the existence of a formal society, or 'Greate Clubb' of thirty members. Consistently with the rules they had '(everyone takeing a portion) gone over all the heads of naturall philosophy & mixt mathematics', collecting scientific data from the literature and themselves performing as many of the experiments as possible. As well as the main meetings, a smaller group of eight persons was involved in regular chemical experiments. Ward reported, and other evidence confirms, that members of the 'Greate Clubb' were establishing both a laboratory and an observatory.[205] From Ward's description it is apparent that the society was numerous and its activities varied. In spite of the idea of membership expressed in the rules, it is probable that no definitive list of members was prepared. In the absence of records of membership, impressions of the Oxford club have tended to be formed on the basis of information about those individuals who later played a part in the foundation of the Royal Society. Considerable identity of personal and intellectual outlook has been assumed to exist between the Royal Society and the Oxford club. But even the limited overlap between the two organisations was far from complete. Members of the Oxford club certainly joined, and some were founder members of, the Royal Society. However, many of the Oxford club were not active in the Society. It is therefore not possible to produce a balanced view of the Oxford club by simply drawing attention to the early careers of the better-known founders of the Royal Society. It is noticeable that both Wallis and Ward allude to 'divers' unnamed figures who were engaged in the work of the Oxford club. For a proper perspective it is necessary to obtain some impression about this wider membership from the scattered preserved records. It is not possible to compile a definitive list, but Table 1 (pp.166-9) provides a tentative, alphabetical catalogue, which includes associates who might not have been regarded as full members but who are known to have worked closely with the fully-accredited members. Such a provisional list does at least give the impression of a society of the size mentioned by Ward. Inspection of the dates of arrival at Oxford indicates that the list is defective for the earlier and perhaps more active phase of the club. The later members have tended to become known because of their habit of following their teachers and patrons into the Royal Society. Accordingly even this more comprehensive list is slightly unrepresentative.

Since no official minutes survive it is difficult to know which members

205. Letter from Ward to Sir Justinian Isham, Feb. 1652; quoted from *Notes & Records* (249).

participated most in the daily work of the society. Wallis recollected meetings at Petty's lodgings and at Wadham College of a group consisting of himself, Wilkins, Goddard, Petty, Ward 'and many others of the most inquisitive persons in Oxford'. Sprat, who was at the time a student at Wadham College, gave a slightly fuller list—Ward, Boyle, Wilkins, Petty, Matthew and Christopher Wren, Wallis, Goddard, Thomas Willis, Ralph Bathurst and Laurence Rooke. Evelyn's account of the active membership of the Oxford club differs slightly from that of Sprat. According to Evelyn, at the time of Boyle's removal to Oxford a group led by Bathurst, Edmund Dickinson, Christopher Wren, Robert Sharrock, Scarburgh, Ward 'and especially Dr. Wilkins', was active. All authorities affirm the pre-eminence of Wilkins, but Evelyn includes a greater number of members who came to have only a peripheral association with the Royal Society.[206]

Certain tentative impressions may be drawn from the provisional catalogue of members given here. A large number of Oxford club members later subscribed to the Royal Society, but very few were more than nominal Fellows. Ten of the 'active members' and seven of the 'active nucleus' of the Royal Society (as defined in Chapter II, above) had been in some way involved with the Oxford club. But examination of their biographies indicates that this connection with Oxford experimental science was often very limited.[207] Another widely accepted opinion, derived from Sprat, that the Oxford club broke up in 1658 and 1659 owing to the migration to London of its leading members, is certainly incorrect. The Oxford group probably adopted a slightly more informal existence, but activities continued much as before, and indeed they were sustained at a level sufficient to encourage such figures as Boyle, Bathurst, Sharrock, Dickinson, Wren, Lower, Willis, and Mayow to concentrate their major scientific researches in Oxford, rather than to transfer their operations to the Royal Society in London. Thus it could be argued that, from the point of view of modern science, the most important and productive phase of the Oxford Experimental Philosophy Club followed the departure of a section of the membership to London. Boyle effectively divided his energies between the two bodies, but most of the rising talents were located in Oxford rather than in London.

The great prestige of Wilkins is denoted by the predominance of members of Wadham College in the catalogue. Wilkins was able to attract mature scholars like Ward, Rooke and Needham (all originally from Cambridge), or such ambitious young students as Christopher Wren and William Neile. Even the manciple and cook at Wadham owed these appointments to their associations with the scientific move-

206. Scriba (257), p.4; Sprat (266), p.55; Letter from Evelyn to William Wotton, 12 Sept. 1703, BM Add. MS 28, 104, fol. 21. This list is slightly different from the printed version of this letter in Evelyn (96), iii, p.391. I am grateful to Professor P. M. Rattansi for pointing out this variant.

207. See above, pp. 88–99.

ment. The manciple, Christopher Brookes, was a London instrument maker, married to the daughter of William Oughtred, while the daughter of the cook, William Austin, married the mathematician John Collins.[208] In the gardens were plants of botanical curiosity or agricultural relevance, waterworks and experimental beehives. Hence experimental philosophy must have impinged upon most aspects of life at this college.

Many leading members of the Oxford club were extremely young. Boyle, Petty, Wren and Neile made a great impression at an early age. Others were not so obviously precocious, but it is clear that Locke, Lower and Mayow laid the foundations for their later celebrated work during their early education at Oxford. Young men were particularly prominent in the club during the period of Boyle's residence in Oxford.

The Oxford club probably enjoyed two main phases of activity. The first occurred before Boyle's arrival and primarily involved individuals most of whom had participated in scientific meetings in London; this group became less important after 1654. Goddard continued to live mainly in London; Robert Wood and Petty had by then left Oxford for Ireland; Ward and Bathurst became increasingly less involved with science; Lydall died in 1657. The new talent of the later period shifted the perspective of scientific interest towards medicine.

The membership catalogue also confirms Anthony Wood's impression that Cambridge scholars took advantage of preferment opportunities at Oxford, but it does not support his view that the migrating scholars were predominantly puritan.[209] Indeed no generalisation can be made about the religious outlook of the Oxford club. Certain dominant figures were recruited to Oxford because of their parliamentarian and puritan allegiance, while others were openly antagonistic to the new order without necessarily being expelled from the university. If pronounced religious and political toleration had not existed, the members of the club would have been unable to sustain their high degree of collaboration and scientific productivity. For our purposes it is sufficient to note that certain dominant members of the group were puritan and parliamentarian, and that the parliamentary reorganisation of the university established conditions favourable for the acceleration of organised scientific work.

Like the Cambridge Platonists, members of the Oxford club were concerned to establish a sound theological basis for their scientific activity. Wilkins, Ward and Wallis were Doctors of Divinity; they published religious works and their professional careers were largely within the church. Bathurst was only temporarily deflected from the church into medicine.[210] This pattern is duplicated among the minor members.

208. Taylor (278), pp.228, 234. See F.A.D., *The Early Connection of the Royal Society with Wadham College* (Oxford, 1912).

209. Wood *Fasti*, ii, p.106—'call'd the scum of Cambridge'.

210. Ward's letter to Isham (249) sought patronage for someone like Bathurst, who had intended to become a divine, but whom political circumstances had diverted into medicine.

Even the laymen like Boyle and Dickinson were deeply involved with religious issues. Whereas the momentum of day-to-day scientific enquiry was probably maintained by the intrinsic interest of the phenomena under investigation, religious ideas provided an implicit motivation for the whole undertaking, which was therefore much more than a sudden spontaneous expression of scientific inquisitiveness.

By contrast with Cambridge, there was at Oxford little thorough-going Platonism, and no sudden enthusiasm for Descartes—or hasty retrenchment from Cartesianism. The exploitation of natural theology, which came about by indirect means at Cambridge, occurred more directly at Oxford. This difference in theological bias had important implications for the approach to natural philosophy. As might be expected from his Cambridge background, Ward was closest to More's position, reacting to the dangers of Hobbesian materialism by arguing that the Being of God could be demonstrated in nature.[211] Wilkins was more specific about the scientific implications of this position.[212] He shared the Platonist concern to demonstrate the power of providence, but his treatment of this question resulted in a much more positive attitude to experimental science. Since it was necessary to appreciate the minute workings of providence in history and nature, Wilkins called for 'experimental divinity' which would yield an insight into the mechanism of nature and society; it would then be possible to predict the course of events and control the processes of nature.[213] Wilkins asked for a systematic and meticulous investigation of nature, with a strong bias towards technological improvement 'whereby men do naturally attempt to restore themselves from the first general curse inflicted upon their labours'.[214] Thus, like More and Ray, Wilkins sustained his science by reference to natural theology, but the scientific approach which emerged incorporated a Baconian and utilitarian dimension. This extremely liberal approach to natural philosophy, expressed at the outset of the Wadham scientific meetings, persisted in the subsequent activities of the experimental philosophers at Oxford. They were concerned on the one hand with abstract mathematics, astronomy and the classic problems of natural philosophy, and on the other with practical chemistry, and mechanical inventions. The Oxford club accordingly overlapped in its interests both with the utilitarians in Hartlib's circle and with the Cambridge Platonists.

The Oxford group became involved in many areas of scientific research work relevant to modern science. This work often exercised considerable influence on the development of the specialised sciences. Even where the researches failed to gain immediate, widespread recognition, they have often been found to contain insights which forestall

211. Ward, *A Philosophical Essay* (Oxford, 1652) (306).
212. Wilkins, *Beauty of Providence* (London, 1649) (332).
213. *Ibid.*, p.60.
214. *Ibid.*, p.49; *Mathematicall Magick* (London, 1648) (331), p.2.

much later developments. In some cases individual creative work was supremely important, whereas in others group enterprise was significant. In mathematics Wallis was supreme, but he was able to conduct fruitful dialogues on specific problems with Wren and Neile. Otherwise, his world was that of the continental mathematicians.[215] Likewise, with Hooke's assistance, Boyle was able to transcend the confused world of the chemists, and to make considerable progress in the understanding of the physical and chemical properties of air.[216] In the case of the physiological and anatomical work of Willis, Lower and Mayow, collaboration was more important and there was appreciable dependence on the pioneer work of Bathurst and Boyle. The role of the general membership of Wilkins's club is well-illustrated by their conduct of experiments on injection and blood transfusion.[217]

Most of this work originated during the later years of the Experimental Philosophy Club and was completed during the early years of the restoration. For the most part the club itself was involved in the unglamorous labours which served to stimulate interest in science and to provide the basic groundwork for more substantial individual achievements. It would be wrong to believe that the whole group was enlivened by a superior 'modern' scientific methodology and engaged upon rigorous experimental studies comparable with the highest attainments of individual members. There are many scattered reports from Oxford, as well as the more general accounts of Wallis and Charleton, which enable us to build up a more balanced historical picture of this scientific community at work.

The Oxford club gives an impression of wide-ranging curiosity. This was undoubtedly encouraged by Wilkins, 'secundum mentem domini Baconi'.[218] The members subscribed to a broad Baconian programme, which embraced at one extreme the pragmatic investigation of scientific problems, and at the other the comprehensive survey of natural phenomena, the improvement of all forms of communication, and the application of science to utilitarian ends. Inevitably much effort was devoted to examining the flood of recent scientific discoveries made by such figures as Galileo, Harvey, Torricelli and Descartes, so perpetuating the spirit of the meetings of the 1645 Group.[219] Ancient and modern literature was sifted for further information on major topics of interest. The level of proficiency may not have been particularly high among the rank and file, but their Baconian spirit of collaborative

215. Christoph J. Scriba, *Studien zur Mathematik des John Wallis (1616–1703)* (Wiesbaden, 1966).

216. C. Webster, 'The Discovery of Boyle's Law, and the Concept of the Elasticity of Air in the Seventeenth Century', *Archive for History of Exact Sciences*, 1965, 2: 441–502; Partington (205), pp.486–613.

217. Webster, *op. cit.* See below, note 233. For a particularly valuable discussion of this subject, see R. G. Frank Jr., 'Oxford and the Harveian Tradition' (104).

218. Aubrey, ii, p.301.

219. Scriba (257), p.40. Wallis stressed this aspect of their work.

enterprise was of the greatest importance in stimulating public interest, and in recruiting experimenters to investigate novel problems. When approached at this level science was within the competence of the whole group. Seth Ward summed up this approach:

> 'Our first businesse is to gather together such things as are already discovered . . . then to have a collection of those which are still inquirenda and according to our opportunityes to make inquisitive experiments, the end is that out of a sufficient number of sure experiments, the way of nature in workeing may be discovered.'[220]

Ward's statement is consistent with the maxims of Bacon as expressed in Wilkins's *Beauty of Providence*. The utilitarian aspect of this form of experimental philosophy created an area of common interest with Baconians outside the universities, such as the Hartlib circle. Although prejudice has prevented acknowledgment of the intellectual affinities between the Oxford club and Hartlib's associates, Turnbull has given ample evidence to illustrate the free flow of information between the two groups.[221] The correspondences of Boyle, Austen and Robert Wood provide further testimony of amicable exchanges of information on specific problems. Closer association was precluded by disagreements about astrology or Paracelsian medicine, or by more general theological and ideological differences.

Various commentators recorded their impressions about the diversity of activities within the Oxford club. Walter Charleton, who was a visitor to his *alma mater* at this time, made special mention of the mathematical work of Wallis, the geometrical astronomy of Ward, optical experiments, the improvement of optical instruments, and universal language.[222] A quite different perspective is given by one of Hartlib's correspondents.[223] In his two-day visit, the writer discovered 'a Knot of . . . Ingenious & free Philosophers'. Contrary to the impression given Hartlib by other informants, this commentator believed that the heads of college and the professors were not steeped in 'Ancient or the vulgar opinions'. If they opposed new ideas, it was only after careful consideration. Wilkins's garden at Wadham was organised according to the view that 'what concernes Naturall Philosophy in generall must not be thought Irrelative to Husbandry, which is but an application of it to rural subjects'. In this garden the writer saw 'Indian Wheat as good as any in Europe'; 'nasturtium indicum' which was suitable for use as a salad crop since it tasted like scurvy grass; and a rose which had a long flowering season. But his greatest enthusiasm

220. Letter to Isham (249), p.69.
221. Turnbull (287).
222. Charleton (46), pp.43–8.
223. Letter to Hartlib, 14 September 1655, BP XXXVII. This letter was possibly written by Boyle; similar comments by him were recorded (Ephemerides 1655). Robert Child had noted the dominance of Aristotelian philosophy at Oxford (Ephemerides 1650).

was reserved for a newly-invented beehive incorporating a glass wall, which was already known to Hartlib from Wren and Rawlinson. These beehives also attracted comment from Evelyn, and Hartlib introduced them to a wider public in his *Reformed Commonwealth of Bees* (1655).[224] This example underlines the freedom of communication between Oxford and the Hartlib circle on matters of common interest, as well as the closeness of the association between Wilkins and his collaborators. Finally it points to a serious interest in husbandry, a feature of the Oxford club which has received too little attention. A model of an improved plough designed by Wilkins was eagerly sought after by one of Hartlib's acquaintances.[225] John Lydall informed Aubrey that Petty had invented a mechanical device 'to set a field of corne as soone as otherwaies it can bee sowne and harried'.[226] When Austen's book on fruit trees appeared, Lydall purchased sixteen trees from the author in order to establish his first nursery. The culture of fruit trees was obviously one of the main horticultural interests of the Oxford club, finding expression in the important writings of Austen and Sharrock.[227]

The interest of Wilkins in mechanical devices is well known. Already in *Mathematical Magic* he had established himself as a minor heir to the artist-engineers of the Renaissance. Wilkins hoped that his book would explain the dependence of complex devices on the rational laws of mechanics, and thereby undermine the secretive and magical tradition which had previously prevented the full realisation of technological improvements. The eccentric assembly of inventions discussed by Wilkins is reminiscent of a much earlier age. His book aroused the interest of Francis Potter, the well-known clergyman-inventor, who disagreed with Wilkins's contention that small models of submarines and flying machines could guarantee the viability of large versions. However he regarded Wilkins as 'a very ingeniose man' and one who had 'a very mechanicall head'.[228] With the assistance of his collaborators, Wilkins embarked on an ambitious programme which embraced on the one hand perpetual motion, and on the other, the construction of a number of simple but useful devices. These became a major attraction to visitors like Evelyn, who reported:

> 'He [Wilkins] had above in his Gallery & Lodgings a variety of Shadows, Dyals, Perspectives, places to introduce the *Species*, &

224. The beehives were described in letters to Hartlib from—Rawlinson, 30 January 1654/5 (HP x 10); Wren, 26 February 1654/5 (HP xxv 9); Oldenburg, 21 June 1656, *Correspondence*, i, p.102; Robert Wood, August 1657 (HP xxxiii 1). See also Evelyn (97), iii, p.110; Hartlib, *Reformed Commonwealth of Bees* (London, 1655), pp.50–2.

225. Boyle *Works*, vi, pp.97, 99.

226. Bodleian, Aubrey MS 12–13, fol. 308r, 27 May 1651; fol. 317r, 23 June 1655. This was also Cressy Dymock's favourite, of his own inventions.

227. See below, pp.477–9.

228. Letter from John Aubrey to Francis Potter, 10 April 1651, Bodleian, Aubrey MS 12–13, fols. 141–2; Aubrey, ii, pp.299–300.

> many other artificial, mathematical and Magical curiosities: A Way-Wiser, a Thermometer, a monstrous Magnes, Conic & other Sections, a Balance on a demie-Circle, most of them of his owne & that prodigious young Scholar, Mr. Chr. Wren.'[229]

The products of Wren's youthful ingenuity resembled Hooke's early work at the Royal Society.[230] Besides the instruments mentioned above Wren's early inventions included improved wagons, a hygrometer, a perspectograph and a double-writing instrument. Such inventories tend to overlap; in Wren's case there was duplication to the point of competition with Oxford's second prodigy, William Petty. Petty had arrived from London with a growing reputation as an inventor, and he kept up these pretensions at Oxford. Already in 1647 he had invented and patented a double-writing instrument, which was widely advertised and dedicated ostentatiously to Boyle.[231] Some years later, after much pressure had been put on Petty to perfect his invention, Hartlib commented sourly, 'those that know the way which Mr. Wren doth use, say his [Petty's] art of double writing is not worth a rush'.[232] Liability to such unfavourable comparisons, and close similarity of interests might have created friction between the two ambitious inventors, had Petty not vacated Oxford in search of preferment in Ireland.

Wren stayed at Oxford, becoming a Fellow of All Souls College. His reputation increased, and his interests continued to diversify. One of his most spectacular and widely publicised achievements was the injection of ale and medicines into the veins of live dogs. This is possibly the start of a series of experiments which led ultimately to Lower's successful blood transfusions, although an alternative and independent source might have been Francis Potter's transfusion experiments which Aubrey may have publicised in Oxford. Wren seems also to have pioneered the splenectomy operation at Oxford.[233] Such examples are evidence for the increasing participation of laymen in the anatomical and physiological work of the medical faculty.

In the course of their researches the Oxford club assembled a varied collection of apparatus and instruments. Ward singled out chemistry as

229. Evelyn (97), iii, pp.110–11.

230. *Parentalia, or lives of the Wrens,* ed. Christopher Wren (London, 1750), pp.208–9; Sprat (266), pp.313–17; H. W. Jones, 'Sir Christopher Wren and Natural Philosophy, with a checklist of his scientific activities', *Notes & Records,* 1958, *13*: 19–37.

231. *CJ,* v, p.481. Petty's *Advice,* 1648 (210) began with an advertisement for the instrument; letter from Petty to Boyle, 21 June 1648, Boyle *Works,* vi, pp. 136–7.

232. Letter from Hartlib to Boyle, 8 May 1654, Boyle *Works,* vi, p.88.

233. Letter from Wren to Petty [c. 1656] in *Parentalia,* p.228: 'A new anatomy experiment at Oxford to open veins and spout medicines into it'. Ephemerides 1658. C. Webster, 'The Helmontian George Thomson and William Harvey: The revival and application of splenectomy to physiological research', *Medical History,* 1971, *15*: 154–67, p.161; *idem,* 'The Origins of Blood Transfusion: A Reassessment', *Medical History,* 1971, *15*: 387–92.

a particularly popular minority interest. The group of eight was 'furnishing an elaboratory and for makeing chymicall experiments which we doe constantly every one of us in course undertaking by weeks to manage the worke'.[234] Names are not given but the group probably included Ward, Wallis, Dickinson, Willis, Bathurst and Lydall. Their central laboratory was probably at Wadham since Willis recorded the expenditure of £27-4-8d. on chemicals, apparatus and building work, 'laid out at Wadham Coll.' probably between 1650 and 1652.[235] The fashion for private laboratories may have been a reflection of the success of this Wadham enterprise. Wood thought that the laboratory at Clarke's house achieved 'things which the memory of man could not reach'. According to Aubrey, Willis was also involved with a laboratory at Peckwater Inn Chamber.[236] The arrival of Boyle in Oxford undoubtedly increased still further the popularity of chemistry. By the restoration chemistry had become so popular that the German projector and physician, Peter Staehl, was persuaded to give private chemistry lessons in Oxford. According to Wallis he was 'invited hither for that purpose', to conduct for classes of six or eight 'of better rank amongst us . . . a whole course of chymistry'. Staehl's talents had been recommended by Hartlib to Boyle who installed the chemist in his own house at Oxford in 1659.[237]

Charleton's eulogy of Oxford science emphasised the value of contributions to the study of optics. 'Shew me the men in the whole World,' he declared, 'who have more illustrated the nature, affections, and motions of that most subtle and glorious Creature, Light'.[238] The production of curious effects with reflections, lenses and mirrors, which so impressed Charleton and Evelyn, is now scarcely remembered. Of more permanent interest was the work on improving the microscope and the telescope. The Oxford astronomers worked closely with other enthusiasts like Sir Paul Neile and the London practitioners Greatorex and Reeves. Charleton believed that the microscope had been so perfected in the previous four or five years that the smallest parts of insects could be discerned. He optimistically predicted that further improvements would bring the 'Seminal Figures', 'smallest *Moleculae*, or first collections of Atoms' into view. So amazing were the initial findings with microscopes that Wilkins declared that it was not possible to improve further the 'certainty and exactness' of their instruments. Wren claimed to have introduced a method of measuring

234. Letter from Ward to Isham (249), p.69.

235. Wellcome Institute, London, Wellcome MS 799a, 'Liber manuscriptus Cl. Doctoris Thomae Willis Medico Insigno'; rough itemised accounts given on last leaves.

236. Wood, *Life & Times* (47), i, p.290; Aubrey, ii, p.303.

237. Wallis (303), pp.315–16; Hartlib reported that Wallis was exchanging chemical secrets with Boyle's laboratory assistant: Ephemerides 1654. Wood, *Life & Times* (47), i, pp.290, 472–3. G. H. Turnbull, 'Peter Stahl, the first public teacher of chemistry at Oxford', *Annals of Science,* 1953, *9*: 265–70.

238. Charleton (46), pp.46–8.

TABLE 1

THE OXFORD EXPERIMENTAL PHILOSOPHY CLUB

Name	College	Comments	FRS	Source
Ralph Austen		Secretary to Visitors		Burrows, p.viii; Wood *Fasti*, ii, p.174. Letters to Hartlib.
William Austin		Cook of Wadham		Taylor, p.228.
John Backhouse	Wadham 1656	Tutored by William Lloyd		Wood *Athenae*, iv, p.715; Gardiner, p.214.
Timothy Baldwin	Balliol 1635 All Souls 1639			Wood, *Life & Times*, i, p.201; *Fasti*, ii, p.171.
William Balle	Wadham 1656		1663	
Ralph Bathurst	Trinity 1637	S.	1663	
Robert Boyle		Private resident 1655	1663	
Thomas Branker	Exeter 1652	S.		Wood *Athenae*, iii, p.1086; *Life & Times*, i, p.473.
Christopher Brookes		Manciple of Wadham		Taylor, p.234.
George Castle	Balliol 1652	MD 1665	1668	Wood, *Life & Times*, i, p.201; *Athenae* iii, p.998.
Timothy Clarke	Balliol c. 1648	MD 1652	1663	Munk, i, p.315.
Nathaniel Crew	Lincoln 1652	S.		Wood, *Life & Times*, i, pp.290, 473; *Athenae*, iv, pp.886–8.
Joshua Crosse	Lincoln 1631 Magdalen 1648	Sedleian Professor		Burrows, pp.506, 516.
Edmund Dickinson	Merton 1642	MD 1656	1667	Wood *Athenae*, iv, pp.777–8.
Joseph Glanvill	Exeter 1652 Lincoln 1656		1664	Wood *Athenae*, iii, pp.1244–55.
Jonathan Goddard	Merton 1651		1663	

Name	College	Comments	FRS	Source
Nathaniel Hodges	Christ Church 1648	MD 1659		Munk, i, pp.361–3; Wood *Athenae*, iv, p.149.
Robert Hooke	Christ Church 1653	Assistant to Willis, then Boyle	1663	
George Joyliffe	Wadham 1637	Left Oxford 1650; MD Cambridge 1652; died 1658		Munk, i, pp.280–1; Venn, ii, p.483.
Gerard Langbaine	Queen's 1626	Provost of Queen's College; Custos Archivorum; died 1657.		Wood *Athenae*, iii, pp.446–9.
John Locke	Christ Church 1652	S; MB 1675	1668	
Richard Lower	Christ Church 1649	S; MD 1665	1667	
John Lydall	Trinity 1644	Died 1657		Frank, *Notes & Records*, 1973, *27*: 193–217.
John Mayow	Wadham 1658		1678	
Thomas Millington	All Souls 1649	S; MD 1659		Wood, *Life & Times*, i, pp.201, 273; Venn, iii, p.190.
Caspar Needham	Wadham 1654		1663	Venn, iii, p.238; Gardiner, p.206.
William Neile	Wadham 1655	Son of Sir Paul Neile; collaborated with club members.	1663	Gardiner, p.210.
Henry Oldenburg		Private tutor 1656–7	1663	
Samuel Parker	Wadham 1657		1666	Wood *Athenae*, iv, pp.225–35.
Peter Pett	Pembroke 1647 All Souls 1648		1663	Wood *Athenae*, iv, pp.576–80; *Life & Times*, i, p.201.
William Petty	Brasenose 1650	MD 1649. Left Oxford 1651	1663	

Name	College	Comments	FRS	Source
Walter Pope	Wadham 1648	Wilkins's half-brother	1663	Gardiner, pp.177–8. Wood *Athenae*, iv, pp.724–30.
Richard Rawlinson	Queen's 1636	Friend of Wren	Proposed for R.S. 1661	Wood *Fasti*, ii, pp.60, 257; letters to Hartlib.
Laurence Rooke	Wadham 1650	Left Oxford 1652		Wood *Athenae*, iii, pp.587–9; Gardiner, p.191; *Notes & Records*, 1960, pp.113–18.
Robert Sharrock	New College 1649			Wood *Athenae*, iv, pp.147–8.
Thomas Sprat	Wadham 1651		1663	Purver, *Royal Society* (1967);
William Sprigge	Lincoln 1652			Wood *Athenae*, iv, pp.727–30. Wood *Athenae*, iv. pp.560–1.
Peter Staehl		Itinerant chemist	1659	Wood, *Life & Times*, i, pp.290, 472–5.
Francis Turner	New College 1655	S.		Wood, *Life & Times*, i, pp.290, 472; *Athenae*, iv, p.545.
John Wallis	Exeter 1649	Savilian Professor of Geometry; S; Custos Archivorum	1663	
Seth Ward	Wadham 1650	Savilian Professor of Astronomy	1663	
John Wilkins	Wadham 1648	Warden of Wadham	1663	
Joseph Williamson	Queen's 1650	S.	1663	*DNB*; Wood, *Life & Times*, i, p.470.

Name	College	Comments	FRS	Source
Thomas Willis		Medical practitioner	1663	
Robert Wood	Merton 1642 Lincoln 1650		1681	Wood *Athenae*, iv, pp.167–8; letters to Hartlib.
Benjamin Woodroffe	Christ Church 1656	S.	1668	Wood *Athenae*, iv, pp.640–2; *Life & Times*, i, p.472.
Christopher Wren	Wadham 1649 All Souls 1653	S.	1663	
Matthew Wren		Private resident	1663	Wood *Fasti*, ii, p.819; *Life & Times*, i, p.201.
Thomas Wren		Private resident	1663	Wood, *Life & Times*, i, p.201.
Henry Yerbury	Magdalen 1646	S; MD 1659		Wood, *Life & Times*, i, p.473; *Fasti*, ii, p.217.

This list includes Peter Staehl and more persistent members of his chemical classes.
The dates for Fellowship of the Royal Society are taken from *The Record of the Royal Society*, 3rd edn. (London, 1912).
Comments refer to the period pre-1660; S. = member of Staehl's class.
MDs are for Oxford unless otherwise stated.
Sources are given for minor figures only.
Of the Oxford Club, 12 came from Wadham; 5 from Christ Church; 4 from All Souls and from Lincoln; 3 from Queen's; 2 from Balliol, Trinity, Exeter, Magdalen, Merton and from New College, and 1 from Brasenose.

small objects under a microscope. Hence it is just possible that he was investigating the application of the micrometer to both the telescope and the microscope.[239] But his most important known contribution was to draft illustrations of microscopical objects which were later used by Hooke in the preparation of his *Micrographia*.[240] Microscopy became a preoccupation with the Baconians. The microscope was a valuable research instrument, but it also provided them with considerable entertainment. Their use of it was at once a means of attracting publicity, and an object of satire. Especially incisive was Harrington's reflection, directed particularly at Wilkins, that the Oxford scholars were 'good at two Things, at diminishing a Commonwealth and at Multiplying a Louse'. This insult called for a prompt response on behalf of Wilkins. On the scientific question, Harrington was reminded of the high-minded motives of the Wadham philosophers: their microscopical work was not trivial since it was a highly appropriate way of magnifying the 'Wisdome of the great Architect of Nature'.[241]

Besides cultivating geometrical astronomy, Ward, Rooke and Wren were eager to establish an observatory, as originally intended by Savile. Pressure from this source was probably responsible for the decision by the university to sanction expenditure on instruments, books and an observatory. £25 was approved by a committee, which included Wilkins and Wallis, for assisting astronomical work by the building of a portable observatory (*Observatorio mobile*) on the tower of Wadham College.[242] Ward reported that he was constructing a 'slight observatory' and procuring telescopes and other astronomical instruments.[243] The records also show that during the 1650s a declinatory instrument was constructed, and a sextant repaired, for this observatory. At this time the observatory also benefited from instruments donated by the Greaves family in memory of the first two Savilian astronomy professors, John Bainbridge and John Greaves. Thus a modest collection of instruments was recorded when a catalogue was prepared at the end of the century. Conspicuous in this list were three telescopes, the largest being a fifteen-foot instrument with three lenses. Telescopes appear to have been a major preoccupation with the Oxford astronomers. Stimulated by the findings of Hevelius and Huyghens, they worked with assistants to improve lens-grinding techniques, and to construct larger and more powerful telescopes. In 1655 it was reported that Wilkins and Wren

239. Ephemerides 1655; Matthew Wren, *Monarchy Asserted* (Oxford, 1659), sig. A8r.

240. Ephemerides 1655, for the first reference to Wren's illustrations; R. Hooke, *Micrographia* (London, 1665), sig. g2r–v.

241. James Harrington, *The Prerogative of Popular Government* (London, 1658), Preface. Matthew Wren, *Monarchy Asserted*, dedication to Wilkins, sig. A7v–8r.

242. R. T. Gunther, 'The First Observatory Instruments of the Savilian Professors', *The Observatory*, 1937, *60*: 190–7.

243. Letter of Ward to Isham (249), p.69.

244. Ephemerides 1655.

were constructing an eighty-foot telescope.[244] A more modest one of twenty-four feet seems to have been the outcome of this work. With the aid of this instrument Wren was preparing 'a Selenographia which will be far more accurate than that of Hevelius, doing all by rule & demonstration which hath been hitherto done by guesses'.[245] He also intended to improve on Hevelius's theory of the moon's libration. But his most successful astronomical venture was to collate the observations on Saturn which had been made by Oxford astronomers since 1649, and to propound a new theory to explain the 'phases' of this planet. His hypothesis of an elliptical corona was probably first publicly announced at his Gresham College lectures in 1658. Wren was probably unaware that Huyghens had independently evolved a similar, but superior theory of a circular corona.[246]

The successful establishment of the Wadham observatory, the improvement of telescopes, the systematic collection of data to solve astronomical problems, and the assembly of a collection of mechanical inventions, established a basis for a more ambitious enterprise. Again Wilkins was the prime mover. Late in 1653 Hartlib noted:

> 'They are now erecting a College for experiments et mechanicks at Oxford, towards which Dr. Wilkins hath given 200 lib. It is over the Schooles or in the long gallery, where all the models of inventions, arts etc, are to bee reserved with a treatise added to each of them shewing the structure and use of it.'[247]

According to this plan Wilkins hoped to establish a repository for the scientific instruments and inventions of the Oxford circle, which would be placed under the superintendence of Ralph Greatorex, the London instrument maker, who had strong associations with Oxford. Commenting on the same project, Ward wrote of a 'reall designe' to erect a 'Magneticall, Mechanicall and Optick Schoole, furnished with the best instruments, and Adapted for the most usefull experiments in all those faculties'.[248]

In 1657 the scheme was still under consideration. Evelyn intimated that his writings on art techniques were appropriate to 'that Mathematico-Chymico-Mechanical School designed by our noble friend Dr. Wilkinson [sic]'. In a much later reminiscence, Evelyn assumed that this school had actually existed, furnished with an 'elaborator, and

245. Ephemerides 1655. In 1658 Boyle claimed that a 35-foot telescope had been successfully produced at Oxford: letter from Robert Wood to Hartlib, 9 February 1658, HP XXXIII 1. In 1650 Hevelius sent Hartlib copies of his *Selenographia* (1647) for deposit in the Oxford, Cambridge and Dublin libraries. Wren himself claimed to have used telescopes of 6, 12, 22 feet and 35 feet: Albert van Helden, 'Christopher Wren's *De Corpore Saturni*', *Notes & Records,* 1968, *23*: 213–29.

246. A. van Helden, *op. cit.* For the interest in this question in Ireland, see T. C. Barnard (*op. cit.* above, p.66, n.112), pp.136, 141.

247. Ephemerides 1653 [after 7 November].

248. Ward (307), p.36.

other instruments', until it was dispersed at the restoration.[249] However, as an ardent royalist during the interregnum he had not given such optimistic accounts of the success of Wilkins's project: there prevailed, he had then complained, an 'uncharitable and perverse' climate of opinion which was uncongenial to the establishment of institutions modelled on Solomon's House.[250]

The evolution of scientific activity at Oxford under the aegis of the Oxford Experimental Philosophy Club was not greeted with universal approbation within the university. As will be seen below, the educational reformers believed that the new science deserved more formal recognition, while traditionalists feared that the informal club was evolving too rapidly towards a collegiate form of organisation. Although Wilkins and his associates left their ultimate goals undefined, they undoubtedly aroused suspicion among those orthodox academics who vigilantly maintained the traditions of Oxford against all innovation. Anthony Wood attributed this opposition to men of 'the old stamp', who remained faithful to ancient authority, scholastic and polemical divinity, disputations and polite learning. These persons stigmatised the members of Wilkins's club as 'Vertuosi', and the work of the members as more suitable for quacks and apothecaries' boys than for serious academic philosophers.[251] All projects, even the laudable schemes for educating poor theology students, were likely to be suspected of being attempts at undermining traditional scholastic standards. Hence, in spite of their seeming to evince proper feeling, for example by their attacks on radicals such as John Webster, the agents of the 'Mechanical College' were suspected of sympathising with the programme of the external critics, or with the Durham projectors. An additional complicating factor was the personal animosity which the Wilkins circle aroused because of its Cromwellian sympathies and career successes. Their rivals were willing to misrepresent the intentions of the experimental philosophers, in order to discredit them before their conservative colleagues. Among even the Puritans at Oxford, the members of the Wilkins circle were subjected to the disapproval of 'peevish People', to whom they were 'mere Moral Men without the power of Godliness'.[252]

Either these unspecified critics employed Henry Stubbe to make articulate their grievances, or alternatively he systematically set about discrediting the natural philosophers on his own initiative.[253] This com-

249. Letter from Evelyn to Boyle, 9 May 1657, Evelyn (96), iv, pp.92–3. Letter from Evelyn to W. Wotton, 12 September 1703, *ibid.*, iv, pp.391–2. Shapiro (259), pp.138–9, wrongly conflates this project with Hartlib's Office of Address.

250. Letter from Evelyn to Boyle, 3 September 1659, Evelyn (96), iii, p.116.

251. Wood *Hist. & Antiq.*, ii, pp.663–4. On the increasing scholastic resentment of the natural philosophers, see above, pp.143–4.

252. Pope (223), p.43.

253. For Stubbe, see *DNB;* Wood *Athenae,* iii, p.1068; Wood *Fasti,* ii, pp.175, 193.

plicated man began his career, as it was to end, in total and uncompromising opposition to everything associated with the Royal Society and its Oxford progenitors. In an extensive series of pamphlets, Stubbe lampooned the enemy from every angle, the central target for his accusations being John Wallis. First he supported Hobbes against Wallis in an ostensibly mathematical dispute about squaring the circle. Then, a specific and singularly appropriate opportunity to discredit Wallis arose when Wallis sought to accumulate, with the office of Savilian professor of geometry, that of Custos Archivorum. There was clearly strong feeling against Wallis's holding both offices, enough to lead him to compose a broad-sheet justifying his position. He was elected, but Stubbe put out a pamphlet arguing the unstatutory nature of the appointment and accusing Wallis of manipulating the election. He asserted that Wallis was motivated by avarice and that by this manoeuvre the mathematician had engrossed for himself a much higher salary than that received by other distinguished, European mathematicians.[254]

Stubbe produced in 1659, the year which was marked by renewed criticism of the universities, some of his most effective and subversive pamphlets, striking at the Puritans from left and from right. The venom of the satire of one of these 'pestilential' books earned for him his expulsion from Christ Church by the Presbyterian Dean Edward Reynolds. It is a tribute to the subtlety of Stubbe's writing that its satirical purpose has generally been overlooked by modern writers, who have found in disconnected excerpts from Stubbe appropriate illustrations of a variety of conflicting points of view. Stubbe's circumstances necessitated an ambiguous stance; he attempted to serve an anti-clerical, republican patron, Sir Henry Vane junior, while cautiously exhibiting his own social and religious conservatism and convictions about the anarchistic tendencies of radical reformation. For the immediate purpose of discrediting the Presbyterians then in power however, separatists and Anglicans were united.

A temporary ally for Stubbe in this debate was James Harrington, whose *Commonwealth of Oceana* (1656) caused immediate consternation in the universities. The principal apologist for the latter was the royalist Matthew Wren, who was a pupil of Wilkins; this connection prompted republicans to scorn the Oxford Experimental Club, its activities and political allegiances. As in earlier debates, reference to science in the universities was made in the context of the general assault on the learned ministry. To Harrington and Vane, Wilkins was a convenient representative of the learned ministry and anti-republican

254. Wallis, *Reasons shewing the consistency of the place of Custos Archivorum with that of a Savilian Professor* [1658]. The Bodleian copy, Wood 515, has a note: 'Published by Dr. Joh. Wallis 1657/[8] Febr.' Stubbe, *The Savilian Professours Case Stated. Together with severall reasons urged against his capacity of standing for the publique office of Antiquary in the University of Oxford,* 1658; preface dated 10 March 1657/[8].

government. Therefore his entire circle and activities were subject to censure. In the interests of higher priorities it became necessary to overlook the originality and effectiveness of Wilkins's scientific endeavours.

Stubbe took up various points which could be found in the writings of such figures as Harrington or Milton at this time. Stubbe's long tract *A Light Shining out of Darkness* (1659) contained a fanatical attack on the universities and learned clergy, but it employed a language and style more eccentric and disconnected than that used by any of the mechanick preachers. The tract was anonymous, but the preface bore a clear sign of Stubbe's authorship, as detected at the time by Anthony Wood. Stubbe's tract had little contemporary influence, but recently it has been cited as a serious quaker criticism of learning and the universities. The author indeed rehearsed the whole repertoire of historical and biblical arguments against the learned clergy, with the explicit intention of supporting the priesthood of all believers; but his mode of expression was instead calculated to expose the destructive consequences of the abandonment of learning and the established church. He dwelled repeatedly on the desirability of a ministry of 'Weavers, (or Combers of Wool) Coblers, Fullers, and Illiterate and Exceeding Rusticke'.[255] The universities and their degrees were scrutinised and ridiculed.[256] Specific proposals were made to abandon degrees in theology, discourage celibacy, forbid the reading of heathen authors and abolish tithes. Reorganisation of the universities by the state was demanded.

Such proposals were unexceptionably part of the sectarian programme. It is not until the language and the style of the work are examined that Stubbe's double purpose is exhibited. Particularly in the conclusions he fully exposed the inconsistencies of the opinions he was reciting. Long quotations from the most celebrated critics of classical learning were given in such a way as to underline their degree of familiarity with pagan writing and classical languages. Contradicting the claim he had just made for a ministry financed by voluntary contributions, he demanded that all clergymen should support themselves by 'some petty handy-crafts'—a remark meant to be reminiscent of Dell. Finally he pleaded for the dispersal of the goods of the church to the poor. This provided occasion for reference to the rich canons of Christ Church, whom he proceeded to pillory as unlawful monsters and hypocrites for their ostentatious mode of living, which involved accumulating wealth and riding in coaches.[257] This concluding portion underlines Stubbe's concern to create dissension among the Puritans by contrasting a caricature of the illiterate and humble primitive church with the corrupt and powerful scholastic ministry in control of Oxford.

255. Stubbe, *A Light Shining out of Darknes* (London, 1659), p.18.
256. *Ibid.*, pp.139–52, 157–63.
257. *Ibid.*, pp.169–86.

The canons of Christ Church, his own college, were singled out for particular censure here and elsewhere in this book, and indeed throughout his early writings.

Stubbe experimented with another style of criticism in *Sundry Things from several Hands concerning the University of Oxford* (1659), a work which has attracted some notice because of the suggestion that it represented a genuine proposal by Henry Wilkinson to establish a Mechanical School at Christ Church.[258] As with *Light out of Darkness,* the identity of the author must be determined from incidental references in the text. Wilkinson is easily eliminated; the evidence for his authorship comes from a reference to his name by Evelyn which was obviously a slip of the pen, Wilkins being clearly indicated by the context and by associated letters.[259] Once the satirical nature of the text is recognised, Stubbe is the obvious candidate for authorship. He was associated with Westminster School and Christ Church, the two institutions discussed; he was a critic of the experimental science and systematic divinity outlined in the central section of *Sundry Things;* his particular enemies, the canons of Christ Church and John Wallis, are singled out for criticism in the final section; finally, the only marginal note in the text is a laudatory reference to his own contribution to the Custos Archivorum debate.[260]

The form of the pamphlet is suggestively reminiscent of the petitions on university reform framed by Hartlib and Thomas Gilson a few years earlier; reference also seems to be made to the various proposals for specialist colleges. There is no reason to believe that the work genuinely represents the views of 'Several' different hands, and the author was certainly not 'well affected' to parliament. But he was clearly extremely well-informed on all aspects of the interregnum debate on the universities. Complete familiarity with context is a characteristic feature of Stubbe's writings.

The final section of *Sundry Things* is the most explicitly malicious. In twenty-five brief sections, the author parodied a wide range of features and personalities of the parliamentary regime in Oxford. Among those attacked is Henry Wilkinson, the putative author of the piece. Many leading intruded academics were named and attacked, primarily for incompetence and personal avarice. The whole parliamentarian government of the institution was regarded as detrimental

258. *Sundry Things* is dated by Thomason, 29 June 1659; reprinted in *Harleian Miscellany,* 1810, vi, pp.86–91. The sources for the mechanical school hypothesis are R. F. Jones, 'Puritanism, Science and Christ Church', *Isis,* 1939, *31*: 65–7; J. I. Cope, 'Evelyn, Boyle & Dr. Wilkinson's Mathematico-Chymico-Mechanicall School', *Isis,* 1959, *50*: 30–2. The suggestion that *Sundry Things* was a satire was originally made by Professor P. M. Rattansi in a personal communication.

259. See Purver (230), p.40; Shapiro (259), p.138. See above, p.171.

260. Wood noted in his copy of the pamphlet (Bodleian, Wood 515), 'Reputed to be written by Joh. Wagstaffe of Oriel Coll. but false'. Also in Wood *Fasti,* ii, p.220.

to its academic traditions. Even the Oxford petition against Durham College was only applauded because it was 'incumbent upon parliaments not to multiply asses'.

Stubbe's pamphlet began with an apparently exemplary address of loyalty to Richard Cromwell's parliament, but even this was betrayed by its exaggeratedly subservient tone, and the author's malicious intent is made apparent by suggestions about general disloyalty within the university.

The central and most important part of *Sundry Things* proposed the reform of Christ Church and its sister institution, Westminster School. In this section the enemy was precisely identified. The canons were openly abused for 'their frauds, dilapidations, mal-administration of discipline, disaffection, and general worthlessness'. The only solution was complete reconstitution of the college, under completely new statutes which would be framed to implement certain *avant-garde* educational ideas. Since parliament had been particularly vigilant to enforce the conformity and puritan associations of Christ Church, this choice of institution would have appeared singularly inappropriate. The proposals would also have seemed an amalgam of the utopian, the impracticable and the undesirable. The college was to be governed from its junior partner Westminster School, which would supply all students. The traditional relationship between the two institutions would thereby be reversed. The intention of this suggestion would have seemed at least ambiguous, since Westminster School, in spite of its popularity with the parliamentarian families, was under a staunch royalist, Richard Busby, who had been on bad terms with the recently retired Independent Dean of Christ Church, John Owen.

Once selected, the students would submit to a rigorous training in preparation for a self-sacrificing service of the commonwealth. In their political studies, they would be made fully acquainted with the reasons for their general 'subjection'. The projected staff of the college was an eccentric collection of public teachers and tutors. Professorial appointments were to cover civil law and politics, Descartes's philosophy, Gassendi's philosophy, physic, anatomy and finally 'useful logic and civil rhetorick'. The professor of politics was appointed to instruct students 'to prefer a commonwealth before monarchy'. With respect to practical work in science, Stubbe proposed that laboratories be erected for the study of magnetism, optics, mechanics and chemistry. The specialities chosen for the science professors were probably intended to parody intellectual fashions among Oxford natural philosophers: there was indeed interest in the new philosophies of Descartes and Gassendi. The laboratory proposals were probably designed to mimic Wilkins's proposed scientific school. Characteristically Stubbe introduced anomalous elements into these proposals. For instance, the chemistry laboratory was to be financed partly by the state, partly by a levy on students of medicine and partly by the Apothecary to the College of Physicians.

Any such suggestions were bound to stir up resentment among the parties so named.

The dominant element in the new college would have been a body of sixty Fellows, forty of whom were to be engaged in training men for the puritan ministry. Again characteristically, Stubbe showed close familiarity with contemporary thought on university reform, appearing to share the widely-felt enthusiasm for the training of the ministry, the construction of scientific laboratories, and the teaching of new philosophy. However, the exaggerated political partisanship with which these proposals were presented, and their juxtaposition with what the reader was likely to find unpalatable, were guaranteed to create an impression of unhealthy departure from the recognised academic functions. Although new philosophy was in favour, the Platonists had fully awakened the public to the materialistic dangers of Gassendi and Descartes. It would have been acceptable for professors to consider new philosophies, but advocates of *philosophia libera* were opposed to partisanship as much in modern as in ancient philosophy. Most reformers had produced innocuous and modest proposals for new institutions to supplement the existing university structure. By suggesting the total reconstitution of the colleges, under strict supervision from London, Stubbe called for a reaction from the colleges, which traditionally had jealously and successfully protected their autonomy. No doubt remembering the manner in which the colleges had fiercely resisted the recommendations of the parliamentary boards of visitors, Stubbe now introduced the even more dictatorial agency of parliamentary 'censors', who would supervise every aspect of academic life.

The different circumstances of modern education make it possible for us to regard *Sundry Things* as an enlightened and straightforward practical proposal for the reorientation of higher education. But from the vantage point of the seventeenth century this pamphlet would have served rather to generate disquiet among academics about the consequences of innovation. Stubbe was therefore merely exploiting a conservative sentiment which he knew to be prevalent among his colleagues. Even the Wilkins circle scrupulously avoided becoming identified with the advocates of educational change. In this light, the failure of the Oxford Experimental Club, Wilkins's 'Mechanical College', or even the College for Ministers referred to below, to develop a settled institutional basis is unsurprising. There was a universal willingness, once the dangers of innovation were revealed, to withdraw under the institutional carapace of the colleges and to maintain educational traditons. It was Stubbe's function in *A Light Shining out of Darkness* and *Sundry Things* to stir up anxieties about religious or educational reform and to frighten his audience into renewing their faith in Anglican and scholastic values. Only in private rooms and as a personal diversion, his writings implied, was science an acceptable element in university life.

The Wilkins proposals for a Mechanical School enabled the experimental philosophers to test reactions to the incipient institutionalisation of science within the universities. The response signalled by Stubbe indicated the desirability of seeking an alternative institutional basis for further scientific development. The diversion of a certain amount of scientific activity to London was perhaps an immediate reaction to this climate of opinion at Oxford; as a trend it was greatly accelerated by the ejection, at the restoration, of most of the parliamentarian nominees from their comfortable academic positions.

(vi) The Throne of the Beast

Detailed examination of the place of science and medicine in the universities during the interregnum vindicates the view that parliamentary interference and puritan intellectuals provided favourable conditions for the expression of the new philosophy. Both the intruded academics, and their fair-minded royalist opponents, were aware of the significance of this movement. For the first time since the Middle Ages the English universities appeared to have become the focal point for developments in medicine, science, mathematics and philosophy. Thus successive later generations of reformers have turned to this period when seeking precedents to support their proposals for innovation. Perhaps particularly during the concerted effort to modernise the institutions of nineteenth-century Oxford, the interregnum was adopted as a source of inspiration by reformers.[261] Currently, the work of historians of science amply vindicates this record of creative scientific achievement on the part of the academics of the interregnum.

It is therefore somewhat surprising that this intellectual revolution was not greeted with universal applause within the puritan movement.[262] Not only extreme separatists, but also a wide range of moderate Puritans, were deeply dissatisfied with the university settlement; and paradoxically they fixed upon the neglect of the sciences as one of the main weaknesses of the new academic order.

There was hence little unanimity among the parliamentarians and Puritans concerning university reform. They all believed that higher education should reflect the religious values of the Reformation, but at

261. Burrows (42); 'Oxford under the Puritans', *Quarterly Review,* 1882, *154*: 469–94.

262. For general discussions of puritan attitudes to learning see James Conant, 'The Advancement of Learning during the Puritan Commonwealth', Massachusetts Historical Society *Proceedings,* 1936, *61*: 3–31; Richard Schlatter, 'The Higher Learning in Puritan England', *Historical Magazine of the Protestant Episcopalian Church,* 1954, *23*: 166–87; Leo Solt, 'Anti-Intellectualism in the Puritan Revolution', *Church History,* 1956, *24*: 306–16; Barbara K. Lewalski, 'Milton on Learning and the Learned Ministry Controversy', *HLQ,* 1961, *24*: 267–81; *idem, Milton's Brief Epic* (London 1966), Chapter XI; Shapiro (259), Chapter IV; Greaves (122), Chapters II & IV.

a practical level there were sharp differences of outlook; every group within the puritan movement aspired to gain control of the universities and their divinity faculties. Sectional interest tended to assume priority over intellectual goals. Most Puritans favoured the extension and reform of ministerial training in the universities, while the separatists demanded the complete abolition of theological education. Sectarian divisions prevented the Puritans within the universities from agreeing on any positive course of action, and the external critics were themselves divided about certain basic issues. But on secular matters the puritan reformers outside the universities exhibited a much greater degree of consensus. Moderates and radicals urged the state to modify university statutes in order to introduce a much greater representation of studies which would directly relate to the economic life of the nation. Furthermore, neither the radical nor the moderate interest limited its horizons to the current institutional arrangements. In contemplating desirable reforms, they quickly concluded that radical change was necessary at all levels in education. This prospect was anathema to the Puritans in power in the universities. They regarded their critics as opponents of civilised values, whereas the reformers came to regard the academics as agents of Antichrist.

Because the proponents of reform were obliged to disparage informal intellectual developments within the universities, they have been too readily dismissed as well-intentioned but ignorant pedlars of pseudoscience. However, on questions of scientific methodology and natural philosophy there existed more common ground than either the intruded academics or their outside critics could afford to admit without sacrificing to their opponent some credit on social and religious issues. Such a compromise was unthinkable for parties convinced that their attitudes to education were completely consistent with their religious premises.

Both universities were briefly brought into confrontation with popular religious movements during military occupation in the Civil War. At Cambridge the effects of military occupation were slightly less severe, since the academics were never given the opportunity for military action, but there were many signs of antagonism between the army and the university. Religious practices provided an obvious point of conflict; common soldiers asserted their spiritual authority, and their prejudices were supported by parliamentary ordinances designed to reorganise chapels along lines acceptable to the new puritan order. In one characteristic incident a suspected papist, the Lady Margaret preacher at Cambridge, was chased through the streets after attempting to deliver a Latin sermon.[263]

At Oxford the friction between academics and the army was, if anything, more pronounced. The close association between the royalist

263. Tatham (277), pp.105–10. The preacher was William Power, the uncle of Henry Power.

party and the university stiffened the army's belief that there was a strong correlation between university education and alien religious and political beliefs. To the parliamentarians conducting the siege, Oxford was an epitome of all forms of malignancy; and there was no shortage of religious enthusiasts able to expound the labyrinthine depths of these transgressions to the soldiers. Once the root cause of iniquity was known, solutions suggested themselves. The first necessity was to solve the military dimension of the problem, but it was appreciated that this must be followed by the more difficult exercise of political and social reconstruction.

One of the most important influences on popular opinion within the army was William Dell who, along with Webster, became one of the most active writers on the educational dimension of spiritual religion.[264] Of one of his sermons preached to the besieging army it was reported that

> 'many soldiers were at each sermon, divers of them climbing up trees to hear, for it was in the orchard before his excellency's [Fairfax's] tent, and it is very observable to consider the love and unity which is amongst the soldiers, Presbytery and Independency making no breach.'[265]

Many of the humble climbers, like Zacchaeus, came down from their trees increased in religious stature, and convinced that the 'Kingdom of God should immediately appear'.[266] The substance of Dell's teaching is found in a sermon preached a few days later to a similar audience.[267] This sermon stressed the sufficiency of spiritual faith provided that this was assisted by the 'clear and evident' teaching of the Word. In Dell's view the army exemplified the qualities of righteousness; its tour of duty had resulted in the spread of 'assemblies of saints'. 'Humane wisdom and learning' was regarded as irrelevant to religious experience; Dell also drew attention to the evil consequences of the division of the puritan movement into Presbyterian and Independent factions, and the degrading influence of the 'old professors', who were hampered by their scholastic equipment. Dell, although having much in common with other puritan writers, differed from the majority in carrying his arguments to an extreme conclusion, with the result that his doctrines were deeply offensive to the powerful Presbyterian faction as well as to the more obvious Anglican enemy. However in spite of protests, voiced even in parliament, Dell emerged unscathed, owing to the support which he enjoyed from all ranks of the army. He was selected to officiate at the wedding of Henry Ireton to Cromwell's

264. For Dell see Walker (299); Webster (323).

265. *Perfect Occurrences*, 24 May 1646. The preacher of the other sermon was Sedgwick. Walker (299), Chapter IV.

266. Luke 19: 9–11.

267. *The Building, Beauty, Teaching* (75); Walker (299), Chapter V.

daughter at a church outside Oxford, and he was chosen to deliver the articles of surrender for Oxford to the House of Commons.[268]

Soldiers entered the university town on 24 June, fortified by their chaplains with scriptural armaments and eager to assert their authority over the learned clergy. They 'thrust themselves into the pulpits, purposely by their rascally doctrine to obtain either proselytes, or draw off from their loyal principles and orthodox religion the scholars and inhabitants'.[269] Both soldiers and chaplains disputed with academics, disrupting normal university functions and substituting attacks on 'human learning' for normal lectures.[270] The most popular handbook of the assailants was Samuel How's *The Sufficiency of the Spirits Teaching, without human Learning* (1640), a tract which enjoyed great popularity among separatists for the rest of the century. This work opened with verses which included lines comparing university education unfavourably with the experience of the author, who was a cobbler by profession:

> 'Cambridge and Oxford, may their glory now,
> Vail to a Cobler if they know by How:
> Though big with Art, they cannot overtop
> The Spirits teaching in a Coblers shop.'

The vigour of this onslaught, which was directed specifically against the divinity faculty, was represented by Anglicans and Presbyterians alike as a threat to all learning and universities. But it is noticeable that, of the four chaplains singled out for criticism by Anthony Wood, Dell and Peter were conspicuous for their interest in secular education while Saltmarsh was a sophisticated Cambridge scholar who incorporated the Platonist position into his general religious attitude. It is clear therefore that the opponents of the universities were highly selective in their criticisms, although the vigour of their denunciation of scholastic divinity and their total commitment to spiritual religion might superficially be mistaken for an aversion to learning itself. When seen in context, it is apparent that the opponents of scholastic divinity recognised the need for a positive approach to higher education, consistent with the programme of social reconstruction which it was hoped would be implemented after military victory. Vigorous action in this area of social reform was urged in the thanksgiving sermon on the surrender of Oxford. In violent language the preacher, Henry Wilkinson, urged parliament not to fall back into complacency. It was the duty of parliament to 'purge and reforme that place [Oxford] above others', if necessary by recruiting new men from abroad. John Dury addressed parliament in similar terms, calling for the restoration of the 'purity of spiritual learning' in the universities and the abolition of 'the giberidge

268. *CJ*, iv, pp.587–8, 24 June 1646.
269. Wood *Fasti*, ii, p.100.
270. *Ibid.*, p.101.

of Scholastical Divinity' which was the product of corrupt human reason. He further appealed to the state to provide schools for 'all sorts of children and youths'. There would be no protection against future dissoluteness, if formal education were disregarded.[271]

Once the universities had come firmly under the influence of parliament preparations were made for reform. Parliament had interfered in various ways since 1640, and it had accepted an obligation to instigate more positive and comprehensive changes. The Remonstrance of 1641 contained the first of many expressions of an intention 'to reform and purge the fountains of learning, the two Universities, that the streams flowing from thence may be clear and pure'. A parliamentary committee was promptly established to consider appropriate policies.[272] Then in 1646 the articles for the surrender of Oxford guaranteed the rights of academics and the protection of university property, but only pending 'any reformation there intended by the Parliament'.[273] Gradually a complex machinery evolved for regulating the universities; the rhetorical language of reform continued, but political and religious aims predominated, and most aspects of education were largely overlooked. At first the authorities limited themselves to such elementary objectives as the control of religious observation and chapel furnishings; they then turned to the more difficult task of enforcing political conformity among academics and scholars. Regulation of the personnel of the universities during the political turmoils of the interregnum became an all-absorbing problem. This emphasis satisfied the major religious and political groups, whose academic representatives, once installed, favoured a return of the universities and colleges to their traditional autonomy. Furthermore, there was little enthusiasm for reforming to any significant degree either college or university statutes. Gradually control and initiative slipped away from the state and its participation in the management of Oxford and Cambridge became limited to sporadic acts of sponsorship such as its grant of financial aid to Cambridge for the acquisition of oriental books and the extension of its library.[274] Educational reformers gained little comfort from the supplementations of salaries which were another striking feature of parliamentary intervention.

None the less, even when expectations of major reform had been disappointed, there was as we shall see no relaxation of pressure for a state educational initiative from a considerable body of activists ranging from Dury to Winstanley. There is also evidence that these reformers commanded a significant degree of respect both within the army and in parliament. They produced a tide of pamphlets which, if

271. Wilkinson, *Mirand, Stupend* (London, 1646), 21 July 1646. Dury, *Israels Call* (85), 26 November 1645.

272. Rushworth (252), iii, pp.437–51; article 187. The Committee was established on 22 April 1642—*CJ*, ii, pp.126, 167, 233.

273. Burrows (42), p.lvi.

274. See above, p.152.

not successful in promoting their practical objectives for the universities, was at least sufficient to keep the idea of educational change alive. Politicians sympathetic to reform exercised a small, but noticeable influence on university appointments; they also prevented the universities' becoming complacent, by repeatedly raising the question of university reform in parliament, particularly in 1653 and 1659. Finally, they worked for the extension of higher education, their exertions leading eventually to the foundation of the Cromwellian college at Durham. But they were more successful at a general level; significant financial assistance for elementary education was introduced, in the context of the work of the committees established to promote 'godly learning'. These positive achievements, although not amounting to an educational revolution, indicate that the reformers were not entirely without influence at a public level, while as conspicuous advocates of new educational doctrines their informal influence was very considerable indeed.

It is noteworthy that the puritan critics of scholastic education found little place in universities, even after the wholesale ejection of royalist academics. For instance the leading army chaplains, who had performed such an important service during the war, were largely passed over in favour of more orthodox divines. Other prominent spokesmen on educational reform were also scrupulously avoided by the universities.

The Visitors supervising the reorganisation of the universities conducted this operation with the greatest caution, whereas parliament, and the commission controlling the universities headed by the mystic Francis Rous, were inclined to be more adventurous. Immediately after the fall of Oxford, an order to provide Hartlib with a suitable place there was passed in the House of Commons.[275] But no action was taken on this. In 1647, Cudworth preached his celebrated sermon to the House attacking scholastic divinity and defending the spiritual faith. He appealed for parliament 'to promote Ingenuous learning, and cast a favourable influence upon it', arguing that secular learning deserved the support which was traditionally accorded to religion. It was again immediately ordered that Hartlib should be found 'some Place of Benefit in the University of Oxon'.[276] However in spite of influential support from London neither he, nor Dury, nor Pell succeeded in obtaining university preferment, although all three were exemplary scholars concerned with the improvement of higher education.

In a few exceptional cases, known educational reformers were intruded into the universities. With the aid of prominent army officers and of John Sadler, Dell secured the Mastership of Caius College, Cambridge—an appointment which would have amazed the college's founder, the catholic humanist physician, John Caius. Hartlib's associates Sadler and Worthington also became heads of Cambridge col-

275. *CJ*, iv, pp.587–8; 25 June 1646.
276. Cudworth (64), preface. *CJ*, v, pp.131–3.

leges, but neither played any notable part in educational debates.[277] Parliament and the army also recorded some successes at a junior level; for instance Petty and Robert Wood were granted fellowships, which were used as stepping-stones for preferment into the Irish civil service. But in spite of such parliamentary intervention, most of the proponents of educational change were excluded from university positions. From this position of independence, they exercised to the full the role of university critics. Moderates and sectarians were united on a diagnosis of the defects of higher education, and they evolved similar programmes of reform. A wide range of authors, including Milton, Hartlib, Dury, Hall, Peter, Biggs, Dell and Webster, maintained the pressure of criticism on the universities, their efforts reaching a peak in late 1653 during the Saints' Parliament. Each writer brought a slightly different perspective to the problem and their combined influence prevented the universities from attaining any sense of security. Academics were driven into alignment with the conservative clergy outside Oxford and Cambridge, who maintained that any departure from the pattern of traditional education would undermine piety and learning.

For their part, the reformers were able to appeal to the general sentiment in favour of revealed religion. The Cambridge Platonists were at one with the army chaplains in emphasising personal revelation, and in their objection to scholastic divinity. But the implications for education of this position could differ radically. The Platonists had no desire to shake the foundations of traditional education: they merely sought to draw attention to its limitations and to create a favourable climate for a more critical and erudite philosophy. By contrast more radical thinkers used the indictment of scholastic education as a convenient platform for an assault on the learned ministry and as the basis for their plans to reorganise higher education according to secular criteria.

'All the learning I had at Oxford, I layd out and improved in opposing truth' was Pinnel's estimate of his university education.[278] The attempt to bind up the mystery of Christ in 'Schoolmen and Common-place-books', or in sermons couched in 'Logicall definitions, divisions and sub-divisions', had been a positive hindrance to his salvation and useful service in the ministry. Most clergymen were never able to transcend this defective education to obtain a true religious insight; his own spiritual enlightenment was attributable to the influence of 'simple countrey people, husband-men, weavers' rather than to any formal education.[279] Similarly Dell claimed that Christian virtue was better exemplified by the rank and file of the army than by learned divines.

The reformers left some role for the minister, but proposed that he should have a different intellectual and economic relationship with

277. *CJ*, vi, p.204; 4 May 1649. Walker (299), p.105.
278. Henry Pinnel, *A Word of Prophesy* (214), p.49.
279. Pinnel, *This Years Fruit* (215), pp.24–5.

the rest of the community. Because of the democratisation of spiritual experience, the minister was only an equal rather than superior participant in the religious life of his flock; but he could assist them over scriptural interpretation and with education, and possibly provide vocational guidance. His income could be derived from subscriptions, or possibly from useful work, but not from tithes. This would bring about a much closer and more harmonious relationship between the minister and his flock. But Pinnel and his associates appreciated that this arrangement would only succeed, if there was a higher general level of education. Pinnel's views were representative of a large section of the puritan movement, of whom it is evident that their attitudes to education and the learned ministry were determined by their approach to the doctrine of salvation.

It was therefore necessary for the reformers to mount the strongest possible defence of their soteriological position, in order to establish the premises from which to conduct arguments about secular issues. Views on educational reform were as they realised most appropriately expressed as a corollary of their theological ideas. Accordingly it is often found that even brief and unspecific comments on education were preceded by long preparatory theological discourses. At the climax of the educational controversy, in 1653, the sermons delivered by Dell and Webster on the power of grace greatly exceeded in volume their better-known proposals for educational reform. In replying, their opponents also concentrated on religious issues. Thus attitudes to the educational role of science can only be understood in terms of the standpoints adopted in the wider religious debate.

Unlike most of his colleagues in the universities, Dell refused to come to terms with the scholastic system. His connection with Caius College was never more than tenuous and what connection he had he used primarily to add weight to his censures of the learned clergy. The substance of his views remained consistent with the sermons which he delivered to the army besieging Oxford. If anything the tone of his writing became more extreme; Dell realised that his siege of the universities from within had become single-handed, owing to the surrender of his former clerical allies. Dell's major sermons were delivered in 1653. *The Stumbling Stone* was preached to a congregation which consisted partly of academics and partly of townspeople. The sermon was not designed to give comfort to the scholars, being explicitly directed against '*All* Universities' as well as any citizens 'baptized into the University Spirit'.[280] The central aim of this sermon was to justify the view that the reformation of the church necessitated the removal of the clergy. On theological and historical grounds Dell argued that the true faith had been most fruitfully cultivated in communities of poor men, without a segregated ministry. The learned ministers, with their 'dull and drowsie Divinity of Synods, and Schools, degrees, caps and gowns'

280. Dell (76), sig. A2r–v.

could not be defended upon scriptural authority; indeed they were less well-equipped from a religious point of view than common men infused with the Spirit of God.[281] Since these views might be construed as implying opposition to all learning, Dell emphasised:

> 'If the Universities will stand upon an Humane and Civil account, as Schools of Good Learning for the instructing and educating Youth in the knowledge of the Tongues, and of the liberal Arts and Sciences, thereby to make them usefull and serviceable to the Commonwealth . . . then let them stand, during the Pleasure of God.'[282]

This was a sentiment acceptable to both the mechanick preachers and more moderate reformers. In this sermon Dell gave no further intimation of his views on university education, but the preface announced his intention of delivering a 'Two-fold Testimonie' on the reform of the church and state. This sequel to *The Stumbling Stone* was published in the same year under the title *The Trial of Spirits,* and was another two-part sermon addressed to an academic and local congregation. Here Dell delivered his most bitter indictment of the puritan academics, who were 'now so full gorged with the flesh of Kings' that they were content to 'take their ease, and comply with the world and worldly Church and the teachers thereof'.[283] In an appendix he replied to the spokesman of the puritan establishment, Sidrach Simpson, the Independent Master of Pembroke College, who had been preaching against Dell at Cambridge.

The Trial of Spirits contained sentiments about the deficiencies of the learned clergy and scholastic divinity which were by then extremely well-rehearsed. Universities earned the ultimate in condemnation: 'the throne of the Beast in these Nations; are the Universities, as the fountaine of the Ministery.'[284] Dell reiterated that his own enlightenment had occurred only after his emancipation from scholastic education. Sermons sprinkled with 'Hebrew, Greek, Latine, as with a perfume acceptable to the Nostrills of the world' were condemned, along with related 'fleshy wisdome, Rhetorical Eloquence, and Philosophical Learning'.[285] Heathen philosophy was singled out as the most pernicious aspect of higher education; this had reduced theology to subjection under an artificial, false and incomprehensible philosophical system. Pagan influences had been allowed to have their effect, with the result that certain heathen authors had 'more credit in the University, then Moses, or Christ himself'.[286]

281. *Ibid.*, p.19.
282. *Ibid.*, pp.26–7.
283. Dell (77), sig.aa2v; see also p.36 and J. Webster, *The Judgement Set* (325), p.86.
284. Dell (77), p.43.
285. *Ibid.*, pp.31, 60.
286. *Ibid.*, Appendix, 'A plain and necessary confutation of . . . Simpson', p.14.

These extreme pronouncements were inevitably reflected in Dell's general educational programme. It was difficult to see how 'daily converse with the Heathens, their vain Philosophers, and filthy and obscene Poets', so damaging to the divinity student, could be wholesome in any educational context.[287] Accordingly Dell concluded that disciplines which corrupted the minds of youth, segregating them from society and productive economic participation, were totally inappropriate foundations for higher education. A brief exposition of a more acceptable curriculum, entitled 'The Right Reformation of Learning', was given as a short final appendix to *The Trial of Spirits*. This appendix on education was Dell's last significant published work and although little more than a sketch, it is valuable in demonstrating his general sympathy with the Baconian reformers. Thereafter hostility within the university and his own temperamental inclinations caused Dell to withdraw into 'fellowship with poor plain Husbandmen and Tradesmen, who believe in Christ'.[288]

John Webster, perhaps the best known critic of the universities, approached the problem in the same manner as Dell. Again, specific educational recommendations were only expressed after careful theological preparation, in a series of sermons delivered by Webster at Allhallows Lombard Street. Webster's writings have greater clarity and breadth of intellectual interest than Dell's, and they are less repetitious. A convenient synopsis of his ideas is provided by *The Saints Guide,* a sermon preached in April 1653. Webster opened with a statement of an epistemological position, which was ascribed to patristic authors. This distinguished between 'acquired' and 'infused' knowledge. For religious purposes only the latter, revealed 'evidential and experimental knowledg' of the Holy Spirit, had validity. Acquired knowledge, the legacy of debased human civilisations, was irrelevant to religion, but it was acceptable in the secular sphere when sanctified by providence 'for the good of [God's] People'.[289] Taking this dichotomy as a basic premise, Webster attacked the universities, the learned clergy, and the system of tithes used to 'maintain an hive of Drones, Wasps and Hornets in their Monkish Cells'.[290] Their 'Academick and Scholastical Learning (the rotten rubbish of Ethnical and Babylonish ruines)' was irrelevant to the true ministry or to secular life.[291] Webster found that spiritual enlightenment brought total dissatisfaction with traditional intellectual standards. In the introduction to a collection of his sermons he declared an intention of ignoring debased learning: 'Here thou shalt not find Terms of Art, nor quirks of humane Learning, Fallen Wisdome . . . but naked truth declaring it self through an earthen

287. *Ibid.*, p.55.
288. *Ibid.*, Preface, sig. aa3v.
289. Webster (324), pp.1–5.
290. *Ibid.*, p.30.
291. *Ibid.*, p.13.

vessel in simplicity and plainnesse of speeche.'[292]

The educational implications of this religious position were defined in detail in *Academiarum Examen*, a tract composed shortly after the above sermons.[293] For the purposes of academic controversy Webster made somewhat clumsy use of the erudite manner of his adversaries, employing classical quotations and references to patristic sources which had been conspicuously absent from the sermons. The major defects of the universities were blamed on their association with the established church. The universities had abandoned their legitimate secular purpose and, as training centres for the ministry, they had assumed a function which was vain and doomed to forward antichristian ends. Spiritual knowledge flowed solely from a spiritual source and scholastic labours only served to impair receptivity to true illumination. The study of biblical languages was of little spiritual use when conducted in a scholastic atmosphere.[294] Languages were intrinsically harmless, but scholastic divinity and logic were intellectually debilitating.[295] From this 'putrid and muddy fountain doth arise all those hellish and dark foggs and vapours that like locusts crawling from this bottomlesse pit have overspread the face of the whole earth, filling men with pride, insolency, and self-confidence . . . and so become fighters against God, and his truth, and persecutors of all those that speak from the principle of that wisedome'.[296] Of all subjects scholastic divinity provoked Webster and a large chorus of reformers to a height of indignation.

In 1659, during the second peak of anti-university feeling, Milton gave even finer expression to puritan anti-scholastic feelings. He claimed that scholastic learning and disputations were 'such as tend least of all to the edification or capacitie of the people, but rather perplex and leaven pure doctrin with scholastical trash then enable any minister to the better preaching of the gospel'.[297] William Sprigg, in terms strongly reminiscent of Milton, prefaced his proposals for educational reform with an extensive attack on the learned ministry, the national church, and tithes.[298]

Opposition to scholastic theology, emphasis on the primacy of personal revelation, and an inclination to accept the equality of believers established considerable common ground between Dell, Webster, Milton, the Platonists and a broad range of Puritans. Although violent critics of the learned clergy, tithes and the national church, both Dell and

292. *The Judgement Set* (325), Preface, sig.A3r–v. For a similar statement see Sprat (266), p.113.

293. Preface dated 11 October 1653. The British Museum copy of *Academiarum Examen* (E.724(14)) has a note, '19 Dec. 1653'. For a facs. edn. with an introduction giving a comprehensive guide to Webster's scientific background, see Debus (72).

294. Webster (326), pp.3–9.

295. *Ibid.*, pp.9–18, 32–40.

296. *Ibid.*, p.12.

297. Milton, *Likeliest Means to Remove Hirelings* (London, 1659), p.138.

298. Sprigg (267), pp.21–44.

Webster were ministers and never relinquished this office until their ejection. Apart from extremists like the Quakers, most spiritual reformers accepted that the ministry could exercise an important function providing that the education, outlook and social role of the clergy were redefined. It would be an over-simplification to believe that the reformers were dedicated to a complete secularisation of education. The abolition of divinity degrees, and the abandonment of scholastic divinity and its rhetorical, logical and metaphysical appendages would have radically altered the complexion of the universities; theology would have enjoyed a less formal status in the university structure, but in another sense religion would have become a more pervasive influence, owing to the consecration of all activity to Christian ends.

Very few sections of puritan opinion advocated a complete retreat from higher education into a life entirely dominated by religious intuition and habit. The Quakers gradually became less iconoclastic about learning, and began to share the opinions of more moderate groups.[299] Even the mechanick preachers, a group castigated for 'being voyd of all learning, tongues, logick, arts, sciences, and the literall knowledge of the scripture' accepted that learning was acceptable 'in its proper place, which is for the repairing of that decay which came upon man for sin'.[300]

Plans for higher education were often elaborated in considerable detail, in anticipation of major reforms of the universities. Although the numerous educational reform programmes addressed to parliament and to influential political figures had a characteristically utopian flavour, they also included clear statements of policies appropriate for the contemporary situation. Science, particularly in its Baconian form, came to play an essential role in these proposals owing to the emphasis on education as a preparation for participation in economic affairs.

Experimental philosophy appealed to the puritan reformers for various reasons. First, it lacked some of the obvious defects of the scholastic system. Baconian science was basically anti-authoritarian; its criteria of proof rested on an appeal to experiment which was seen as analogous to personal revelation. Then, unlike Aristotelian natural philosophy, experimental science had no rigid associations with scholastic metaphysics and divinity. Accordingly Baconian science appeared to be an exemplary field of intellectual enquiry, which could be harmoniously reconciled with the puritan theological position. Secondly, because of its relevance to natural theology experimental science could be elevated to become an important ancillary to spiritual religion. Finally, the sciences could be applied to practical purposes, and in accordance with the social ethic of puritanism they could improve vocational proficiency and assist in the important task of social amelioration.

299. R. L. Greaves, 'The Early Quakers as Advocates of Educational Reform', *Quaker History*, 1969, *58*: 22–30.

300. Samuel Rutherford (253), p.38; Samuel How (154), p.17.

Thus the puritan reformers were not condemned to a negative approach to education. They adopted an iconoclastic attitude to the established curriculum, but put forward the experimental sciences as a viable substitute. The writings of Bacon, Comenius, Descartes, van Helmont and the Paracelsians, proved abundant sources from which to derive materials to fill the vacuum left by the abandonment of the scholastic curriculum. Thus science gradually emerged as the common denominator, even the central element, in positive plans for university reform.

(vii) Piety, Equity and Public Spiritedness

The growing dominance of Bacon, Comenius and Paracelsus is evident from the tracts composed in the wake of Milton's *Of Education* (1644). Milton's celebrated essay was an entirely humanistic product. In tone it was not greatly dissimilar from the writings of the Renaissance writer on education, Juan Luis Vives. The tractate was aggressively critical of scholasticism, and it advocated a more liberal approach to knowledge. There were indeed clear traces of the influence of Comenius and Bacon, but their views were completely assimilated into a humanistic framework. No other writer associated with Hartlib was able to maintain this strong humanistic bias against the growing tide of new ideas.

John Hall, a younger Cambridge contemporary of Milton, illustrates the rapid shift of opinion among the puritan educational writers. Whereas Milton discussed the general principles of humanistic education, Hall addressed himself to the immediate problem of the function of universities under the new regime. His *Humble Motion Concerning the Advancement of Learning and Reformation of the Universities* (1649) was addressed to parliament. Milton's stylistic influence was dominant to the point of imitation, particularly in the general introduction. By contrast Hall's educational programme was conceived in the spirit of the new philosophies of Bacon, Descartes and Comenius. Like the army pamphleteers he demanded that social reform should follow military victory. Otherwise the reformation would not be secure. After a lengthy appeal for parliament to accept this wider obligation, Hall turned to the deficiencies of the universities; these were outwardly distinguished, but inwardly corrupt and subversive. He reiterated familiar criticisms about 'jejune barren Peripatetick Philosophy' and disputations which baptised broods of 'ignorant mercenary Divines'.[301] Public teachers were accused of negligence and their students of failure to attend statutory lectures. The list of neglected subjects commenced with chemistry 'which hath snatcht the keyes of Nature from other sects of Philosophy, by her multiplied experiences'. This was followed by anatomy, botany, practical mathematics, experimental philosophy, history,

301. Hall (127), pp.26–7.

antiquities and the 'ready and generous teaching of Tongues'.[302] Mathematics had hitherto been disorganised and inconsequential, but Hall believed that it had recently become sufficiently perfected to provide an instrument capable of solving all problems. Equally natural philosophy had hitherto not been adequately appreciated, because of ignorance of the principles of induction.[303] With the reform of education sound knowledge would triumph, enabling the useful arts to multiply and to establish a firm foundation for reconstruction of the commonwealth.

These proposals demanded drastic institutional reforms. Hall proposed to replace college Fellows by professors, a change which would have replaced general arts tutors by specialists, thereby increasing the range of subjects taught. College revenues were to be deflected into 'examining and pursuing experiments, encouragements of honour, compleating and actuating some new inventions, supplying the needy ones, relieving strangers; and lastly, provoking some sydereall and flaming soules to display themselves.'[304]

Hall found an imitator in Noah Biggs. In the address to parliament of his medical reform tract, *Mataeotechnia medicinae* (1651) Biggs paraphrased many of Hall's sentiments about general reform and the defects of university education, underlining those points relevant to the medical profession. This work marks a further conspicuous dilution of Milton's style and humanistic bias. The universities were accused of neglect of public lectures and recalcitrancy over the reform of statutes. In almost identical language, Biggs repeated Hall's catalogue of the defects of the university curriculum, emphasising the neglect of chemistry, experimental philosophy, practical mathematics, anatomy and botany.[305]

In order to dispel complacency and provoke alarm, Hall claimed that the English universities had fallen behind even poorly endowed Jesuit colleges and 'many trans-marine Universities'. The justice of this adverse comparison must have been apparent to numerous English medical students, or visitors to the low countries during the rise of Cartesianism and experimental science in Dutch universities. Among the English reformers, Dury spent considerable time abroad; Pell had taught at Breda and Amsterdam; Petty studied at Leyden; and Worsley went to study the work of Dutch inventors. Hall almost certainly drew upon the letter on education composed by William Rand shortly after he had returned from an extended visit to the Dutch universities; appended to this document was 'A Description of a Transmarine School'.[306] While Rand was not specifically concerned with universities,

302. *Ibid.*, p.27.
303. *Ibid.*, pp.39–42.
304. *Ibid.*, pp.29–30.
305. Biggs (25), preface, sig b1r, derived from Hall (127), p.27.
306. Letter from Rand to Joshua Rawlin, 5 March 1648/9, BM, Sloane MS 649, fols. 57r–81v. The 'Description' has been attributed to Dury, by Corcoran (59), pp.229–47 and A. C. F. Beales, *Education under Penalty* (London, 1963), p.72. Corcoran also misdates Rand's letter.

he outlined the main elements of Hall's proposals, albeit shorn of Miltonian rhetoric. He described a science-based curriculum in considerable detail; this was intended to replace the languages and 'vaine ostentation in discourse' with 'principles of pietie, equitie, publique Spiritedness, despising of wealth and worldly superfluities'.

A similar approach was adopted, but with even greater elaboration, in Dury's *The Reformed School* (1650). Like Rand, Dury avoided direct reference to universities, outlining in exhaustive detail the curriculum and pedagogy suitable for higher education. But the relevance to universities was so obvious that Hartlib persuaded Dury to add an apologetical supplement on this subject to the second edition. In this supplement, Dury disclaimed that his discourse implied universities were superfluous; he had merely wished to argue that it was pointless to reform elementary education if universities were not modified according to the same principles. Dury believed that the public professors should concentrate on developing the natural aptitudes of students, who would then become socially useful and able to elaborate 'some desiderata of useful knowledge'. An overriding concern should be the subordination of the universities to the 'well-reformed Commonwealth'.[307] Like Hall, Dury believed that neither the college tutors nor the university teachers were assisting this function. It was imperative that the colleges should show greater sensitivity to general social needs, rather than a tendency to retreat into 'a monkish life in popish cloisters'—a comparison calculated to create unease. In contrast with the conciliatory tone of the opening passages of his book, Dury's concluding analysis underlined the failure of the universities to adapt to the requirements of the new age of reformation.[308]

In defending the need for an Office of Address, Hartlib summarised the reformers' grievances against the universities. Notwithstanding the excellent advice of Bacon, they had become insensitive to the public good:

> 'How little they have endeavoured that the knowledge of those things, which they profess might bee made more certaine and lesse full of idle dispute or contention. Or that the principles and Arts which they commonly teach might bee indeed of some solid use, profitt, or service to mankind; noe choice, or singular experiments for Arts, for Education, or for the facilitating or Advancement of any Part of learning having usually flowed from the Universityes or Publickly maintained Professors.'[309]

Hugh Peter, chaplain to the Council of State, and a longstanding member of the spiritual brotherhood, suggested that Cambridge Uni-

307. Dury (89), 'The Supplement', pp.5–6.
308. *Ibid.*, pp.9–10.
309. Papers relating to the 'Memorial for Advancement of Universal Learning', HP XLVII 14.

versity should pay equal attention to secular as to religious teaching. He proposed that eight colleges should be responsible for ministerial training, with appropriate emphasis on scriptural analysis and cases of conscience. The remaining eight were to embrace 'whatever any out-Landish Academie can teach'.[310] Although he made few specific recommendations, Peter was clearly in sympathy with Baconian reform of education. He commented favourably on schemes for the advancement of learning; and he believed that some tutors should be dispatched abroad, like the Merchants of Light of New Atlantis, to ensure that the universities were acquainted with the most recent discoveries.[311] Graduates of the reformed universities were expected to take up useful employment; physicians and lawyers were expected to provide free medical or legal advice to needy citizens; clergymen were to preach wherever required.

The initiative for university reform came primarily from outside critics who were described by commentators like Anthony Wood as vindictive and ignorant sectaries. However, the major exponents of reform were university-educated. Dell, although existing in self-imposed isolation, was the head of a Cambridge college. The major critics were well-informed about university education and they were not entirely unsuccessful in recruiting sympathisers from among the academics. Webster himself retired to a living in Yorkshire, but his friend Joshua Sprigg, the author of the preface to Webster's collected sermons, was rewarded for his services to Fairfax with a fellowship at All Souls College. Joshua Sprigg did not pronounce on educational matters, but his younger brother, William Sprigg of Lincoln College, wrote a tract on educational reform which adopted some of Webster's ideas. At Oxford Hartlib gradually built up a small party of adherents. He even enjoyed the good opinion of Francis Rous, chairman of the London Parliamentary Committee for the Universities. But Hartlib's influence did not extend to the university Visitors, although eventually he corresponded with Ralph Austen, registrar to the Oxford Visitors.

Perhaps the most influential supporter of the reformers at Oxford was Henry Langley, the intruded Master of Pembroke College. From his correspondence with Hartlib it is apparent that he took an active interest in Comenius and in schemes for reform.[312] At Langley's instigation Hartlib was granted the income from the Pembroke College augmentation and he was offered accommodation at this college, pending his appointment as Bodley's Librarian.[313] During the final illness of John Rouse, the non-submitting librarian, Langley was extremely

310. *Good Work for a Good Magistrate* (208), addressed to 'The Supreme Authority', p.11.

311. See Bacon, *New Atlantis* (14), p.44.

312. Letters from Langley to Hartlib, HP xv iii.

313. *CSPD 1653/4*, pp. 53, 206 (27 July & 18 Oct. 1653). *Ibid., 1653/4*, pp.44, 249 (24 March & 11 July 1654). These proceedings record the efforts of Rous to enforce regular payment of the augmentation to Hartlib.

active in pressing Hartlib's candidature before the London Committee. He also proposed a substantial augmentation in the librarian's stipend. In April 1652 he confidently announced that Hartlib's nomination was imminent. As already indicated, both Hartlib and Dury believed that a major library would form the best foundation for a national communications agency and this plan was probably responsible for securing Langley's support for Hartlib's appointment. But this scheme aroused suspicion and opposition from other academics, who were anxious to prevent the university from becoming involved in the puritan programme for social reform. Accordingly the post of Bodley's Librarian was deflected to the academically orthodox Thomas Barlow, who was widely known to be a royalist sympathiser. The failure of Langley's patronage perhaps inspired the alternative proposal of Philip Parsons, Principal of Hart Hall, who offered the use of his hall (which was adjacent to the library) as an Office of Address.[314] But neither these, nor efforts to secure for Hartlib the headships of Oriel or St. John's, were successful. However, they do indicate the existence within the university of a small faction working for more unorthodox appointments and greater involvement with national social policy.

Letters from Thomas Gilson, a young Fellow of Corpus Christi College, illustrate the outlook and associations of Hartlib's supporters. Upon his appointment at Corpus, Gilson expressed his determination to 'act *ad extremum rerum* to do you and your commonwealth of Learning any service'.[315] He appreciated that any substantial reform of the university depended on revision of the statutes. A brief set of reform proposals, probably composed by Gilson and entitled 'Ut felix et fausta fiat Reformatio Statutorum Academiae Oxoniensis', was sent to Hartlib. Many of the ideas from this document were embodied into a longer petition which was probably composed by Hartlib, entitled 'To the Supreame Authority of Parliament of the Commonwealth & of England. The humble petition of Severall Members of the Universitie of Oxon.'[316] Both petitions were probably directed at the London Committee.

These petitions may have been prompted by the increased attention being paid by the Committee to the question of statutory reform in the summer of 1649. The Visitors ordered strict compliance with existing statutes 'untill the Statutes of everie House can be received, reformed, and settled'.[317] But within the university there was too little initiative for change for it to persist without further outside promptings from the London Committee. After a brief pause, Rous sent to Oxford some

314. 'A motion for the public good of religion and learning', HP LIII 24. For Parsons, see Wood *Fasti*, i, pp.411, 414; *DNB*; S. G. Hamilton, *Hertford College* (London, 1903), pp.329–30.

315. Letter from Gilson to Hartlib, 10 Aug. [1649], HP X 1.

316. The Latin petition (HP X 1) is dated 9 Oct. [1649]; the English petition (HP XLVIII 17) is undated. The texts of both are given in Appendix I, below.

317. Burrows (42), p.259; 8 Aug. 1649.

specific proposals in 'A Modell' concerning the further reformation of the universities. This document was entered into the register and presumably accepted in principle, although no action was taken to implement its provisions.[318] The *Model* pressed for continuing ejection of 'scandalouse persons', the reform of the statutes to 'promote pietie and good learninge', the initiation of lectures on biblical exposition and the introduction of terminable fellowships. Hence Gilson's impression that a general reform of statutes was imminent, a notion which was further confirmed by an order of the London Committee for its delegates to report on the University Statutes and for the heads of colleges to report on theirs.[319] The authors of the *Model* are not named but they were probably a group of London ministers, mainly Independents, three of whom were mentioned in the text of the document. Of these, Thomas Goodwin and Joseph Caryll were later approached by Gilson to support his petition, which may well have been designed to carry a stage further the process of reform initiated by the London Committee.

Both Latin and English petitions were probably consciously framed to appear consistent with the *Model*. The provision for limited tenure was praised as a means of hastening the dissemination of new ideas. The English petition appealed for a completion of 'your worke' by 'new Moulding our constitutions in severall Colledges to a more ingenious and lesse tedious way of Learning [than] what is already'.

Although the two petitions are similar in many respects, their bias is strikingly different. Gilson was more concerned with the curriculum and with teaching. He appealed for the cultivation of *Philosophia libera,* based on reason rather than authority. Instead of their relying on tradition and authority, as boundaries beyond which the intellectual could not penetrate, he urged the public teachers to enter into the spirit of Bacon's philosophy, and to give serious regard to research and the promotion of recent discoveries. Consistently with these aims, the Custos Archivorum and Bodley's Librarian would be employed to collect and publish approved documents.

Hartlib's petition emphasised the research and communication aspect of Gilson's proposals, although it was undoubtedly assumed as a matter of course that statutory reform would bring teaching into line with the most recent state of knowledge. Hartlib repeated the widespread demand for an increase in the number of public teachers. He called for the professors to undertake a 'practicall pursuit of Nature in all Luciferous experiments' and to produce regular research reports. This work would be facilitated by a board of trustees holding sufficient funds to collect books, manuscripts, mathematical instruments and models, from both English and foreign sources. Furthermore the trustees would also be permitted to print select abstracts and documents. The most important provision was for the augmentation of the office of librarian to become

318. *Ibid.*, pp.261, 264; 30 Aug. & 18 Sept. 1649.
319. Univ. Oxon. Arch., Reg. Convoc. T. 27 Sept. 1649.

that of an agent who would serve the commonwealth and university by foreign correspondency. Thus Gilson's original petition was considerably revised by Hartlib to become a thinly veiled proposal for the establishment of an Office of Address at Oxford. Gilson's ideas on curricular reform, and the communications agency, would have been equally unpalatable to the academic establishment.

The later letters of Gilson show that there was a disinclination in Oxford to accept the need for a revision of statutes. He complained to Hartlib what

> 'slender designements our Academicall witts are, the order procured for reforming statutes, and constitutions, is by them interpreted to search no further then takinge away of holy dayes, the oathe of Allegiance and such like *crepuscula et* the Advancement of Learninge *ne Gry quidem*. Quis talia fando temperet a lachrymis.'[320]

Any hopes for action rested on outside initiative. But Gilson noted that of their list of potential supporters, only Thomas Goodwin was an Oxford graduate.[321] Later he detected increased support from 'many heere, lovers of your ingenuous designes, but they are as yet very lothe to appeare upon the stage as professed Antagonists to the present pedantry'.[322] Others were undecided whether it was best to invite Dury and Hartlib to join the Visitors, or to serve as directors of a separate agency located within the university. The emphasis on the Office of Address in the English petition aroused fears about the cost of reform; the office was clearly unpopular among academics. Gilson hoped that Petty would be a valuable ally, but Petty's days as an active educational reformer were over. However other young adherents were Elisha Bourne and Thomas Danson of Corpus, the latter being a pupil of Hartlib's friend the orientalist Christian Rave. Danson had attracted attention as an orientalist, being described by Hartlib as '18 years of age of very pregnant and extraordinary parts', when he was maintained by Sir David Watkins before going up to Oxford.[323] Danson was a friend of Langley and he married the daughter of Tobias Garbrand of Gloucester Hall. John French referred to Garbrand as a reformer, and appealed to him to support the introduction into the curriculum of chemistry, since this was the 'true naturall philosophy; which most accurately anatomizeth nature and naturall things', thereby supplanting 'that empty naturall philosophy which is read in the Universities'.[324]

320. Letter from Gilson to Hartlib, 1 Jan. 1649/50, HP x 1.

321. Apart from Goodwin, Gilson named Hartlib, Dury, Sir David Watkins, William Petty, John Sadler, John Selden and Joseph Caryll.

322. Letter from Gilson to Hartlib, 12 March 1649/50, HP x 1.

323. Ephemerides 1648 and 1650; Wood *Athenae*, iv, pp.591–4.

324. French, *The Art of Distillation* (109), dedication, sig. A2v–3r.

Although the evidence about Gilson's collaborators is not extensive, it points to the close personal and intellectual association between Hartlib's supporters at Oxford. Their insistence that commitment to experimental philosophy implied a radically different approach to university education was consistent with the argument of Dury's *Reformed School.* This doctrine was certainly not attractive to the more conservative academics, or even to such active Baconians as John Wilkins. Hence the reformers appear to have been indifferent to the Oxford Experimental Philosophy Club, which they would not have regarded as a satisfactory substitute for statutory promotion of the *philosophia libera.* Hence Hartlib's protégés were not conspicuous in the lists of the club and they never came to exercise political influence within the university. This divergence of outlook on the principles of education was the source of enmity between the two groups of advocates of the new science, causing Hartlib to receive conflicting reports from Oxford; one party was stressing the backwardness of formal education, while the other publicised the fruitful enterprises of the Experimental Philosophy Club.

The zenith of the reformers' efforts and expectations came during the Saints' Parliament of 1653. Samuel Herring, Webster, Dell and the Hartlib circle produced significant writings at this time. They undoubtedly hoped to influence the parliamentary Committee for the Advancement of Learning which was known to include sympathisers with educational reform. The Speaker of this parliament was Hartlib's patron, Francis Rous. The parliamentary debate on the role of universities was probably held as a result of the reformers' pamphleteering. Subsequently this initiative came to be regarded as an unsuccessful attempt at suppressing 'Universities and all Schools for Learning, as heathenish and unnecessary'.[325] But despite the heat of this debate, there was probably only negligible support for the radical position caricatured by Anthony Wood. By those opposed to change, any interference with the universities was regarded as a retreat into barbarism.

Events proved that these fears were unjustified. The Oxford Visitors exercised their authority to promote 'godlinesse and learning', without interfering with normal academic routines; the writings of the outside critics show little trace of the anti-intellectualism described by Wood. In their submission to the parliamentary Committee, 'Proposals towards the Advancement of Learning', Hartlib and Dury were primarily concerned with universal education, but the final sections included an unequivocal statement of their strictures on universities, in terms reminiscent of the supplement to *The Reformed School.*[326] The universities were censured for maintaining a monkish aloofness; they pretended to uphold humanistic standards, while actually displaying an

325. Wood *Hist. & Antiq.*, ii, p.657; *idem.*, *Life & Times* (47), i, pp.291–6.

326. 'Some Proposalls towards the Advancement of Learning', 1653, HP XLVII 2. Given in full in Webster (320), pp.166–92.

indifference to genuinely useful higher studies. Only by displaying an 'engagement towards the publick concernements of the Commonwealth of learning' could they exercise a genuinely fruitful function. The *Proposals* appealed to the chancellors to direct academics into 'usefull parts of learning', both secular and religious, and requested them to take as one of their main aims the training of teachers who would improve the educational standards of other sections of society. This general dissemination of knowledge would have been assisted by the introduction of fellowships with limited tenure.[327]

Dell advocated a more rigorous exclusion of divinity studies, but he shared Dury's tolerance of grammar, rhetoric and logic, providing that they were applied exclusively to secular topics. Mathematics was to be positively encouraged since 'Arithmetick, Geometry, Geography, and the like, which as they carry no wickedness in them, so are they besides useful to humane Society'.[328]

One of the fullest expressions of the reformers' standpoint is Webster's *Academiarum Examen,* composed during parliamentary discussions on educational reform, and published just before the dissolution of the Saints' Parliament. Its intrinsic qualities, and its publication at a moment of crisis both recommend *Academiarum Examen* as a representative document of reform. The effectiveness of this tract is suggested by its contemporary notoriety and by the vehemence of Webster's critics. But *Academiarum Examen* was not an isolated product; Webster had much in common with the other university critics and it was perhaps some of his obvious weaknesses which provoked such a hostile response. It is certainly arguable that critics were unwilling to assail Hall, Hartlib, Dury or Peter because of their acknowledged political influence and stature as respected exponents of puritan educational and social ideas. On the other hand Dell's eccentricity, Hobbes's unsound political associations, and Webster's personal obscurity, rendered them safer targets for attack. In addition, Webster's detailed criticisms involved obvious and pronounced inaccuracies on specific points of fact. But it would be a mistake to overlook Webster's positive qualities, or to underestimate the intellectual sophistication of the movement of which he was a single representative.

Of all the educational reformers Webster had the greatest direct interest in science and medicine. However this enthusiasm was recent and his knowledge uneven; he was not well-informed about the universities and he seems to have been unaware of the recent growth of interest in experimental science among the academics. Nevertheless he impulsively undertook a detailed censure of the scholastic curriculum, rather than following Dury, who concentrated on the positive aspect of reform. Webster subsequently made numerous erroneous accusations and his constructive suggestions were obscured by polemic. Thus his well-

327. *Ibid.*, p.191.
328. Dell (78), p.27.

intentioned efforts were crowded with anomalies; he exposed inconsistencies in the position of the reformers and he opened the door to counterattacks by the opponents of change. He became an ideal target for the sophisticated academics, whose rejoinders have convinced most modern writers that it was Webster's misfortune to condemn university science at the very point of its greatest accomplishment. By concentrating on his failure to appreciate the extent of academic involvement in scientific research, historians have tended to ignore the more central tenets of the reformer's position. Webster was not primarily concerned with the informal cultivation of new subjects, but with the question of their formal status. Thus the recent achievements of the Oxford club, or other individual cases of philosophical enlightenment, were irrelevant to his purposes. But in the heat of polemic *Academiarum Examen* failed to make it clear that its author's censures related specifically to the statutory mechanism of university education.

In spite of this defect, Webster produced a damaging caricature of the scholastic education generally practised in the universities. Bacon or Milton would have concurred with many of his sentiments. Then, whatever the limitations of his positive proposals from a modern point of view, they were at least consistent with his religious and social premises. Webster's approach to the new philosophy was highly selective; like other reformers he felt the strongest sympathy for experimental philosophies which were most relevant to social reform. Although he shared the Oxford club's enthusiasm for Bacon, Webster's Baconianism was infiltrated with ideas taken from the Paracelsians, van Helmont and other authors conformable with his religious and social aims. This bias led Webster and other reformers to become enthusiastic about chemistry, the subject which had provided Webster's own initiation into science.[329]

Academiarum Examen took up an extreme position about the extent of reform needed in the university curriculum—'the great part of it doth deserve eradication, some of it reformation, and all of it melioration.' The abandonment of scholastic divinity and philosophy, and traditional academic exercises, was demanded. Wherever possible academic discourse should be in English; ancient languages were to be accepted only if taught by Comenius's simplified methods. Divinity was to be radically attenuated; its few essential ingredients could be incorporated into natural philosophy. It was difficult to suggest an effective reform of logic; the most fruitful area for expansion was induction, while 'Syllogizing Sophistry' which dominated logic was superfluous, since it had no constructive function. The chemist who prepared a new compound was superior to the logician who merely reorganised information under the pretence of practising 'invention'.[330] Likewise metaphysics was castigated for leading the mind into idle and vain speculation. Only the system

329. Rightly stressed by Debus (72), Introduction.
330. Webster (326), p.38.

of Descartes exhibited a meaningful and certain application of metaphysics.[331] Otherwise, along with the scholastic forms of ethics, politics, economics, poetry and rhetoric, metaphysics was a candidate for complete extirpation.

The range of subjects canvassed to replace the scholastic subjects was determined by utilitarian considerations. Subjects which were 'speculative' had no place since they were 'of no use or benefit to mankind'. Consequently natural philosophy and mathematics enjoyed the greatest esteem since they were most obviously 'profitable, excellent and usefull'.[332] These subjects were even allowed to dictate the approach to other studies; language reform was expected to benefit by following the model of algebra, or a universal character might evolve from chemical symbolism and the doctrine of signatures developed by Jacob Boehme.[333]

Whereas scholastic logic carried 'no certitude, nor evidential demonstration . . . and makes men Parrat-like to babble, argue, . . . but still to remain nescious, and ignorant', the 'superlative' mathematical sciences were transcendent in 'perspicuity, veritude and certitude, and also in their uses and manifold benefits'. Although this subject was formally included in the scholastic curriculum, Webster believed that each branch was treated superficially, with reference to a limited range of ancient texts, while taking too little account of modern authors, new theories, or practical application. The productive aspects of geometry were not cultivated by scholars, but by merchants, mechanics, and other manual operators.[334] Scholastic astronomy and optics were indicted for their failure to absorb new theories and instrumental methods from Galileo, Kepler and Hevelius. Besides these subjects which received only token recognition, or were misapplied, Webster listed numerous parts of mathematics which were totally ignored in the universities. He considered that certain of these subjects should be obligatory, particularly if they were relevant to navigation, 'one of the most necessary employments and advantages of our Nation'. Even more strenuous pleas were made for astrology, in view of its recent 'resuscitation' by English practitioners.[335]

Despite objections against Aristotle and peripateticism, a continuance of the authority of Aristotle's writings was anticipated, especially in such subjects as zoology. None the less in all subjects there would be a continual reassessment in the light of the findings of both ancient and modern authors. This would promote a freer spirit in philosophy and allow much greater attention 'to the compleating of Physical knowledge'.

331. *Ibid.*, p.107.

332. *Ibid.*, p.18.

333. Webster's enthusiasm for Boehme was shared by Samuel Herring, who proposed that the 'Teutonic Philosopher' should be prescribed reading in the universities for those who inquired into 'the true ground and depth of all things'. Herring (148), p.100.

334. Webster (326), pp.40–52.

335. *Ibid.*, pp. 50–2. No doubt Webster was thinking of the recent active exploitation of astrology by the parliamentarian astrologers.

Philosophy would then be emancipated from its 'verbal, speculative, abstractive, formal and notional' nature.[336]

In his proposals for a more active and experimental approach to natural philosophy, Webster displayed his own strong scientific predilections. The first object of attention was that 'almost divine Science of natural Magick'. Its sphere of operation was not precisely defined, but natural magic was expected to be relevant to a wide range of phenomena, and to produce explanations which would provide the key to the widespread practical exploitation of nature.[337] Equally important was chemistry, which had been rescued from impostors by such reformers as Paracelsus and van Helmont. Chemistry had recently become an 'openly known' subject, capable of yielding important discoveries, but before its virtues could be fully appreciated it was necessary for academics to abandon their prejudice against 'the coals and furnace'.[338]

In medicine Galen was an even more unsatisfactory authority than was Aristotle in natural philosophy. The Galenic system was unsound and incomplete. A new system, having the advantage of sound empirical foundations, could be based on the sciences of botany and anatomy. Harvey had demonstrated the potentialities of practical anatomy, but the nature and treatment of diseases could only be understood by reference to 'Mystical Anatomy', which was the creation of the iatrochemists, Paracelsus, van Helmont and Fludd. By following their example, 'the whole Theatre of nature' could be searched for medicines suitable for every disease. Further desiderata in academic studies relating to medicine, discussed more briefly, were physiognomy, the doctrine of signatures, the three principles of Paracelsus, magnetism (for sympathetic cures) and the various atomic theories.[339]

In spite of obvious signs of hasty composition, poor organisation, and many ill-digested notions, *Academiarum Examen* was the most extensive critique of scholastic education produced by the reformers. It also drew together many positive proposals from earlier writings, to demonstrate the fertility and comprehensiveness of the reformers' programme for the reconstitution of university education. The experimental sciences and the new philosophies supplied the unifying factor in the positive programme which was evolved in correspondence, petitions and tracts on reform produced between 1649 and 1653. But the underlying motive for the reform of the scholastic curriculum was a total dissatisfaction with the existing social and religious order. The sermons of Dell and Webster show particularly clearly that educational issues were treated in a manner dictated by revealed religion. Their sentiments were widely shared, albeit with disagreements on the exact training and role of the ministry. But ministers, whatever their type, were expected to

336. *Ibid.*, pp.52–84; 104–8.
337. *Ibid.*, pp.68–70.
338. *Ibid.*, pp.70–2.
339. *Ibid.*, pp.72–8. See below, pp.282–8.

undergo an elaborate education in institutions closely involved with the secular functions of the state, rather than in the isolated divinity faculties of the unreformed universities. Religious, pedagogical and philosophical arguments pointed to the necessity for major reorientation and expansion of secular studies in the universities. Webster's summary of educational objectives would have received almost universal approbation among the puritan reformers:

1. The sciences were to be cultivated according to Bacon's axiom that all theories must be supported by diligent observation, luciferous experiments, and natural histories. By this means knowledge would be established on firm and lasting foundations.
2. As suggested by Comenius and Fludd, a synthesis of rational, inductive and scriptural knowledge should be constructed.
3. All systems of philosophy, ancient and modern, should be subjected to disinterested scrutiny, doctrines being accepted or discarded according to their merits.
4. The universities should no longer rely on disputation, but turn to manual experience, with a view to obtaining an exhaustive understanding of 'natures hidden secrets, which can never come to pass, unless they have Laboratories as well as Libraries'. Chemistry was the model for the new empirical disciplines.
5. In medicine the Galenic system was to be abandoned in favour of ideas derived from van Helmont and Paracelsus; this reorientation would promote a systematic search for the causes and cures of all diseases.[340]

The works of Bacon, Comenius, van Helmont, Boehme and the Paracelsians were found to accord with the religious, philosophical and social objectives of the reformers. Hence these works were interpreted, actively publicised and translated by the educational reformers, whose efforts undoubtedly assisted the reception of new philosophical and scientific ideas, as well as creating a body of opinion favourable to educational innovation. Although the reform movement was never influential inside the universities, its growing influence in the country and vigorous expression in the 1653 parliament called for an equally vigorous response. The derisory tone adopted by numerous defenders of the *status quo* could not disguise the deep anxieties which were felt about the revolutionary social implications of educational reforms proposed by the advocates of spiritual religion.

(viii) Authentic Messengers of God

The strong linkage forged between experimental philosophy and spiritual religion in the writings of the reformers drove their critics to dwell

340. *Ibid.*, pp.105–7.

on the dependence of the learned ministry on the scholastic curriculum. If it could be argued on theological and historical grounds that the more recondite ministerial duties were essential, the whole edifice of scholastic education might be defended as a necessary preparation to sustain the linguistic, rhetorical and theological skills of the pious clerk in holy orders. It was crucial for the clergy to carry this debate, since the case for tithes and a beneficed clergy, even for a national church, relied on the concept of the learned ministry. Thus for reasons of self preservation, as well as out of intellectual conviction, it was necessary for the clergy to rush to the support of traditional university studies. Their writings were strikingly uniform, being mainly distinguished by differences in length. In number and extent they greatly exceeded the tracts on university reform. 1653 generated a torrent of these apologetical works. Robert Boreman was primarily absorbed with counteracting the claims of mechanick preachers in his neighbourhood, or the petition from Bedfordshire against tithes. Thomas Blake defended the traditional duties of the clergy, arguing against their active involvement in secular matters. It followed that their education had to be literary—'A School for Tongues and Arts cannot be a shop for Trades'. This sentiment was also expressed in John Gauden's defence of tithes, which asserted that it was wrong to 'yoke the Minister and Mechanick together'. The longest defence of traditional studies came from Edward Waterhouse, who also defended tithes, calling for the maintenance of the ministry and universities in 'comfort and plentie', in order to encourage the recruitment of diligent ordinands.[341] Attacks on the universities by Dell and Webster provoked fierce censures from the clerical apologists. Webster was the target of a very ineffective polemic by Thomas Hall, written shortly after the latter's slightly more substantial *Vindiciae Literarum* (1654), which was primarily concerned with refuting the cobbler Samuel How.[342] Dell had a more effective adversary in Joseph Sedgwick of Christ's College Cambridge. Along with many other apologists Sedgwick was obliged to concede the validity of personal revelation, but this belief was 'stretch'd too farre' by such authors as Dell. The pitfalls of enthusiasm, was the theme used by Sedgwick to undermine the position of his adversaries.[343] He was quickly followed by his Cambridge colleagues Henry More and John Arrowsmith, who were equally concerned to pro-

341. Boreman, *The Triumph of Learning over Ignorance* (London, 1653); Blake, *Vindiciae Foederis* (London, 1653); Gauden, *The Case of Ministers Maintenance by Tithes* (London, 1653); Waterhouse, *An humble Apologie for Learning and Learned Men* (London, 1653).

342. *Histrio-Mastix: A Whip for Webster* (London, 1654); facs. reprint in Debus (72). Hall had produced an earlier criticism of How, *The Pulpit Guarded* (1652); answered by Thomas Collier, *The Pulpit Guard Routed* (1652). Webster was also attacked by Edward Leigh, *A Treatise of Religion & Learning* (London, 1656).

343. Joseph Sedgwick, *An Essay to the discovery of the Spirit of Enthusiasme and pretended Inspiration that disturbs and strikes at the Universities* (London, 1653).

tect traditional learning from the excesses of the enthusiasts.[344] Sedgwick diagnosed the major defect in Dell's position as 'a puffing up the minds of men with aiery fancies' which were far from the true spirit of godliness instilled by the educated ministry.[345] More supported this view by pointing to the philosophical eccentricities of Paracelsus and the theosophists, who falsely believed that they were 'Authentick messengers from God Almighty'.[346] Thus the authors who claimed to hold the key to puritan educational reform were castigated as dangerous 'nonconformists'. The clergy saw no need for the reform of their own education. Sedgwick argued that while increased provision for the training of ministers was required, traditional linguistic, rhetorical and philosophical subjects were an indispensable part of this education.[347] But as a small concession to Dell, it was admitted that the state or private individuals should endow some chairs having 'Politicall and more Temporall usefullness'.[348]

Sedgwick's theological position resembled that adopted in *Vindiciae academiarum,* the most distinctive and effective reply to the criticisms of Webster, Dell and Hobbes. Apart from the introductory letter by John Wilkins, the text was composed by Seth Ward.[349] Consequently the *Vindiciae* represented an authoritative academic opinion and the views of two of the best informed members of the Oxford Experimental Philosophy Club. This skilful composition had little in common with more pedantic defences of 'humane learning'. It avoided any detailed defence of the scholastic curriculum, learned ministry or tithes—territories on which the Puritans were deeply divided. Instead, Wilkins and Ward pooled their scientific knowledge to demonstrate Webster's lesser acquaintance with modern science; and at the same time they publicised their own scientific work, which was represented as one of the manifestations of the liberal intellectual atmosphere at Oxford. By showing that an academic community could assimilate, teach and advance any new sphere of learning through informal initiative, they hoped to preclude radical curricular reform. Substantially the same arguments were advanced by Wallis fifty years later, by the opponents of the Victorian Royal Commissions on the universities, and even by more recent generations of academics dedicated to sabotaging the

344. More, *Enthusiasmus Triumphatus: or, A Brief Discourse of the Nature, Causes, Kinds and Cure of Enthusiasm* (Cambridge, 1656); Arrowsmith, *Tactica Sacra . . . Accesserunt Orationes aliquot anti-Weigelianae* (Cambridge, 1657); for similar views from an Oxford Presbyterian, see Edward Reynolds, *A Sermon Touching the Use of Humane Learning* (London, 1658).

345. Sedgwick, *op. cit.,* p.9.

346. More, *op. cit.*; quoted from More (191), pp.29–36.

347. Sedgwick, *op. cit.,* pp.49–56.

348. *Ibid.,* p.36.

349. Cambridge University Library and British Museum (E.738(5)) copies are dated 26 May. Reprinted in Debus (72). The authors are given as 'N.S. & H.D.'—generally identified as the last letters of the names of John Wilkins and Seth Ward. However, Wood, *Life & Times* (47), i, p.296 suggests that the author of the introduction was John Wallis, not Wilkins.

modernisation of university institutions. None has exceeded Wilkins and Ward as effective exponents of this position.

The success of *Vindiciae* is probably indicated by the lack of reference within the universities to the reform of statutes after the initial moves in 1649 and 1650. The universities convinced the parliamentary authorities that they could promote piety and learning without such changes. Wilkins and Ward could claim to share many of the basic aims of the reformers (interpreted with necessary discretion), without wishing to modify the traditional social function of the universities.[350] Theology was as indispensable as other professional studies, while the 'very great numbers of youth' from the nobility and gentry had no taste for tuition in chemistry, agriculture or mechanics:

> 'Their removall is from hence commonly in two or three years, to the Innes of Court, and the desire of their friends is not, that they be engaged in those experimentall things, but that their reason, and fancy, and carriage, be improved by lighter Institutions and Exercises that they may become Rationall and Gracefull speakers, and be of an acceptable behaviour in their Countries.'[351]

Not one student in many hundreds was thought to desire acquaintance with natural philosophy. Thus Wilkins and Ward refused to concede that puritan theology or the new sciences necessitated radical educational change, so long as current social attitudes persisted. The scientific and mathematical components of the arts curriculum were thought to be quite sufficient for normal purposes in academies 'of a more generall and comprehensive institution'. Science was relevant to mature philosophical reflection, which belonged to the period after the completion of formal education. Nevertheless it was conceded that natural philosophy and medicine could be perfected only if 'instead of verball Exercise, we should set upon experiments and observations, that we should lay aside our Disputations, Declamations, and Public Lectures, and betake our selves to Agriculture, Mechanicks, Chymistry, and the like'.[352] But despite this admission, Wilkins and Ward believed that it was inappropriate for the sciences to be 'as a generall rule imposed upon us' in view of the overriding social obligation of the universities to provide a polite education for the sons of the gentry.

This social outlook was probably increasingly adopted by the intruded Puritans. Reacting against the reformers they became guardians of the form of university education inherited from Laud and ultimately passed on to grateful successors at the restoration. From a less comfortable standpoint, their critics, accepting an obligation to promote social and ecclesiastical reform, were more willing to modify the universities in order to supply more effective public servants and an economically

350. Ward (307), p.(4).
351. *Ibid.*, p.50.
352. *Ibid.*, pp.49–50.

productive gentry. The introduction of a scientific curriculum was an obvious desideratum. Assimilation of science into the universities would stimulate technological and agricultural innovation, provide means for the relief of the poor, establish a more effective system of medicine and accord better with the 'experimental' spirit of the age.

The events of 1653 placed the reformers in a distinct minority. Authority continued to be insensitive to new models of society. Thus, the great educational reform initiative was gradually dissipated. During the remaining years of the interregnum Oxford and Cambridge were relatively secure. During 1659 there was a faint echo of the events of 1653, when there were further criticisms and defences of the learned clergy and the universities, the most celebrated contribution of the critics being Milton's *Likeliest Means to Remove Hirelings*. Republican political issues were central to this debate; ideas on education were merely abstracted from previous writings. A parliamentary debate was provoked on a proposal to establish the universities according to the Dutch model, with colleges specialising in each of the three professional subjects. But within a few months parliament reaffirmed its traditional obligation to uphold and encourage all universities and schools.[353] One of the topical issues of this period among puritan clergymen was the religious complexion of universities. Many Puritans were not convinced that the purges had proceeded far enough, and there was a constantly shifting balance between the various religious factions within the universities. A group of Independents put forward a scheme to establish St. Mary Hall as a college for ten divines engaged in preparing a synopsis of the 'true reformed Protestant Christian Religion professed in this Commonwealth'.[354] This project would have been directed by Locke's tutor, Thomas Cole. After the completion of these duties the college was to be used for supporting exiled protestant ministers from the continent. A more broadly based plan emanated from John Worthington's pupil, Matthew Poole, who proposed a scheme for financing poor students at the universities. During their eight years at university these students would be expected to undertake the traditional course of studies. However, there was an interesting provision for any gifted divinity graduate to remain in the university to specialise in one of a range of subjects, including mathematics and philosophy.[355] Thus the light of

353. Wood *Hist. & Antiq.*, ii, p.695; *CJ*, vii, pp.662, 819, 22 May 1659 & 23 Jan. 1660. Universities were supported by petitions from Oxfordshire and Leicestershire, 30 Jan. 1659/60 & 13 Feb. 1660; *CSPD 1659/60*, pp.335–6, 361.

354. I. G. Philip, 'A proposed refoundation of St. Mary Hall', *Oxoniensia,* 1957, *22*; 93–7.

355. Matthew Poole, *A Model for the maintaining of students of choice abilities at the university principally in order to the Ministry* (London, 1648 [actually 1658]). A revised edition, more cautious in tone, is dated 1658. Attacked from the sectarian viewpoint by E.M., *A Brief Answer unto the Cambridge Moddel* (London, 1658). An earlier scheme establishing 40 trustees to control funds to support poor scholars was announced in a broadsheet headed 'London, Anno Dom. 1647', HP LIII 1.

university reform was not completely extinguished, even at the eve of the restoration.

(ix) Universal Education

The educational expansion of the century before 1650 indicates an ever-increasing demand for education from all classes, and the reformers were determined to expand educational opportunities still further.

It has already been noted that the Puritans had traditionally attached considerable importance to education. Reliance on individual responsibility in religious matters, a point emphasised by the spiritual reformers whose writings dominated the literature on education of the Puritan Revolution, greatly increased the demand for a high standard of general literacy. The puritan reformers believed that all members of society should receive sufficient education to enable them to exercise their religious function independently, pursue their callings effectively and defend their liberties when necessary. They realised that the universities and their 'nurseries' the grammar schools, were completely inadequate to meet these requirements. These institutions seemed to be too much associated with outmoded religious and social values. The reformers accordingly turned against scholastic education and they looked for substitutes which would give acquaintance with things rather than words. They evolved a comprehensive range of school, college, and academy proposals in which the sciences and technology increasingly took precedence over linguistic subjects. These models, which were initially conceived in a supplementary context, soon came to be regarded as an alternative to the traditional universities and grammar schools. Although new schemes were often conceived in idealistic and impracticable terms, they caused considerable offence to the academic establishment and were treated as a form of subversive criticism.

The onset of the Puritan Revolution was marked by a substantial increase in pressure for universal education, so reviving an ideal which had been first promulgated by Martin Bucer during the Edwardian reformation. The architect of the reformation at Strassburg, Bucer believed that the state had an obligation to pay great attention to education. He agreed with other protestant reformers that children from even the poorest homes required instruction in reading, writing and the elements of the reformed faith. He also recommended that they should be given vocational instruction by skilled practitioners of trades or agriculture.[356] Thus it was established that the formal education of all citizens was essential for the efficient management of the religious and secular life of a reformed state, and this ideal was never completely forgotten. Generations of puritan ministers like Richard Greenham took their educational duties extremely seriously. Their lay counterparts

356. Bucer, *De Regno Christi* (39), pp.135–6. Allan H. Gilbert, 'Martin Bucer on Education', *JEGP*, 1919, *18*: 321–45.

endowed 'free schools' on an extensive scale, a provision which was taken for granted by theorists like Richard Mulcaster.[357] However, both educational writings and endowments overwhelmingly related to those social groups which could hope to benefit from humanistic studies. Apart from rudimentary literacy, attained in a haphazard manner, the lower classes were not educated systematically or treated to the vocational guidance envisaged by Bucer.

Dissatisfaction with this state of affairs was expressed by Samuel Harmar in *Vox Populi, Or Glostersheres Desire: With the Way, and means to make a Kingdom Happy . . . By setting up of Schoolmasters in every Parish* (1642), which scheme for national education would have been financed by taxation levied by parliament. Agitation for schools found spontaneous expression in petitions from widely different sources, and eventually the Levellers' social programme included a demand for sufficient free schools to ensure universal literacy.[358] Parliament was mildly sympathetic to these proposals. After much debate it was declared that the substantial income from the abolition of Deans and Chapters would be applied for 'the Advancement of Learning and Piety'.[359] John Hacket complained at the time that this would undermine the endowments of many grammar schools, but parliament went on to protect educational endowments, while securing further resources for the support of schoolmasters and preachers. The Committee for Scandalous Ministers was ordered to examine the state of all free schools and hospitals.[360] Much later an order was made for proposals on school reform to be submitted for the urgent consideration of the Council of State. Then the Saints' Parliament set up a Committee for the Advancement of Learning, which operated between July and December 1653. Although the activities of this committee are not recorded, its sympathy with educational expansion was likely, owing to the association between its members and Samuel Hartlib.[361]

To the disappointment of reformers, this succession of committees produced no coherent national educational policy. However schoolmasters became incidental beneficiaries of national grants made primarily to assist the propagation of the gospel. Official agencies such as the County Committees, the Commissioners for the Propagation of the Gospel in New England, Ireland, Wales and the Four Northern Counties, and Commissioners for Charitable Uses, often became agents for the maintenance of schoolmasters and the establishment of small local

357. M. M. Knappen, *Tudor Puritanism* (Chicago, 1939), Chapter XXVI; Joan Simon (260), Chapters VI & XIII; W. K. Jordan, *Philanthropy* (167), pp.279–97; *idem, London* (168), pp.206–50; *idem, Rural England* (169), pp.52–60; K. R. M. Short, 'A Theory of Common Education in Elizabethan Puritanism', *Journal of Ecclesiastical History,* 1972, *33*: 31–48.

358. Corcoran (60), pp.31–3, 69–70; James (158), pp.318–26; Vincent (297), pp.30–3. Richard Overton, *An Appeal from the Commons* (204), p.104.

359. *CJ,* ii, p.176; 15 June 1641.

360. *CJ,* ii, p.317; 16 November 1641. Webster (320), pp. 27–8.

361. *CSPD 1650*, p.33; 7 Sept. 1650. Webster (320), p.61.

schools.[362] Other regional studies will probably provide confirmation for Richards's view that 'the propagation period [in Wales] saw . . . the new type of Puritan preaching schoolmaster, State subvention of Learning, schools for all classes, and a restricted experiment in the co-education of the sexes.'[363]

These grants were made for general pious uses, without specific regard for educational bias. Equally most of the petitioners, whether the citizens of Durham, for a 'College or School of Literature', those of Lincoln for 'some Schools for the better education of youth', or *Vox Populi's* pleas for poor schools in Gloucestershire, were silent on specific educational goals, beyond insistence on a high moral and religious tone.

As within the universities, there was a tendency to lapse into traditional forms, which produced weak imitations of the humanist grammar school foundations of the previous century. Westminster and St. Paul's maintained the Erasmian educational tradition and they were followed by a whole succession of later foundations, such as Felsted School, and by the numerous private tutors who played such an important part in preparing students for university entrance.[364] The single-minded and for the most part overriding devotion of the grammar schools to classical studies represented a tenacious tradition, which was given fresh authority by such enlightened schoolmasters as Ascham and Brinsley. Under their aegis, Latin and Greek grammatical studies were codified, perfected and rendered painless, but the dedicated schoolmaster was not expected to advance far into the liberal arts curriculum. Brinsley was silent on the educational value of the sciences and mathematics, while Ascham warned against overmuch attention to music, arithmetic and geometry. Mathematics was thought to render men solitary and unapt 'to serve in the world'.[365] Wallis at Felsted was probably exceptional in acquiring a knowledge of mathematics before entering university. John Langley's enterprising teaching at St. Paul's ironically provided a leading puritan divine with a basis for the argument that the grammar schools should be encouraged.[366] Such effective teachers laid the foundations for many successful undergraduate careers, by introducing the elements of the liberal arts curriculum. The better schools would have provided fluency in Latin and wide experience of classical authors; never-

362. Firth & Rait, ii, pp.144–5, 199, 377, 392–8. Watson (310); Corcoran (60), pp.31–3; Richards, *The Puritan Movement* (242), pp.222–39; *idem, Religious Developments* (243), pp.54–68; Vincent (297), pp.58–81, 94–108.

363. Richards (242), p.233.

364. For grammar schools in the seventeenth century, see J. Sargeaunt, *A History of Felsted School* (Chelmsford & London, 1889); G. F. Russell Barker, *Memoir of Richard Busby: with some account of Westminster School in the Seventeenth Century* (London, 1895); D. L. Clarke, *John Milton at St. Paul's School* (New York, 1948); W. A. L. Vincent, *The Grammar Schools: their continuing tradition 1660–1714* (London, 1969).

365. John Brinsley, *Ludus Literarius or the Grammar Schoole* (London, 1627); Roger Ascham, *The Scholemaster* (London, 1570), p.34.

366. Edward Reynolds, *A Sermon Touching the Use of Humane Learning* (London, 1658), pp.25–34.

theless Milton was probably correct in describing normal practice as 'seven or eight yeers meerly in scraping together so much miserable Latin and Greek, as might be learnt otherwise and delightfully in one yeer'. Similarly Hall characterised the university entrants as 'raw striplings, come out of some miserable Country-school, with a few shreds of Latine, that is as immusical to a polite ear as the gruntling of a Sow'.[367]

The reformers cultivated the general puritan commitment to education, but they also sought to bring about a complete intellectual reorientation by encouraging support for institutions with quite different intellectual and social aims from the grammar schools and universities. Hartlib expressed the widely-held view that 'this endeavour or nothing, will be able to work a Reformation in this our Age'.[368] A leading part in the propagation of the literature on education was played by Hartlib, whose protégés drafted schemes on all aspects of education. Hartlib was thus able to provide parliament with plans for a complete system of education, embracing research, teacher training, inspection, schools and workhouses for all social classes and both sexes. During the central and most productive phase of this enterprise, between 1648 and 1653, Hartlib regarded himself as the official parliamentary agent for educational affairs.[369]

The older ideal of universal education was reaffirmed, elaborated and translated into Baconian and Comenian terms. The blueprint for a national educational system, which had been gradually evolved by Hartlib and Dury, was presented to the Committee for the Advancement of Learning in 1653.[370] The reformers' first priority was given as the establishment of Common, and Mechanical Schools to serve the educational needs of the lower classes. By a serious and liberal approach to education the reformers believed that the 'common men in this Commonwealth will be so changed that few commoners in the world, or none in any Nation will be found like unto them for publick usefulnesse'. In a similar vein Winstanley pressed for each district administration to pay particular attention to education and to the supervision of the manners and vocational training of all children.[371] Hartlib's associates, Petty and Robinson, took up this call for national education. Petty proposed a system of *Ergastula literaria,* or 'literary work-houses' for all children above seven, none being excluded by poverty. Like Harmar, he proposed that poor children should earn their living by labour pro-

367. Milton, *Of Education, CPW,* ii, pp.370–1; Hall (127), p.25. For similar sentiments see Dury (89), pp.38–40; and letter from Wood to Hartlib, 10 June 1657, where the writer claims that the grammar schools do 'more hurt than good': HP XXXIII 1.

368. Dury (89), Preface, sig. A3r–v.

369. Webster (320), pp.50–3.

370. 'Some Proposalls towards the Advancement of Learning', HP XLVII 2; given in full in Webster (320), pp.166–92.

371. *Ibid.,* p.189. Winstanley (336), pp.15, 68. For a more eccentric statement of Winstanley's scheme see William Covel (62).

vided in the workhouse schools. The workhouses projected by Hartlib also had this educational dimension although the vocational aspect was more prominent. Robinson petitioned for the establishment of a system of state schools designed to provide free education for all boys and girls. No specific curricular recommendations were made, but elsewhere he supported vocational training schemes in accordance with the projects elaborated by other members of the Hartlib circle. An original item in Robinson's writings was a repeated insistence that the nation's maritime obligations rendered it essential that all children should be taught to swim.[372] Subscription to the idea of general educational expansion, not always with specific regard to curriculum or organisation, is found in a wide variety of sources, including Overton's *An Appeal from the Degenerate Representative Body* (1647), *Tyranipocrit* (1649),[373] Snell's *Right Teaching of Useful Knowledge* (1649), Dell's *A Reformation of Schools* (1653), Harrington's *Oceana* (1656), Humphrey Barrow's *The Relief of the Poor* (1656), Milton's *Likeliest Means to Remove Hirelings* (1659) and Plockhoy's *A Way Propounded to Make the Poor in these Nations Happy* (1659).

Care must be exercised not to exaggerate the democratic intentions of these writers. However they looked forward to a great expansion in the number of schools, which were to be staffed by lay teachers paid by the state or by the local community. This would at least have guaranteed basic literacy in the male population. Some theorists went further, to suggest formal education for both sexes. In principle these state schools would have broken the ecclesiastical control of education, giving much greater flexibility for religious expression and further opportunities of developing secular education.

Owing to their optimistic view of human abilities, and appreciation of the intrinsic worth of craft experience, the ideas on elementary education of Petty, Hartlib and Dury, completely transcended Bucer's more limited expectations. The puritan reformers followed tradition in designating reading, writing and arithmetic as the first requirements for Common Schools. Thereafter in normal practice the catechism and Anglican religious exercises would have completed this education. By contrast Petty's *Advice*, or *Some Proposals*, framed an education which was religious in spirit but non-sectarian in approach. Apart from the basic subjects, the puritan Common School curriculum included: a description of the natural world, the history of civilisation and Christianity, elementary rules of reasoning, the principles of natural justice and the constitutional history of England.[374] This ambitious foundation for elementary education came from Dury's pen, but its

372. Petty (210), pp.4–7; Hartlib, *The Parliaments Reformation* (1646) and later writings on workhouses; Robinson, *Certain Proposalls* (247), pp.24–6.

373. *Tyranipocrit, Discovered with his Wiles, wherewith he Vanquisheth* (Rotterdam, 1649)—attributed to Walwyn.

374. 'Some Proposalls', in Webster (320), pp.178–9.

ultimate source was probably Comenius's *Didactica Magna*, which was known to Dury in manuscript. The *Proposals* of Hartlib and Dury followed the example of Comenius's Vernacular School closely, except for the significant omission of reference to religious instruction. Comenius had given great prominence to music, psalms, hymns, the catechism and scriptural studies.[375]

Petty's *Ergastula literaria* had an overwhelmingly practical orientation. In early education priority was to be given to training in manual arts, with recreation to ensure a sound physique—a feature also found in Comenius. Reading and writing were to be followed by 'artificial memory'. Drawing would have inculcated a secure knowledge of the objects under consideration. With respect to mathematics Petty reversed the judgement of Ascham, arguing that this subject was useful in human affairs; it was also a sound guide to reason and a remedy for 'volatile and unstedy' minds. Petty's system of basic education concluded with participation in one of a wide range of listed crafts, although in cases of special aptitude, students might learn music or languages.[376]

Thus from the very first stages of education the English writers placed the emphasis on practical life. Comenius's explicit religious, aesthetic and literary provisions were largely sacrificed, owing to the reformers' concern to awaken interest in the study and exploitation of the natural environment. The student would then be equipped for more specialised scientific and technical education in Mechanical Schools. These were to be adapted according to local circumstances, specialising in either husbandry, navigation, mineralogy, surveying, architecture, painting, or metal-working.[377] The regular supplementation of elementary education by formal technical instruction was widely advocated; and vocational training became a common denominator of a wide range of projects, whether workhouses for the destitute, or colleges for the gentry. Bucer had hoped to encourage skilled practitioners to disseminate their knowledge, but he had not envisaged the evolution of this practice into the systematic provision of formal technical education.

Hartlib and Dury believed that the lower classes could not perform their social role efficiently unless they were provided with a comprehensive education. These planners did not expect the poor to benefit from social mobility, but envisaged that they would enjoy greater security, independence, wealth and esteem.

It was thought that once general education was introduced, a desire for even higher educational attainment would inevitably follow. Hence there was a widespread call for the recruitment of gifted poor scholars into the ministry, and it was a common complaint that the universities, which had been founded for this purpose, had virtually become closed to the lower classes. Thus Hartlib, Dury, Peter and Poole urged the

375. *ODO*, i, pp.172–6; *Didactica Magna* (56), pp.266–73.
376. Petty (210), pp.4–7.
377. 'Some Proposalls', in Webster (320), pp.179–80.

establishment of scholarships to restore the social balance among theological students. More importantly, they wished to realise the potentialities of the lower classes to advance secular knowledge. In particular the skilled artisans could be expected to make an invaluable contribution to the compilation of Baconian natural histories and to the improvement of technology, agriculture and trade. Petty went even further. He was convinced that 'many are now holding the Plough, which might have beene made fit to steere the State'. Likewise Robinson recommended that his national system of elementary schools should be organised to enable gifted poor scholars to enter university.[378] Winstanley wished to employ education as a means to promote even more radical social equality. But such ambitious objectives were not generally acceptable. The relief of poverty, and promotion of effective economic participation were generally applauded goals, but social rise through education, or utopian egalitarianism, were not always regarded with complaisance even as ideals. Snell and Milton firmly stated that vocational training should instil a sense of public service but preclude men 'soaring above the meanness wherein they were born'.[379] Sprigg pointedly contradicted Petty, warning that good ploughmen would make bad scholars; higher studies should not be 'sullied by the rude embraces of every Mechanick Son', since this would bring learning into ill repute with the gentry.[380]

An important step towards narrowing the educational gulf between the upper and lower classes was provided by the programme for Noble Schools announced in the *Proposals*. Since active economic participation was considered an object of the education of all classes, the Noble Schools outlined by Petty and Dury took on many of the qualities of Common or Vernacular Schools. Comenius had warned against regarding 'vernacular' education as appropriate to one class, and 'classical' education as most befitting their betters. If vernacular education was sound pedagogically and socially, it was appropriate to all children.[381] This attitude was accepted by his English followers. Since classical studies were irrelevant to the programme of education for the lower classes, they were also not central to the Noble Schools. The latter were expected to build on the Vernacular School foundation, developing each subject to a higher level and introducing a wider range of topics in the greater time available for studies. Noble Schools were also expected to parallel Mechanical Schools by providing appropriate vocational training during the later stages of education. Whereas the proposals for Common and Mechanical Schools were directed to parliament, as the agency required to finance educational expansion, the plans for Noble Schools were primarily addressed to the educated pub-

378. Petty (210), p.4; Robinson (247), p.24; see also Peter (208), p.6.

379. Milton, *Likeliest Means to Remove Hirelings* (1659), pp.96–7; Snell (262), Preface.

380. Sprigg (267), pp.92–4.

381. Comenius, *Didactica Magna* (56), pp.266–8; *ODO*, i, pp.172–3.

lic. Great skill would have been required to convince this audience to abandon its customary educational habits, to embrace institutions having little in common with grammar schools or universities and employing a pedagogy suited equally to the needs of the lower classes.

William Petty's *Ergastula literaria,* although not primarily intended for the élite, were designed to meet the educational requirements of all children. Even the crafts which were introduced in the final phase of this education were thought appropriate for 'all Children, though of the highest ranke'. The curriculum embraced practical mathematics, watch-making, art, optics, botany, music, ship design, architecture, confectionery, chemistry and anatomy; the teaching methods would have included reference to techniques and instruments.[382] Many of these subjects, particularly the sciences, had already achieved a firm place among the cultural interests of the 'virtuoso'. Petty no doubt felt that the virtuosi might be sympathetic to a science-based education, which would also have encouraged accomplishment in the crafts; he argued that this would be to their intellectual and material advantage. Scientific and technical education would give them intellectual satisfaction, advance learning, and lead to the improvement of their estates. By subtle modification, the workhouses of the poor had become Noble Schools for the rich.[383]

The plan for a Noble School produced by Dury was the most detailed educational project produced during the Puritan Revolution. This work displayed the same exhaustive and systematic approach which Comenius was simultaneously developing in his *Pampaedia*. Dury's Noble School emphasised complete and direct commitment to the ideals of the active life, designed to direct students

> 'into profitable employments which may fit them to be good Commonwealths men, by the knowledge of all things which are fundamentall for the settlement of a State in Husbandry, in necessary Trades, in Navigation, in Civill Offices for the Administration of Justice; in Peace and War; and in Oeconomicall Duties by which they may be serviceable to their own families, and to their neighbours.'[384]

Nothing was to be accounted 'true learning' unless it was directly serviceable to mankind. Superficially this approach might be identified with the educational objectives of many Renaissance advocates of the active public life. However Dury reacted against the humanistic curriculum of the schools and universities, which 'neither containe any substance or solidity of Matter; or give them any addresse by way of Method to make use of that which they know for the benefit of Mankind'. It was therefore necessary to undertake a complete recon-

382. Petty (210), pp.4–7.
383. *Ibid.,* p.6.
384. Dury (89), p.21.

struction of education according to a 'new method'.[385] Dury's organisation of his school and curriculum resembled that of Comenius's *Pampaedia,* but there were important differences of emphasis.

Entrants to the Noble School were expected at the age of eight or nine to have obtained, under ushers attached to the school, a working knowledge of a curriculum very like that of the Vernacular School.[386] Thus the Noble School was in the place of the Mechanical School of the lower classes. In its first stage (lasting from eight or nine to thirteen or fourteen years of age) the education to be provided was predominantly vernacular and scientific. The only linguistic exercises were: an introduction to the names of familiar objects in classical languages; simple Latin sentences relating to everyday experience; and the most elementary exercises in translation from an edition of the *Janua linguarum* of Comenius. Otherwise the subjects for study were a natural development of the Vernacular School curriculum, involving further investigations into natural history, applied science, the branches of pure and practical mathematics, husbandry, gardening, fishing and fowling, and anatomy. The non-scientific area was represented by secular and ecclesiastical history.[387]

The last stage of the Reformed or Noble School would have taken the student to maturity and this was clearly intended to supplant university education by providing a full vocational training. Fluency in the ancient languages would have been attained through the study of classical authors selected according to their relevance to particular aspects of the curriculum. There was very little overlap with the university arts curriculum even if this was conceived in its broadest terms. On the other hand the Reformed School aimed to perform some of the functions of the higher faculties, although their literary bias, teaching methods, formal academic exercises and disputations would have been avoided. Of the ten major divisions of the curriculum, one included logic, rhetoric and poetry, two embraced moral philosophy, economics, and legal studies, and six were concerned with the natural sciences, medicine and mathematics.[388] The scientific subjects were outlined as follows:

'1. The Latine Authors of Agriculture Cato, Varro, Columella may be put into their hands by parcels, to be an enlargement unto that which they have alreadie been taught concerning Husbandry.

2. The Natural History of Pliny and Others, by choice parcels are also to be perused by them; and brought home to what they have formerly seen; together with the Histories of Meteors, Minerals, etc.

385. *Ibid.,* pp.39–41.
386. *Ibid.,* pp.52–4.
387. *Ibid.,* pp.55–7.
388. *Ibid.,* pp.57–61.

3. In the like manner some Models and Books of Architecture, Enginry, Fortification, Fireworks, Weapons, Military Discipline, and Navigation are to be lookt upon . . .
6. The Theory of all the Mathematicks, with the full Practice of that which was deficient in their former Institution; where the Opticks with Instruments belonging thereunto and the Art of Dialing is to be entertained; and in Arithmetick the way of keeping Accounts.
7. The principles of Naturall Philosophie and the main grounds of Medicine, with the Instruments of Distilling and other Chimicall Operations, and the Art of Apothecaries, are to be offered unto them partly in books, partly in the Operations themselves by an ocular inspection thereof, and of their drugges.
8. The Art of Chirurgery described in books, with an ocular inspection of all their tooles, and Compositions of plaisters and ointments, and the use thereof.'[389]

These subjects completed the education of the élite in a manner thoroughly consistent with the education envisaged for Vernacular Schools. In the final stages classical authors were utilised, but they were assimilated according to their merits, in the manner recommended by Bacon. Thus the overall bias of this education was non-humanistic, its content was determined according to the puritan social ethic and its methods were consistent with the new psychological theories of learning.

Adoption of this educational formula for the élite was expected to have repercussions throughout the educational system. One of the main aims of the reformers was to train 'Reformed School-Masters'. Neither the magistrate nor the minister would 'prosper or subsist long without him'.[390] Yet, it was lamented, schoolmasters occupied a lowly social position. By increased attention to their education, increased influence and status would be achieved. Accordingly various plans for national education included special provision for teacher-training colleges. The puritan educational literature emphasised the complementary relationship of the minister and the teacher. Their partnership would not be completely effective without greater parity of status.[391] Joshua Rawlin, a teacher from Kent, proposed that each county should establish a committee of ministers to appoint grammar school teachers; approval would only be given to those able to teach according to the methods of Comenius. In 1649 Hartlib visited Cromwell's physician, John Bathurst, who announced to him an ambitious scheme for a high-level training college, having a structure resembling a university college. This was to be financed by local taxes and it would serve as 'an Inspector

389. *Ibid.*, pp.58–9.
390. *Ibid.*, Preface, sig. A4v–5r.
391. For example, Dury (86), p.22; 'Some Proposalls' (320), p.191.

and Seminarie of all schoolmasters of all free-schooles throughout the kingdome'. Bathurst's scheme was expected to cost £4,000.[392]

The Reformed School undoubtedly appealed to the university critics and advocates of educational expansion. Its humanistic element was probably too slight to meet with Milton's approval, but most moderate and sectarian reformers would have regarded it as a practical expression of their objectives. There was soon demand for an expanded edition, to which Dury added an appendix criticising the universities.[393] The main principles were reiterated in *Some Proposals towards the Advancement of Learning* in 1653. *The Reformed School* became a leading influence on puritan educational thought and its effect was apparent on many college proposals which emerged from a variety of sources during the 1650s. These ranged from schemes for technical and agricultural colleges (discussed below, in Chapter V) to ambitious plans for new universities.

(x) Practical Projects

During the 1650s there emerged from the provinces a variety of requests for local colleges. Provincial towns became more assertive and petitioners hoped for a decentralised system of education of the type prevalent in the Netherlands. Hugh Peter called for the establishment of 'Illustrious schools' in such areas as Yorkshire, Cornwall and Wales, to replace the 'very rotten' older universities. Their function would be 'the preparing and fitting younger people for som service, in reference to their Counties'.[394] After maintaining a discreet silence on university expansion in his earlier writings, Dury proposed in 1653 that 'the teaching of Noble Sciences' should not be confined to universities and made unlawful elsewhere. Everyone who was able and willing should be allowed to establish institutions of higher education.[395] Dell stigmatised the current situation as a distasteful 'Monopoly of Humane Learning'; he called for the provision of specialised universities and colleges 'in every great town or City in the Nation, as in London, York, Bristow, Exceter, Norwich'. This decentralisation would reduce the cost of education to parents, who were currently faced with substantial fees for sending their children to distant Oxford and Cambridge. Furthermore it would prevent their children's exposure to unwholesome influences, as well as facilitate the integration of general education with local vocational training. By spending part of each day in study and part at work, students would be deflected from unprofitable knowledge

392. Letter from Rawlin to Hartlib, 9 Feb. 1645/6, HP x 11; Ephemerides 1649. A similar scheme is given by Snell (262), pp.310–13. Bathurst founded two schools in Yorkshire; attention to accountancy was a notable feature of the curriculum outlined in their statutes: Watson (311), p.305.

393. Dury (89).

394. Peter (208), pp.3–5.

395. 'Some Proposalls' (320), p.190.

and scholasticism.[396] William Sprigg, Fellow of Lincoln College, Oxford, turned Dell's proposals to the advantage of the virtuosi. He proposed that the colleges of the universities should be dispersed to the provinces, Durham being specifically mentioned as a suitable location. The curriculum outlined for these colleges echoed Dury's enthusiasm for science, but it lacked his earnest sense of social purpose. Sprigg aimed at a strange hybrid between the sciences (anatomical exercises, husbandry, and laboratory chemistry) and traditional gentlemanly accomplishments such as horseriding, fencing, vaulting, dancing and music.[397] Reference to such diversions indicates a distinct dilution of principle, and compromise with popular gentlemanly taste within the ranks of the puritan reformers.

Sprigg's ideas confirm the presence of continuing middle-class interest in a form of education modelled on the French Academies.[398] These academies paid considerable attention to experimental science and other modern subjects; before the Civil War this ideal of higher education was offered tentatively as an alternative or complement to the liberal arts curriculum of the universities. One advocate of this form of education was Sir Francis Kynaston, who established his Musaeum Minervae in Bedford Street, Covent Garden. This college was guided by an intelligently conceived constitution, which provided for languages and other gentlemanly pursuits, but also emphasised surveying, navigation, architecture and cosmography. The staff of six included the physician Edward May; the astronomy professor was Nicholas Fiske, a well-known astrologer; and the geometry professor was John Speidell, a mathematical practitioner. The inventor de Berg was also associated with Kynaston.[399] Although Kynaston's academy failed, the kind of education which he advocated was available elsewhere in London on an informal basis. Association with the Inns of Court was often a means of access to tutors who could provide the embellishments offered by the French Academy. If this was not sufficient, the young gentleman could absorb the academy curriculum at source during a tour of the continent.[400]

After 1640, various proponents of the French Academy emerged to reap the fruits of puritan educational enthusiasm. John Humphrey

396. Dell, *The Right Reformation* (78), pp.28–9.

397. Sprigg (267), pp.38–55.

398. F. A. Yates, *French Academies in the Sixteenth Century* (London, 1947); Watson (312), pp.xxxii–xxxiv.

399. Kynaston, *The Constitution of the Musaeum Minervae* (London, 1636); BM Add. MS 6269, fols. 11–17, 'Diploma Regum Regenti et Professoribus Musei Minervae'. See *VCH Middlesex,* i, p.242; G. H. Turnbull, 'Samuel Hartlib's connection with Sir Francis Kynaston's "Musaeum Minervae"' *Notes & Queries,* 1952, *197*: 33–7.

400. C. Howard, *English Travellers in the Renaissance* (London, 1914); J. W. Stoye, *English Travellers Abroad 1604–1667* (London, 1952). Mr. Randall Caudill of Christ Church Oxford is preparing a major study on this subject. See also below note 411.

petitioned parliament to provide him with a house to teach the sons of gentlemen, in order to counteract the common practice of travelling abroad for education. He proposed to teach ancient and modern languages, history, oratory, poetry, experimental philosophy and mathematics. Hartlib suggested the addition of calligraphy, double-writing, stenography and 'the history of the most principall things obvious to the sense'.[401] As an alternative to their economic projects Hugh l'Amy and Peter le Pruvost proposed to establish a French Academy either in London or at one of the university colleges. This would have taught the characteristic assortment of French, divinity, the sciences, economics, music, art and military skills.[402]

The most ambitious and enterprising academy projector was Sir Balthazar Gerbier who made contact with Hartlib from Paris in 1648, with a view to settling in England as a teacher. In the hope of preventing hostility from the universities, which it was believed had undermined Kynaston's Musaeum, he claimed that his academy would avoid the university curriculum except for Latin and philosophy. A prospectus was prepared setting out a curriculum which was based on Latin, other, modern languages, experimental philosophy and mathematics. Recreational subjects were also offered. Gerbier arranged for this prospectus to be distributed throughout England by Hartlib. In a revised version of the prospectus he removed Latin in order further to appease the universities. Having made careful preparations, Gerbier arrived in England in March 1649 and opened his Academy at Bethnal Green in July of that year. Prominent public figures were invited to inspect the Academy and an advertisement appeared in each of two newspapers.[403] Representative lectures delivered in 1649 and 1650 were published. Those on military architecture, navigation, cosmography, geography, law, 'the art of well speaking' and 'all languages, arts, sciences and noble exercises which are taught in Sir Balthazar Gerbier's academy' have been preserved.[404] Despite the originator's great gifts as a publicist, it is doubtful whether his academy had more than the briefest life.

In the course of the educational proposals very little reference was made to the education of women. Generally, where positive conviction was absent, it may be assumed that no serious plans for women's education were contemplated. The most notable exponent of women's education was John Dury. Throughout *The Reformed School* it is apparent that his Noble School was designed for adaptation to the requirements of

401. 'The Petition of Col. John Hunfrey', HP XLVII 8b.

402. HP XII 1e.

403. Gerbier, *To All Fathers of Families.* At least four editions were produced in 1648 and 1649, one form bearing the title, *The Interpreter* (London, 1648). *Perfect Occurrences,* July 13–30 1649, No. 133; July 27–Aug. 31 1649, No. 135. *Man in the Moon,* July 25–Aug. 2 1649, No. 15. Hartlib's relations with Gerbier are discussed by Turnbull *HDC,* pp.59–63. See also Watson (312), p.64 & *passim.*

404. For details of these lectures see Wing (335), ii, p.103; Fortescue (101), ii, p.57.

both sexes. They were to be educated separately, and according to their different vocational requirements. The girls were primarily intended to become 'good and carefull housewives' but those 'found capable of Tongues and Sciences' were to be given every encouragement. This liberal attitude to women was consistent with their important role in the Hartlib circle.[405] The involvement of Mrs. Dury in a project for girls' education is indicated by a letter to Lady Ranelagh, in which she included general strictures on female upbringing, and hinted that she was composing a longer treatise on this subject.[406]

Education for girls from the lower classes was discussed by Winstanley and Robinson, and in the workhouse schemes of Hartlib. Their primary aim was to equip girls for their domestic tasks and to train them in cottage crafts, such as weaving. For the more wealthy families, private girls' schools were already flourishing in London. These were very conventional and no doubt distasteful to strenuous Puritans.[407] An ambitious alternative was Gerbier's Bethnal Green academy, which was established to pioneer co-education, but which was probably not successful in attracting either sex for more than a short time. Adolphus Speed proposed parallel academies for young men and women. The male curriculum epitomises the educational fashions against which Dury was competing. Speed proposed to use new methods which would facilitate the teaching of French and the classical languages. Improved efficiency in language teaching would leave ample scope for heraldry, art, music, dancing, horsemanship and fencing. The 'true experimentall naturall Phylosophy and what is most necessary of the Mathematics' were optional extras, to be taken at parents' discretion. This curriculum completely reversed the priorities of *The Reformed School*. Speed's project is particularly valuable as a source of information about fashionable tastes in girls' education. Its ample provision for vanities such as 'the most excellent wayes to make the Hands, and Face faire, and to take out wrinckles, fleckles, etc', might have been the specific instigation for Dorothy Dury's counterproposals. More innocuous subjects in the curriculum included natural history, practical medicine, distillation and winemaking.[408] Mrs. Dury would have been more attracted by the methods of Bathsua Makins, the sister-in-law of John Pell and one of the most able women teachers of the period. Her outline of female education praised Comenius and approached the spirit of Dury's *The Reformed School* and the nonconformist academies.[409]

405. Dury (89), pp.18–20; 'Some Proposalls', (320), p.190.
406. 'Of the Education of Girls', BM Sloane MS 649, fols. 203–5; given in full in Turnbull *HDC*, pp.120–1.
407. Watson (313), ii, pp.711–14; M. Bryant in *VCH Middlesex*, i, pp.251–5.
408. Speed (264). A variant in HP LVII 3d, is given in Turnbull *HDC*, pp.117–19.
409. Bathsua Makins, *Essay to Revive the Ancient Education of Gentlewomen* (London, 1673); based on Anna Maria Schuran, *The Learned Maid, or whether a Maid may be a Scholar* (London, 1659). For Bathsua Makins, see Vivian Salmon in *Pelliana*, N.S., *1*, No. 3: 19–20; Watson (312), pp.419–20.

The reformers were aware that it was necessary to work out their schemes at a local level. In the counties most initiative was devoted to the re-establishment of schools and maintenance of schoolmasters, but headway was also made on plans for more advanced and prestigious institutions. It was this challenge to break the university monopoly and experiment with new forms of higher education which particularly excited the theorists. Dell and Webster did little to translate their ideas into practical terms but others were more active in outlining specific projects and in generating public support for them.

London was the most obvious location for developments in higher education. Even the opponents of the establishment of new universities in small provincial towns were obliged to concede that London was large enough to support institutions of higher education. London already had societies which took on certain educational functions. These included the Inns of Court, the College of Physicians, Chelsea College, Sion College, and Gresham College, as well as other, craft organisations. There were also many active individual teachers and practitioners in such specialities as mathematics or even oriental studies. The capital had already been called the 'third university of England'.[410] At Gresham professors were appointed to lecture on many aspects of the liberal arts curriculum. This college had been conspicuously successful as a centre for mathematical studies. Chelsea and Sion were Anglican foundations which had supported theologians and scholars. The mathematician, Nathaniel Torporley, had lodged at Sion. At the outset of the Long Parliament Chelsea had been considered as the location for Comenius's College of Light. Both the Inns of Court and the College of Physicians acquired educational functions by virtue of their professional obligations. The Inns during the sixteenth and early seventeenth centuries attracted large numbers of young gentlemen; some of these studied law, but a sizeable percentage used the residential facilities in London to take advantage of a French Academy type of education. This could be adapted to individual taste, by appropriate selection from the ranks of the specialist tutors available in the vicinity. Often this education was undertaken after a brief spell at university. The College of Physicians sponsored lectures and its members became increasingly engaged in research. The Barber-Surgeons' Company undertook similar activities at a slightly less sophisticated level.[411]

In view of the vigour of London intellectual life and the assertiveness of its merchants and politicians, it is somewhat surprising that only scattered evidence exists about proposals to establish a university in the capital. But it is clear that many groups were sympathetic to

410. Sir George Buc, 'The Third Universitie of England' (1612), appended to Edmund Howe's edition of Stow's *Chronicles* (London, 1615).

411. K. Charlton, *Education in Renaissance England* (London, 1965), pp.169–95. W. Prest, 'Legal Education of the Gentry at the Inns of Court 1560–1640', *Past and Present,* 1967, No. 38: 20–39; *idem, The Inns of Court under Elizabeth I and the Early Stuarts 1590–1640* (London, 1972). Hill (149), pp.14–84.

the idea, although there is no indication that professional organisations or Gresham College shared this enthusiasm; they had an established relationship with the old universities and were satisfied that their aspirations could be realised within the existing institutional framework. One discordant voice from the professions was that of William Rand, the advocate of a College of Graduate Physicians, which he hoped would lay the foundations for a new university of London.[412]

The first significant reference to a university of London was made in 1643, during discussions at the Westminster Assembly on the expansion of ministerial training. Soon afterwards a more ambitious proposal emerged, for the use of ecclesiastical endowments to finance both 'a glorious university' in London, and replicas of Eton College in each bishop's residence.[413] An anonymous pamphlet gave a more expansive account of the proposed university, repeating the Westminster Assembly's concern to improve the stock of well-trained ministers. It argued that the old universities had never housed more than six thousand students; furthermore only ten per cent of these completed the seven-year arts course. Hence the author doubted the capacity of the old universities to supply the estimated deficit of 20,000 ministers. Upon that estimate there was scope in London for a university of considerable size. In addition to its primarily theological function, the new university was expected to cultivate modern languages and contribute to the promotion of trade.[414]

Hartlib and his associates drafted various schemes, either for the reform of individual London institutions, or for their amalgamation into a university. Anxiety was expressed about the condition of Gresham College, which had greatly declined from its position as a centre of the mathematical arts. In an essay on Gresham, Petty argued that the traditional university method of lecturing on texts was worthless; Gresham should confine its lectures to topics capable of experimental demonstration. Accordingly, the chairs of divinity, civil law and rhetoric were inappropriate to the College; they were also superfluous, since these subjects were more efficiently taught elsewhere. The remaining professors, of physic, geometry, astronomy and music, needed to reorientate their lectures to pay maximum attention to experimental philosophy, practical demonstration and social application, while four new chairs were proposed: for magnetism, optics, mechanics and chemical technology.[415]

Hartlib drafted proposals for a major federal institution which would have included the reformed Gresham College. The new university of London would have been controlled by an 'agency' or committee. This was to examine schemes, determine an appropriate form of collegiate

412. See below, pp.306–8 and Appendix III.
413. *LJ*, vi, 319. Cooper (58), iii, p.361. *A Good Motion*, 1646, BM 669 f 10 (108).
414. *Motives grounded upon the word of God*, 1647 (193).
415. No title; HP XLVII 18. This document is given in full in Appendix VII, below.

organisation, and negotiate with the Court of Aldermen and the Common Council, the bodies which would undertake the building or 'perfecting of the publick schooles or Gresham College and compleating the Membership of Professors'. Locations considered for colleges included bishops' houses, Charterhouse, Christ's Hospital and Hatton House; Gresham College 'should bee made the Publick Schooles for Professors to read daily, to confer, to dispute, to make orations; both for Strangers, Natives and Citizens; the Professors to bee outlandish and English men'.[416]

The final draft involved eleven colleges, most of which may be related to projects announced by the Hartlib circle between 1647 and 1649:

'University of London to consist of severall Colledges by way of Eminence besides training up of Ministers and Scholars.

1. For an Office of Addresse. [under Robinson, established at Threadneedle Street]
2. For a Seminary for Plantations and the Churches beyond Seas. Irish Colledge. [Dury, and anon., *Motives grounded upon the Word of God* (1647), had stressed missionary training]
3. For Education or an Academy of Nobility and Gentry. [Dury's Noble School]
4. For Advancement of Universal Learning. [Hartlib's Agency for the Advancement of Universal Learning]
5. For Conversions or correspondency of Jews and advancement of Oriental Language and Learning. [for Dury's college for 'oriental Languages and Learning' see his *Seasonable Discourse* (1649), pp. 15-17]
6. For Verulamian Experimental Philosophy. [Gresham College]
7. For Inventors and Advancement of all Mechanical Arts and Industries. [Vauxhall House]
8. For State Studys or Politics *ad Verulamium*.
9. For Controversies and Pacification or Chelsey to bee that Colledge. [Chelsea College]
10. For Plantations and Conversion of the Gentiles. [cf. item 2, above]
11. A seminary or one College for all Foreigne churches. [originally suggested in Dury's *A faithful and seasonable Advice* (1643)]'[417]

From this sketch it is evident that Hartlib and his associates were making elaborate plans for a university of London. This institution would have drawn together many different foundations, and these would

416. No title; HP XLVII 8. (Other notes suggest the addition of colleges for medicine and agriculture.)

417. HP XLVII 8; Webster (320), p.60. Burnet (41), i, p.139, believed that Cromwell's favourite project was for the establishment of a council of seven members of Chelsea College for the administration of protestant affairs.

have been brought into line with the religious and social aims of the Puritans. In subsequent years efforts tended to be devoted to specific aspects of this programme, although the idea of a metropolitan university was not entirely forgotten, as witnessed by Rand's reference to it in 1656.

The ample supply of ministers, schoolmasters and educational institutions in London may have led to complacency, and hence resistance to the grandiose and utopian amalgamation proposed by Hartlib. In view of the already diverse educational provisions in the capital, a university probably appeared to be superfluous to the needs of the élite. By contrast there was deep concern about the shortage of teachers and pastors in the provinces, a problem which was particularly critical in Wales, Ireland and the Northern Counties. Consequently these areas were accorded special priority when parliament applied the long-promised ecclesiastical revenues to the support of ministers and schoolmasters. There was significant local enthusiasm for the appropriation of these resources, and the educational reformers appreciated that this policy provided an opportunity for the realisation of some of their goals.

The Welsh Puritans were primarily concerned with the expansion of elementary education. There was no obvious centre in which to develop advanced studies, and local enterprise was not greatly affected by London intellectual fashions. Whitelocke's claim that schoolmasters were settled in every Welsh town was an exaggeration, but the short-term achievement was certainly considerable.[418] Hugh Peter had proclaimed the desirability of a Welsh university, probably in response to the suggestion of John Lewis, who became an important member of the Welsh Gospel Propagation Commission.[419] Lewis's primary concern was to improve recruitment into the ministry. Wealthy Welsh patrons were sought for academies which would teach 'the most necessary kind of Arts and good literature'. Little was achieved, although others sympathised with Lewis's aims—notably John Ellis of Dolgelly, who offered his services as a teacher. A further adherent, John Humphrey, earlier a pupil under Langley at Pembroke College Oxford, informed Lewis that Richard Baxter was also an advocate of university extension in Wales. Baxter claimed that he had canvassed this idea as early as 1646. However, no general support had been forthcoming, although in 1657 Baxter was more confident that the scheme would be patronised by the Protector and parliament. He favoured the establishment of the college in England; Shrewsbury was thought to be particularly suitable, but various Welsh sites were more agreeable to his correspondents. Tentative estimates were made about endowments and size, but Ellis remarked despondently that, despite his and his coadjutants' assurances

418. Richards (242), pp.222–34; *idem* (243), pp.54–68.

419. John Lewis, *Contemplations upon these Times, or the Parliament explained to Wales* (London, 1646), p.32; *idem, Some Seasonable and Modest Thoughts in Order to the Furtherance of Religion and the Gospel, especially in Wales* (London, 1656), p.30 (dedicated to Cromwell).

about respecting the privileges of English universities, 'for their special Interests, they will oppose us'. Like Baxter he believed that the support of Cromwell was indispensable for the further promotion of a Welsh university. They were probably correct in anticipating his support, but their efforts were made too late to achieve practical expression under the Protectorate.[420]

By contrast with Wales, Ireland required constant and vigilant supervision from London. In 1649 John Owen was appointed as parliament's delegate charged with examining the spiritual condition of the inhabitants of Ireland. In an impassioned sermon to parliament preached upon his return he pleaded for the provision of ministers to rescue the 'gospelless' people of Ireland.[421] Prompt action was taken to supply preachers, and this was followed by various orders, to regulate the grammar schools, settle new schools and introduce apprenticeship schemes.[422] One of the resultant committees, appointed in 1651 to order Irish schools according to 'the Rules and Discipline used in the free-schooles of Literature in England or Holland, known to any of the said Committee', was dominated by Hartlib's associates, Anthony Morgan, Henry Jones, Petty and Worsley.[423] The last two had direct experience of Dutch education and were probably responsible for the reference to Holland.

Dublin provided a natural centre for Irish educational ventures. Immediately following Owen's sermon an influential committee was appointed to develop a comprehensive educational foundation on the basis of Trinity College. This committee was ordered to supervise the

> 'maintenance of the Colledge now in or near the city of Dublin commonly called Trinity Colledge, and of a Master, Fellows, Scholars and Officers there; and for the erecting setling and maintenance of one other Colledge in the said City of Dublin, and of a Master, Fellows, Scholars and Officers therein, and of publique Professors in the University there; and also for the erecting, establishing and maintenance of a Free-school; and of a Master, Ushers, Scholars and Officers there.'[424]

Once again, the trustees for this scheme included known sympathisers with intellectual and educational reform, Sir Robert King, Henry Jones and John Cook. Since these names occur on later smaller

420. G. F. Nuttall, 'The Correspondence of John Lewis, Glasrug, with Richard Baxter and with Dr. John Ellis, Dolgelly', *Journal of the Merioneth Historical & Record Soc.*, 1953/6, 2: 120–34.

421. W. Orme, *Memoirs of the Life and Writings of John Owen* (London, 1826), pp.86–93; Toon (282), pp.34–7. Owen, *The Steadfastness of the Promises and Sinfulness of Staggering* (London, 1650), preached 28 Feb. 1650.

422. Corcoran (60), p.78; Dunlop (83), ii, pp.494, 578–85.

423. Corcoran (60), pp.76–7, 30 March 1655/6.

424. 'An Act for the better Advancement of the Gospel and Learning in Ireland', Firth & Rait, ii, pp.355–7.

lists of Dublin trustees, King, Jones and Cook were perhaps active in framing the constitution of the new university. Furthermore they appear to have enjoyed the sympathy of Henry Cromwell and John Owen, two of the most powerful of the trustees.

The trustees saw that Trinity College, which had previously functioned at the level of a small college in the English universities, was virtually extinct. John Owen was invited to initiate discussions with his colleagues on revised constitutions for the college.[425] During these consultations Trinity was invested with a staff more acceptable to the Commonwealth, headed by the conscientious puritan preacher Samuel Winter. Besides playing a prominent part in propagating puritanism in Ireland, Winter seems to have revived the fortunes of the college, even attracting 'several hopeful young Schollars' from England.[426] Most of the teaching staff of about six Fellows were also dedicated Puritans, who supplied adequate if conventional guidance for the small body of students.[427] Characteristically, in view of their interest in ministerial training, one of the few new academic regulations introduced by these puritan preachers stipulated increased attention to Greek, Hebrew and rhetoric.[428] Two other of the appointments at Trinity College were more adventurous. Miles Symner, a friend of Hartlib and Petty, was established as professor of mathematics with an explicitly utilitarian brief, 'forasmuch as there is a great occasion for surveying of lands in this Country, and that there are divers ingenious Persons, Soldiers and others who are desirous to be instructed and fitted for the same'.[429] Besides playing a leading part in the Irish survey, Symner was an enthusiastic experimental philosopher, so that at least one senior member of Trinity was intimate with the scientific affairs of the English Baconians.

An even more significant appointment for the institutional strength of Trinity was John Stearne, who had been educated under Samuel Ward at Cambridge. Stearne settled in Dublin as a medical practitioner and worked assiduously for the establishment of a College of Physicians to regulate medicine in the city. His broad humanistic interests probably recommended him to Trinity, where he was one of the first new Fellows. This versatile figure served as Senior Fellow, registrar, and at different times as professor of civil law, of Hebrew, and of medicine. His permanent achievement was the acquisition of Trinity Hall, previously a small student residence, which was repaired at his own expense and established as an independent college 'for

425. Urwick (295); J. P. Mahaffy, *An Epoch in Irish History, Trinity College* (Dublin, 1903), pp.293–324. Dunlop (83), i, pp.10–11, 2 July 1651.

426. J.W. [John Winter], *The Life of Dr. Samuel Winter* (London, 1671), pp.10–13.

427. Urwick (295), pp.73–83.

428. *Ibid.*, p.62.

429. Trinity College Dublin, MS General Registry from 1626, fol. 95. Quoted from T. C. Barnard (*op. cit.* above, p.66, n. 112), p.130.

accommodating Physicians with a convenient place to meet in'. Gradually, Trinity Hall developed as a teaching and professional centre, awarding its first medical degrees in 1659. After the restoration Stearne's position as professor of medicine was confirmed. As in the English universities, medical education provided an uncontroversial area for expanding the scope of formal studies. The initial participants in Stearne's college are not identified, but Dublin held many resourceful figures having medical qualifications, including Petty, William Hill, Robert Wood, Worsley and William Currer.[430]

The trustees made extremely slow progress with their ambitious scheme for the new college in Dublin. Soon after arriving in Dublin in 1656 Robert Wood reported that Henry Cromwell 'is about a very noble Designe, of making another Colledge in this City, and putting things into a better way for the Advancement of Learning'.[431] The resuscitation of this project was assisted by Henry Cromwell's keenness for the purchase of Archbishop Ussher's library. Immediately after Ussher's death in April, 1656, when the sale of his library seemed imminent, parliament established a committee to consider purchasing the collection for the nation. Henry Cromwell's officers and soldiers contributed £2,200 to secure the purchase. Official orders reporting the transit of the library to Ireland were recorded during the summer of 1657.[432] Wood described Cromwell's great enthusiasm for the new college:

> 'I have heard my Lord often speak of it, who is indeed a passionat & great lover of Learning & a person of a very pious & noble mind, though his hands at the present be full of other publick business in setling the Nation. But because you shal understand that the Interest of Learning is not altogether unregarded here in Ireland, . . . be pleased to know that on Friday last the Officers of the Army here, upon my Lord's recommendation of the business unto them, very willingly assented to allow out of their pay so much as to purchas that great Magazeen of Learning the Archbishop of Armagh his library, contracted for . . . by Sir Theoph. Jones at 2,500 lb, & not only so, but also to defray the charge of transporting them hither (which will be don this spring) & to build a Theca for them &c. Thus you see how well Soldiers may be employed in times of peace.'[433]

430. J. D. H. Widdess, *A History of the Royal College of Physicians of Ireland 1654–1963* (Edinburgh, 1963), pp.7–32; Mahaffy, *op. cit.*, pp.318–24.

431. Letter from Wood to Hartlib, 23 Nov. 1656, HP XXXIII 1.

432. Urwick (295), pp.90–4.

433. Letter from Wood to Hartlib, 3 March 1656/7, HP XXXIII 1. This places the acquisition of the library slightly later than the documents cited by Urwick; it also gives a different figure for the purchase price. For further information on this subject, see T. C. Barnard, 'The Purchase of Archbishop Ussher's Library in 1657', *Long Room,* 1971, No. 4: 9–14.

This generous and constructive action of the army established what it was hoped would be a precedent for the active participation of the army in peacetime social reconstruction.

Progress was also made at the site of the university in Dublin. A location was selected for the new college and arrangements were made for the necessary land transfer; Cork House was designated for the library and schools.[434] About the same time Henry Cromwell and the Irish Council appointed William Hill as the head of a new grammar school, which was presumably the 'free-school' of the original Act.[435] They also detailed £500 for 'propagating civilitie as well as Religion among the Irish'. When Robert Wood visited Oxford in the summer of 1657 he conveyed a request from Henry Cromwell for the loan of the Oxford statutes. Naturally these were regarded by Cromwell as a model which would assist Dublin to become a 'university to the interest of piety and learninge'. Owen's reply was remarkably despondent; he pleaded that the statutes of the English universities were framed according to the 'road of studys in former days'. They would therefore be of little assistance to Cromwell's design for 'Godlinesse and solid literature'. Owen's considered advice was to frame entirely new constitutions appropriate to 'the present light, interest of state and advantageous discourse of literature'. If this course was followed, the 'inveterate prejudice' of the English universities against reform might itself be broken down.[436] Owen, at the point of his being removed from the vice-chancellorship, felt no confidence in the statutes of his university. He accordingly pressed for the new university to become a model for the reform of the old.

In December 1657, Cromwell submitted his plans to the trustees, who probably introduced only small modifications before attaching their signatures to the final detailed document. This completed the first stage of their administration of the original commonwealth order.[437] The new university was to comprise Trinity College, a new college, a staff of public professors, a library building with schools, and finally a free-school. Extremely detailed proposals were announced for the reorganisation of Trinity College; the original pattern was followed in many respects, but there were to be additions to the tutorial staff, the most notable being a lecturer in English. The new college was to receive the same endowments as Trinity, but no details of its structure were given. But it is clear that there was some response to the reformers' demands for increasing the representation of public teachers, in order to promote advanced research and tuition in new disciplines. The proposals included

434. Urwick (295), p.63; 20 March 1657. But Cork House had been under consideration for this purpose in 1654. In a letter to Hartlib, 4 Jan. 1658/9, Wood valued Cork House at £3,000: HP XXXIII 1.

435. Letter from Wood to Hartlib, 8 April 1657, HP XXXIII 1.

436. Letter from Owen to Henry Cromwell, 9 Sept. 1657, BM Lansdowne MS 833, fol. 179. Printed in Orme, *John Owen*, pp.423–4; Toon (282), pp.100–1.

437. Urwick (295), pp.62–8, 18 Jan. 1658/9.

provision for professors of divinity, civil law, mathematics, rhetoric, and a 'Physick Professor who is to read Natural Philosophy'. Their lectures were intended for students of Trinity, the new college and any future accretions to the emergent university. All of these subjects had been taught sporadically at Trinity by the Fellows; Symner probably taught the various branches of mathematics. The new proposals would have regularised this procedure and established medicine and natural philosophy as teaching subjects. There would have been six professors, compared with, at Trinity, seven tutorial Fellows, a balance incomparably more favourable to the public teachers than at the English universities. The professors would also have had the advantage of the use of Cork House for schools, its gallery and armoury being intended for conversion by the army into a library. Provision was made for keepers to maintain the library and schools. The free-school mentioned in the plan was probably to be the grammar school already established under William Hill, who would have been assisted by an usher in teaching forty scholars. No reference was made to Trinity Hall, which Stearne was developing as a medical college.

The grammar-school master was by no means a negligible scholar. After a short period as a Fellow of Merton College he became master of the Free School, Sutton Coldfield, later moving to London as a medical practitioner, for which purpose he applied to accumulate for medical degrees at Oxford in 1649 and 1652. Hill's major energies were devoted to preparing a Greek-Latin edition of Dionysius Periegetes's *Orbis descriptio commentario critico & geographico* which was published in 1658 and dedicated to Henry Cromwell, the author describing himself as 'jamvero Gymnasiarcha Dubliniensi'. In the dedicatory letter, Cromwell was praised for services to the ministry and learning in Ireland; the purchase of Ussher's library and the provision of liberal salaries for the Dublin School, its Master and his assistant, received specific mention. Hill's book was designed to promote geographical studies in universities and schools. His translation was supported by lavish ancillary sections, including a grammar, commentary, an introduction to geographical terms, and indices. One introductory poem was provided by a fellow schoolmaster William Dugard, another by the orientalist and lawyer Sir Dudley Loftus, described as the public professor of law at Dublin. Loftus, the editor of an Armenian philosophical work, was probably introduced into the college in a similar manner to his friend Symner; both were primarily involved in public affairs, but their special talents called for association with the expanding university.[438]

438. For Hill see Wood *Athenae,* iii, pp.800–2; Burrows (42), p.521; *DNB.* After his expulsion in 1660 Hill kept a private school near Dublin. For Dudley Loftus see Wood *Athenae,* iv, p.428; *DNB;* G. T. Stokes, 'A Dublin Antiquary of the Seventeenth Century', *Jnl. Roy. Soc. Antiquaries of Ireland,* 5th Series, 1890, *1*: 17–30. Loftus translated *Logica seu Introductio in totam Aristotelis philosophia ab Armenico idiomate in Latinum* (Dublin, 1657); Symner was mentioned in the introduction.

The new Dublin statutes are silent as to curricular developments. That there was active discussion of this question seems probable from the letters of John Beale, who, shortly after the Dublin statutes were framed, wrote to the stationer Joshua Kirton expressing a desire to publish a small treatise on the 'Advancement of literature', which would be of particular interest to their friends in Ireland. Shortly afterwards he apologised for delays in completing this treatise.[439] Like so many of Beale's projected works, his educational tract was not published, but a draft set of fifteen rubrics, headed 'For a Colledge', may have been a synopsis. No specific reference to Dublin was made, but this connection is suggested by the second rule, which stated that its members must be bound to the English interest. On the other hand another rule referring to the Office of Address, mentioned possible amalgamation with a college established in London. All the other rules could have applied to the new college at Dublin. Like those of the Dublin professors, the salary of each teacher in Beale's scheme was to be 'proportioned to the excellency of his Science or Art'. The college would have had many unusual features. Places at the college table were to be arranged with a view to encouraging useful exchanges of ideas. Certain times of the day were to be reserved for conversations in foreign languages. Finally it was intended that the college would attract adults who had lacked educational opportunities at an earlier age.

On the curriculum, Beale's suggestions were reminiscent of the Oxford petitions of Hartlib and Gilson. The college was to offer theology, classical and oriental languages, ancient and modern history, and natural philosophy. Beale's most extensive specific comments concerned the sciences. The students should be

> 'allowed freedome to engage in the way of Aristotle, or of the Academics or Sceptiques, as far as to notion of Chimityes & Principles or elements. or in the way of Democritus & any moderne proposalls of Ld. Bacon, Gassendus, Synertus &c. And descending to the practise of Physique, believe Methodists, or Secreteryes of Chymistry &c. Herbarists &c. some with encouragements in Anatomy & Elements of Chirurgery. Some to bee Mathematicians, to give Accompt of Ancient & Modern Astronomy, of the ancient & modern Geography & Topography, of Optiques, Engines & the great effects of the ancient Mechaniques.'[440]

Although this proposal was framed in Beale's usual rambling prose, it was clearly in the spirit of *philosophia libera*. An equally strong tie with other reformers was his insistence on the relevance of education to the secular functions of the state. The college was expected to provide advice on the framing of national laws; it was to be closely asso-

439. Letters from Beale to Kirton, 22 May 1658, and n.d. [c. June 1658], HP LI.
440. HP XXXI I.

ciated with the Office of Address, which was itself a government agency. The 'founders of such a Colledge may bee founders of generall Accomodation to advance Trade, literature, & husbandry, To correct manners, To devise fit lawes, To invent Arts, Trades & Sciences. And may soone bee a Mother Colledge not only to many others in this nation but allso to very many abroade, even in the utmost borders of the world'. Beale's views on the social function of education were likely to have had a considerable appeal for Henry Cromwell. Very similar ideas would have been expressed by some of Cromwell's most able young advisers recruited from the universities. Thus Petty, Wood, Worsley or Symner might have urged support for Beale's ideas when the Dublin scheme was under discussion. It is therefore possible that Cromwell intended the expanded university of Dublin to take in certain of the features of Dury's Reformed School.

Petty's plans for the reform of Gresham College suggest that he was sympathetic to many of Beale's ideas; Wood was a critic of the grammar schools. Symner believed that 'most of the good wits, that come to our Universities, suffer shipwrack. For after a young Schollar hath got a little prayse for beeing able to wrangle in the Schooles about a *Universale a parte rei,* that puff fils his sayles and makes him steere his course to find out nothing but vanity'. Hence philosophy had not progressed since the time of Aristotle, despite strenuous efforts by the scholastics and 'a readines in wrangling'. In reaction he declared his support for the schemes of Petty and Hartlib, since he was in favour of 'reall and experimentall Learning'.[441]

After ten years of preparation the blueprint for university education in Dublin was drawn up. Further negotiations took place during 1659, but the tenure of Cromwellian authority was at an end. At the restoration, this project was erased from memory, its only memorial being Ussher's library, which was deposited at Trinity College. In the development of informal scientific activity in Ireland during the Protectorate, Trinity was probably of only incidental importance. Although Symner was professor of mathematics, his main associations lay outside the university; the major advocates of the new sciences were in the army and the civil service, which were better able than Trinity to attract 'hopeful young scholars' from the English universities. The failure of the constitutions of the new university to specify a precise curriculum gave every opportunity for the tutors to lapse into traditional practices. Accordingly, the success of mathematics, natural philosophy and medicine depended entirely on the calibre of the public professors, whose standing was certainly sufficient to give them considerable authority in the development of their specialities, as witnessed by the success of John Stearne.

Plans for education in the northern counties of England followed the Welsh pattern. The Commissioners for Propagating and Preaching the

441. Letter from Symner to Sir Robert King [1648], HP XLVIII 1.

Gospel in the Four Northern Counties were active in supplementing incomes, founding new posts and endowing primary schools.[442] A general awareness of the importance of education in the northern counties is indicated by local initiatives to restore the grammar schools after the disruption of the civil wars. Earlier, for example, John Webster had vacated his post as schoolmaster at Clitheroe, which was situated in an area of royalist control, to enter the parliamentarian army. At Newcastle-upon-Tyne, the substantial grammar school was partly destroyed. Then, when the city fell into parliamentarian hands, it was necessary to remove the royalist schoolmaster. The city council exhibited considerable resourcefulness in the search for a replacement. The first candidate considered was Hezekiah Woodward, the prolific Presbyterian author and advocate of the language reforms of Comenius. Eventually the appointment went to Georg Ritschel, who had been delegated by Comenius to prepare a treatise on metaphysics at Oxford. The post at Newcastle, which may have been obtained through his patron Hartlib, solved Ritschel's financial difficulties. With the active assistance of the Newcastle council he was successful in restoring the fortunes of the school. Its buildings were repaired and there was a great increase in the entry of Newcastle exhibitioners at Oxford and Cambridge.[443]

The Civil War had enhanced the sense of isolation from the universities, felt in the northern counties. Not only was teaching and residence disrupted, but the journey to Oxford and Cambridge became hazardous. Many must have been tempted to follow Robinson's decision to travel further north for higher education, to Edinburgh.[444] Accordingly the war led to a revival of interest in schemes for a northern university. The distant ancestor of this movement was a petition of 1604 from the corporation of Ripon, for a college 'after the manner of a university'. There is no indication that this proposal was widely supported but in 1641 a more general petition from 'Northern Parts' for a university at Manchester, was directed to Fairfax. Whitelocke reported in 1647 that the north was again petitioning for a university, this time at York. Two petitions to parliament expressed the desire for a 'University, College, or colleges' for 'the Education of Scholars in Arts, Tongues, and all other learning'.[445] A further obvious location for a northern university was Durham, with its rich resources of ecclesiastical revenue and extensive cathedral precincts.

The first formal intimation of the Durham university proposal came

442. The Commission was established 1 March 1650. For details, see Lambeth Palace, Lambeth MS 1006.

443. Howell (155), pp.322–8.

444. *The Autobiography of Matthew Robinson,* ed. J. E. B. Mayor (Cambridge, 1856), pp.8–16.

445. F. Peck, *Desiderata Curiosa,* 2 vols. (London, 1779), ii, pp.283–91; J. T. Fowler (ed.), *Memorials of the Church of SS. Peter and Wilfred, Ripon,* vol. 2. (Surtees Soc. Durham, lxxviii, 1886), p.257. *Fairfax Correspondence,* ed. C. W. Jackson, 2 vols. (London, 1848), ii, pp.271–80; Whitelocke, *Memorials* (329), p.275; Rushworth (252), vii, pp.854–5.

in 1650, when the gentlemen, freeholders and inhabitants of Durham petitioned parliament for the appropriation of the buildings of the dean and chapter to higher education. Parliament was tactfully reminded of its war debts to the northern counties and of its longstanding pledge to apply the revenues of Deans and Chapters for the advancement of learning. The petitioners wished to establish 'some Colledge or schoole of Literature, or Academy' to serve the remote northern counties.[446]

Launched with serious regard to the advancement of piety and learning, but having only the vaguest terms of reference academically, the proposed Durham College appeared sufficiently innocuous to escape opposition and indeed to attract some share of the general approbation which greeted the Dublin project. The Durham petitioners also had the advantage of the support of Oliver Cromwell, who commended the college as 'soe good & pious a worke I could not but willingly & hartily concur'.[447] As in the case of Dublin, the active sympathy of a Cromwell was essential to overcome the inertia of interregnum bureaucracy. Even then it required six years of petitioning and the work of various committees of state, before the letters patent were granted for the 'College in Durham of the Foundation of Oliver, Lord Protector'.[448] The petitioners were assisted by two powerful allies, John Lambert and Sir Arthur Heselrig, figures who had certain other connections with university reform; Webster had dedicated his *Academiarum Examen* to Lambert, while Heselrig was approached to support the Welsh university project. Lambert was the major common factor in the committees which established the Cromwellian college. He was one of the committee of four members of the Council of State appointed to report on the local petitions and produce acceptable guidelines for procedure. It was decided that the new college should be organised according to statutes drawn up by a larger committee of trustees; Lambert was one of the four members of the Council of State appointed to select the trustees. He then served as a trustee, and submitted their draft constitution to the Council of State; finally he supervised the concluding amendments to the statutes.[449] At the local level a committee of north-countrymen was empowered to advertise the college and to collect subscriptions for the

446. 'The humble Desires of the Gentlemen, Freeholders and Inhabitants of the Countie of Durham, delivered in by the Grand Jury at the Session of Peace holden at Durham the xxiiii April 1650 to be presented to the Honorable Parliament of the Nation', Bodleian, Tanner MS 56, fol. 207. General sources on Durham College include:—*CJ*, vi, pp.389, 410, 589–90; W. H. Hutchinson, *The History & Antiquities of Durham,* 3 vols. (Carlisle, 1785–94), i, pp.514–19; W.H., 'Cromwell's College at Durham', *Durham Univ. Jnl.*, 1880/1, *4*: 7–8, 16–17, 30–1, 41–2, 54–5; J. T. Fowler, *Durham University* (London, 1904), pp.15–21; C. D. R. Ranson, *Oliver Cromwell's College* (Durham, 1913); C. E. Whiting, *The University of Durham 1832–1932* (London, 1932), pp.18–29; G. H. Turnbull, 'Oliver Cromwell's College at Durham' (285).

447. Letter from Cromwell to Lenthall, 11 March 1650, Abbott, ii, pp.347–8.

448. Text in Hutchinson, *op. cit.*, pp.518–27; 15 May 1657.

449. *CSPD 1655/6,* p.140, 29 Jan. 1656; p.156, 1 Feb.1656; pp.213, 218, 6 & 10 March 1656. *CSPD 1656/7,* p.50, 1 Aug. 1656; p.100, 5 Sept. 1656.

'new college for the advancement of learning and piety'. But their funds were to be controlled from London.[450]

The letters patent indicate that the college was sufficiently well endowed for it to become operational. It was to be housed in the ample complex of buildings associated with the castle and cathedral, and its possessions were to include the library and mathematical instruments of the bishops. Furthermore the college was to have the privilege of licensing and printing books.

Cromwell's college had a surprisingly large staff. The senior members were: the provost, Philip Hunton; two preachers and Senior Fellows, William Spinedge and Joseph Hill. There were twelve Fellows, in three categories: Thomas Vaughan, 'John Kifler', Robert Wood and John Peachill were professors; Ezerel Tong, Richard Russell, 'John Richel' and John Doughty were tutors; Nathaniel Vincent, William Corker, William Sprigg and Leonard Wastel were schoolmasters. Two later recruits reported by Calamy were Richard Frankland and William Pell, both of whom were local ministers.[451]

From the evidence of the petitions, negotiations and letters patent, it is apparent that the Cromwellian college project had affinities with the Dublin model; Durham also indicates the likely outcome of the projects for new colleges in Dublin and Wales, had the restoration not intervened. Its official terms of reference were unexceptionably vague—'promoting of the gospel, and the religious and prudent education of young men'. Like the staff of Trinity College, the provost, Senior Fellows and certain other members of Durham College were expected to take an active part in propagating the gospel in their area. As with the educational complex at Dublin (or Dury's Reformed School), the Durham Fellows were expected to teach students of various ages. However, the curriculum and exact purpose of the education to be offered were not specified. No doubt the university representatives among the trustees expected the college to prepare students for Oxford and Cambridge; others would have adhered to the aims of the Welsh projectors, and seen the college as a seminary for the puritan ministry; the local gentry might have favoured more secular education including elements from the French Academy curriculum.

The actual establishment of the new college in 1657 was an occasion for remedying this lack of definition of purpose. The great rarity of state experiments in higher education before the nineteenth century adds particular interest to this question. In the absence of official statutes, the complexion of Durham College must have depended on the educational outlook of its Fellows. Surprisingly their endeavour has elicited virtually no comment from historians, perhaps owing to the extremely short life of the college and the absence of direct information about its academic

450. *CSPD 1655/6*, p.262, 10 & 12 April 1656.

451. Whiting, *op. cit.* pp.25–6. For a corrected identification of the Durham Fellows, see Appendix II, below.

work. Nevertheless the college was established; its friends and enemies alike believed that it was fulfilling a distinctive educational function. Many of the appointed staff took up residence, and rapidly framed ideas about the educational objectives of the new college.[452] According to an account probably derived from Sprigg or Tong, even in its second session the college seemed destined for great achievements:

> 'The College here is in a very hopefull way, and seems to be favoured both by God and man, and is prospered by many eminent Providences; it hath lately received a considerable augmentation of its Revenue viz. of 200 lb. p. an. and is daily improving, so that the present Revenue is 600 lb. p. an. clear (of which it was endowed with 400 lb. p. an. by our renowned Founder the late Lord Protector) and there is almost as much more in reversion after the expiration of some yeares. For the present situation, gallant air, and faire prospect we may compare with most places in England, as also for plenty of the most necessarie accommodations of life, fewell and food, especially all sorts of good fish. Here is a great resort of very hopefull youth and young gentlemen for the shortness of the time. And as here already present some of the Fellows men of worth and gallant spirits, so we want nothing but more able men to carry on the work and bring forth the designe which is now come to the birth. And if this College be well setled at first on the good constitution thereof the good complexion and health of the North of England will much depend.'[453]

After the death of Oliver Cromwell, the Durham Fellows sought to consolidate their position by gaining the support of his son. Like numerous other pressure groups, they submitted a 'humble Address of the Provost and Fellows of the College of Durham', pleading for a continuation of Oliver's policies.[454] William Sprigg dedicated his *Modest Plea* to parliament, outlining his ideas on university reform and including explicit reference to the suitability of Durham for an experiment in higher education.[455] Informal moves were made by Sprigg's colleagues to secure full university status for Durham. This occasioned strong and successful counter-petitioning by the universities of Oxford and Cambridge, which believed that the new college was about to be given licence to confer degrees in all faculties. Even after the failure of the petitions from Durham, Tong composed a plea for the systematic employment of cathedral precincts and incomes for higher education.[456]

452. There is evidence of residence at Durham for Hunton, Peachill, Spinedge, Sprigg, Tong and Hill. Ritschel, Frankland and Pell were already in the vicinity.

453. Quoted in a letter from Wood to Hartlib, 4 Jan. 1658/9, HP XXXIII 1.

454. Hutchinson, *op. cit.*, i, pp.528–9; 4 Sept. 1658. *Mercurius Politicus*, 2–9 Dec. 1658, No. 44, pp.559–61.

455. Sprigg (267), pp.49–55.

456. 'To the Honorable Lords St. S.T.W.L.H. et all Members of the Honorable the House of Commons assembled in Parliament. Humbly sheweth that the

The above evidence suggests that Durham was regarded as a significant educational venture by its supporters and a dangerous precedent by its enemies. In the absence of direct records about educational practices at the new college, it is necessary to rely on circumstantial evidence about the general intellectual attitudes and opinions on education of the Fellows. In general terms, Durham had similarities with the colleges of the old universities, or Trinity College Dublin, especially as the latter was intended to evolve, under Henry Cromwell's plan. The Durham Fellows had strong puritan loyalties and they were expected to play a leading role in the evangelization of the northern provinces, in accordance with the general aims of the Commissioners for Gospel Propagation. However, Durham had distinctive characteristics, which increase its educational significance. By contrast with Dublin or most of the colleges at Oxford or Cambridge, Durham included not only diligent puritan divines, but also intellectuals appointed with respect to other qualifications. The lesser-known Fellows were probably typical puritan ministers,[457] but leading members of the college are generally remembered for other reasons, including their interest in educational reform.

Although the Durham project was prompted by local initiative, the ultimate outcome was determined entirely by trustees operating from London. The puritan educational reformers located in London were therefore able to influence the relevant committees and there is every indication that they assumed this role, once the new college became a practical possibility. Lambert was acquainted with the reformers, but although a number of its members were correspondents of Hartlib, the large committee responsible for the statutes was not conspicuous for its interest in educational reform. In August 1656 Hartlib and Tong were added to the statutes committee, probably in recognition of their previous behind-the-scenes involvement.[458] Tong was an activist who had firm ideas about the development of education at Durham, and he exerted pressure on the various committees from 1655 onwards. Hartlib played his usual role of intelligencer and publicist. Early in 1655 he reported that Tong's Durham scheme was 'very much advanced', enjoying the support of both Lambert, Tong's 'very great friend', and other petitioners from the Northern Counties. Early in 1656 (before the statutes committee was formed) Tong noted the Council of State's decision on the Durham revenues and suggested that 'a draught of new reformed statutes is most desired to avoid errors in the foundation'.[459] Tong may even perhaps have been involved in the selection of the Fellows. He felt

---

Cathedral & other Churches of England . . . were by them intended for nurseries & seede plottes of learning & Religion', HP X 4 & XLVII 5.

457. For example William Corker, John Doughty and Leonard Wastel.

458. *CSPD 1656/7*, p.50, 7 Aug. 1656. The statutes committee was formed on 10 March 1656. Hartlib excused himself from attending at the committee on the grounds of ill-health.

459. Ephemerides 1655 & 1656.

himself to have been cheated out of the headship of University College Oxford by Owen and Goodwin, with the result that he vacated his fellowship and probably acted as a focus for disgruntled and reforming academics at Oxford. In view of this association, it is not surprising that almost the entire original staff at Durham was recruited from Oxford. Thomas Vaughan was a particularly close friend of Tong, while Vincent, Wood and Sprigg were young, promising, and noted for their receptivity to new ideas. Tong probably hoped that Hartlib's friends, who were given so little opportunity to promote educational innovation at Oxford, would succeed better in the new framework of Durham.

The letters patent for Durham included no instructions about academic matters, a lapse disappointing to the historian, but invaluable to the Fellows, who were, at least initially, given a free hand to develop education in the college without reference to statutory limitations, or fear of censure from the universities for trespassing into their territory. In 1657 Tong commented on the abilities of his colleagues:

> 'One Sprig is a fellow of Durham Colledge excellent for drawing and painting and very optical also.
>
> Mr. Vaughan an other Fellow undertaking in two years to fit schollars for University for Latin and Hebrew.[460]
>
> Hinton the Master of it an indisputable schollar.
>
> Also a Fellow of Magdelene Colledge [Joseph Hill] a universal schollar, one of the Professors or Fellows.'[461]

This vignette probably gives a fair impression of the intellectual atmosphere at Durham. Traditional linguistic studies were not abandoned, but new methods of language teaching were introduced, making it easier to find time for study of the oriental languages to which the Puritans attached such importance. Tong was primarily celebrated as a teacher of Latin. Anthony Wood reported of him that at Durham 'he followed precisely the Jesuits' method, and the boys under him did by that course profit exceedingly'.[462] Tong planned the construction of a *Janua linguarum,* while his friend Vaughan proposed tabular and 'harmonical' grammars.[463] Hill augmented the Greek lexicon of Schrevelius and his pupil, Pell, was esteemed as an orientalist.[464]

The Fellows were as well-equipped to teach modern subjects. There is little direct information, but much circumstantial evidence suggests that the Durham Fellows were concerned to pay attention to utilitarian considerations and recent intellectual developments. Tong proposed 'the

460. A similar claim was made for Sprigg: Ephemerides 1657.
461. Ephemerides 1657.
462. Wood *Athenae,* iv, p.1261.
463. Ephemerides 1655.
464. Cornelius Schrevelius, *Lexicon manuale Graeco-Latinum et Latino-Graecum auctum et adornatum Josephi Hill* (London, 1663), and many later editions.

foundation of a Mechanical Schoole and acquainted mee [Hartlib] with the whole designe of founding a College of Sciences with severall Schooles and a Library, [and] a workhouse in Durham'.[465] This is strongly reminiscent of the Dublin proposals, or Beale's ideas on the scope of a college. Tong's letters from Durham described the interest of Hunton and Vaughan in new medical and veterinary recipes. Tong himself was an horticultural enthusiast; out of the gardens at Durham he hoped to prepare 'wines and medicines for all seasons and for all tempers'.[466] In discussion with Beale he noted that raspberries and blackberries thrived in the northern climate. Accordingly he was intending to direct the planting of soft fruits in the college gardens. Such pronouncedly utilitarian tendencies met with favourable responses in the neighbourhood, even from such an unlikely source as the Quakers. Their representative Anthony Pierson was persuaded to share the secret of his 'universal compost', which was duly relayed to Boyle and other agricultural practitioners.[467] Given the medical interests of the Durham Fellows, it is not surprising that a Dr. Turnbull appealed for financial support from the Cromwellian college for his plan for a free local clinic to serve the poor, hoping that public subscriptions would be sufficient to pay the salaries of its staff of physicians, surgeons and apothecaries.[468]

Broad sympathy for Tong's educational outlook is apparent in Sprigg's *Modest Plea for an Equal Commonwealth* (1659), which was probably composed at Durham, despite the author's claim that it originated 'before the late Rebellion'.[469] Like Dell and Webster, Sprigg used a tract on education to express opposition to the learned ministry's use of tithes. Like Tong, Sprigg advocated the provision of workhouses, to be established on glebe lands in each district and financed by the revenues from tithes. The old universities were represented as a corrupting influence, inextricably linked with episcopacy and monarchical government. According to Sprigg universities should not aspire to become a school of prophets, but 'should stoop to a more honest civil notion of Schooles of Education and humane literature, for the training up the youth of the Gentry in Learning and good manners'.[470] This view may have been shared by his colleagues, and such a secular bias would have been attractive to the local gentry. But it would have provoked deep opposition from the established universities, which were convinced that the divinity faculty was indispensable, as the only solid guarantee against the spread of heresy. Sprigg accepted that fluency in Latin and other languages was indispensable, but thought that this could be

465. Ephemerides 1655.
466. Letter from Tong to Beale, n.d., BL vii 14.
467. Letter from Hartlib to Boyle, 30 June 1657, Boyle *Works*, vi, p.93.
468. 'Physical Charity, Durham Colledge', 4 Sept. 1658, HP liii.
469. For a discussion of this work, see R. L. Greaves, 'William Sprigg and the Cromwellian Revolution', *HLQ*, 1971, *34*: 99–113.
470. For a similar emphasis, see Sprigg, *The Royal and Happy Poverty* (London, 1660). This was also composed at Durham.

achieved more efficiently by better teaching methods. Other aspects of scholasticism were less welcome: disputations were to be replaced with work in a 'Laboratory for Chymical Experiments, together with frequent Anatomies'; logic was to be supplanted by grafting, planting and other agricultural studies—an aspect of the curriculum undoubtedly inspired by Tong, the advocate of 'Tongue grafting'.[471] Perhaps imitating Petty's Literary Workhouse, Sprigg proposed training in arts and crafts, according to the aptitudes of the young gentlemen. The embellishments of Sprigg's curriculum were such subjects as horseriding and fencing, which would have completed the emancipation from monkish pedantry.

Durham was not given the opportunity to evolve into such a 'Literary Workhouse', but Tong and Sprigg probably had this model in mind. Furthermore their colleagues displayed very great diversity of interests, and were competent to teach a wide range of subjects. Vaughan matched his friend Tong's versatility. During his first visit to Hartlib, he discoursed upon 'his Harmonical Grammar. 2. A way of Commonplaces invented by himself. 3. Of Braithwaits musick. 4. Of a secret recipe to cure the stone. 5. Of a good ancient English book concerning silkworms'.[472] Philip Hunton also displayed wide interests, but his major concern was political philosophy, to which he contributed a classic exposition of the theory of limited monarchy.[473] William Pell's interests may have extended beyond oriental studies; an associate was the celebrated minister and physician, Richard Gilpin, who was one of the Visitors to Durham College. Richard Russell, according to Whiting, was projector of a complete translation of Paracelsus and responsible for several translations of chemical works, published after the restoration.[474] William Spinedge had been a colleague of Hunton in the puritan ministry in Wiltshire; he was described by Calamy as a 'great Philosopher and disputant'. Vincent had been at Corpus Christi College Oxford; it would be interesting to know whether he imbibed there the ideas of Gilson on university reform. 'John Richel' has hitherto escaped identification. I would like to speculate that this is the efficient Newcastle schoolmaster, Georg Ritschel, his foreign name resulting in a clerical error, as in the case of Küffeler ('Kifler'). Ritschel left his Newcastle post in July 1657 in order to take up the living of Hexham. He might well have followed the practice of other Fellows, by combining pastoral duties with teaching at Durham. His abilities as a metaphysician and collaborator with Comenius would have been a great asset to the new college.[475] One of the most significant appointments at Durham was that of the vicar of

471. Sprigg (267), pp.49–55; Birch (26), iii, p.78.
472. Ephemerides 1655.
473. *A Treatise of Monarchy* (London, 1643). For Hunton's political ideas, see J. M. Wallace, *Destiny his Choice: The Loyalism of Andrew Marvell* (Cambridge, 1968), pp.15, 24–5, 205, 230.
474. But for the problem of his identification, see Appendix II, below.
475. Young (347), pp.14–15; Howell (155), p.328.

Bishop Auckland, Richard Frankland. His connection with the college represents the first stirrings of his interest in education. Frankland's sympathy with educational innovation is apparent from his subsequent services to nonconformist education.

Two of the appointments at Durham which were potentially of the greatest importance from the point of view of educational innovation and the development of a substantial scientific component in the curriculum, were those of Robert Wood and Johann Sibertus Küffeler. The former was designated professor of mathematics, the position corresponding to that of his friend Miles Symner at Dublin; while Küffeler was probably professor of medicine. However, the scientific competence of both men extended well beyond their subjects. Unfortunately neither, it appears, took up his chair, although Wood found the prospect appealing, and displayed continuing interest in the Cromwellian college. No doubt he hesitated to leave the service of Henry Cromwell until the security of his new post was guaranteed. He reported with equal enthusiasm, educational developments at Dublin and at Durham; then, in the spring of 1657, he 'had the honor to be proposed for a mathematical Professor'. During a visit to Oxford in the summer of that year, he confirmed that the new charter was being actively implemented, but he returned to Ireland without taking up his new post.[476] Küffeler had an even more tenuous relationship with the college. He had arrived in England as an official guest of the state, to display his 'dreadful Engine' of war. His abilities attracted the notice of Tong and Hartlib, with whom he concluded an agreement to serve the commonwealth as an inventor, in return for financial assistance.[477] Tong probably secured Küffeler's appointment to Durham, in order to exploit further his abilities as a physician and inventor. This arrangement would also have satisfied the Council of State's obligations to its guest. However, given his expectations of generous financial reward for his military inventions, there was little incentive for Küffeler to take up his Durham fellowship.

To the Fellows and to outside observers in the spring of 1659, Durham would have appeared to have reached the threshold of university status. Full maturity would have been marked by the college's being given permission to award degrees, a prospect which brought criticism from both extremes of the religious spectrum. George Fox stigmatised the college as a new source of learned clergy, urging along familiar lines that the Christian minister had no need for 'Hebrew, greeke & latine & ye 7 arts which all was but ye teachinges of ye naturall man'.[478] Fox debated with Hunton, and the influential Durham trustee Sir Henry Vane

476. Letter from Wood to Hartlib, 13 May 1657, HP XXXIII 1.

477. HP XXVI 49; 20 June 1656.

478. Fox, *The Journal of George Fox*, ed. N. Penney, 2 vols. (Cambridge, 1911), i, pp.311–12; also, *Some Quaeries to be answered in Writing or Print by the Masters, Heads, Fellows and Tutors of the Colledge they are setting up at Durham* [1657].

Jr., who was an acquaintance of Anthony Pierson. The Quakers must however have applauded Sprigg's later attacks on the learned ministry and scholastic education. As the college evolved into a secular academy having a strong utilitarian bias, Pierson and other radicals probably became reconciled. Indeed later quaker educational ventures in many ways resembled Durham College.

More intransigent and influential opposition to Durham came from the 'schools of prophets', the universities. Cambridge, having noted that full university status was about to be granted, sent a brief petition to the Council of State appealing for delay until its delegates had had a full opportunity to present objections.[479] Oxford composed a long petition propounding eight 'Reasons to be presented in the name of the University of Oxford against the erecting of an University at Durham'.[480] The arguments used have subsequently become a standard part of the armament of those opposing university extension. For a new university to be tolerated, Oxford stipulated mutually incompatible requirements; it was necessary for the new institution to provide the same facilities as the old universities, while at the same time avoiding being in competition with them. It was asserted that failure to comply with the first criterion would result in a dilution of standards. Durham as a provincial centre and the college as an academic unit were judged too small to support higher education. Failing these arguments, the critics could rely on the legal technicality that the MAs at Durham were breaking their degree oath by teaching outside Oxford or Cambridge. This argument was considerably weakened by the critics' also asserting that some of the Durham Fellows were not graduates at all. Of course, the Durham Fellows were quite as well qualified academically as Fellows in the old universities. Finally, the petitioners pandered to the government's fear of subversion, by alleging that decentralised higher education would encourage the spread of heresy. The state was accordingly urged to prevent Durham rising above the status of such colleges as Eton or Winchester.

Oxford's petition took up arguments which had already been used by Ward to answer Dell's case for university decentralisation. At a still later date, John Wallis expressed the underlying prejudice of the academics that Oxford and Cambridge could satisfy the entire legitimate demand for higher education; the ancient universities were 'as eminent, and as well endowed, as any in the Christian world. And we need no more'.[481] Wallis was one of two delegates selected to carry the Oxford petition to Richard Cromwell in London, where he was joined by the Cambridge representatives. Their combination of academic, legal and political objections immediately produced a satisfactory response from Cromwell

479. Cooper (58), iii, pp.473–4, 18 April 1659.

480. Univ. Oxon Arch. T26 1647–59, fols. 340–3; Wood *Hist. & Antiq.*, ii, pp.687–94, 12 April 1659.

481. Ward (307), pp.63–5; Wallis (303), p.324.

who ordered that the keepers of the Great Seal should 'forebear passing the said grant for Durham Colledge untill further order from us'.[482] This confirms Burton's judgement that Richard recognised no obligation to honour his father's predilections. With Oliver Cromwell's support, the embryonic university could begin to establish itself, unimpeded by objections from the old universities. Once his protection was removed, the universities moved quickly to suppress their adversary, which was unable to mobilise support sufficient for its survival. In July 1659 Tong complained: 'I am here left alone with many youthes, more enemies, great hindrances, noe helpes or helpers but God'.[483]

(xi) Education in Dissent

By the restoration Durham was suppressed, Dublin still-born, and numerous other projects aborted at various stages in their development. State revenues ceased to flow into education and were diverted back to their original ecclesiastical uses. This brought a sudden end to the attempt by puritan reformers to realise their educational objectives through state patronage. The puritan reformers who enjoyed state pensions, academic positions or benefices found themselves ejected and without public influence. Educational expansion or innovation was thenceforward dependent on private initiative. But although circumstances had changed dramatically, the educational impetus established during the Puritan Revolution was sufficiently strong for its influence to continue after the restoration. Indeed, paradoxically, the new conditions provided an ideal opportunity for educational experiment, but only within the ranks of the non-conformist community. Many ejected academics who had not been able to put new ideas into practice in their colleges, or expelled ministers who had been absorbed in pastoral duties, found that this form of teaching was a secure and rewarding occupation. In this capacity, they were free to adopt new educational ideas. Thus the model of educational theory which has been postulated above for Durham College, was given an opportunity to proliferate through the creation of dissenting academies. Not surprisingly the Puritans discussed above played a leading part in the foundation of these institutions. Tong returned to London and established a small academy for girls in Islington; his scientific interests were furthered through association with the Royal Society. William Pell remained in the Durham area and was urged to resume the teaching of 'university learning', but he felt bound to decline by the terms of his MA oath.[484] This appeal for the preservation of higher education in the Durham area was taken to Richard Frankland, who established an academy at

482. Univ. Oxon. Arch. T26 1647–1659, fol. 346; 22–29 April 1659. The other delegate from Oxford was Daniel Greenwood.
483. Letter from Tong to Hartlib, 4 July 1659, HP LXV 3; extract in BL VII 14.
484. Bodleian, Aubrey MS 20, fol. 13. *Calamy Revised,* p.385.

his Rathmell estate, the first of his numerous academic ventures and one which greatly influenced the development of non-conformist education.[485] At one stage during his varied career, Robert Wood served for a short time as mathematics master at Christ's Hospital. The restoration careers of dispossessed Durham Fellows indicate a continuing involvement in education. Furthermore, there was local pressure for them to continue to practise informally the form of higher education officially sanctioned under Cromwell. Richard Frankland's persistence in organising academies in the face of official hostility and persecution, bears witness to the tenacity of the puritan tutors.

This pattern may be traced elsewhere. At least one of the ejected Trinity College Fellows founded an academy.[486] Oxford was a focal point for the development of dissenting education, since many ejected academics sought to employ their talents in the neighbourhood as private tutors. The most important member of this group was Hartlib's old ally, Henry Langley. He began by teaching and preaching in Oxford, but his presence in the city was felt to be odious, and he and his allies were expelled from Oxford, for 'keeping conventicles and meetings in their houses'. They moved into adjacent villages; Langley established himself as a tutor at Tubney, while Thomas Cole went to Nettlebed and Henry Cornish to Stanton Harcourt. Others became ministers and physicians in the same area. Anthony Wood reported that this cadre of dissenting tutors harboured the sons of 'fanaticks' and 'taught them logic and philosophy, and admitted them to degrees'.[487] Hence although the puritan educational reformers from London, Oxford and Durham were expelled from their livings or offices, they quickly adjusted to this situation and were even able to maintain a foothold in higher education in these same localities. This dispersed network of tutors provided an essential continuity between the projects of the Puritan Revolution, and the institutionalised academies of the later part of the century. The latter became the permanent expression of the educational models generated during the period of parliamentary rule. Many echoes of Petty's *Ergastula literaria, The Reformed School* and Durham College are detectable in the first large academies, such as Newington Green, founded by Charles Morton a student of Wadham College during the first active phase of the Oxford Experimental Philosophy Club. Morton's chief interest had been in the 'Mechanic part' of mathematics; subsequently he contributed to the *Philosophical Transactions* on practical husbandry and composed a treatise on games of chance. His academy had a garden, bowling green, fishpond and a laboratory furnished with mathematical instruments.[488] His students acquired cele-

485. Whiting (330), pp.458–9; Ashley Smith (5), pp.17–21, 269.
486. Edward Veal; see Whiting (330), pp.457–8.
487. Wood, *Life & Times* (47), i, pp.499–500; ii, pp.96–7.
488. *Calamy Revised,* p.356; Whiting (330), p.456; Ashley Smith (5), pp.56–61. See Petty (210), p.8; Dury (89), pp.74–5; Cowley (63).

brity for their cultivation in modern languages, experimental science and commercially useful subjects. Such academies were one of the means whereby the dissenting community could turn their adversity to advantage. They could benefit from educational innovation; this opportunity was denied to the orthodox, whose sons suffered the fate of exposure to the decaying scholastic tradition of the universities. Thus the natural sciences, experimental philosophy and Cartesianism became an established feature of English higher education, but only for the non-conformist followers of the puritan reformers.

Because of the strong relationships between English non-conformity and New England, there was considerable interchange of personnel and educational ideas between the two communities. The two ex-Fellows of Wadham, Morton and Samuel Lee, after successfully ministering and teaching in Newington Green, settled in New England in 1686. Intellectuals of this kind carried to the colonies both enthusiasm for Boyle's natural philosophy and valuable libraries. Morton's compendium of physics became widely read at Harvard. Perhaps even better than the early dissenting academies this college represents the educational ideals of Independents like John Owen, who recognised the necessity of reform, without wishing to indulge in radical experiments.[489]

The impressive features of non-conformist academies must not obscure their limitations. Enlightened education was only available to limited sections of the middle classes, and it was confined to certain regions where particularly resourceful tutors were active. Private initiative was not able either to secure continuity for the embryonic system of state-aided elementary schools which had been established before 1660, or to preserve the ideal of universal education which was seen as fundamental by Comenius or Winstanley. The reformers' programme for a well-educated, articulate class of craftsmen and labourers, able to take advantage of vocational training in schools of husbandry or mechanics, was after the restoration relegated to the sphere of utopian phantasy. The only significant revival came with the emergence of workhouse schemes in the later seventeenth century. Increasingly these proposals were motivated by purely economic considerations, rather than by a genuine humanitarian belief in the value of education. The Quaker John Bellers was indeed actuated by a desire to relieve the poor, but Locke and his friends moved in a world of Leviathan political economy. Charles Willoughby expressed the characteristic belief of this group that workhouses 'ought to be the next thing after the improvement of land', as the means

489. It will be recalled that in the 1630s Hartlib's friend John Stoughton was an advocate of education in New England. For the basic literature on this extensive subject, see S. E. Morison, *The Founding of Harvard College* and *Harvard College in the Seventeenth Century*, 2 vols. (Cambridge, Mass., 1936); *idem*, *Puritan Pronaos: Studies in the Intellectual Life of New England* (New York, 1936); L. A. Cremin, *American Education: The Colonial Experience 1607–1783* (New York, 1970); R. P. Stearns, *Science in the British Colonies of America* (Urbana, Ill., 1970).

to achieve national prosperity.[490] Training was conceived merely in terms of economic exploitation. The onset of the industrial revolution further encouraged neglect of lower class education. It survived as a vestigial form in the charity schools, which were designed to instil the basic literacy needed for moral and religious conformity. This was a return to the attitudes of the Laudian period. Consideration of elementary education in terms familiar to Hartlib was not given widespread official expression in England until the middle of the nineteenth century, when advocates of state education again appealed for a more humanitarian attitude to universal education.[491]

490. M. G. Mason, 'John Locke's Proposals on Work-house Schools', *Durham Research Rev.*, 1962, No. 13: 8–16. Letter from Dr. Charles Willoughby to Locke, 17 April 1691, Bodleian, Rawlinson MS C.406, fols. 69–81.

491. For the characteristic sentiments of Kay-Shuttleworth and his inspectors on elementary education, see Minutes of the Committee of Council on Education, 1840–1; quoted by M. Sturt, *The Education of the People* (London, 1967), pp.172–4. Kay's earlier statement, *The Moral and Physical Condition of the Working Classes . . . in Manchester* (London, 1832), is extremely restrictive in its educational outlook.

IV

The Prolongation of Life

'I would have you understand my Prognostication of the true universal Medicine, which shall serve not onely Men, but also all Flesh; namely, that there growes in Paradice a Tree, which is, and is called the Tree of Life, which in the glorious and long expected coming of Jesus Christ our God and Saviour shall be made manifest, and then it shall be afforded to men, and the fruits of it shall be gathered, by which all men and all flesh shall be delivered from death, and that as truly, solidly, and surely, as at the time of the fall, by gathering the fruit of the forbidden Tree, we together with all flesh fell into sin, death and ill. And this glory and great joy hath God reserved for Us, that live in these latter dayes, and hath kept his good Wine until now . . . I do foretell all Physitians, that then their Physick shall be worth nothing; for another Garden will be found, whence shall be had herbs, that shall preserve men not onely from sickness, but from death it self.'

Samuel Hartlib, *Chymical Addresses* (1655), Appendix

(i) Introduction

Whatever their attitude to medical theory, protestants believed that there was an integral relationship between spiritual guilt and physical corruption. Man had been created in the garden of Eden without physical imperfections. He was designed for longevity, although such authors as Milton were doubtful whether the gift of immortality was ever granted by the Supreme Architect. Roger Bacon on the other hand asserted that 'man naturally is immortal'; even after the Fall he had retained a residual capacity to live for a thousand years.[1]

After the creation the creatures were brought before Adam; among other things man was given an immediate and intuitive knowledge of their properties, including medicinal qualities. This perfect equilibrium between man and nature had been sacrificed at the Fall. Man's immortality (however conceived) was forfeited; he was destined to endure unremitting punishments and to suffer from physical degeneration and

1. Roger Bacon, *Epistola de secretis,* trans. by T.M. as *Frier Bacon his Discovery of the Miracles of Arts, Nature and Magick* (London, 1659), p.30. Williams (334), pp.102–4. See also Sir John Pettus, *Volatiles from the History of Adam and Eve* (209), pp.35–6.

disease. The lower animals were left with an intuitive ability to cure their own ailments, as a constant reminder to man of the powers sacrificed at his transgression. Something of this capacity remained in the life of unlettered peasants, but scholarly medicine was destined to be 'more professed, than laboured; and yet more laboured than advanced'.[2] Nevertheless God offered spiritual redemption through Christ and one anticipated aspect of His grace was the conservation of health and prolongation of life. Christ was not only a teacher but also a worker of miracles, 'Physician both of Soul and Body'.[3] Thus medicine was influenced by protestant religious aspirations; and the Puritans came to regard a medical restoration as a corollary of their spiritual regeneration.

As in the case of the church, history was expected to reveal the causes of decline and indicate the reforms necessary for a return to primitive purity in medicine. Historical grounds were used to justify any degree of departure from traditional practice. In general, primitive Hebrew or Hippocratic medicine was thought to possess spiritual and scientific merits which were not to be detected in subsequent periods. Hippocrates, Pythagoras and Democritus were described as expert anatomists and proponents of empirical medicine, whose inspiration derived from the sages of the east. Their approach to medicine was religious, and as practitioners they displayed a strong sense of public duty. Primitive medicine was accorded the virtues of the primitive church, and its subsequent decline was attributed to authoritarianism, dogmatism, exclusiveness and insensitivity to public needs. Hence the medical profession came to suffer from the same defects as the Roman Catholic church. The Latin language provided the final, conclusive bond between these two 'heathenish professions'.

The form of indictment of traditional medicine depended very much on the bias and degree of radicalism of the critic. Vesalius, the restorer of anatomy, found the root cause of decline in later Roman medicine, which had developed an aversion to human dissection. This lesser regard for anatomical knowledge resulted in the relegation of anatomy and surgery into the hands of uneducated barbers. Physicians had subsequently come to adopt a priestly disdain for dissection, which was looked down upon as a manual craft. While not wishing to undermine Galenic physiology and humoral pathology, Vesalius, inspired by the example of Renaissance artists, instigated a movement for the restoration of practical anatomy in medical education. Vesalius became the leader of this movement, which led to a return to anatomy by academic physicians throughout Europe. The intellectual vigour of the medical profession was restored, and the foundations were laid for the rise of scientific physiology in the seventeenth century. The ultimate medical significance of this development was enormous, but in the short term the practice of

2. Francis Bacon, *De Augmentis Scientiarum* (13), p.121; Roger Bacon, *op. cit.*, p.29; Pinnel (216), pp.81, 98; Williams (334), pp.143–8.
3. Bacon (13), p.119.

medicine was very little changed by improved anatomical knowledge.

By contrast, the movement which crystallised around the versatile mystic and polemicist, Paracelsus, detected deeper inconsistencies in ancient medicine, and advocated more radical solutions. The neglect of anatomy characteristic of Roman medicine was not regarded as its most crucial weakness. More serious was the failure of physicians to retain an active interest in therapeutics. They had become 'quill-doctors', writing prescriptions without any practical knowledge of the materials dispensed by apothecaries; thus abandoning their basic skill to artisans. The Paracelsians believed that even old women and empirics had come to possess more reliable knowledge than physicians.[4] It was asserted that Galen had relied on the practical assistance of empirics, while elaborating theoretical works which were divorced from reality. His system was dismissed as a fiction, along with the rest of scholastic natural philosophy.[5]

Contempt for the classical medical inheritance was shown in a wide range of vernacular medical works in the sixteenth century. Paracelsians gave this movement more systematic and articulate expression. Even before the seventeenth century, Petrus Severinus produced a Latin Paracelsian textbook, designed to appeal to academic audiences.[6] Although ancient medical texts continued to serve as the basis for professional studies, the educated public came to adopt an increasingly sceptical attitude to Galenism. Deficiencies in the ancient knowledge of anatomy were exposed by the followers of Vesalius; Galenic physiology was questioned; the potentialities of alternative explanatory models were illustrated by Harvey's discovery of circulation. With the investigation of the chemical properties of inorganic substances and the exploration of the flora of Europe and the New World, new horizons opened up for pharmacology and nutrition. Concern for the better regulation of diet and interest in new medicines were already well-developed in the Tudor period and these trends greatly increased in the seventeenth century.[7] At all levels, from university disputations to popular compendia, there was a growth of interest in empirical medicine and a diminishing concern with the details of humoral pathology or the intricacies of Galenic physiology. Galenic medicine was less and less conceived as a closed and authoritative system. Such influential voices as those of Bacon and Montaigne appealed for a suspension of judgement on theoretical matters, and a change of direction involving a more pragmatic approach to

4. Bacon (13), p.125. Similarly Biggs asserted that physicians, 'contracted by the opium of dull ignorance and sloth, are now slipp'd into the hands of Apothecaries, and old women': *Mataeotechnia Medicinae* (25), p.24. Starkey, *Helmonts Vindication* (268), pp.12–14.

5. Biggs (25), p.29.

6. *Idea Medicinae Philosophicae* (Basel, 1571).

7. Jane O'Hara May, 'Foods or Medicines?', *Transactions of the British Society for the History of Pharmacy*, 1971, *1*, No. 2. J. C. Drummond & A. Wilbraham (82), pp.65–90.

nature. In *De Augmentis Scientiarum* Bacon claimed that the improvement of diet and the promotion of husbandry would prolong life and prevent disease. The experimental chemist should test the validity of drugs and discover new remedies. Bacon predicted that through the systematic collection of medical data, physicians would come to a new understanding of the mechanism of the body and the nature of disease.[8]

These ideas for a restoration of medicine found expression in the utopian literature. Both Comenius and Campanella gave instructions for the prolongation of life, but both operated within the conventional framework of dietary regulation and balneotherapy. Andreae by contrast was more familiar with contemporary alchemy and iatrochemistry. In *Christianopolis* the laboratory, drug supply house and anatomical theatre were important institutions of the state. The properties of 'metals, minerals and vegetables, and even the life of animals are examined, purified, increased and united, for the use of the human race and in the interests of health'. Andreae realised that scientific medicine offered enormous potentialities for progress, providing that its practitioners could avoid the faults characteristic of unscrupulous innovators, quacks, and the dubious Rosicrucian brotherhood.[9]

Bacon's utopian fragment, *New Atlantis,* was published posthumously as an appendix to *Sylva Sylvarum* in 1626. Both of these works had a definite medical bias and both had a strong appeal during this period, eight editions appearing between 1626 and 1658. The general public were probably more familiar with these works than with any of Bacon's more philosophical writings.[10] The mines, laboratories and gardens of Solomon's House were designed to perfect man's control over the environment, and provide advice on diet and medicines, so preparing the way to the prolongation of life. Like Andreae and the Paracelsians, Bacon attached particular importance to mineral and metallic cures. This was a distant echo of a medieval natural magic tradition; Roger Bacon had advocated finding 'the secrets, of Stones, Herbs, Sensibles &c. both for the knowledge of Nature and especially the Prolongation of Life'. He predicted that the life span could be augmented by one hundred years, the limit set at the Fall. Beyond this man was not permitted to go, until the resurrection, which would reveal his propensity to achieve immortality.[11] Such ambitious goals were appropriate to utopian literature, but subsequent writings indicate that the Puritans seriously believed man's natural life was capable of more effective regulation than had

8. Bacon (13), p.121.

9. Campanella, *Civitas Solis: Idea Reipublicae Philosophicae* (Frankfurt, 1623), pp.445–8; Comenius, *Didactica Magna* (56), Chapter XV; Andreae, *Christianopolis* (146), pp.196–200.

10. R. W. Gibson, *Francis Bacon, a Bibliography* (Oxford, 1950), pp.149–51.

11. R. Bacon, *op. cit.*, pp.30, 33–4. Both he and Campanella anticipated the life span could be extended to 200 years in exceptional cases. See also G. J. Gruman, 'A History of Ideas about the Prolongation of Life', *Trans. American Philosophical Soc.*, 1966, *56,* Part 9.

been attained under traditional medicine. Thus the medical reform tracts of the Puritan Revolution carried a marked imprint of the utopian ideals of *New Atlantis*. Correspondingly, an obvious medical dimension was apparent in such utopian writings as *Macaria* (1641) by Gabriel Plattes, Chamberlen's *Poor Mans Advocate* (1649), Winstanley's *Law of Freedom* (1652) and Peter Cornelius Plockhoy's *A Way Propounded to Make the Poor Happy* (1659).

The innovative writings of Bacon and his continental counterparts suggested that medical reform would occupy an important place among the achievements of the Great Instauration. Although the immediate practical achievement was limited, there was a conviction that experimental science could achieve a transformation of medicine. Paracelsian iatrochemistry and Harveian physiology provided a stimulus to medical reform, and both emerged as powerful forces in England during the Puritan Revolution. Both served to widen the gulf between classical authority and current scientific opinion. Once the intellectual inheritance was undermined, reformers turned to questioning the traditional organisation of medicine, which was increasingly seen as a limitation to further progress. Reformers urged medical practitioners to return to Hippocratic standards and to exercise medical skills which were commonly divided between physicians, surgeons and apothecaries. But this return to primitive efficiency could not be readily accomplished, since the lower medical ranks were so likely to infringe the traditional privileges of physicians. Attempts during the early Stuart period to define the roles of the medical organisations along traditional lines resulted in an unstable compromise which ran counter to the social conditions and intellectual aspirations of the age.

(ii) The Medical Monopolies

In the organisation of the medical profession in early seventeenth-century England there was a great contrast between London and the provinces. Outside the capital, medical facilities were rudimentary. In the network of small towns and rural communities in which the great majority of the population lived, medical services were supplied by a motley assortment of practitioners who operated under a loose system of licensing organised by the bishops and the universities. Only a small minority of these practitioners possessed medical qualifications; the majority held neither degree nor licence, and many must have been almost illiterate. In London, amongst a population which had increased from c.200,000 in 1600 to c.400,000 by the middle of the century, rewards were higher and professional rivalries sharper. Metropolitan medical services were less primitive, but that a crisis situation existed was strikingly apparent from the condition of the poor and the epidemics which claimed thousands of victims. During the Tudor and early Stuart period, the various groups controlling London medicine formed into corporations which negotiated charters designed to preserve their rights and define their boundaries of operation.[12] Gradually an order was established giving adequate protection to the physicians, surgeons and apothecaries, although the rigidly hierarchical nature of this arrangement was an affront to ambitious practitioners from the lower echelons. The structure of medical organisation evolving in London followed the pattern adopted much earlier in major cities of the continent. It was a rational, symmetrical and well-regulated system, which had operated smoothly in smaller communities under more stable intellectual and social conditions. But in London it was not given the opportunity to reach an equilibrium.

The dominant force in London medicine was the College of Physicians which, since its foundation in 1518, had acted as the guardian of humanistic medical standards. Its members constituted an extremely well-organised and vigilant medical élite. Membership was restricted to medical graduates of the two English universities, at a time when the MD was supposedly obtained after a long course of studies in the arts and medical faculties.[13] Even so, four years of practice were required before a candidate was eligible for a fellowship. Before 1640, a convenient and congenial method of qualifying for membership of the College was to spend a brief period abroad, taking an MD at Padua or some other popular continental medical centre, and then incorporating at an English university. As a slight disincentive triple fees were charged to graduates of foreign universities applying for any form of membership at the College.[14]

Apart from correcting anomalies and strengthening clauses relating to inferior organisations, very few changes were made in the college statutes until after the restoration.[15] Despite the growth of London, the number of Fellows was not increased, remaining at thirty until after 1660; the four Royal Physicians were additional to this number between 1618 and the Civil War.[16] When the College was required to submit a complete list of its members in 1614, its Fellows, candidates and licentiates totalled only forty-one.[17] Since an optimum number of six candidates was permitted, the numbers indicate that few availed themselves of licences, partly because of the initial fee of £8 and subsequent fee of £4 per annum, but more likely because unlicensed medical practice was not

12. For a summary of estimates of London population see E. A. Wrigley in *Past and Present,* 1967, No. 37, p.44. R. S. Roberts, 'The personnel and practice of medicine in Tudor and Stuart England', *Medical History,* 1962, *6*: 363–82; 1964, *8*: 217–34. For an excellent brief discussion of social conditions in early seventeenth-century England, see Thomas (281), pp.3–21.

13. For the early history of the College, see my 'Thomas Linacre and the Foundation of the College of Physicians' in the forthcoming volume, *Linacre Studies*. For the actual length of English medical studies, see above, p.121.

14. Clark (50), i, pp.134–5.

15. Clark (50), i, pp.172–81, 'Statuta Vetera', pp.376–92.

16. Clark (50), i, pp.132, 188, 190.

17. Clark (50), i, p.133.

under effective control. Under these circumstances the College was constantly seeking legal sanction for stronger powers against empirics. However, it was not at all successful in drawing physicians under the authority of its statutes. Between 1640 and 1660 there were only just over forty Fellows, candidates and licentiates: about one for every 10,000 of the population. Inevitably the increased demand for medical care far exceeded the capacities of the authorised practitioners. Hence the conditions were ripe for the proliferation of unauthorised medical activity.

The Barber-Surgeons' Company had been established in 1540. It excluded barbers from surgery and gave surgeons a monopoly in the London area. The Company was both protected and controlled by the College of Physicians.[18] Surgeons, particularly those engaged with the navy, naturally tended to increase the scope of their activities, effectively arguing reasons of state whenever the College attempted to prevent such developments. The surgeons were also quick to recognise the value of the Norman Yoke weapon. The College was able to prevent any formal recognition of the rights of surgeons to practise medicine, but they were obliged to grant *ad hominem* licences to allow surgeons limited rights to practise. Indeed the Barber-Surgeons' Company attracted many allies who possessed formal medical qualifications. Such London surgeons as John Gerard, George Baker, William Clowes, Richard Surphlet and John Bannister demonstrated their competence by making a substantial contribution to vernacular medical literature. One of the most celebrated of the surgeons, John Woodall, besides writing a pioneer manual of surgery, was an early exponent of Paracelsian medicine. There is firm evidence that the anatomical lectures given at the Barber-Surgeons' Hall had a considerable following. One of the lecturers, Alexander Read, described by Anthony Wood as 'brother of the Barber Churgeons', became one of the most widely-read of medical writers during the Puritan Revolution.[19]

The apothecaries were the last major medical group to become institutionalised.[20] In 1614 they petitioned the king for separation from the Grocers' Company, hoping to secure a division of labour analogous to that effected between barbers and surgeons in the previous century. Like the surgeons, the apothecaries obtained the support of the College of Physicians, which was confident that a well-defined apothecaries' organisation would be more open to supervision. The Society of Apothecaries

18. Clark (50), i, pp.154–5, 206–7; Roberts, *op. cit.* (1964), p.226; J. F. South, *Memorials of the Craft of Surgery in England,* ed. D'Arcy Power (London, 1886); S. Young, *Annals of the Barber Surgeons of London* (London, 1890).

19. Munk (195), i, pp.183–4; Hill (149), pp.74–6; C. E. Raven, *English Naturalists from Neckam to Ray* (234), pp.204–17; *New Cambridge Bibliography of English Literature,* vol. I, ed. G. Watson, pp.2365–73.

20. C. R. B. Barrett, *The History of the Society of Apothecaries of London* (London, 1905), pp.1–11; E. A. Underwood (ed.), *A History of the Worshipful Society of Apothecaries of London,* vol. I (London, 1963), pp.8–22; Clark (50), i, pp.218–26; Roberts, *op. cit.* (1964), p.227.

was awarded its charter in 1617; it was granted a monopoly for dispensing drugs in the London area, to the exclusion of the grocers who had fiercely opposed an apothecaries' grant. In return for the co-operation of the physicians, the new Society was made subject to inspection by the College of Physicians, which issued the *Pharmacopoeia Londinensis* (1618) for the guidance of dispensers.[21] As indicated below this Latin manual, which was intended to constrain and regularise the apothecaries' craft, became in the hands of its translator a medium for the liberalisation of medicine.

Members of the Society of Apothecaries tended to trespass into medical practice quite as much as their brother surgeons. Their effective exploitation of the newly imported drugs and plants from the New World gave them a proprietary interest in an important branch of knowledge which was at that time inadequately appreciated by the physicians.[22] Besides enjoying the commercial benefits of such novelties as tobacco, scammony, senna, spikenard, guaiacum, china root and sarsaparilla, the apothecaries developed a conscientious interest in botany. James Garrett became a leading authority on exotic plants, assembling specimens collected on Ralegh's voyages, including the sensitive plant (*Mimosa pudica*) which subsequently excited the curiosity of botanists. The comprehensive herbals of the apothecaries Thomas Johnson and John Parkinson were the product of gardens and botanical excursions patronised by the Society.[23] These encyclopaedic works were a great advance on the simple botanical lore of the *Pharmacopoeia Londinensis*. A logical development of this interest on the part of the apothecaries was more serious attention to the British flora; under Johnson's leadership botanical excursions became a regular part of the discipline and training of many London apothecaries.

It was therefore from the standpoint of scientific competence and professional authority that the apothecaries made inroads into medical practice, claiming an even broader freedom of action than did the surgeons. Although the Apothecaries' Bill claiming sole rights to compound medicines was not successful, the College was not able to curb their ventures into general practice. As a result physicians and apothecaries fought a continuous legal and parliamentary battle which was still unresolved at the outbreak of the Civil War.[24]

A final feature of official medicine was the Distillers' Company, which obtained its charter in 1638. This represented a further breakdown of the Grocers' Company. The Distillers' Company was objectionable to the

21. Underwood, pp.227–8, 314–15.

22. R. S. Roberts, 'The Early History of the Import of Drugs into England', in *The Evolution of Pharmacy in Britain*, ed. F. N. L. Poynter (London, 1965), pp.165–85.

23. John Gerard, *The Herball or Generall Historie of Plants. Very Much Enlarged and Amended* [by Johnson] (London, 1633); John Parkinson, *Theatrum Botanicum: The Theater of Plants* (London, 1640); H. W. Kew & H. E. Powell, *Thomas Johnson Botanist and Royalist* (London, 1932); Underwood, pp.88–9; C. E. Raven (234), pp.248–97.

24. Clark (50), i, pp.265–72; Barrett, *op. cit.*, pp.12–62; Underwood, pp.41–57.

apothecaries, who claimed sole rights to prepare and sell distilled products.[25] It was also opposed by other companies which alleged a traditional involvement in distillation. The distillers fought an intense battle for separate rights.[26] Little was achieved until interest in the distillation monopoly was exhibited by the two Royal Physicians Sir Theodore de Mayerne and Thomas Cadyman, who were granted a monopoly for their method of distilling strong waters and vinegars in 1636, upon payment of a £10 rent to the king. This monopoly matured into the Distillers' Company in 1638, under the direction of de Mayerne, Cadyman and Sir William Brouncker.[27] At the time the Distillers' Company might not have appeared as having a serious interest in medicine; the petitioners probably recognised the commercial profitability of strong drink. But it is also important to note that, owing to the great rise of distillation iatrochemistry, the distiller was becoming a key figure in chemical therapy. The Paracelsian de Mayerne would have been well aware of these potentialities. Hence it is possible that his shrewd exploitation of the monopoly system was instigated by the College of Physicians, in order to prevent the apothecaries from controlling one of the most effective methods of preparing chemical medicines; thereby also the distillers would be more readily regulated by the College.

From the above account it is apparent that the carefully constructed edifice of medical monopolies established under the Stuarts was highly unstable. As in the commercial world, the logical delineation of functions, even if guaranteed by monopoly rights, was no protection against natural expansion when market conditions were favourable.

Each of the three medical bodies was constantly evolving plans to infringe the liberties of its professional neighbours. At the same time official medicine was eroded by other companies, or by practitioners lying outside organised medicine. The system was a pyramid, surmounted by an élite of not more than fifty members and licentiates of the College of Physicians. Beneath them was a larger number of apothecaries and surgeons. But as far as the majority of Londoners were concerned, the medical profession consisted mainly of a large and ill-defined assembly of independent practitioners. These ranged from itinerant foreign physicians with formal medical qualifications, to illiterate herb women. Medicine was also practised as a method of supplementing income by poor clergymen or artisans. William Trigge discovered his own aptitude for medicine while working as a cobbler at Canterbury. He then conducted a successful practice for many years in London, suffering

25. Barrett, *op. cit.*, pp.54–7, 76–7; Underwood, pp.55–7, 314–16.
26. *CJ*, i, p.529; 27 Feb. 1621.
27. *CSPD 1635/6*, p.318. *Specification of Patent 1636, No. 81.* In recognition of their 'skill and great industrie, after many chargeable experiments', Cadyman and Mayerne were given a 14-year patent for distilling strong waters and vinegars from cider, perry, etc. (25 March 1636). *Specification of Patent 1636, No. 90,* gave Brouncker a patent for a method of improving the yield in the distillation of malt liquors.

continuous harassment from the College of Physicians. Noah Biggs commented that medicine had largely fallen into the hands of old soldiers, or 'Priests and poor Scholars, that have nothing else to do must now turn Physitians'.[28]

In rural communities, where professional medical assistance was frequently not available, each family was obliged to undertake responsibility for basic medical care, exploiting traditional herbal cures and cordials according to local tradition. The comments of Edward, Lord Herbert of Cherbury suggest that knowledge of the virtues of plants and herbs 'made for the use of man' was an essential part of a gentleman's education. A particularly important medical role was assumed by gentlewomen and clergymen, who would dispense medicine for their neighbours as an expression of charity. A celebrated aristocratic practitioner was Elizabeth Grey, Duchess of Kent, the originator of 'Kent's powder', a much-favoured cure. At a lower social level Elizabeth Ray, the blacksmith's wife at Black Notley, was reputed to have been an able medical adviser, and it is thought that she introduced her son, John Ray, to botany. A parallel instance is provided by Dorothy Burton, mother of the author of the *Anatomy of Melancholy,* who was reported 'to have excellent skill in chirurgery . . . and such experimental medicines, as all the country where she dwelt can witness, to have done many generous and good cures upon divers poor folks'.[29] Herb women were drawn from an even more humble social group, but their intuitive expertise with a well-tried, if narrow range of cures earned them general respect.

Apart from local gentlewomen or old wives, clergymen were the common purveyors of medical lore. Indeed medical practice by the priest and his wife was specifically advocated by George Herbert in his celebrated advice to the Anglican clergy.[30] One extreme in competence was Timothie Bright, who entered the ministry after a formal medical education and service at St. Bartholomew's Hospital; he had even published substantial medical writings.[31] The monumentally erudite Robert Burton confessed that he had occasionally trespassed into medical areas. More commonly the minister was like Richard Baxter, having no formal medical education, but attaining by trial and error a medical competence not inferior to that of local physicians. Baxter reflected with satisfaction that 'God made use of my Practice of Physick among them [the people of Kidderminster]'.[32]

28. Biggs (25), p.25. For a similar statement, see Burton, *Anatomy of Melancholy* (Everyman edn.), i, pp.36–7.

29. Lord Herbert, *Autobiography,* ed. S. L. Lee (London, 1886), pp.57–9; C. E. Raven, *John Ray Naturalist* (235), p.9; Burton, *Anatomy of Melancholy* (Everyman edn.), ii, p.250.

30. George Herbert, *Priest to the Temple, or, the Countrey Parson* (Cambridge, 1633), Chapter XIV.

31. G. Keynes, *Timothie Bright* (London, 1962).

32. F. J. Powicke, *A Life of the Reverend Richard Baxter,* 2 vols. (London, 1924–7), i, pp.104–5.

In an age of idealism this arrangement could give little ground for satisfaction, despite the success of pious individuals. Anxiety about health is a frequent topic in private correspondence of the period. Increasingly, the educated public came to hope that the new science would lead to an improvement in the quality of medical judgement. Especially when backed by this rational scientific basis, medical innovators were assured of a sympathetic audience. They lost no opportunity of castigating tradition and they were neither cautious nor modest in their advocacy of reform.

To the extent that there was a settlement of the medical profession under Charles I, it was dictated more by the interests of the entrenched professional parties than by any concern to expand the services available to the public. Particularly during the revolutionary decades, medical reformers tended to blame the monopolistic system for the failure of physicians to control epidemics. With hindsight it is apparent that limitations of knowledge precluded effective action by the medical profession in these situations, but contemporary critics were confident that certain basic reforms would greatly increase the efficiency of medical services. Consequently the medical profession was subjected to prolonged public scrutiny along with other uncongenial social institutions, ranging from industrial patents to the national church. At this public tribunal, neither the church, nor the law, nor the medical profession was able to stem the tide of critical literature.

(iii) The Poor Man's Physician

'Monopoly' became the watchword for the social critics. The outburst of popular sentiment against monopolies was one of the most characteristic features of the economic and social history of the Puritan Revolution.[33] This was one of the few issues which united puritan opinion, with the result that it was possible for the Long Parliament to intervene promptly to remedy some of the most flagrant abuses. Industrial monopolies were abolished and the rights of large commercial companies curtailed. The radicals sought to exploit popular resentment by publicising the extreme ramifications of the monopolistic system, their concern extending from the more familiar industrial monopolies to the professions and universities. Scornful of their claims to be considered higher 'callings', the clergy, lawyers and physicians were designated as practitioners of 'trades', motivated like tradesmen by desire for personal gain, and their practices protected by the powerful courts, the Anglican church, or College of Physicians. Through legal or medical fees, and clerical tithes, the maximum profit was extracted from the public, who received neither satisfaction nor the right of access to more efficient alternatives.

33. M. James (158), p.131.

Pamphleteers argued that the clergy sought to mulct their benefices, rather than to provide genuine spiritual guidance for their flocks; the lawyers spawned on the complexities of law without regard for justice; physicians cultivated expensive practices which served only to perpetuate illness and disease. There was a close interrelationship between the monopolistic professions: 'The Liberty of our Common-Wealth . . . is most infringed by three sorts of men, Priests, Physitians, Lawyers; . . . The one deceives men in matters belonging to their Souls, the other in matters belonging to their Bodies, the third in matters belonging to their Estates.'[34] Similarly, Dell, who devoted considerable energies to undermining the learned ministry, believed that medicine and law should be brought 'to that Reformation which a wise and godly Authority will cause them to pass under, both being now exceedingly corrupt and out of order, both for practice and fees'. Starkey saw the entire medical system as a part of a conspiracy to 'monopolize the lives of men . . . that so they [physicians] might maintain themselves, their Bakers, Apothecaries, and Druggists after a Lord like way'.[35] The general context for this critique of the professions was provided by the puritan demand for liberty of conscience, which in turn led more radical groups to press for the abandonment of a national church. Only then would the clergy cease to be a caste apart from their congregations, representing an alien cultural tradition derived from scholastic education and largely pagan authors. These views were reflected in the policies suggested for the reform of the academic, legal and medical professions.

The medical reformers took their immediate cue from the movement for law reform. Winstanley expressed generally accepted priorities: 'the main Work of Reformation lies in this, to reform the Clergy, Lawyers and Law; for all the Complaints of the Land are wrapped up within them Three, not in the person of the King'.[36] Not only were there obvious similarities between the legal and medical professions, but the physicians depended very much upon their legal advisers. It was realised that changes in the legal system might directly affect the status of the medical organisations, and that a receptivity in influential politicians and lawyers to the need for law reform could also bring about a more unsympathetic attitude towards physicians.

The movement for law reform was spearheaded by the Levellers; their numerous manifestoes were complemented by sermons and tracts from other sources. Although the greatest commitment to this issue was shown by the radicals, many of their aspirations were shared by prominent lawyers and by such laymen as Oliver Cromwell.[37] Law reform was seriously considered by an active and influential committee of the

34. Culpeper, *A Physicall Directory,* 1649 (65), sig. A1r.

35. Dell, *Right Reformation* (78), p.27; Starkey, *Helmonts Vindication* (268), p.24.

36. Winstanley, *Law of Freedom* (336), p.7.

37. D. Veall (296); S. E. Prall (227); C. Hill, *God's Englishman* (150), pp.122, 140–5.

House of Commons, which prepared an elaborate 'System of the Law'. This was a professional attempt at a legal code. The termination of the Long Parliament brought a temporary halt to this commission, but the Saints' Parliament of 1653 established a similar committee for law reform, and parliament itself passed a motion calling for 'a new body of the law'.[38]

Pamphleteers made widespread use of the Norman Yoke doctrine to substantiate their demands. According to this historical reconstruction the free people of Anglo-Saxon England had been reduced to slavery under the degenerate tradition of common law imposed by 'William the Bastard'. This law, written obscurely in Latin and Norman French, was the monopoly of a legal profession which was under the control of the Norman aristocracy. Thomas Collier, in a sermon to the army, pointed to the injustice 'in writing our laws in an unknown tongue, that the most part of our national inhabitants cannot understand their own laws, that the French should be better-read in our English laws than those to whom they pertain'.[39] In similar vein, an anonymous Leveller tract complained :

> 'that considering its a Badg of our Slavery to a Norman Conqueror, to have our Laws in the French Tongue, and it is little lesse then brutish vassalage to be bound to walk by Laws which the People cannot know, that therefore all the Laws and Customs of this Realm, be immediatly written in our Mothers Tongue without any abreviations of words, and the most known vulgar hand'.[40]

There were appeals for a return to a system of decentralised local courts, free from obstruction by a highly centralised legal system under rigid crown control. In framing proposals for the reform of common law, attention was increasingly paid to the practical implications of the rights of the individual, rather than to traditional legal precedents. It was held that a vernacular, codified system of law could be composed, by which all citizens would be able to determine what were their rights. The books embodying this code, annotated by legal experts, would be available for inspection in each parish church. Whatever legal system was practised, it was assumed that decentralisation would occur and that lawyers would have to accept greater public accountability.[41]

This widely publicised programme for law reform provided a natural starting point for the debate on the medical profession. The works of Galen had been translated from Greek into Latin, not English; in the

38. Veall (296), pp.83, 86; Mary Cotterell, 'Interregnum Law Reform: The Hale Commission of 1652', *EHR*, 1968, *83* : 689–704.

39. Thomas Collier, *A Discovery of the New Creation* (London, 1647), quoted from 1651 edn., p.407.

40. *To the Supreame Authority of England* [Jan. 1648], quoted from Wolfe, *Leveller Manifestoes* (339), pp.266–7. For similar statements, see John Lilburne, *The Just Mans Justification* (1646); John Warr, *The Corruption and Deficiency* (1649).

41. *The Representative of Divers well-affected persons* [6 Feb. 1649].

hands of the medical humanists, Galen's system seemed to rival the law in its complexity. The College of Physicians, with its long-standing interest in the centralising of medical institutions, was seen as an agency for perpetuating the authority of Galen and for maintaining medical discourse in an alien tongue. In view of these similarities—which were often exaggerated for polemical purposes—it is not surprising that law reformers like Overton, Cook and Robinson turned part of their attention to the medical profession. They first proposed greater public control over the professional bodies, in order to ensure a more economical, comprehensive and humanitarian service; this was also to be facilitated by a less restrictive approach to medical practice. The success of this last measure depended on the degree to which the public could be protected against unscrupulous practitioners. Secondly, a vernacular system of practical medicine could be compiled, which would free the population from most of its dependence on physicians. This reform would have been particularly valuable for those sections of the public which normally had no access to medical practitioners. It was envisaged that the individual would assume greater responsibility for himself and become as effective a guardian of his health as of his legal rights.

The first significant comments on medical reform to appear during the Puritan Revolution were made by Gabriel Plattes in his utopian sketch *Macaria* (1641). In Plattes's ideal community, the king and his counsellors governed wisely, conscious that the vigilant and well-educated citizens could not be exploited, because they were fully aware of their legal rights. In this thinly-veiled reform tract Plattes translated the general medical aspects of Solomon's House into more practical terms. Like other Puritans, he believed that clergymen should take an active part in secular affairs. In particular he sought to regularise their involvement in medicine:

> 'In *Macaria,* the parson of every parish is a good physician, and doth execute both functions, to wit, *cura animarum & cura corporum,* and they think it as absurd for a divine to be without skill of physick, as it is to put new wine into old bottles; and the Physicians being true Naturalists, may as well become good Divines, as the Divines doe become good Physicians.'[42]

Social service was one of the roles which Dell envisaged for reformed ministers, who would 'grow up to teach the people, whilst yet they live in an honest calling and imployments as the Apostles did'. By this means the minister would be emancipated from the 'idleness' of scholasticism, to perform an 'honest' vocation, which would improve his qualifications for spiritual leadership. This view of priesthood continued to be canvassed within Hartlib's circle; in 1655 Ezerel Tong, himself a clergy-

42. Plattes, *Macaria* (219), p.6. Bacon, *De Augmentis* (13), spoke of 'our Saviour, who was a Physician both of Soul and Body': p.119.

man-physician, proposed that the First Fruits Office should be used to communicate information about the latest developments in medicine, husbandry and technology to ministers, who would then dispense advice to their parishioners.[43]

The clergy would have provided an excellent basis for a national medical service, but such obligatory extension of charitable duties was probably uncongenial to most clergymen; and it was a positive anathema to the College of Physicians, which refused to give medical licences to clergymen and exerted pressure on the universities to follow this policy.[44] Nevertheless clergymen continued to practise medicine and gain university licences, although in a more sporadic manner than envisaged by *Macaria*. Plattes also proposed that the state should establish a 'house, or Colledge of experience, where they deliver out yeerly such medicines as they find out by experience'; successful innovators would be rewarded from the public purse. Like Andreae and Bacon Plattes was an undoctrinaire exponent of chemical therapy, and he was himself an expert practical chemist.[45]

Further elaboration of these proposals occurred in the social programmes of the Levellers and the Hartlib circle. Problems which Plattes had discussed in the context of a utopian society became more real and urgent as a result of the Civil War, which left a legacy of severe social distress. This social crisis exposed the inadequacy of the hospitals and poor relief system, particularly in London.[46] A wide range of authors contributed plans for more effective poor relief, aimed at easing the plight of wounded soldiers, the elderly and distressed poor, orphans, and victims of the epidemics which were rife in the under-nourished population. Such phenomena as the rapid increase in the incidence of rickets, led to the view that new diseases were being generated during this period—royalists were inclined to attribute such developments to the unwholesome spiritual condition of the population.

In this situation, the problems of poor relief and medical care were inter-connected. The social reformers who were concerned with these questions showed little inclination to adopt conventional views about the organisation and training of the medical profession, or about the administration of poor relief. There was a conscious desire to convert the utopian aspirations of *New Atlantis* and *Macaria* into practical programmes. Projectors varied greatly in their ability to evolve economically feasible schemes, but all contributed to stimulate popular interest in medical reform.

The Levellers presented the problem almost exclusively in political and economic terms, although the 'cries of the starving poor' were un-

43. Dell (78), p.29; Ephemerides 1655.

44. Clark (50), i, pp.240, 247–9, 260–1.

45. Plattes (219), p.5. The obvious source for the 'Colledge of experience' was the 'dispensatories or shops of medicines' in Bacon's Solomon's House, or Andreae's *Christianopolis,* Chapters XLIV & XLV.

46. M. James (158), Chapter VI.

doubtedly a useful adjunct to their political platform.[47] The most significant excursion into general social policy in Leveller literature was a brief appendix to Overton's *Appeal from the degenerate Representative Body*. This contained a series of suggestions relating to parliament, the law, the clergy, education, enclosure and hospitals. Better-maintained hospitals were regarded as an important factor in poor relief.[48]

More detailed proposals on poor relief came from Hartlib and his colleagues. They appealed to public authorities to take on an obligation to maintain the sick poor and William Petty described a model teaching hospital, which will be discussed below. But they placed their main emphasis on preventative measures and rehabilitation. For the urban poor they designed a national system of workhouses which were to be financed on a local basis. By being taught to operate the new textile trades, the urban poor could be made economically self-sufficient. For the agricultural poor, Plattes described a series of simple innovations which would enable agricultural workers' families to be supported in comfort and produce a surplus from extremely small acreages. Plattes and Blith urged that measures of this kind, rather than the provision of hospitals, were the most effective means to improve the conditions of the poor.[49]

These general ideas were taken up by Peter Chamberlen, the physician and entrepreneur, who revived long-standing differences with his colleagues at the College of Physicians by petitioning parliament for the right to establish public baths under his own surveillance. Baths were merely one of a whole constellation of his projects, which ranged from imitations of Hartlib's workhouses to a scheme for law reform.[50] Although he was soon expelled from the College, there was no decline in his medical fortunes. With a sensitive appreciation of the anti-monopolistic sentiments of the period, the College wisely refrained from acting against Chamberlen and other unlicensed physicians. In their turn the legal authorities adopted a less restrictive attitude to medical licensing. An indication of this changing situation is given by the influential parliamentarian barrister John Cook, a moderate exponent of law reform, who was greatly disturbed about the state of the poor.[51] Cook believed that the poor received insufficient legal protection, and he suggested various means to redress major grievances. In general his pamphlet on these

47. *The mournfull Cryes of many thousand poor Tradesmen, who are ready to famish through decay of Trade* [22 Jan. 1648], Wolfe (339), pp.275–8; Brailsford (33), p.534.

48. Overton's appendix was entitled 'Certain Articles for the good of the Commonwealth', Wolfe (339), pp.189–95.

49. The first of Hartlib's workhouse proposals was *The Parliaments Reformation*, 1646 (135). This was followed by many others; see below, pp. 360–3. Petty, *Advice of W.P.*, 1648 (210). Plattes, *Infinite Treasure* (217), sig. a1v; Blith, *English Improver* (27), sig a1r–a2v.

50. Letter from Chamberlen to Cromwell, 14 Dec. 1650, in Nickolls (200), p.36. Chamberlen, *Legislative Power in Problemes*, 1659 (45); *idem, The Poore Mans Advocate*, 1649 (44).

51. John Cook, *Unum Necessarium*, 1648 (57); for Cook, see Veall (296), p.112.

questions followed the lines of Leveller agitation, but with greater practical insight. One of his main themes was the need for a more liberal attitude to medical licensing. He pressed for a more charitable attitude to the poor within the professions; for instance he thought it would be appropriate for the needy to be allocated a proportion of the tithes currently paid to clergy, as well as to receive free advice from lawyers and physicians. Recognising that the collegiate physicians were otherwise engaged and too few to serve the lower classes, he entreated them not to 'hinder any man that would be the poore man's Doctor'.[52] In particular he made representations on behalf of William Trigge, the shoemaker empiric, who had been imprisoned at the instance of the College under Charles I.[53] The College was now attempting to impose upon Trigge a fine of £115. Cook claimed that Trigge had successfully ministered to the poor in London since 1624, and had treated them for very small fees. Consequently, he was able to assemble many petitions in support of Trigge's abilities. Cook even believed that Trigge was justified in claiming the title 'Doctor'. With reference to Trigge's failure to obtain a college licence, Cook tersely commented: 'It may be he thinks it a Monopoly, for by the Common-Law everyman may Administer Phisick that hath any skill therein.'[54] Cook's memorandum may well reflect a more general opinion in favour of reinstating the notorious 'Quacks' Charter' of 1542/3 as a means to support the position of all reliable but unlicensed practitioners.[55]

Thus Cook, an important voice among the parliamentarian lawyers, was anticipating a more liberal approach to medical licensing than had been acceptable to the College of Physicians at any earlier stage in its history. Other proposals made by Cook became a commonplace in the subsequent reform literature. He advocated that physicians should make up their own prescriptions, and that it should be set down 'in plaine English wordes what they prescribe, and what they [the patients] pay for'. Furthermore, the poor, who particularly in London had lost contact with traditional herbal lore, should be taught simple medicine, in order to prevent their having to rely on apothecaries and physicians.

Such views were consistent with Cook's general outlook on law reform. This integrated approach to the professions was also emphasised in an address to the Saints' Parliament by Samuel Herring, who reaffirmed the obligation of the state to maintain the poor. He proposed that all divines, physicians and lawyers should be state-salaried; they could then be conscripted according to the requirement for their services. Finally, 'all law bookes, physick or whatsoever . . . should be translated into English'.[56]

52. Cook (57), p.61.
53. Charles Goodall, *The Royal College,* 1684 (119), pp.420–2.
54. Cook (57), p.62.
55. Clark (50), i, pp.86–7, 264.
56. 'Mr. Samuel Herring to the parliament', 4 August 1653, in Nickolls (200), pp.99–102.

The social reformers of the Puritan Revolution created a climate of opinion favourable to the expression of ideas about medical reform. Medical practitioners who had remained silent during the period of dominance of the College of Physicians were now able to come forward and announce their views on all aspects of medicine. They propagated unorthodox medical theories and they appealed for the reform of medical organisation and education. This movement gained the sympathy of a wide range of intellectuals, some of whom came from outside the central puritan tradition. The College of Physicians was particularly offensive to the medical reformers. For polemical purposes, they characterised the College as the guardian of Galenic medicine: an authoritarian and socially degenerate medical organisation appeared to be linked with a dogmatic and intellectually debilitating body of medical doctrine.

A major statement of the position of the medical reformers was made by Noah Biggs, an author who has so far escaped identification. From the context it is probable that Biggs was young and well-educated; his writings display familiarity with the iatrochemical medical literature and with the general puritan literature on social reform. The sentiments expressed might well represent the views of the young Robert Boyle. If his style had been more laborious, or his opinions more impenetrable and convoluted, the author might well have been Boyle himself.[57]

Biggs addressed his book to parliament, appealing in the manner of Milton for that body's support for a general social and intellectual reformation following on from the successful defeat of episcopacy and Presbyterianism. The Commonwealth, having established a healthier spiritual climate, was urged to reform medicine in order to bring about a physical regeneration of the nation. Like Comenius, Biggs believed that physical health was a necessary precondition for spiritual well-being. He noted that the College of Physicians had so far not been reformed, and warned parliament of the dangers, if

> 'we should pin our faith and knowledge upon the Cabin of an Amen-corner, when the Rialto, or Palace Royal of Galenical Physick, where they have crown'd him with the Title of Parent and Monarch thereof, stands unhung with any experiment of real good, and divested of all real, solid and substantial vertue of Medicine'.[58]

57. Biggs, *Mataeotechnia medicinae,* 1651 (25). Introductory poems were by 'R.B.iatrophilos', W.R., and James de Villiers. It would be interesting to speculate that the first two were Robert Boyle, and William Rand. For the influence of Milton on Biggs, see above, pp.190–1. 'Dalepater Mendemus' composed *Lex Exlex: or the Downfall of the Law, and the Gospell. Being a Warning-piece to the Colledge of Physitians* (London, 1652). Ostensibly this repeats many of Biggs's criticisms of the College, but it is really an attempt to ridicule the reformers.

58. Biggs (25), sig. a4v.

An equally severe attitude was taken to the universities. In an age of great enthusiasm for Baconian learning, the ancient institutions were found unresponsive or positively reactionary. Biggs hoped that parliament would take the initiative to reform learning and restore medicine to the central place which it had occupied in the Hippocratic age. His summary of reform proposals exhibited a strong medical bias. He advocated:

1. The establishment of an academy where free philosophy and reformed knowledge would be practised.
2. The reform of the universities; their failure to train the medical profession was to be heard in 'the Clamours of the Sick, and the cries of Widows and Orphans'.
3. The reform of abuses in all professions.
4. The construction of a clear and simple system of practical and theoretical medicine, unobscured by Galenic or Aristotelian theory.
5. The production of a new pharmacopoeia, which would take full account of the value of chemical therapy.
6. The promotion of chemistry, the '*terra incognita*' of traditional medicine.[59]

Biggs produced a wide-ranging plan for reform, which was the counterpart for medicine of the platform discussed by the law reformers. But no parliamentary action was taken on medical reform, although freedom from interference made it possible to develop on an informal basis some of the schemes mentioned by Biggs. The promotion of chemistry, the revision of the pharmacopoeia, the production of a system of practical and vernacular medical works, and the more liberal organisation of the medical profession could proceed without active parliamentary intervention. By contrast law reform was not possible without parliamentary initiative. But regardless of the degree of impact of these social reform movements, the Commonwealth and Protectorate proved to be a highly fertile period for debate in both law and medicine. In medicine, numerous authors worked towards the goals set in *Mataeotechnia medicinae*.

(iv) A Whole Model of Physick

It was not until 1649 that George Thomason added a medical work to his exhaustive collection of books and pamphlets, which was begun in 1640. Thomason's first medical tract, obtained on 11 September, was an inauspicious collection of forty medical recipes and a few notes about cosmetics put together by the 'Neopolitan operator' Salvator Winter, who was at that time practising medicine in London. Hartlib noticed that *The New Dispensatory* was produced in two forms, a

59. Biggs (25), sig. b3r–v.

standard edition of fifteen pages, and a nine-page cheap edition for the poor. Thomason collected the former. The pamphet was evidently successful. Winter then combined forces with a similarly Italianate colleague, Francesco Dickinson, to produce *A Precious Treasury, containing 70 approved physical rare receits.* Before the end of the month Dickinson separately put out *A Precious Treasury of twenty rare Secrets.*[60] Individually these works are of little interest or originality, but they are valuable indicators of the demand for popular vernacular medical literature. Immediately the conditions were favourable to such productions, a class of authors emerged to satisfy the market. Winter and Dickinson were the heralds of a great flood of medical literature which appeared between 1650 and 1660, produced in an atmosphere charged with enthusiasm for every aspect of medical speculation, which

TABLE I

MEDICAL WORKS CONTAINED IN THE THOMASON TRACTS

Year	English	Latin	TOTAL
1649	4	—	4
1650	4	—	4
1651	13	—	13
1652	5	2	7
1653	11	—	11
1654	3	1	4
1655	11	—	11
1656	8	1	9
1657	8	—	8
1658	3	—	3
1659	4	2	6
1660	3	4	7
TOTAL	77	10	87

These totals are compiled from G. K. Fortescue, *Catalogue of the Pamphlets collected by George Thomason, 1640–1661* (London, 1908).

was given ample room for expression with the collapse of censorship and the liberation of London medicine from the authority of the College of Physicians.

Before the Puritan Revolution a stringent centralised procedure for censorship had been established by Laud. It applied not only to political

60. Winter, *A New Dispensatory* (337); Dickinson, *A Precious Treasury* (80); Winter & Dickinson, *A Pretious Treasury* (338); Ephemerides 1649.

and religious literature, but also to medicine, philosophy and even poetry. There was also rigid control of imported books.[61] The College of Physicians had no direct right to license books, but its opinions were sought by the ecclesiastical censors; a mutual confidence subsisted between the physicians and the church over this procedure. Even though it was not used to interfere actively with the content of medical works, this mechanism was sufficient to inhibit any expression of hostility towards the College, or the development of a co-ordinated medical reform movement. Consequently the vernacular medical literature of the Laudian period was largely a relic of Elizabethan medicine. It was dominated by reprints of popular collections of recipes, although a few original writers and translators like the surgeon Alexander Read and the apothecary Thomas Johnson, also made use of the vernacular.

The rise of vernacular literature in medicine is indicated by Thomason's collection and the wider statistics of London medical publishing between 1640 and 1660.[62] Thomason's annual intake of medical books rose sharply, to reach a peak of thirteen in 1651. Seventy-seven vernacular medical works were acquired between 1649 and 1660, compared with only ten Latin works. Of the latter, six were obtained over 1659 and 1660. The impression obtained from the Thomason collection is confirmed by more general statistics. Of the 238 medical works published in England between 1640 and 1660 which have so far been recorded, only twelve per cent are in Latin, which was still the dominant vehicle of communication among European academic physicians. The Latin works published in England are found particularly for 1660, the year of the restoration. These data also show how little medical publishing occurred between 1641 and 1648, explaining why Thomason collected no medical tracts before 1649.[63]

The great growth in medical publishing which began in 1649 was partly a reflection of the return to normal conditions after the inhibition of non-political publishing during the Civil War. But this cannot be the whole explanation, since the rate of production of medical works in the 1650s greatly exceeded that of the 1630s as well as that of the 1640s. Sixty-three medical works were published in the ten-year period from 1630 to 1639, at an average of six per annum. Between 1650 and 1659, 182 medical works were published, which gives an average of eighteen per annum. This does not represent merely a quantitative increase; as will be seen below there was a marked difference in the general character of the higher-level medical literature produced during the Puritan Revolution.

61. H. S. Bennett, *English Books and Readers 1603 to 1640* (Cambridge, 1970), pp.40–54; F. B. Williams, 'The Laudian Imprimatur', *The Library*, Fifth Series, 1960, *15*: 96–104.

62. See Table 1 for details of the medical works in the Thomason collection.

63. See Table 2 for details of general medical publishing between 1640 and 1660.

TABLE 2

MEDICAL WORKS PUBLISHED IN ENGLAND 1640-1660

Year	English	Latin	TOTAL
1640	4	—	4
1641	—	2	2
1642	2	—	2
1643	—	—	—
1644	1	—	1
1645	—	—	—
1646	1	—	1
1647	2	—	2
1648	5	2	7
1649	13	3	16
1650	13	3	16
1651	19	2	21
1652	21	2	23
1653	16	2	18
1654	13	2	15
1655	18	1	19
1656	14	1	15
1657	20	—	20
1658	15	1	16
1659	17	2	19
1660	13	8	21
	—	—	—
TOTAL	207	31	238

These totals are compiled from lists provided by bibliographical sources, which have been checked, wherever possible, against the works themselves.

Among the factors which stimulated the growth of medical publishing was the collapse of both censorship and medical licensing. Salvator Winter is typical of the class of authors who were quick to take advantage of such opportunities. However this again is only a partial explanation, which relates particularly to works of the type produced by Winter. Other authors entered into vernacular medical publishing because of their concern for medical reform.

Ideological commitment to the vernacular is well illustrated by the example of Nicholas Culpeper, whose first work, the *Physical Directory,* appeared within a few weeks of Winter's *New Dispensatory.* It represented a much higher plane of vernacular medical literature than Winter's work. Culpeper rapidly established himself as the most aggressive and prolific medical editor of the period; he and his disciples were responsible for forty-one issues of thirty different works between 1649 and 1660.[64] Many of these books remained popular into the next century and a few have persisted until the present day. Culpeper's writings indicate that he was not merely concerned with the straightforward task of translation. He spent a short time at Cambridge University before becoming apprenticed to a London apothecary; during service in the parliamentarian army, he came under the influence of William Lilly, the popular parliamentarian astrologer. Culpeper combined these experiences to become an exponent of astrological medicine, styling himself 'Student of physick and astrology'.

His first exercise in translation was that of the *Pharmacopoeia Londinensis,* produced with considerable pride in 1618 by the College of Physicians, as the authoritative and obligatory source of guidance for London apothecaries. This compilation was maintained in its Latin form by the College of Physicians and its translation was not contemplated. Culpeper accordingly undertook the responsibility for producing an unauthorised translation, an act which was calculated to antagonise the College. Fully aware of the implications, Culpeper introduced the *Directory* with a brief but deliberately provocative political preface, predicting the imminent and inevitable victory of 'THE LIBERTY OF THE SUBJECT', which would be marked by the collapse of the monopolistic professions.[65] He identified the College of Physicians with the papists, on the grounds of their resistance to the use of the vernacular in medicine. Culpeper produced a complete translation of the *Pharmacopoeia*; and he inserted much additional matter which included astrological notes, or interjections abusing the College. His greatly expanded alphabetical list of drugs with their properties, formed the basis for his famous *Herbal.*[66]

The *Physical Directory* was sufficiently noteworthy to arouse comment in the parliamentarian press by Henry Walker, who described it as 'an excellent translation'.[67] Walker himself performed a direct service to medicine by instigating the regular publication of the London Bills of Mortality in *Perfect Occurrences,* this practice being soon imitated by various rival newspapers. Hartlib was similarly impressed by Culpeper's work, which received prompt and favourable mention in his Ephemerides.

This parliamentarian approval provoked an immediate response from the royalist press, which violently attacked the *Directory,* using the occasion to indulge in a character assassination of this satellite of its

64. October 30 was the date recorded on Thomason's copy of Culpeper's *Physicall Directory*. For a list of Culpeper's works, see F. N. L. Poynter, 'Nicholas Culpeper and his Books', *Jnl. Hist. Med.*, 1962, *17*: 152–67.
65. Culpeper, *Physicall Directory* (65), sig. A1r; capitals as in the original.
66. *Ibid.*, pp.1–77.
67. *Perfect Occurrences*, No. 139, 31 Aug.–7 Sept. 1649.

arch-enemy William Lilly. The strength of this denunciation, which the newspapers usually reserved for important public figures, is a manifestation of the importance attached to Culpeper's translation of the *Pharmacopoeia Londinensis.* It was probably anticipated that Culpeper's work heralded further translations and more general interference by the sectaries in medicine.[68]

The royalist warnings about the dangers of the *Physical Directory* had little effect, since Culpeper and his publisher Peter Cole decided to issue another edition in the following year. The original quarto was replaced by a substantial folio edition, little different in general content, but with a new preface, again attacking the use of medical Latin. The strident opening sentence asserts Culpeper's intention of relating this issue to the general theme of the Norman Yoke: 'William the Bastard having conquered this Nation . . . brought in the Norman Laws written in an unknown tongue, and thus laid the foundation to their future, and our present slavery.'[69] The use of Latin was a scholars' conspiracy, ensuring that theology, law and medicine would be unintelligible to laymen, and accessible only to those who could afford an expensive professional education. The effect of this linguistic convention had been the sacrifice of productive knowledge and the perpetuation of scholastic education, which served to stupefy the mind by the placing of 'faith upon the sleeve of that monster Tradition'.[70] Replying to the *Pragmaticus* attack on the sects, Culpeper countered with specific criticisms about the dishonesty of the London Presbyterian ministry. Despite the objections of the College of Physicians, he expressed a devotion to the systematic translation of medical works in order to provide the English with 'the whol Moddel of Physick in their Native Language'.[71] By this means, his countrymen could be familiarised with the medicinal qualities of common local plants. This practical function had only been served to a limited degree by the expensive encyclopaedic herbals of Parkinson and Gerard. The College of Physicians was criticised for not giving adequate attention to practical botany. This censure had some foundation since the physicians in the seventeenth century played little part in the investigation of the English flora, or in the medical application of these data. This defect is made even more apparent by the careful attention of the apothecaries to botany, their discoveries being incorporated in the editions of Gerard's *Herbal* prepared by apothecary Thomas Johnson, or in William How's *Phytologia Britannica*

68. *Mercurius Pragmaticus Part 2,* No. 21, 4–11 Sept. 1649. The author has generally been identified as Marchamont Nedham (following Lee's *DNB* art., 'Culpeper'). However, Needham's association with *Pragmaticus* seems to have ended in June 1649. Subsequently he wrote on behalf of the parliamentarians and became a critic of the College of Physicians. The *Pragmaticus* attack may have been the work of George Wharton. Frank (103), pp.194–5.

69. Culpeper, *Physical Directory,* 1650 (66), sig. B1r.

70. *Ibid.,* sig. B1r.

71. *Ibid.,* sig. B2r.

(1650). How practised medicine in London without academic medical qualifications.

Yet a third, further augmented edition of the *Directory* appeared in 1651, again in folio and with a fresh Preface. Here Culpeper made his most direct attack on the College of Physicians, which he stigmatised as an inefficient monopoly, motivated by financial self-interest, and displaying no sensitivity to more enlightened attitudes on medicine and society. Accordingly Gresham College, rather than Amen Corner was canvassed as a prospective centre for reformed medicine. Culpeper was not quite finished with the London *Pharmacopoeia.* This handbook was slightly revised by the College in 1650, and the revision was in due course translated by Culpeper, again without authorisation, as *Pharmacopoeia Londinensis: or the London dispensatory further adorned* (1653). The latest amendments were thus made available to the English reader as a further step to 'the pulling down Monopoly'. This latest revision had yet another preface (Culpeper's fourth version) which subordinated polemic to a useful discussion of the theory of astrological medicine.[72] Until the nineteenth century frequent reissues of Culpeper's edition of the London *Pharmacopoeia* completely overshadowed the authorised editions produced by the College of Physicians.

This initial success was consolidated by embarking on a wider range of translations, which were continued with undiminished vigour in Culpeper's name after his premature death in 1654, by his wife Alice in conjunction with Culpeper's former assistants, Peter Cole and William Rowland. Eventually 'Culpeper' became a hallmark for a variety of compilations the contents of which bore little relation to the founder's astrological physic. His name came to have considerable commercial appeal, as witnessed by the longstanding popularity of his works, and the numbers of pirated editions.

The medical books issued by Culpeper himself represent various medical viewpoints. He was certainly not attracted to the works of the pioneers of modern physiology who are the main interest of modern historians. Although Harvey, Descartes, Bartholin and Pecquet were translated during this period, their works were designed for an audience concerned with issues which had little relevance to practical medicine. Culpeper was motivated by pragmatic considerations; his aim was to raise the standards of vernacular medicine, which had hitherto been dominated by the random compilations of such authors as Winter and Dickinson. Their recipe books had a long ancestry and were to continue as a cheap ancillary to quack medicine, but Culpeper made them subordinate to major pharmacopoeias, or to translations of the writings of influential European physicians. Through Culpeper's work the literate public had access to reliable contemporary opinions on many aspects of medicine. His increasingly comprehensive range of translations approximated to the 'whol Moddel of Physick' which he had sought to com-

72. Culpeper, *Pharmacopoeia Londinensis,* sig. A3r; see Thomas (281), p.332.

pile for the English reader. The pharmacopoeia was the foundation for this system of medical knowledge. Culpeper shared the widely-held view that providence had endowed local plants with considerable medical potentialities. The use by upper-class physicians of exotic herbs was dismissed as a fraudulent practice. He was deeply impressed by a vision he experienced in which 'All the sick People in England presented themselves before me, and told They had Herbes in their Gardens that might cure them, but knew not the vertues of them'.[73]

The systematic exposition of the medical properties of freely available local plants was regarded as the most rational basis for empirical medicine. This would guarantee the health of the poor and break their dependence on apothecaries and Galenic practitioners. To assist this development Culpeper produced a new work based on the alphabetical list of drugs with which he had prefaced his translations of the *Pharmacopoeia Londinensis.* The resultant *English Physician* (1652), his most celebrated work, amplified the alphabetical lists of herbs to provide a complete guide to the medicinal properties of English plants. The *English Physician* (eventually known as *Culpeper's Herbal*) counteracted the trend established by the herbals of Gerard and Parkinson, of emphasising botany at the expense of medical information. Instead of multiplying species Culpeper preferred to concentrate on supplying astrological hints which would enable the properties of common herbs to be used to their maximum effect.

Other popular and unorthodox dispensatories produced by Culpeper were his own *Treatise of Aurum Potabile* (1657), and an augmented translation of Jean Prevot, *Medicaments for the Poor* (1657). Chemical remedies were given in George Phaedro, *Physical and Chymical Works* (1654). With regard to general medicine Culpeper issued the works of the standard continental authorities, Lazar Riverius and Jean Riolan; he also put out a work by the Paracelsian Simeon Partlicius, and one by Comenius's collaborator John Jonston.[74] Daniel Sennert, who assimilated elements from orthodox and Paracelsian medicine, was influential abroad and popular with Culpeper and his colleagues who even translated his systematic digest of natural philosophy, *Thirteen Books of Natural Philosophy* (1659). After 1660 many of Sennert's medical and chemical works were issued by Culpeper's successors. In obstetrics, Culpeper contributed an original work, the *Directory for Midwives* (1651).

73. Culpeper, *Physical Directory* (66), sig. A2r. This view is very similar to that of the prefaces of William Turner's pioneer herbals composed a century before. Turner abandoned his plans to publish a Latin *Herbarium* and published a three-part English *Herbal* (1551–8). Timothie Bright re-echoed this opinion. See also William How, *Phytologia Britannica* (1650), Preface; Biggs, *Mataeotechnia medicinae,* 1651 (25), pp.59–64; Robert Turner, *ΒΟΤΑΝΟΛΟΓΙΑ The British Physician* (1664). For a similar French debate, see Howard Stone, 'The French Language in Renaissance Medicine', *Bibl. d'Humanisme et Renaissance,* 1953, *15:* 315–46.

74. For details, Poynter, *op. cit.,* and *idem,* 'Nicholas Culpeper and the Paracelsians', in Debus (73), i, pp.201–20.

This became extremely popular. Among other specialist writings translated, were Veslingius's *Anatomy* (1653), which was one of the first anatomical textbooks to incorporate Harvey's theory of circulation; also the monograph on rickets by Harvey's follower Francis Glisson, which was the first pathological monograph to apply the theory of circulation.[75] Glisson's work was first published in 1650 by a committee of the College of Physicians; it was regarded as one of the ornaments of interregnum medicine. The rapid appearance of such unauthorised translations may have stimulated Harvey's disciples at the College of Physicians to adopt a more positive attitude towards translating his writings. In 1653, after a lapse of 25 years, a translation of Harvey's *De motu cordis* was issued. By contrast his last major work, *De Generatione* (1651), was translated without delay, also appearing in 1653.

Generally, the pressure for vernacular medicine came from the medical reformers and amateurs; the academic physicians continued to publish predominantly in Latin for the benefit of audiences on the continent. For the same reason they often used continental publishing houses. The College's major concession to the English language was the employment of its chemist, William Johnson, to produce English editions of iatrochemical works, which it was hoped would stem the tide of unauthorised Paracelsian literature.

Between 1640 and 1660 thirty-one Latin medical works were published in England. They were not without significance, and it is interesting to note that it was gradually becoming acceptable to publish a serious Latin medical work in London, rather than on the continent. This development was partly due to the influence of Harvey, whose anatomical and physiological researches were continued by Ent, Glisson, Willis and Wharton. None of these authors published in English, and when Glisson's *De Rachitide* was translated, it was owing to the activities of pirates such as Culpeper. Two progressive academic physicians, Charleton and Highmore, who were not associated with the College of Physicians, had a greater interest in the vernacular. In 1651 Highmore dedicated to Robert Boyle his *History of Generation,* a small book which explained embryology in terms of Democritean atomism. More substantial medical works by Highmore were published in Latin. Walter Charleton, physician to Charles I, became a temporary advocate of van Helmont, translating two of his works into English. Charleton also composed a not unimportant physiological textbook, *Oeconomia animalis* (1659), which appeared concurrently in a slightly abbreviated English form.[76] Such vernacular medical writings from academic physicians were somewhat unorthodox and philosophical in bias; they were composed for the benefit of a wider and possibly non-medical audience. In general the research enterprise of academic physicians continued in the tradition of the Renaissance anatomists and William Harvey. The

75. *A Treatise of the Rickets* (London, 1651), 2 issues.
76. *Natural History of Nutrition, Life and Voluntary Motion* (London, 1659).

exploitation of Harvey's techniques and discoveries made this period the golden age of English anatomy and physiology. Notwithstanding the ultimate scientific importance of this work, it was not addressed to immediate social problems, and the physiologists themselves were not involved with either the religious or the social dimension of puritanism. The reform of general medicine became the concern of an entirely different group of laymen and physicians, who were predominantly outside the traditional medical organisations, and not concerned with current developments in anatomy and physiology. Their outlook became increasingly identifiable with the medical theories of Paracelsus and his followers: they were also more closely in tune with the puritan social reform movement.

(v) The Chemical Evangelists

Harvey's discoveries led to no immediate reaction against Galenic medicine among his disciples. New anatomical discoveries and physiological ideas were absorbed into the traditional mechanism of medical practice. Galenic texts and tenets were retained as the requirement for admission into the College of Physicians under its revised statutes of 1647.[77] This training was a natural continuation of classical education, and it made conspicuously few concessions to modern developments. One apparent departure from tradition was the incorporation of chemically prepared medicines into the London *Pharmacopoeia.* This assimilation was assisted by a small number of cosmopolitan physicians who were responsive to Paracelsian ideas. But it is highly doubtful whether this movement was sufficiently extensive for it to be claimed that a 'Paracelsian compromise' within the medical profession had been achieved by 1640.[78] In the decades before 1640, Paracelsianism had attracted only isolated English adherents; these came mainly from the lower echelons of the medical profession, but Paracelsus was also supported by two notable physicians, Theodore de Mayerne and Thomas Mouffet.[79] In addition Robert Fludd absorbed Paracelsian doctrines into a wider hermetic framework. By contrast with Germany and France there were published in England no important literary expositions, or popular handbooks of Paracelsian medicine and chemistry. It is also noticeable that there were no translations of the prolific and popular continental Paracelsian authors. Indeed the only Paracelsus item available in English before 1650 was a single supposititious work, translated by John Hester in 1587.

77. Clark (50), i, pp.410–11.
78. The 'compromise' view is defended by A. G. Debus in his excellent survey of the influence of Paracelsus before 1640, *The English Paracelsians* (71).
79. Manfred E. Welti, 'Englisch-baslersche Beziehungen zur Zeit der Renaissance in der Medizin', *Gesnerus,* 1963, *20*: 105–30.

Even chemical therapy, often taken as the hallmark of Paracelsianism, owed much of its success to the ancient distillation tradition, which was revived by and had widespread appeal among non-Paracelsians in the sixteenth century. Indeed there was nothing in Galenic medicine to restrict the use of chemically prepared products, or of drugs introduced from the New World. Galenic physicians applied these remedies without disturbing their belief in humoral pathology. Chemical therapy was accordingly gradually assimilated from various sources, without any sense of this implying any degree of affiliation with Paracelsus.

Thus evidence from various directions, including the painstaking investigations of Debus, suggests that Paracelsian medical theory and natural philosophy had made no particular headway before the Puritan Revolution. Certainly nothing resembling a conscious and organised compromise between Galenic and Paracelsian medicine had been attained.

This situation changed dramatically after 1640. Paracelsian medicine was transformed from a dormant force into a coherent social movement, which claimed a substantial share in the vernacular medical literature. The influence of this movement was sufficient to threaten established medical authorities and cause alarm in the universities. The keynote of the movement was the assertion of an *incompatibility* between Paracelsian and Galenic medicine. Any compromise claimed by the Galenists was denounced as a fraudulent device aimed at stemming the Paracelsian tide, or as uncomprehending misappropriation of the fruits of scientific medicine. It was asserted that chemical therapy could only be exploited effectively within the context of Paracelsian medical theory, which in turn required reference to the whole system of Paracelsian natural philosophy. This would involve the complete abandonment of traditional medical theory and practice, and a corresponding transformation of intellectual values.[80]

The sudden surge of Paracelsian medicine and philosophy was intimately related to the social and religious trends of the Puritan Revolution.[81] By 1640 an influential audience existed which was intrinsically suspicious of classical authorities, and receptive to new approaches to social institutions and to different ideas about man's role in nature. It was realised that the established church and traditional medicine had not in their centuries of dominance succeeded in ministering to man's spiritual and physical needs. In the time of 'generall labour of reformation', a medical reformation consistent with the contemporary religious reformation was demanded by puritan medical writers. It was argued that medicine was second only to religious experience in 'restoring of the defects of decaying Nature'.[82]

In theology and law the ground was already well prepared; there

80. Starkey, *Helmonts Vindication* (268), pp.244–5; Biggs, *Mataeotechnia medicinae* (25), p.14.

81. Rattansi (232), pp.26–8.

82. Biggs (25), p.16; Starkey (268), p.4.

had been widespread objection to scholasticism, classical languages and the dominant authorities. Medical men in their turn were as we have seen accused of maintaining their lore in the language of the Roman church, and of obstructing translation into the vernacular. If they acquiesced to translation, their Greek authors were attacked as heathens. Medical education seemed to share the defects of the arts curriculum, engendering 'many fruitless wrangling disputes in which Scholars are chained up, that tend to nothing but strife, and rendering men factious, morose, and troublesome in the Commonwealth'.[83]

These opinions were trenchantly expressed by Bacon before the Puritan Revolution, but he was less confident about alternatives to traditional medicine. As in the case of astronomy, he was content with general maxims on the importance of accumulating data, in this instance about disease and human anatomy. Ever anxious to prevent a premature acceptance of Copernicus or Gilbert, he was also deeply suspicious about Paracelsus. Only the empirical aspects of Paracelsian medicine appealed to him.

By 1650 these doubts were resolved. Paracelsian medicine was judged to have proved its superiority. The appeal of Paracelsus to the religious reformers was greatly assisted by the trends in the Paracelsian movement during the first half of the century. The genuine medical and philosophical works of Paracelsus remained a deep mystery; many defied translation, and they lacked in direct appeal to all but the most erudite readers. But such was the compelling lure of his ideas that he attracted swarms of continental adherents, many of whom were devout protestants. Among them were effective codifiers of Paracelsian natural philosophy, chemistry and medicine.

The Dane, Petrus Severinus, produced an influential exposition of Paracelsian medicine which was admired by Bacon.[84] A different approach was adopted by the popularisers who composed manuals of chemistry, or collections of chemical remedies, together with abbreviated introductions to Paracelsian medical theory and natural philosophy. The best examples of this genre were such frequently reissued handbooks as Oswald Croll's *Basilica chymica* (1609) and Jean Beguin's *Tyrocinium Chymicum* (1613). Such works stimulated a fresh enthusiasm for practical chemistry which was increasingly directed to preparing Paracelsian specific or universal remedies. Fresh impetus was given to this movement during the Puritan Revolution by Johann Rudolph Glauber, whose writings had a strong practical bias, enabling chemists to undertake more sophisticated operations and investigate a wider range of problems in applied chemistry.[85]

A contrasting, but equally fertile trend in Paracelsian thought was that of the pansophic exploitation of his ideas by such authors as

83. William Sprigg, *A Modest Plea* (267), p.58.
84. Bacon *Works*, i, p.564; iii, p.533.
85. For Glauber, see below, pp.386–8.

Valentin Weigel, Robert Fludd, Comenius and Jacob Boehme. Their writings were only indirectly concerned with medicine, but they were highly effective in exposing the harmonic relationship between biblical doctrines and Paracelsian natural philosophy and medicine. These authors led the more spiritually inclined protestants to regard Paracelsus and his followers as sanctified interpreters of nature and medicine. As a reaction, critics of this religious position sought to deny the special wisdom of Paracelsus.[86] Hence the spirit of Paracelsus became drawn into the centre of theological debate during the Republic, achieving prominence for his ideas, at the cost of inspiring highly partisan reactions.

The final spur to the adoption of Paracelsian ideas within the English medical community was provided by the writings of Joan Baptista van Helmont, whose reticence as an author caused a considerable delay in the publication of his works.[87] Ultimately this proved of advantage to the puritan reformers. Unlike the scattered and rare first editions of Paracelsus, Franciscus Mercurius van Helmont presented the public with a convenient collected posthumous edition of his father's rich and varied essays. This work, *Ortus medicinae* (1648), made no claims to impartiality; it delivered sweeping indictments of Galenic medicine and humoral pathology, and included van Helmont's ingenious clinical observations and medical theories. Van Helmont appealed immediately to a wide audience. A complete English translation of the *Ortus medicinae* was produced by John Chandler in 1662.[88]

Van Helmont's influence was by then firmly established. During the Republic his reputation rapidly increased, soon eclipsing that of Paracelsus himself; the 'Helmontian' physicians became the most articulate and active opponents of Galenic medicine. While van Helmont had carefully distinguished some of his major theories from those of Paracelsus, his English adherents adopted an amalgam of opinions, the term 'Helmontian' as then applied occasionally indicating an author who derived his ideas primarily from Paracelsus.

The appeal of van Helmont is indicated by comments made by correspondents from the low countries. Medical students who followed the common practice of studying in the medical school at Leyden or at other Dutch universities were rapidly introduced to his works. Even before the publication of the *Ortus medicinae,* Dury's brother-in-law

86. Margaret Lewis Bailey (15), pp.49–51, 79–90. Rattansi (232), pp.28–32.

87. Major sources on van Helmont are Walter Pagel, 'Religious and Philosophical Aspects of van Helmont's Science and Medicine', *Bull. Hist. Med.*, Supplement 2 (Baltimore, 1944); *idem*, 'J. B. van Helmont seine Lehre und seine Stellung in der heutigen Wissenschaftsgeschichte', Appendix to Christian Knorr von Rosenroth, *Aufgang der Artzney-Kunst* (Reprint, Munich, 1971); Partington (205), ii, pp.209–43.

88. *Oriatrike Or Physick Refined* (London, 1662); reissued 1664. The translator John Chandler is almost unknown, apart from his work on this translation. He matriculated at Magdalen Hall Oxford, in 1641 (Foster (102), i, p.260). There was a quaker author of the same name active around 1660.

Henry Appelius, an acquaintance both of Franciscus Mercurius van Helmont and of Glauber, advised that 'none will repent his cost, time & labour bestowed' on the works of van Helmont. He applauded this author as being the ally in medicine of the protestant movement for intellectual reform:

> 'Joh. Baptista van Helmont who lately dyed at Brussell, having been an ancient and expert Physician hath sett forth 4 treatises in 8°; de Lithiasi. 2. de febribus. 3. de IV humoribus; 4. de Peste: wherein he hath many paradoxes, corresponding that kind of Philosophy which Verulamius, Comenius, Cozak and others require: to take notice of the book: and labour that whether his other writings may come to light; which will worke more upon the Papists, then many bookes of learned Divines.'[89]

In 1647 Appelius was able to report that the *Ortus medicinae* was half printed. Once the work was published van Helmont's adherents reacted as if he was a spiritual leader like Jacob Boehme. When George Starkey arrived from New England in 1650 he was immediately greeted by Hartlib as a 'pure Helmontian'. This characterisation was encouraged by Starkey's writings. In autobiographical references he referred to van Helmont as 'Paracelsus's Great Interpreter', from whom 'I have reaped more real Benefit . . . then from any that I have read'.[90] In a dedication to Robert Boyle he declared: 'Helmont in particular, (to both Your Honour and myself a deserved Favourite) whom I formerly made my Chimical Evangelist, but do now believe, not convinced by his Arguments and Reasons, but by Experimental Confirmation, and Practical Ocular Demonstration.'[91] Starkey expressed a common attitude among the Helmontians. In terms of affected piety, he argued that though Galenic medicine was the source for its adherents of financial reward, it was intellectually debilitating, as well as ineffective in practice. After searching through the major Renaissance medical authorities for assistance, he had adopted van Helmont as the only reliable guide to scientific medicine.[92]

Glauber, who was at the height of his literary productivity during the 1650s, was almost as popular as van Helmont. The day-to-day progress of his *Furni Novi Philosophici* was reported by correspondents

89. Letter from Appelius to Hartlib, 5 February 1645, HP XLV 1. Joachim Polemann similarly asserted 'that the botomlesse mercy of God hath set up this Jacob Boehme and also this our Philosopher Helmont, as two bright torches for this present age', *Novum lumen medicum* (222), p.116.

90. *Pyrotechny Asserted,* 1658 (269), p.78.

91. *Ibid.,* p.iii.

92. Van Helmont also appealed to various medical thinkers who were antagonistic to puritanism. George Thomson was converted to van Helmont while studying at Leyden. He believed that van Helmont was 'ordained in these last times by especial providence of God, for the comfort and relief of distressed Man', *Galeno-pale* (London, 1665), p.4.

from the low countries. This work was expected to provide instruction in a wide range of chemical processes, not the least of which were those involved in the preparation of chemical remedies.

As Starkey defined it: 'Chymistry is the Art of preparing Simples, Animal, Vegetal, and Mineral, so as their crasis or vertue being sequestred from its superfluities, and its virulency overcome, its crudities digested, it may be an apt medicine to perform what God and nature hath granted to it.'[93] Starkey was probably not far wrong in representing van Helmont as Boyle's favourite author. At an early stage in his scientific career, Boyle was intimately involved with a group which displayed the greatest enthusiasm for the newly-published works of van Helmont and Glauber. The combination of religious and scientific elements in the writings of these two experimental philosophers and intellectual reformers was most attractive to Boyle. Their tenets appealed to his deep religious sensibilities and contributed to the dynamic motivation evident at the outset of his career as a natural philosopher. His closest colleague, Benjamin Worsley, shared this point of view and the approach to medicine and practical chemistry of their Invisible College was essentially that of the evangelical chemists. The influence of this early experience was never completely counteracted, even by later affiliation with the 'mechanical philosophy'.

Interest in Glauber's distillation methods, van Helmont's medical theories, and the Paracelsian pharmacopoeia soon achieved a literary manifestation. Culpeper and his translator associates took very little part in this movement; most of their translations were of more orthodox works. Provision of standard works in the vernacular was the main aim of their 'Model of Physic'. Nevertheless, Culpeper's introductions and astrological writings reveal much common ground with Paracelsus, particularly in the use of the macrocosm-microcosm analogy. But apart from generally approving of chemical therapy, Culpeper exhibited little direct interest in the new medicine.

The first major promulgation of Helmontian medicine was issued by the ardent royalist and Anglican Walter Charleton. His translations of two works by van Helmont (the only direct translations before 1662), were furnished with prefaces extolling van Helmont in characteristic quasi-religious terms.[94] Charleton was very much the intellectual barometer of the age, and his numerous works are a valuable index to contemporary fashions. In this case Charleton is almost certainly reflecting a curiosity about van Helmont which was affecting all sections of the medical community. In 1650 it may not have been apparent that Helmontianism would develop strong bonds with separatist and anti-monopolistic factions. Immediately this association became apparent Charleton recanted his former allegiance to van Helmont, composing

93. Starkey, *Helmonts Vindication* (268), pp.109–10.

94. Walter Charleton, *Deliramenti Catarrhi* (London, 1650); *idem, A Ternary of Paradoxes* (London, 1650); *idem, Spiritus Gorgonicus* (Leyden, 1650).

treatises in the Cartesian style in 1652 and in the Gassendian in 1654.[95] No further translations of van Helmont appeared during the Republic, although John Chandler would have been working on his edition of the complete works, which appeared in 1662. Van Helmont's disciples, the 'Philosophers by Fire', relied primarily on popular expositions to publicise his ideas. By contrast numerous works by Paracelsus and Paracelsian authors were issued as translations, produced by such little-known figures as John French, Henry Pinnel, John Harding and William Dugard. This group will be found to have had extremely strong parliamentary and puritan associations.

John French was from Broughton, near Banbury; he was a protégé of Lord Saye and Sele of Broughton Castle, who persuaded him to enter the parliamentary army of Fairfax as a physician. French had previously studied at New Inn Hall Oxford, graduating BA in 1637 (on the same day as Marchamont Nedham), and as MA in 1640.[96] After the cessation of military hostilities French remained in the state's service as physician to the Savoy Hospital. In 1650 he issued a collection of writings by Sendigovius and Paracelsus, together with a brief 'Chemical Dictionary' derived from Dorn.[97] This was the first of a series of compilations and translations produced by French; he also wrote an original work on the virtues of spa waters. The majority of his works were concerned with distillation. *The Art of Distillation* (1651) was dedicated to his friend Tobias Garbrand, the puritan physician and Principal of Gloucester Hall Oxford, and was derived from sixteenth-century works, with sections from Glauber.[98] In the same year he issued a full translation of the first complete edition of Glauber's *Furni Novi Philosophici*.[99] The promptness of this translation suggests that French had been working on this subject for some time, using the earlier forms of Glauber's work. He may well have taken over a translation originated by the Hartlib circle: in letters dating from 1647, Sir Cheney Culpeper describes himself as correcting a badly translated version of the *Furni*.[100] From Culpeper's comments it is apparent that this work was nearing completion, but no mention was ever made of the outcome. French was well acquainted with the Hartlib circle; hence he may have taken over the commission. French also issued a translation of Cornelius Agrippa's famous *De Philosophia Occulta,* which he dedicated to Hartlib's friend Robert Child, who was at that time engaged in completing Boate's Natural History of Ireland.[101]

95. Rattansi (232), p.30; N. R. Gelbart, 'The Intellectual Development of Walter Charleton', *Ambix,* 1971, *18*: 149–68; L. G. Sharp, 'Walter Charleton's Early Life 1620–1659', *Annals of Science,* 1973, *30*: 311–40.

96. Wood *Athenae,* iii, pp.436–7; *DNB.*

97. *A New Light of Alchymie* (108); Sudhoff (274), No. 365.

98. Later editions, 1653, 1664, 1667. Garbrand and French were granted MDs at Oxford on 14 April 1648: Wood *Fasti,* ii, p.115.

99. *A Description of New Philosophical Furnaces,* 1651 (117).

100. HP xiii; see below, p.387.

101. *Three Books of Occult Philosophy* (London, 1657).

A second important puritan translator was the former army chaplain Henry Pinnel. Pinnel was a graduate of St. Mary Hall Oxford. After leaving the army he became a minister at Brinkworth in Wiltshire, which was the parish in which his family lived. His first excursion into medicine was *Five Treatises of the Philosophers Stone* (1652), derived from various alchemical authors, mainly pre-Paracelsus. More important was *Philosophy Reformed & Improved in Four Profound Tractates* (1657), a translation mainly composed of the lengthy preface to Croll's *Basilica chymica* and the shorter work by Paracelsus, *Philosophia ad Athenienses;* numerous marginal annotations were added by Pinnel.[102] Although largely overlooked by modern commentators, the Croll preface provides one of the most succinct and effective introductions to Paracelsian natural philosophy and medicine. Owing to Pinnel therefore, the English reader had access to a reasonably comprehensible account of the rational basis for the various practical Paracelsian treatises published during this decade. The Croll preface also gave valuable clues to the interpretation of the numerous hermetic works which were published at this time.

Advocates of spiritual religion like Pinnel were increasingly attracted to the writings of Jacob Boehme. His works were carefully translated and published as substantial volumes, which were better printed and designed than most of the medical literature. Humphrey Blunden took on the publishing side of this enterprise, while the introductions and translations were begun by John Elliston and continued after his death in 1652 by a younger relative, John Sparrow. Sparrow was in the parliamentary civil service and a lawyer at the Inner Temple; he played an active part in the movement for law reform.[103] Works such as *De Signatura Rerum* (1651), *Of Christs Testament* (1652), and *Mysterium Magnum* (1654), indicated the pervasive influence of Paracelsian natural philosophy and medicine on the theosophy of Boehme. The introductions reinforced this impression and underlined the analogy between Paracelsian medicine and spiritual religion; indeed the editors asserted that 'Chimick Philosophers' would be best equipped to understand Boehme.

The writings of the spiritual reformers served to generate greater interest in the works of Paracelsus. *Paracelsus His Dispensatory* (1654) was a large collection of medical writings by Paracelsus issued and possibly translated by the versatile puritan stationer William Dugard, who was also involved in publishing works by Hartlib and Comenius.[104]

102. Sudhoff (274), No. 378. Foster (102), iii, p.1167.

103. For Elliston and Sparrow, see *DNB; Notes & Queries* 1931, *167*: 312; Veall (296), p.81; *Essex Review,* 1939, *48*: 214–17. For Boehme's influence see S. Hutin, *Les Disciples Anglais de Jacob Boehme* (Paris, 1960).

104. Sudhoff (274), No. 376. Dugard was a schoolmaster who became Headmaster of the Merchant Taylors' School. In 1648 he began publishing and produced mainly educational, medical, scientific and grammatical works. Dugard was extremely active in politics: see *DNB*; Rostenberg (251), i, pp.130–59.

An even more active puritan translator of Paracelsus was the Presbyterian minister, John Harding, who has previously escaped identification since he signed his works 'J.H.Oxon'. Harding, rector of Brinkworth in Wiltshire since 1642, must have known Henry Pinnel as a minister there; Pinnel's major work *Philosophy Reformed & Improved* was signed at Brinkworth in 1656.[105] In earlier writings Pinnel had signed himself 'H.P.', or 'H.P.Oxford'. Hence, his works also have often escaped identification.

Harding issued three collections of Paracelsian writings. The first contained 'Aurora' and 'The Treasure of Treasures' by Paracelsus, and a translation of Ambrosius Siebermacher's *Wasserstein der Weisen* (1619).[106] The second and more important collection was based on Paracelsus's 'Archidoxes', with many smaller treatises.[107] Harding's translations were dependent mainly on Huser's Latin edition, but with material from later Latin and perhaps even German sources. His final translation was of Basil Valentine, the *Triumphant Chariot of Antimony* (Oxford, 1660).[108] Then as 'a most violent presbyterian' he was ejected from his living, retiring to Northampton for a short time, before his death in 1665. This interrupted the plans announced in the *Archidoxis,* of publishing a complete translation of Paracelsus's *Paramirum*. However Harding's work is sufficiently extensive to be considered as the first serious attempt to provide an English edition of Paracelsus. The project was later revived by Richard Russell, but he met with even less success than Harding.[109]

While most of the Paracelsian works were direct translations, there were some more original writings. Biggs and Webster incorporated Paracelsian ideas into their reform programmes. Hartlib's *Chymical, Medicinal & Chyrurgical Addresses* (1655) was a miscellaneous collection of alchemical writings, which contained Boyle's first published essay. James Thompson produced a clumsy dialogue generally favourable to van Helmont,[110] while George Starkey's books contained detailed, if badly-organised statements of Helmontian chemistry.

With Starkey the invective against Galen and the professional organi-

105. Most authors follow Sudhoff in identifying J.H. as John Hester. However, the same translator was responsible for *The Triumphant Chariot of Antimony* (Oxford, 1660) and the Bodleian Library copy of this work is inscribed 'Ex dono interpretis D.Jo: Harding'. See Madan (184), No. 2534. Harding was the son of the President of Magdalen College Oxford. He graduated at Magdalen College and was a Fellow before entering the church: *Calamy Revised,* p.247.

106. *Paracelsus His Aurora,* 1659 (131); Sudhoff (274), No. 389.

107. *Paracelsus His Archidoxis,* 1660 (132); later editions 1661, 1663. Sudhoff (274), Nos. 392, 393, 395.

108. Madan (184), No. 2534; later edition 1661.

109. In 1686 in his preface to *The Works of Geber* Richard Russell announced that he had largely completed the translation of Paracelsus's works. This was probably not the Richard Russell of Durham College; see Appendix II, below.

110. *Helmont Disguised: or the Vulgar Errors of Empericall and unskilfull practisers of Physick confuted* (London, 1657).

sations reached a climax.[111] By this stage, Paracelsian and hermetic writings had come to occupy a prominent place in the medical literature; half the medical works published in 1657 fell into the Paracelsian category. Not all of this literature emanated from puritan sources. Just as Neoplatonism had traditionally appealed to a broad religious spectrum, so those attracted to the hermetic philosophy during the Puritan Revolution included such Anglican authors as Elias Ashmole, Sir Thomas Browne, and Henry and Thomas Vaughan. The Anglican Hermeticists felt no immediate sympathy for the political and social ideas of the puritan Paracelsians. They also tended to concentrate on a less practical and more esoteric range of hermetic writings. However their subscription to unorthodox philosophical systems brought them into conflict with established medical opinion, which created some common ground with the puritan writers. Thus Henry Vaughan expressed strong disapproval of Galen and applauded the experimental methods of the Hermeticists.[112] The royalist physician George Thomson held similar views and he developed an acute antipathy to the College of Physicians. After the restoration he took over Starkey's role as the most active Helmontian pamphleteer.[113]

(vi) Physick and Divinity

Paracelsus was popular during the Puritan Revolution for various reasons. He appeared to offer a viable substitute for the 'heathen' Galen, and his ideas were compatible with the philosophical and theological outlook of the Puritans. The Paracelsian literature published in England was sufficiently extensive to provide a coherent body of medical doctrine which could be used to counteract Galenism. Paracelsianism also developed an increasingly experimental bias; hence the Paracelsians could claim to represent the medical dimension of the experimental philosophy of Bacon. Most important of all the Paracelsian writings were framed in religious terms, and the theological viewpoint they expressed was thoroughly congenial to a puritan audience. There was complete harmony between the medical texts edited by Henry Pinnel, his own specifically theological works, and the writings of such puritan mystics as John Saltmarsh and Francis Rous. A similar unity existed between the religious and medical ideas expressed in Webster's *Academiarum Examen*. These authors recognised that a return to the state of grace was a pre-condition of man's return to the state of nature. They took up the call for the minister to imitate Christ by paying attention to both bodily and spiritual needs; their aim being that 'Nature,

111. *Natures Explication and Helmonts Vindication,* 1657 (268); *Pyrotechny Asserted,* 1658 (269).

112. *Hermetical Physick: or, the right way to preserve and restore health* (London, 1655). From Heinrich Noll.

113. For a sketch of Thomson's career, see Webster (322).

grace, physick and Divinity, so returning to their first unity'.[114] Webster was both minister and physician and this combination of duties would have been regarded as an ideal expression of puritan virtue: he would be ensuring that the restoration of 'inward' or 'spiritual' man would be accompanied by a physical renewal of his 'outward' body.

Medicine was accordingly the area of scientific activity which would most directly show the benefit of a return to grace; hence its immediate appeal to those spiritual reformers who often took less interest in other aspects of experimental science.

As far as the puritan medical reformers were concerned, in spiritual and material things man had not succeeded in progressing beyond superficialities. Despite successive attempts at reformation, society remained in bondage to a cultural heritage which had placed insurmountable obstacles between man and the rich treasury of the spiritual and material world. The first essential was for an experience going beyond 'the shell and cover of things' to achieve an 'Inward, Spiritual' revelation or '*inward Experience,* Examination or Experimenting of Spiritual things'.[115]

This doctrine of salvation had the greatest implications for Paracelsian and Helmontian medicine as presented to the English reader during the Puritan Revolution. Pinnel described Paracelsianism as a 'Theological Phylosophy wherefore the New Birth is first to be sought for, and then all other Naturall things will be added without much labour'.[116] Although grace was the free gift of God within reach of all men, its benefits would be wasted on the unworthy. All men accordingly had an obligation to labour unceasingly to imitate the life of the Saviour, and to remain always on guard against intellectual degeneration and corruption.

Paracelsus was presented as an exemplary advocate of these standards. He castigated decadent scholastic medicine, sacrificing fortune for a wandering existence in search of true knowledge; he gathered his information from whatever source seemed promising; he communicated both with humanist scholars and the illiterate peasantry. His biography served as a model for imitation by generations of Paracelsians, the image being embellished and modified according to the needs of the situation. Croll for instance described his own *Basilica chymica* as the result of nearly twenty years of arduous labour; peregrinations throughout Europe had been undertaken at great expense, as the author indefatigably collected evidence from all reliable sources. Private gain had been scorned, and the sick poor were treated without charge.[117] Such was

114. Pinnel, *Philosophy Reformed* (216), prefatory poem.

115. Boehme, *Mysterium Magnum* (London, 1654), preface by John Sparrow, sig. A5r; Boehme, *Of Christs Testament* (London, 1652), preface by Sparrow, sig.A4v.

116. Pinnel (216), p.132.

117. *Ibid.*, pp.12–13. For Croll see R. J. W. Evans, *Rudolf II and His World* (Oxford 1973), p.142 and *passim; DSB,* iii, pp.472–3.

the life of a Paracelsian apostle. Physicians were admonished to lead ascetic lives displaying the qualities of penitent industry: 'in the sweat of our browes, that . . . by laying the Cross upon us which we should bear with patience, it might stir up our industry in this LAND of LABOUR to attain the fruits of Terrene and Coelestiall Wisdome'.[118] But industry and faithful vocational service were not sufficient. It was also necessary to evolve an objective methodology which would arrive at knowledge as sound as that given by inward revelation. In the search for suitable criteria a direct analogy was detected between the 'experience' of personal revelation and the practical experience of the manual arts:

> 'All the Arts and Trades in the world are *Mysteries,* and are not truly knowne, but by those that have had *Experience* in them; we are able to learne them *all* by Experience, but without that, wee know *nothing* of them, more than the very beast.'[119]

Puritan authors followed Paracelsus in regarding the sound empirical practices of the manual arts as an actual equivalent to spiritual 'experience' or 'experiment'. Accordingly they saw a definite relationship between experimental science and religious experience. By following the way of experience, an efficient and productive vocational life could be combined with intense spiritual understanding. Croll's spagyric mysteries had been attained by 'manuali experientia', 'in manualis operationis', or 'laboribus manum & Practica operatrice'.[120] The operations of 'Collier-like Physicians', although their labours would be despised by the intellectuals such as the Galenists who daily 'hammered out' ancient knowledge, were ordained to give rise to a more successful system of medicine. Increasingly the alchemists identified themselves with the collier (*carboniana*), searching relentlessly to uncover treasures in the mine of nature. The favourite Helmontian slogan, *philosophia per ignem,* suggests a similar association of ideas.[121]

Chemistry offered an ideal illustration of the potentialities of this method. Natural products were ordained by God for man's use, but their properties would not be revealed directly, since Adam's transgression had sacrificed our rights to direct experience of nature's purity. Medicines were 'imprisoned', and they could only be isolated by the 'artificial Anatomy of Chymists'; their labour would show that God had created an inexhaustible supply of specific remedies, each country furnishing sufficient for its own requirements.[122] The Paracelsians drew

118. Pinnel (216), p.96; see also p.140, 'without paines-taking none is fit to injoy that Art'.

119. Boehme, *Of Christs Testament* (London, 1652), preface by Sparrow, sig. B2v–3r.

120. Croll, *Basilica chymica* (Cologne, 1631), pp.4, 9, 134.

121. Biggs, *Mataeotechnia medicinae* (25), p.14; Pinnel (216), pp.19–20; French, *A New Light* (108), pp.92–3.

122. Pinnel (216), p.76; Starkey, *Helmonts Vindication* (268), sig.a7r, pp.43–4.

a comparison between fruits and medicines: just as the seminal and most nutritious part of the fruit lay in the middle, surrounded by husks of protective material, so the quintessence or active medicinal principle was surrounded by 'the Rinds, and Membranes, the Covers, Shells, Husks, and dreggs'.[123] Separation performed by such processes as distillation isolated the spiritual principle or *astrum* of a species from its material substratum, leaving behind the dregs or *caput mortuam*. This theory was regarded as an application of the religious view that the 'Body is but the Shell or Vessel of the Spirit'.[124]

The obvious and traditional subjects for chemical preparation were organic products, such as plants, which had been the subject of a considerable distillation literature in the sixteenth century. An obvious improvement had taken place in techniques of preparing strong wines, cordials and medicines. More varied methods were required for the preparation of reasonably pure samples of inorganic substances. The chemists of the seventeenth century were very much concerned with the improvement of techniques in inorganic chemistry. From the time of Paracelsus, inorganic preparations were regarded with ever increasing favour as a complement to the organic components of the pharmacopoeia. Certain inorganic substances were thought to have extremely active medical qualities. Even such poisonous substances as the compounds of arsenic or mercury were investigated, since it was believed that their virulent properties could be neutralised in order to expose medicinal virtues.[125] Minerals 'rightly prepared doe much excell all vegetables in effecting cures'.[126] All species had a part in a single world-soul by virtue of their common origin. Since at the Creation minerals had been derived from elements which were also the antecedents of the substances in man's body, they could be expected to have some basic function in his life. Each chemist had his favourite element; gold had a universal appeal; antimony enjoyed a long period of popularity. By the mid-seventeenth century, the compounds of such cheap and readily accessible substances as copper and iron were widely prepared for medicinal use. Although this enterprise yielded medical results of only limited value, it provided valuable experience in practical chemistry.[127] Gold, precious stones, or indeed any substances with celestial associations were thought to have particularly great medical potentialities. Hence there was considerable interest in *aurum potabile;* it was also believed

123. Pinnel (216), p.98.

124. Helmont, *Oriatrike* (London, 1662), preface by Chandler, sig.a2r.

125. For mercury compounds, see Starkey, *Helmonts Vindication* (268), pp.100–3; Boyle, *Usefulnesse* (32), Part II, pp.177–8.

126. Pinnel (216), p.100; also, 'God hath written with his own sacred finger in sublunary things, but especially in perfect Metalls': p.23.

127. Starkey and Polemann were advocates of copper; Boyle, *Usefulnesse* (32), Part II, pp.154–6, 330–8. For the discussions about *ens veneris,* see R. S. Wilkinson, 'George Starkey, Physician and Alchemist', *Ambix,* 1963, *11*: 121–52; pp.129–33.

that investigation would ultimately uncover a universal medicine. This achievement was indeed claimed by many chemists.

While elixirs or panaceas were objects of popular curiosity, the success of iatrochemistry depended primarily on the production and use of large numbers of 'specifics', compounds which were anticipated to act as an antidote for a single condition or small group of conditions.[128] In explaining the basis for the action of these remedies the Paracelsians sought to undermine Galenic humoral pathology; and they regarded the traditional Galenic therapeutic techniques as ineffective, or positively harmful. Criticism of the humoral theory and of such practices as phlebotomy reached a climax with van Helmont. The Paracelsians believed that humoral pathology had been, 'in the schoole of Paracelsus, and writings of Helmont, where the anatomy of humans hath been most rationally and fully discussed, . . . sufficiently confuted'.[129] The reformers consistently stated that it was necessary to abandon Galenic physiology, pathology and therapy, before the advantages of chemical therapy could be fully enjoyed. Chemicals could not be conceived as ancillaries to bleeding or purging, but as a substitute, their practical application being determined upon a completely different rational basis. The medical reformers introduced extensive polemical sections into their works, which contained attacks on humoral physiology and the Galenic repertoire of blistering, cupping, scarification, cauterising and bleeding. This kind of criticism was certain to elicit a sympathetic response from readers, who could have given cheerful assent to the view that more died by such methods than were killed in war.[130]

The Paracelsian attitude to man and his diseases was unsympathetic not only to Galen, but also to the research bias developed by the anatomists of the Renaissance. Croll asserted : 'It is not the Locall Anatomy of a man and dead corpses, but the Essentiated and Elemental Anatomy of the World and man that discovereth the disease and cure.'[131] Even after the great discoveries of Harvey, this view was not substantially changed. Thomson approved of Harvey's discoveries and himself conducted vivisection experiments, but he did not regard such activity as a significant aid to therapy, which could only be assisted by 'Pyrotechnical Anatomy'.[132]

The views of Paracelsus on human nature, disease and therapy were founded upon complex and obscure cosmological and cosmogonical theories which were rooted in gnostic, hermetic and biblical sources. The three principles of Paracelsus, salt, mercury and sulphur, were only one aspect of a theory of matter which was designed to provide a comprehensive synthesis of scriptural, philosophical, and empirical

128. Starkey (268), sig.a7r.
129. French, *Art of Distillation* (109), sig. *2v.
130. Biggs (25), pp.65–108, 136–8; Hartlib, *Chymical Addresses* (144), pp.159–60; Boyle, *Usefulnesse* (32), Part II, pp.109–14.
131. Pinnel (216), p.43.
132. Thomson, *Galeno-pale* (1665), pp.25–8.

themes. This theory was the basis for a unified representation of man and nature. Man was a microcosm, a 'Deified glass' (*Deifico speculo*), the centre of creation, reflecting the nature of God and the universe and able to direct the outer world for his own benefit. 'Man hath the true and Reall possession of all things and Natures in himselfe, as also the speciall and perfect Image even of the Creator of all things.'[133] Man was therefore the centre of a complex system of correspondences between the terrestrial and celestial worlds: 'In the lesser world Man there is no member or part that doth not answer to some Element, some Planet, some Intelligence or other, and to some measure and number in the Archetype or first pattern.'[134] This line of thought might be expected to have led to the acceptance of astrological determinism in medicine. Astrological medicine was indeed widely in vogue, as is witnessed by the Culpeper writings, which rested on the general macrocosm-microcosm theory.[135] Surprisingly, the astrological element in Paracelsian medicine was not always exploited, partly owing to Paracelsus's anthropocentric outlook, which emphasised the ability of man to influence his environment: 'Whence it is requisite that the starres should follow him, and obey him, and not he the starrs.'[136] Bacon had expressed exactly the same opinion of astrology.

The active relationship between the human body and external elements was determined by the *astrum,* a specific life force impressing formal and vital characteristics upon its material substratum. The physical body was nothing but an 'excrement' of the astra.[137] Such semina or astra, partaking of the nature of the stars, represented a potent creative force. As Creation had unfolded, every species, animate or inanimate, had developed as an actualisation of its characteristic *astrum.* The hierarchy of astra maintained an ordered universe as agents of the general world-soul.[138] This theory had important implications for the Paracelsian attitude to disease. Disease was not caused by an imbalance of humours, but by the semina of disease agents. These alien semina were thought to exist in large numbers, perhaps equalling the number of species of growing things.[139] They afflicted the body, settling at some location, rather in the manner of a parasite; the human astrum then became undermined.

This ontological theory of disease dictated attitudes to therapy. A disease could only be cured by the preparation of an astrum which

133. Pinnel (216), p.48. For the medical theories of Paracelsus, which formed the basis for the synopsis produced by Croll, see Walter Pagel, *Paracelsus* (Basel, 1955); *idem, Das Medizinische Weltbild des Paracelsus* (Wiesbaden, 1962).

134. *Ibid.,* pp.58–9.

135. Culpeper, *Pharmacopoeia Londinensis* (London, 1653), preface, For astrological medicine, see Thomas (281), pp.300, 334–5.

136. French, *A New Light* (108), p.109. For an attack on astrology see Biggs (25), pp.25–6, 40.

137. Pinnel (216), p.67.

138. *Ibid.,* p.34.

139. *Ibid.,* p.44.

would act as an antidote. An analogy was drawn with venom, a specific substance introduced into the body, and causing a condition which animals cured intuitively by taking an appropriate herbal antidote. Particularly after van Helmont an impression existed that a disease was a specific growing entity which had to be removed at its source, rather than the symptoms being treated: 'The root of the disease is eradicated, and as it were cut off with a knife.'[140] It was hoped to isolate 'specifics' which could cure any known disease. The Galenists were accordingly constantly chided for their belief in a class of incurable diseases.[141]

In separating specifics from their organic or mineral bases, and in testing such remedies, the Paracelsians were led to play an active role in experimental chemistry and various branches of medicine. By the time of the Protectorate Paracelsian practitioners had become sufficiently numerous and influential to compete openly with the orthodox physicians.

The rise of Paracelsianism was not merely a matter of the appearance of a new fashion in medicine. The new movement changed the relationship between the physician and the patient. Galenic therapy could only be practised properly by a physician familiar with the complex lore of the humoral theory. Furthermore considerable skill was required in the administration of the painful treatments used by the Galenists. For this expertise substantial fees could be charged. By contrast the methods and treatments of the Paracelsian physicians were relatively cheap and simple. While full acquaintance with Paracelsian natural philosophy and medical theory was a condition not readily achieved, the routine practical procedures were much more straightforward. Accordingly it was possible for the intelligent layman to practise self-help using Paracelsian methods. In addition the cheap and simple Paracelsian remedies appeared to offer a means of relieving the medical problems of the growing population of the poor.

(vii) Public Health

Before the Civil War utopian writers had speculated about the organisation of medicine in an ideal state. In such literature it was common to suggest that the state should sponsor comprehensive medical services. Laboratories in a utopian society would produce new drugs and test those brought from the New World, before releasing them for use by the public. Physicians were characterised as devout public servants, or as 'ministers of nature'. The state was expected to provide adequate institutions for those having special disabilities, such as orphans, the

140. Joachim Polemann, *Novum Lumen Medicum* (Amsterdam, 1659); English edition 1662 (222), pp.186–7.

141. 'A Conference whether or no each several Disease hath a particular and specifical remedy', in Hartlib, *Chymical Addresses* (144), pp.89–99.

sick, the poor or the aged. By an intelligent and charitable approach to all social contingencies, the prince or ruler would be able to preside over a harmonious and grateful community. Such ideals, as expressed by Campanella, Andreae or Plattes, must have appeared ironically inappropriate and irrelevant, as the already inadequate social relief agencies of Stuart England gradually broke down during the Civil War. The armies were never able to set up adequate medical services for themselves; the major part of the population was plunged into distress. These problems were magnified in London, where an ill-fed population was swelled by an unwelcome influx of destitute poor and wounded soldiers.

Many of the utopian planners temporarily set aside their fictional schemes to face these adverse conditions realistically; they analysed the situation rationally and suggested practical solutions to the manifold problems they isolated. Thus social medicine became firmly established as part of the wider programme for poor relief.

John Cook illustrates the traditional approach to this problem, appealing for local acts of charity, and the enforcement or extension of Elizabethan poor law regulations at the parish level. The magistrate could act by controlling the price of grain or restraining the use of grain for malting. The clergy and rich parishioners could assist by directing various small funds to the benefit of the poor. Nevertheless it was recognised that such preventative measures were unlikely to provide sufficient guarantees against ill-health. Medical assistance of some kind was a necessity. In conditions when a poor man might receive only 6d. per day to support a family of seven, little could be expected of physicians, who might charge 10s. for a single visit.[142] Even apothecaries' bills were beyond the means of the poor. Cook declared that these conditions had effectively disqualified the poorer classes from receiving professional medical assistance. Even market towns were frequently without a physician. Hence it had become necessary for the local clergy to take on medical responsibilities. This situation provided the basis for Cook's insistence that the 'Quacks' Charter' of Henry VIII should be respected, allowing all able practitioners to exercise their vocation. Wiliam Trigge, the London practitioner, who had been in conflict with the College of Physicians for twenty years, was a test case. It was alleged in 1648 that he had treated 30,000 patients since 1624; many were treated *gratis,* while others had paid only nominal fees. Cook considered that in view of their social importance in districts never visited by academic physicians, this class of physician should be freed from fine or restriction. In addition Cook recommended that physicians should make up their own prescriptions, which were always to be written in English; the patient would know 'what they prescribe, and what they [the patients] pay for'.[143] Finally, the poor living in areas where no medical assistance was available should be taught enough in the

142. Cook, *Unum Necessarium,* 1648 (57), p.61.
143. *Ibid.,* pp.64–5.

way of medical preparations to make them self-sufficient. These views undoubtedly commanded wide popular support, but they were particularly significant when expressed by Cook, who was appointed Solicitor-General in 1649. Cook probably reflects a disinclination among the legal authorities to adopt a vigorous policy in favour of the London medical monopolies. Thus the 'lastmaker' Trigge and his medical associates, former weavers, pewterers and poor gentry, were left free to practise and advertise their patent remedies in numerous ephemeral pamphlets.

The Revolution also saw the termination of ecclesiastical licensing, which related to midwives in London and to all medical practitioners elsewhere. Before the Civil War the resourceful Peter Chamberlen had attempted to emancipate the midwives from clerical control. Chamberlen was well-equipped to make this move; he possessed a Padua MD, which was incorporated at both Oxford and Cambridge; he was also a Fellow of the College of Physicians. Having obtained these qualifications, he followed his father's vocation by specialising in midwifery. Chamberlen hoped to establish an organisation for training and licensing midwives under his own sponsorship. The scheme caused resentment among the Fellows of the College of Physicians, who persuaded the Bishop of London to reassert his rights over the licensing of midwives. To escape censure Chamberlen adroitly transferred his activities to the low countries, but re-emerged with further schemes for the education and government of midwives in 1647.[144] Both at this time and in later writings Chamberlen exhibited general agreement with the views expressed by Cook. He appears to have employed an apothecary at his house, and he claimed to have provided a free medical and midwifery service for the poor. In 1647, his midwives project could be revived without fear of opposition from the church or the College of Physicians. But the new atmosphere of toleration encouraged Chamberlen to dissipate his energies by producing a whole range of projects, which included various public health measures. His most ambitious scheme sought to employ the poor on a large scale. This publicly financed venture suggested appropriating church property for the settlement of colonies of poor families. In return for their labour, they would be provided with all social facilities, including hospitals.[145]

Chamberlen's project was not as realistic as the various schemes for rehabilitation propounded by the Hartlib circle. However both illustrate the social reformers' concern with public health. As Gerbier declared: 'charity cannot be confined within the walls of hospitals or almshouses, nor under the gowns of a small number of old men or women'.[146]

144. *A voice of Rhama: or, the Crie of Women and Children* (London, 1647). For Chamberlen, see Munk (195), i, pp.194–7; J. H. Aveling, *The Chamberlens* (London, 1882); Clark (50), i, pp.253–4.

145. *The Poore Mans Advocate,* 1649 (44), p.23.

146. Balthazar Gerbier, *A New Years Result in Favour of the Poore* (London, 1652), p.5.

According to this view it was necessary to extend the concept of charity to embrace all aspects of social planning. Thus projects aimed at reversing the economic misfortunes of the poor included the provision of medical care and hospitals. This was a concern of much higher priority with Hartlib and his associates than with the Levellers, whose greatest rhetoric was employed on questions of political and legal rights. Overton's *Appeal from the degenerate representative body* (1647) is exceptional among the Leveller tracts in containing a brief plea for free hospitals.[147]

Robinson's *Certain Proposals* terminated in a very similar manner to Overton's tract, by outlining schemes for the erection of workhouses for training the able-bodied poor, schools for their children, and medical care for the sick and aged. But Robinson's plans were announced in greater detail. On the problem of public health, he proposed:

> 'That physicians and Chyrurgions be appointed in every County throughout the Nation, particularly to every proportionable division of this great Citie of *London,* at the Publick charge, who may be obliged once a day to visit and administer according to their respective Professions, to whomsoever in that Division shall desire it, without any other fee or consideration, but what the State allowes them.
>
> And lastly, that Hospitals be erected, and endowed, in every County and proportionable Division, to which it may be free for all poore people to repaire for taking Physicke, as well to prevent sicknesse before it comes, as when it hath seized on them, at the sole charge and attendance of the Hospitall.'[148]

Thus Robinson believed that the state should set up comprehensive preventative and curative medical services, operated by state-salaried officials. These services would have been completely free for the majority of the population. This ideal not only outstripped the imagination of his contemporaries, but has scarcely approached realisation in the modern welfare state. Robinson's views were very much in sympathy with the social welfare proposals contained in Gerrard Winstanley's *Law of Freedom,* published in the same year as Robinson's tract. Winstanley was however less explicit on the organisation of the medical services for his communes, than on other aspects of social organisation. No doubt he envisaged that ill-health would become a less severe problem in the ideal environment which he hoped to create. He made no reference to a specialist class of physicians; he believed that lectures on medicine, to be given on the sabbath, would ensure that the population was sufficiently well-informed about routine medical matters. They were already expected to maintain a lively interest in scientific questions

147. Brailsford (33), pp.232–3, 534.
148. Robinson, *Certain Proposalls* (247), p.26.

and to report any useful observations relating to medicine or technology to the community.[149]

The social realities of the interregnum were a far cry from the tidy models of social organisation produced by the idealists. The general failure to evolve an efficient mechanism for poor relief was a grievance mentioned in petitions from all parts of the country.[150] The relaxation of medical licensing regulations produced only a minor ameliorating effect, which was offset by the problems created by the disruption of hospital revenues and the drastic increase in the number of wounded requiring treatment. A paradoxical situation was reached in which the London hospitals were treating smaller numbers of patients as the need for their services was increasing. St. Bartholomew's and St. Thomas's did not regain the level of their pre-war turnover of patients until 1650 and 1655 respectively. Similar statistics apply also to the numbers of destitute poor kept by Christ's Hospital and Bridewell.[151] Statements from the hospitals indicate that inadequate revenues were the cause of this deterioration in their services.[152] The gradual return to normal civil life was probably the main factor in the revival of the hospitals, but this was also assisted by legislation. From 1643 onwards, a series of doubtfully effective measures embodied attempts to deflect the revenues from ecclesiastical and delinquents' estates into colleges, schools and hospitals. More important were the ordinances freeing the hospitals from assessment for taxes, and enforcing the full payment of their rents, in view of the 'great numbers of sick, wounded, and other Soldiers . . . constantly kept in the said Hospitals, at very great and extraordinary Charges, especially for their Cure and Dyet'.[153] In order to reduce this burden a direct subsidy of 2s. per day was paid to the hospitals for each wounded soldier in their care. In London the situation was also eased by the creation in 1647 of a Corporation for the Poor. This was a response to pressure exerted jointly by the hospital trustees and the social reformers. The Corporation was primarily intended to support the large number of destitute poor requiring rehabilitation rather than medical treatment. As a result of the measures designed to meet the Civil War crisis, the four great London hospitals were brought into closer administrative relationship with local and national authorities, but otherwise there was little interference with their routines. As indicated below, this contrasts with the direct manner in which even the medical routines of the 'nationalised' London hospitals were supervised.

From the examples cited in Chapter II, it is apparent that the mili-

149. Winstanley, *Law of Freedom* (336), pp.56–7.

150. M. James (158), pp.241–54.

151. Lists of 'Costs & Charges' of the four London hospitals, derived from the Thomason tracts, tabulated in James (158), pp.399, 405.

152. *Ibid.*, pp.247–8.

153. Firth & Rait, i, pp.570–1, 16 Nov. 1644. See also i, pp.984, 1077; ii, pp.57, 318, etc. James (158), pp.295–302.

tary medical services provided attractive career opportunities for ambitious young intellectuals. Medical service was lucrative for the conscientious practitioner, and it offered the possibility of association with powerful patrons. Even lesser practitioners could expect an honorary MD and a minor public office.[154] With respect to the armed forces, the parliamentary attitude to the medical profession was in keeping with its general anti-monopolistic policy. The various professional associations were consulted where appropriate, but none was allowed to exercise a monopoly. The College of Physicians stood largely aloof from the war and was rarely consulted on medical questions, although such members as Goddard and Bate offered their services to the army. The Barber-Surgeons continued to supply surgeons for the navy, but physicians and apothecaries were also involved in naval service. The physician Daniel Whistler had outstanding success in organising the provincial naval medical corps.[155] An increasing part was played in military medicine by physicians who had only the remotest connection with the professional organisations. Hence they often remain extremely shadowy figures from a biographical point of view. The Irish army was a particularly attractive field for physicians. Of the better-known physicians, Arnold and Gerard Boate, Jonathan Goddard, William Petty and Benjamin Worsley, obtained posts in the Irish army at various times. Such minor physicians and surgeons as John Waterhouse and Thomas Trapham were rewarded with Oxford MDs. Interest in medical reform and iatrochemistry had spread to such chaplains as Webster and Pinnel, who have already been mentioned in the contexts of Paracelsian translation and educational reform. It is highly likely that such chaplains took on medical responsibilities within their regiments.

One of the most practical and constructive proposals for medical reform was put forward in William Petty's first publication *The Advice of W.P. to Mr. Samuel Hartlib* (1648). Petty had obtained his medical education in Holland; after a brief spell as Anatomy Reader at Oxford, he followed Goddard as Physician-General to the army in Ireland. Petty probably aimed at designing an institution to spearhead medical reform, a plan which would have completed other institutional schemes produced by his friends in the Hartlib circle. He was also probably inspired by the first tentative but successful attempts to introduce clinical medicine at Leyden and Utrecht.[156] Although the *Advice* is now remembered for its sections relating to general educational reform, it also contained an elaborate plan of a teaching hospital or 'Nosocomium Academicum'.[157]

154. C. H. Firth, *Cromwell's Army* (London, 1902), pp.253–77; Keevil (172), ii; see above, pp.79–83.

155. Keevil (172), ii, p.13 and *passim*.

156. Albert Kyper, *Medicinam rite discendi et exercendi methodus* (Leyden, 1643), pp.112, 255–6. See also G. A. Lindeboom, 'Medical Education in the Netherlands (1575–1750)', in C. D. O'Malley (ed.), *The History of Medical Education* (Berkeley and Los Angeles, 1970), pp.201–16.

157. *The Advice of W.P.* (210), pp.8–17.

Petty paid great attention to detail. With characteristic practical insight he utilised elements from diverse sources to produce a design for a medical centre which could conceivably be developed from the hospitals familiar to his readers. He emphatically repressed any inclination he might have had to 'frame Utopias', or elaborate impracticable, comprehensive programmes. Rather he set out to describe a structure which could be brought into existence without great expense, possibly 'out of one of our old Hospitals'. The staff would be no larger than normal and their salaries would not be excessive. He hoped to recruit a staff of unmarried men whose major reward would be the opportunity of public service and intellectual endeavour.[158]

The Nosocomium was to be controlled by a committee of four. The administrator, or *Steward,* would be a mathematician, who would receive a salary of £80 per annum. Someone like John Collins, who arrived back from naval service at about this time, would have been Petty's choice for this post. The Steward was to be skilled in arithmetic, accountancy, 'measuring of Land, timber, board, Architecture, frugall contrivances and the like'. He was also expected to assist the medical staff by investigating judicial astrology, meteorology and medical statistics. The medical staff would be headed by a *Physician,* 'who would be expected to display great virtuosity'—a description of the prodigious Petty himself. His salary would be £120. He was to be skilled in classical and modern medicine; his duties were, to visit all patients twice each day, supervise their treatment by his colleagues, and conduct the education of junior staff. By embracing all facets of medicine, he would be able to give sound guidance to specialists. He would be required to conduct dissections, and to prepare chemical remedies. The ultimate aim of his work was the compilation of an experimentally based system of medicine. The *Vice-physician,* paid £50, would assist the Physician, but have very little power of independent action, being primarily responsible for close clinical study and the compilation of case-histories. This was exactly the kind of function later advocated by Sydenham. The *Students* would have had five or six years' university education; presumably they would have completed the liberal arts course and qualified as MAs. This was the normal point of departure for medical studies in the university medical faculty, but at the Nosocomium, the students would work in the hospital and receive a salary of £25. They would assist the surgeon, apothecary and even the nurses. When necessary they were to act as amanuenses to the Physician, who would in return direct his pupils' reading and practical training in 'herbs, drugs, Compound Medicaments, Anatomy, Chirurgicall Instruments, bandages, operations &c.'. The *Surgeon* (paid £60) would also teach anatomy, to the medical students as well as to the *Surgeon's mate* (paid £20) and the *Apprentices* (paid £10). The surgeon was expected to be proficient in Galenic methods, but he was also to be skilled in the new arts of

158. *Ibid.,* pp.9–10.

comparative anatomy, including the mounting of animal skeletons, and to be familiar with chemical ointments obtained from the Apothecary. The *Apothecary* was to be a proficient botanist, keeper of the botanical garden, an expert on *materia medica* and an experimental chemist. The salary of the Apothecary, his mate and apprentice were the same as those of the surgeon and his staff. *Nurses,* with salaries of £4, were charged with the routine care of patients. When the medical students had served five years, and the apothecaries' or surgeons' mates four, the Nosocomium would issue a certificate giving them permission to practise in any locality 'notwithstanding any former law to the contrary'.[159]

As outlined by Petty the Nosocomium could easily have come into competition with university medical faculties and the London medical organisations. From a professional point of view it would have been regarded as a dangerous adventure, notwithstanding the benefits of combining medical education and clinical experience. This was the kind of education which had attracted generations of English medical students to Padua. Despite the acknowledged value of clinical studies, the Oxford and Cambridge medical faculties were not able to offer clinical experience, whereas in London the hospitals were isolated from the teaching establishments. Even anatomical dissection was not an established feature of medical education at the universities. The implementation of Petty's plan might well have completely extinguished the small English medical faculties, which had dwindled to the point of extinction during the Civil War. Medical education in England might thus have been transferred to a context more viable as a centre of clinical study; it could then have taken on many of the features of the best continental medical schools. In determining the content of medical education, Petty undogmatically absorbed fruitful ideas from various sources, retaining Galen as the foundation of preliminary studies, but also including practical botany, anatomy and chemistry. The emphasis was accordingly shifted from literary to scientific medicine, very much along lines recommended by Bacon or Browne : Petty himself felt that his scheme was faithful to the ancient Hippocratic tradition of enlightened empiricism.

Little is known about the specific reaction to Petty's proposals, but an anonymous commentator on the *Advice* probably reflects a general view; he suggested a 'new moulding of one of the larger and richer of the old Hospitals' to form a teaching hospital.[160] It would be interesting to know if this view elicited a sympathetic response from the London hospitals. In this context it is relevant to examine developments at the two nationalised hospitals, Ely House and the Savoy which, more than the older hospitals, responded to changing medical needs. Although initially established for only limited military purposes, they came to take

159. *Ibid.*, pp.10–16.
160. 'A Remonstrance of the Designes described by W.P. in his Advices to Mr. Samuel Hartlib, concerning the Advancement of Learning and Arts', HP LIII 36.

on certain of the features of the Nosocomium Academicum. They were the immediate responsibility of the Committee for Maimed and Wounded Soldiers which, in 1642, took over the Savoy Hospital, cleared its inmates and replaced them with war wounded.[161] The master was replaced by an overseer, Richard Malbon, a little-known, but competent administrator. In 1646 the Committee also took over the town house of the Bishop of Ely, which was used as the headquarters for payment of war pensions and as a hospital for the wounded. Thenceforth the two hospitals were managed jointly by four commissioners. Many staff posts involved responsibilities at both hospitals. The basic staff for Ely House in 1657 was described as comprising a treasurer, two overseers, comptroller, physician, surgeon, three mates, clerk, chaplain, door-keeper, two messengers and a porter.[162] There were more administrative officers than were included in Petty's Nosocomium; but this was necessary because of the more complex functions of the state hospitals. The two hospitals initially housed about 200 patients, who were cared for by about 30 nurses who were often soldiers' widows.[163] At this time medical cases were directed to Ely House and surgical to the Savoy.[164] Very strict regulations governed the behaviour of the soldiers and their nurses, and there are many indications that the authorities fully enforced these rules in the interests of the orderly management of these hospitals. This contrasts with the situation at the independent hospitals where indiscipline seems to have been a recurrent problem.

The Savoy and Ely House were adequately furnished with material requirements. Equally necessary was the provision of an efficient medical staff : most of the staff appointed were not only competent practitioners, they also took an active interest in the experimental sciences and iatrochemistry. George Starkey mentioned 'Dr. Ridgeley, Dr. Gurdan, Dr. Goddard of Oxford, Dr. French, Dr. Bathurst [sic], Dr. Currar' with special approval as physicians who were 'chymically given' and not guilty of Galenic practices. Most of this group had served in the military medical corps and at least three (Gurdan, Goddard and French) were directly involved with the nationalised London hospitals.[165]

Aaron Gurdan made his initial reputation as a physician at the Savoy. His first appearance in the public records, in February 1646, was as a petitioner engaged in the not unfamiliar quest for arrears of salary : in this case, for the treatment of 'the sick and wounded soldiers brought from the parts of the country belonging to the Parliament into

161. Keevil (172), ii, pp.21–7.
162. *CSPD 1657/8*, p.364.
163. The number of patients increased to 400: *CSPD 1657/8*, p.256.
164. *CSPD 1655/6*, pp.228–9.
165. Starkey, *Natures Explication and Helmonts Vindication* (268), sig.a4v–5r. Thomas Ridgely (d.1656) was an elderly member of the College of Physicians, described by Hartlib as 'the chiefest chymical doctor': Ephemerides 1656. John Bathurst was physician to Cromwell. William Currer was one of the few unlicensed physicians to be censured by the College of Physicians during the Republic.

the Savoy Hospital, as also those lying at their own or friends' houses within the City of London'.[166] From the Savoy, Gurdan moved to the important post of Master of the Mint. More significant was the appointment of John French, who probably succeeded Gurdan after serving in Fairfax's army. French was already at the Savoy when he was awarded an MD at Oxford in 1648.[167] At this time he was already known to Hartlib as a skilled chemist and mineralogist. His work as the major translator of distillation literature has already been mentioned; he was also an enthusiast for mineral water baths, a treatment which he introduced at the London hospitals.[168] The last member of Starkey's group of chemists who was also associated with the London hospitals is Jonathan Goddard. In 1653 he was added to the hospital management committee, while in 1658, just after the death of French, he was actively considering vacating the Wardenship of Merton College Oxford to become master of the Savoy. It is possible that Abraham Cowley, who took an MD at Oxford in 1657, also hoped to obtain this post; he is known to have made an unsuccessful attempt to secure the appointment at the restoration.[169]

Apart from French, the dominant figure at the hospitals was James Rand, a London apothecary and friend of John Evelyn. Rand was a frequent petitioner for arrears of salary; there was obviously considerable official demand for his services.[170] His intellectual bias can be surmised from his patronage of Samuel Hartlib and from the activities of his son William, which will be discussed below. Rand's immediate associate was Thomas Trapham, a successful army surgeon, who entered the Savoy in 1653.[171]

The salaries paid to the staff appear to have fluctuated considerably. The physician was due to receive £150 per annum, thirty pounds more than Petty's recommendation. However John French received £200, while his successor in 1658 was paid only £100.[172] On the whole lower grades received salaries a little higher than those envisaged by Petty; the surgeons and apothecaries were nearer in status to the physicians than he recommended. This was probably a reflection of their generally ascending social position; approximate parity was thereby established between the main sections of the medical profession.

From the financial accounts, and fragmentary information about hospital routine, it appears that the standards pertaining in the nationalised hospitals were humane ones. Patients were comfortably housed, resting on flock mattresses and clothed at the expense of the state. They were

166. *CSPD 1645/6*, p.343; Munk (195), i, p.307.
167. Wood *Fasti*, ii, pp.106, 115; Ephemerides 1648.
168. *The Yorkshire Spaw* (London, 1652); another edition 1654.
169. *CSPD 1652/3*, pp.363–4; Barnett (20), p.120; A. H. Nethercot, *Abraham Cowley* (London, 1931), p.196.
170. *CSPD 1652/3*, pp.333, 341, 445; *1653/4*, pp.44, 66.
171. *CSPD 1652/3*, p.320.
172. *CSPD 1655/6*, pp.228–9; *1658/9*, p.256.

supplied with a good diet, as well as beer, and clay pipes for smoking. Those with smallpox were kept apart in an isolation ward, while the rest received considerable quantities of medicines.[173]

A novel experience for the soldiers was the ward known as the Hothouse. Here two nurses supervised the soldiers while they sat or reclined in cubicles, wearing special caps and coats; the atmosphere of a Turkish bath was created by a copper bath stove. Interest in this treatment was probably prompted by Peter Chamberlen, who had patented an invention for bath stoves while in Holland. In 1648 he reappeared in England requesting a patent for his invention from parliament. The College of Physicians was officially consulted about this project, but despite their vigorous objections which were subsequently published, a patent was granted to Chamberlen.[174] This patent was allowed on condition that it was operated to provide the maximum accessibility to the poor of 'artificial Baths and Bathstoves', and 'hamacco beds and couches'. The College of Physicians promptly announced that public baths were harmful to morals, their argument being supported with choice classical allusions. The College also expressed anxiety about the introduction of dangerous chemical decoctions. The evil influence of Paracelsus was as usual detected at work behind the proposals. Little is known about the fate of Chamberlen's scheme, but this episode had important repercussions for the innovator himself. He was accused of avoiding meeting representatives of the College to defend his scheme; this and his subsequent impenitent behaviour paved the way for his expulsion from the College on the grounds of non-attendance, a misdemeanour which was allowed to pass unnoticed in the case of other absentee members.[175] The application of Chamberlen's invention at the London hospitals indicates one use which presumably avoided the scruples of the College.

Mineral water treatments were increasingly popular among English physicians. The first writer on English baths was William Turner (1562), whose brief essay on this subject was appended to a work designed to publicise the medicinal virtues of English plants. Thereafter a succession of writers praised the virtues of various local mineral springs, while the standard general survey was produced in 1631 by Edward Jorden, a Bath practitioner.[176] John French followed Jorden's scientific approach to this subject in his book on the 'Yorkshire spaw', which proclaimed the

173. Keevil (172), ii, pp.24–6. The soldiers may have been dressed in clothes made by the female inmates of St. Bartholomew's Hospital; see N. Moore, *The History of St. Bartholomew's Hospital,* 2 vols. (London, 1918), ii, p.310.

174. Chamberlen, *To the honorable Committee for Bathes* (London, 1648); *Publique Bathes Purged. Or a Reply to Dr. Chamberlen* (London, 1648). For Chamberlen's patent, see *CJ,* vi, p.27; J. H. Aveling, *The Chamberlens,* pp.60–77; Doorman (81), p.42.

175. Annals, 30 Sept. 1648, 4 June 1649, 23 Nov. 1649.

176. *New Cambridge Bibliography of English Literature,* ed. G. Watson, i, pp.2362–4; see also C. F. Mullett, *Public Baths and Health in England,* Supplement to *Bull. Hist. Med.,* No. 5 (Baltimore, 1946).

potentiality of English spa waters to match their continental equivalents. Shortly after the appearance of French's *The Yorkshire Spaw* (1652), a long series of entries in the public records describe applications made by the overseer of the Savoy Hospital for means to carry 220 wounded soldiers to Bath to take the waters. The Council of State agreed to pay £800 to cover the cost of transport and treatment; and an officer's widow received £20 to enable her to make a private visit to Bath.[177] This expensive expedition was undertaken in 1653, although some difficulty was encountered in recovering the cost.

Such evidence suggests that the physicians at the nationalised hospitals were committed to medical ideas of the kind advocated by Petty. The final dimension required for the London hospitals to match the Nosocomium Academicum was the development of a teaching function and attention to anatomical study. The surgeons and apothecaries in following the normal method of apprenticeship would have made use of the hospitals for training their assistants. John French despised the traditional forms of university medical education and he appealed to his friend Tobias Garbrand, the Principal of Gloucester Hall Oxford, to support university reform. In association with like-minded London colleagues, he may have used the London hospitals as a base for the medical training of graduates in the manner advocated by Petty. It would be tempting to conclude that these graduates were intended to provide the nucleus for the College of Graduate Physicians planned by William Rand. There is a little evidence to support this supposition. The records indicate that dissections were carried on as a matter of routine in the hospitals.[178] These anatomies may have led to the association of French and his colleagues with some of Harvey's followers. In one important instance, the services of the hospitals were acknowledged. In the preface to Wharton's *Adenographia,* the hospitals were thanked for allowing the author access to dissections, thus enabling him to avoid the use of inferior evidence derived from animals. Wharton singled out Edward Emily, John French, 'amico plurimum colendo', and Thomas Trapham for particular mention in connection with this service.[179] In view of this evidence it might have been the availability of corpses in these hospitals which led Francis Glisson to concentrate his researches in London, rather than at his academic post in Cambridge.

The London hospitals were thus well equipped to achieve the final transition into teaching establishments. This outcome was prevented by the abolition of the Savoy and Ely House military hospitals at the restoration, but the necessity of clinical experience was so apparent that by 1662 the staff of St. Bartholomew's Hospital were taking private stu-

177. *CSPD 1652/3*, pp.224, 341.
178. Keevil (172), ii, pp.24–6.
179. Emily was physician to St. Thomas's Hospital; he was succeeded by Wharton. F. G. Parsons, *The History of St. Thomas's Hospital,* 2 vols. (London, 1934), ii, pp.81, 85.

dents. By the end of the century, such clinical education was systematically provided in London.[180]

Apart from the enterprise of the London hospitals, both local and national administrations performed traditional public health duties relating to street cleaning, sewers, and procedures to control epidemics, in much the same manner as their Stuart predecessors. Only in isolated cases were new trends discernible. During the idealistic period of the Saints' Parliament a large and impressive 'Committee for Lunatics' was established. Among the members of the committee were Jonathan Goddard and John Sadler; the latter made this subject his particular concern. The committee appears to have dealt with individual cases, but not to have taken any major decisions.[181] An example of local enterprise was provided by Dr. Turnbull of Durham, who elaborated proposals for a free health service for the poor of his area. This required the collection of subscriptions at a parish level in order to pay the salaries of physicians, apothecaries and surgeons employed under the scheme. On the refusal of the Grand Jury to implement his plans, Turnbull appealed for support from the Governors of the new Cromwellian College at Durham. According to the surviving draft, the College may have intended to adopt his plan.[182] In view of the strong medical and social interests of Ezerel Tong and his colleagues, it was likely to have had considerable appeal among the Cromwellian College Fellows.

(viii) The College of Graduate Physicians

The convergence on London of so many practitioners interested in new approaches to social medicine and responsive to new medical theories, inevitably led to dissatisfaction with the traditional organisation of medicine. Although the medical fraternities no longer exercised their monopolistic powers, the College of Physicians in particular was determined to re-establish the Stuart system of medical organisation at the first opportunity. Warning signs appeared during the last years of the Republic, when the College of Physicians began making tentative but menacing moves against unlicensed practitioners. In these circumstances unlicensed academic physicians sought legal sanction for their position, in order to prevent a return to pre-war conditions when highly qualified practitioners had been suppressed along with empirics. They produced a plan for a 'Colledge of Graduate Physitians' which would protect the rights of physicians who were disqualified from membership of the College of Physicians for technical reasons, or who were disinclined to seek membership. Inevitably the new college would have drawn its strongest support from among the articulate proponents of medical reform. The English candidates for such an organisation might have been physi-

180. Clark (50), i, p.320.
181. *CSPD 1653/4*, pp.215, 237.
182. 'Physicall Charity, Durham Colledge, Septemb. 4, 1658', HP LIII 12.

cians who had completed the full period of arts and medical education at Oxford or Cambridge, but were unable to become candidates for the College of Physicians because there were no vacancies. Even orthodox physicians who enrolled as candidates were annoyed by long delays over promotion to full fellowship of the College. More commonly the practitioner had academic degrees but perhaps no specifically medical qualification. The bishops were no longer in a position to issue medical licences, and few were sought from the universities. A common course of action for graduates was to spend a short time on the continent in order to obtain an MD at Leyden or Padua. George Thomson paid a brief visit to Leyden for this purpose, to return a convinced Helmontian. A longer course of study in the low countries, with similar intellectual results, was undertaken by the architect of the College of Graduate Physicians, William Rand, son of James Rand apothecary to the London nationalised hospitals. After a conventional arts education at Cambridge, Rand spent some years in the low countries, registering at Leyden in 1652.[183] At some stage he received an MD, although not from Leyden. Rand's letters to Hartlib indicate a strong interest in the new philosophy and social reform. His first preserved letter discussed Dury's *Reformed School* and Hobbes's *Leviathan*.[184] This must have been one of the first references to Hobbes's work and is evidence for the rapidity of its dissemination to the continent. Shortly before returning to England, Rand decided upon a medical career and reported that, like Worsley, he had been converted to Helmontianism by Johann Morian. He expressed pleasure at the appearance of an improved edition of van Helmont's works and also propounded a scheme for producing a yet further edition of the *Ortus medicinae,* with the contents arranged topically. This was expected to increase the influence of van Helmont's badly organised medical essays.[185] At this time Rand was associating with Luke Ridgely who, like his father Thomas Ridgely, was an iatrochemist.

The English Helmontians were joined by growing numbers of continental physicians who settled in England either temporarily or permanently, taking advantage of the freedom of medical organisation under the Protectorate. Although these itinerant physicians often took up bizarre intellectual positions, they also had genuine skills and a desire to promote practical and industrial chemistry. They generally also supported Paracelsus and van Helmont. John Webster was introduced to iatrochemistry by the Hungarian Johannes Hunniades, who became chemist to the Earl of Pembroke after settling in England.[186] Johann Sibertus Küffeler was an inventor and chemist in the tradition of his father-in-law Cornelius Drebbel. In the absence of state remuneration for his inventions,

183. Venn, iii, p.418; Innes Smith (157), p.189.
184. 18 July 1651, HP LXII 30.
185. Letter from Rand to Hartlib, 14 February 1652/3, HP XLII 17.
186. F. Sherwood Taylor & C. H. Josten, 'Johannes Banfi Hunyades', *Ambix,* 1953, *5*: 44–52.

he was obliged to turn to medicine, being known to Hartlib as a Helmontian who possessed the secret of the 'arcanum of the celestial liquor'.[187]

Peter Staehl, like Küffeler, was recommended to Hartlib by Johann Morian. He arrived in England in 1658 and settled at Oxford, where he became a most successful physician and lecturer in chemistry.[188] Johann Brun (alias Unmussig) obtained his MD from Franeker; he was attracted to England in 1648 after spending many years journeying in the classic Paracelsian manner through Europe, Transylvania and Turkey. Brun greatly commended van Helmont 'for many reall good experiments intermingled in his books. Most of his specifica are taken out of Paracelsus'.[189] One of Brun's English friends was John French, who might have absorbed his enthusiasm for Glauber from Brun. Boyle applied to Brun for medical advice and on questions of practical chemistry. Hartlib wryly commented that he was impressed by Unmussig's doctoral charter 'but alas! this will cure no distempers or diseases'.[190]

Such settlers greatly increased the rate at which the English became acquainted with continental medical ideas. The changing tone of English medicine was noted by a shorter-term visitor, the Dane Johann Christian Agricola, who described the flourishing state of Helmontian medicine in England after a visit to Frederick Clodius. He told Bartholin about the English Helmontians' reliance on chemical therapy, which it was anticipated would completely supplant the techniques of Galenic medicine.[191] The Brandenburg diplomat Frederick Kretchmar also became involved with the Helmontians during his protracted embassy to Cromwell during 1657 and 1658. Finally, just before the Chemical Council was formed, the Helmontians were visited by the notorious Johann Fortitudo Hartprecht, whose chemical expertise attracted much interest, although his taste for polemic and for secrecy made some suspect his abilities.[192]

Their numbers swelled by this band of cosmopolitan supporters, the London iatrochemists became many and confident. Although they developed an obsessive passion for arcana, an equally strong feature of their work was an attention to practical chemistry. They became familiar with a wide variety of preparations in inorganic chemistry.

The iatrochemists quickly realised the advantages of establishing well-equipped chemical laboratories. During the Republic private laboratories proliferated; even the College of Physicians and the Apothecaries' Society joined the movement to sponsor laboratories, which competed with

187. Letter from Hartlib to Boyle, 19 April 1659, Boyle *Works,* vi, p.121.

188. G. H. Turnbull (286).

189. Ephemerides 1648.

190. Boyle *Works,* vi, pp.81, 85, 87, 94, 96. Maddison (185), pp.83–4. Dr. T. C. Barnard kindly informs me that Brun settled in Ireland during the Protectorate.

191. Letter from Agricola to Bartholin, 19/29 February 1656 in Thomas Bartholin, *Epistolarum medicinalium Centuria V* (Copenhagen, 1664–7), i, pp.631–4. See also Boyle *Works,* vi, p.650.

192. For Hartprecht see Turnbull (286), p.267; Ferguson (98), i, pp.338–41, 368–70.

those developed by the Helmontians and Hermeticists. In *Macaria* Gabriel Plattes outlined a scheme for a state laboratory which would 'deliver out yeerly such medicines as they find out by experience'. Shortly afterwards he petitioned parliament to establish him in a laboratory under conditions of complete secrecy.[193] Shortly after the death of Plattes, chemical laboratories became the focus for the work of the Invisible College. It was probably the College's search for improved furnaces which led Worsley to visit the low countries. Frederick Clodius, who arrived in England in about 1653, established a laboratory in Hartlib's kitchen. This rapidly evolved towards the institution envisaged in *Macaria*. The effects of this were keenly felt by the tolerant father-in-law:

> 'As for us poor earthworms, we are crawling in my house about our quondam back-kitchen, whereof my son hath made a goodly laboratory; yea, such a one, as men affirm, they have never seen the like, for its several advantages and commodiousnesses. It hath been employed days and nights with no small success, God be praised, these many weeks together.'[194]

Even these premises were not sufficient; Clodius was obliged to use a nearby blacksmith's shop for the preparation of the 'Helmontian cinnabar'.[195] This extended laboratory became the basis of a plan for 'a general chemical council', which was to be led by Clodius and the rehabilitated catholic, Sir Kenelm Digby.

The immediate aim of the Council was to prepare specifics, but ultimately they hoped to obtain 'the great medicinal arcana'. This would require a new 'universal laboratory', which was intended to promote the health of the nation and of the whole of mankind. Digby was expected to spend at least £600 on this venture. The promoters were also very anxious to obtain Boyle's support.[196] Various proposals were discussed, one involving Boyle's sponsorship of an entirely new laboratory for Clodius, who would 'be entrusted with a full and entire communication of them all and others, as we shall advise amongst ourselves'.[197]

Boyle's involvement with the affairs of this laboratory is perhaps indicated by his first authenticated essay 'An Epistolical Discourse of Philaretus to Empericus . . . inviting all true lovers of Vertue and Mankind to a free and generous Communication of Secrets and Receipts in Physick'.[198] Since his first introduction to chemistry Boyle had been

193. *Macaria* (219), p.5. 'A Caveat for alchymists' in Hartlib, *Chymical Addresses* (144), pp.44–88.

194. Letter from Hartlib to Boyle, 28 February 1653/4, Boyle *Works,* vi, p.79.

195. Boyle *Works,* vi, p.83.

196. Letter from Hartlib to Boyle, 8 May 1654, Boyle *Works,* vi, pp.86–7.

197. Letter from Hartlib to Boyle, 15 May 1654, Boyle *Works,* vi, p.89.

198. Published in Hartlib's *Chymical Adresses* (144), pp.113–50. For the identification of Boyle as the author of this anonymous essay, M. E. Rowbottom, 'The Earliest Published Writing of Robert Boyle', *Annals of Science,* 1950, *6*: 376–89. The text of Boyle's essay is reprinted by R. E. W. Maddison, *Annals of Science,* 1961, *17*: 165–73.

concerned about the habitual tendency of its practitioners to relapse into secrecy and vain boasting. His essay was composed very much in the spirit of Hartlib's demand for the completely free distribution of intelligence on all matters. Boyle argued on both practical and theological grounds for the free communication of newly discovered chemical remedies. He asserted that by preserving cryptic language and oaths of secrecy, the chemists could never be certain of the quality of their discoveries or ensure the survival of their work in future generations. The laboratory in London was conceived in the spirit of Boyle's proposals; the overseers, like those of Solomon's House, acknowledged a duty to apply their discoveries for the best possible ends.

Entries in Boyle's 'Philosophical Diary' for this period also indicate a preoccupation with chemical and medical preparations derived from Digby, Clodius, Brun, Starkey, French, and Smart, most of whom were probably directly involved in the Chemical Council.[199] Boyle's direct participation in their chemical activities is suggested by Agricola, who referred to meeting Boyle at Clodius's laboratory, probably in 1658. Starkey was undoubtedly the most unstable and meteoric member of the alliance. He had greatly impressed Boyle by his preparation of *ens veneris*, but in 1654 Hartlib described him as 'altogether degenerated', having abandoned his house and been imprisoned for debt.[200] Despite the clear evidence of instability, curiosity about his chemical activities persisted. His Helmontian tracts were significant; one was dedicated to Boyle, who made favourable references to the 'philosopher by fire' in his early chemical writings.

Remeus Franck was an apothecary, probably sent over by Morian, who was maintained at Hartlib's house. He was able to supply chemical balsams for the healing of wounds. These were described in 'A Short and Easie Method of Surgery', translated by William Rand for Hartlib's chemical collection. Rand hoped particularly that these balsams would be 'employed in the publick Hospitals of the Commonwealth'. His translation argued that dangerous and painful surgical practices employed in hospitals could in most cases be replaced by chemical methods. A list of five easily prepared balsams was given for this purpose.[201] Judging by the hospital accounts for chemicals, Rand's father may well have taken this advice seriously. The popularity of Rand's view is indicated by the increasing inclusion of chemical preparations in ship surgeons' chests.

199. Maddison (185), pp.86–7. Thomas Smart was a Vauxhall chemist and chemical assistant to the Marquis of Dorchester. Letter from Hartlib to Boyle, 1 Sept. 1657, Boyle *Works,* vi, p.94.

200. Letter from Hartlib to Boyle, 28 February 1653/4, Boyle *Works,* vi, pp.79–80; Wilkinson (*op. cit.* n.127 above), pp.128–33. *Ens veneris,* a copper compound, is typical of the products investigated by the Helmontians. Another associate of the group, Joachim Polemann, showed considerable familiarity with the chemistry of copper in *Novum lumen medicum* (Amsterdam, 1659); English translation by F.H. (London, 1662).

201. Hartlib, *Chymical Addresses* (144), pp.153–89. Rand's contribution is dated 2 November 1654.

Hartlib's *Chymical, Medicinal and Chyrurgical Addresses* (1655) was produced at the height of the activities of the Chemical Council. This apparently haphazard collection of essays is more intelligible when seen in the context of the London proposals to establish a national laboratory. Plattes's posthumous 'Caveat' provides a link with the original laboratory design described in *Macaria* and with Petty's scheme for the reform of the national hospitals. The essays of Rand and Boyle outlined specific uses for the laboratory and they elaborated the general principles underlying its management. Most of the contributions to the *Addresses* were drawn from foreign sources. Discussions about specific remedies and the Philosopher's Stone came from the French Paracelsian and social reformer Théophraste Renaudot, many of whose ideas on social reform were taken up by Hartlib. A contribution issued under the pseudonym Eirenaeus Philalethes belonged to the increasingly common genre of translations of and commentaries on old alchemical literature; this approach was made fashionable by such dilettantes as Elias Ashmole, who was a recent enthusiastic recruit to hermeticism. The 'Exposition' by Philalethes illustrates all the dangers of subjectivism and of the drift away from experimental and utilitarian medicine, inveighed against in the essays by Plattes and Boyle.[202] Hartlib's collection accordingly indicates the divergent tendencies of the chemical movement at this period. Whereas Boyle and Hartlib were anxious to construct an experimental, utilitarian and objective science of chemistry, strong influences directed practitioners into the occult and metaphysical. In the latter tradition excessive claims would be made with greater confidence and reputations established without recourse to tedious experimental studies. Most of the Helmontians exhibited a tendency to drift away from Boyle's approach. This may have been the cause for the decline of the Chemical Council. Starkey and Clodius became unstable and moved to the fringes of scientific activity. Others concentrated on their private laboratories, which became increasingly common in London, at the universities, and even in country houses. Boyle's removal to Oxford insulated him from the excesses of Helmontianism; but he remained closely associated with the experimental chemists of the type involved with the Chemical Council, as is witnessed by his patronage of Peter Staehl at Oxford. He may well have wished to import into Oxford the best elements of the work of the Chemical Council.[203]

William Rand identified himself with the aims of Hartlib and Boyle. He translated material for the third edition of Hartlib's *Legacy* (1655) and then embarked on a major translation, *The Life of Peiresc,* which

202. 'An Exposition upon Sir George Ripleys Epistle', signed 'Eirenaeus Philalethes'. This has been regarded by Kittredge and Turnbull as a pseudonym adopted by Starkey, but Wilkinson has favoured Winthrop: R. S. Wilkinson, 'The Problem of the Identity of Eirenaeus Philalethes', *Ambix,* 1964, *12*: 24–43. But see *Ambix,* 1972, *19*: 204–8, where Wilkinson accepts the Starkey hypothesis.

203. See Turnbull (286).

was dedicated to John Evelyn, a family friend.[204] From the preface it is apparent that Rand hoped that the virtuous life of Peiresc would stimulate the English gentry to follow his example by turning away from vain diversions to the serious study of antiquities and philosophy. Peiresc, like Bacon, was offered as a model to Rand's public-spirited compatriots.

As an unlicensed London medical practitioner with a foreign medical degree, Rand appreciated the defects of the traditional system of medical organisation. He wished to secure the benefits of unrestricted practice for able physicians, regardless of their connection with the College of Physicians, while protecting the medical profession against the encroachment of mountebanks. Rand believed that this liberalisation could be effected by a College of Graduate Physicians. It was perceptively recognised that the controlled liberalisation of the medical profession should be undertaken during the Protectorate, and before the College of Physicians was given an opportunity to reassert its authority. After a period of judicious leniency, the increasing strength of the unlicensed medical profession in London created pressure within the College for a more aggressive approach to the enforcement of its statutory regulations. In response Rand and his colleagues pressed for the formation of a rival college. The draft 'Proposals relating to those Graduate Physicians now resident in London'[205] indicates that a complex mixture of professional, social and intellectual considerations determined Rand's approach to medical organisation. His plan assumed that there existed in London a substantial group of responsible physicians who bore sufficient animosity towards the established College and its regulations, for them to support a completely new professional organisation. Rand argued that the London College was not sufficiently broadly defined to embrace all physicians with acceptable academic qualifications for practice. Discrimination against foreign graduates and English graduates without formal medical degrees, created a large group of practitioners who felt equal to the collegiate physicians but lacked their legal status and were accordingly liable to the same penalties as illiterate empirics. In order to overcome this injustice, Rand's new college was to include all university graduates qualified to practise medicine. They intended to defend their privileges in the customary manner, but the 'Proposals' makes it clear that the main enemy was the old College, rather than the empirics.

An alternative approach to this problem might have been collaboration with the London College in order to secure the minor statutory amendments required to allow full fellowship rights to licensed graduates. But the extremely conservative attitude of the College to its membership qualifications, exhibited as recently as the 1647 revision of statutes, was probably thought to rule out such an approach. As with education, the

204. *The Mirrour of true Nobility & Gentility, Being the Life of the Renowned Nicolaus Claudius Fabricius Lord of Peiresk. Englished by W. Rand, Doctor of Physick* (London, 1657).

205. Given in full, Appendix III below.

reformers increasingly placed their faith in new institutions, which could be more readily adapted to their intellectual and social outlook. Rand contrasted the traditional academic physician with the 'more studious, public and humble spirited' practitioners who would join the new society.[206]

From Rand's comments it is apparent that the Graduate College was expected to embrace the medical ideas of his London associates. It would have been in a position to exercise considerable influence on the military medical services, and on the London hospitals. The College would also probably have been an active participant in the Chemical Council, since it was intended to take advantage 'not only of Physic but of all natural Discoveries'. Rand even hoped that the new college would become the nucleus for a University of London.

Somewhat surprisingly there is no further evidence about the Graduate College. It was conceived and discussed under conditions of secrecy, in order to prevent counter-moves by the old College. It may have lapsed through lack of interest; most graduate physicians were probably over-complacent, in an atmosphere during the Protectorate which was unfavourable to monopolies. To some extent, events justified this attitude. Despite strenuous efforts by the London College to regain its privileges after the restoration, the jealousy of the rival medical organisations successfully prevented a return of the rigid hierarchical system of the pre-war period. The apothecaries and surgeons were supported by the Helmontians, who formed a 'Society of Chymical Physitians' which attracted influential supporters. This society was a partial realisation of the puritan proposal, but it embraced the mountebank element so carefully excluded from Rand's College. By taking in a broader cross-section of practitioners, the Society could command considerable numbers, but it was so heterogeneous that there were soon internal dissensions which were the prelude to its relatively rapid extinction.[207]

Rand's project would not have failed for lack of suitable candidates. Such able English physicians outside the London College as Rand, Worsley, French, Currer, Thomson and Sydenham could have formed a rival organisation capable of making a significant contribution to medical reform and experimental science. By this means Helmontian medicine might have developed in the controlled and scientific manner advocated by Boyle and Hartlib, uninfluenced by unbalanced personalities and pedlars in the occult. Rand's project may have failed owing to legislative inertia, although it would have evoked a sympathetic response from certain influential figures. Rand's father was a trusted state servant, who had successfully secured support for Hartlib's Office of Address.

206. Letter from Rand to Hartlib, 15 August 1656, given in full in Appendix III below.

207. Sir Henry Thomas, 'The Society of Chymical Physitians', in *Science, Medicine and History,* ed. E. A. Underwood, 2 vols. (London, 1953), ii, pp.56–71; P. M. Rattansi, 'The Helmontian-Galenist Controversy in Restoration England', *Ambix,* 1964, *12*: 1–23.

Even more important, William Rand enjoyed the patronage of Robert Boyle's sister, Lady Ranelagh. Rand's College seems to have been conceived during discussions on medical reform held at Lady Ranelagh's home. Through this channel it may well have been brought to the attention of Boyle, Thomas Coxe, Thomas Sydenham, and John Sadler. This would have opened the way to a coherent and comprehensive policy for the reform of the medical profession in accordance with the principles of the new system of law evolved partly by the same group a few years earlier.

(ix) The College of Physicians of London

Although the College of Physicians never achieved complete control over the medical profession, even in London before 1640, its legal authority and social ascendancy were firmly established. As Goodall's records show, it vigorously pursued its enemies and was vigilant in extinguishing any precocious instincts displayed by the surgeons and apothecaries.[208] However, the social realities of the expanding capital would have made it extremely difficult for this neat institutional arrangement to succeed for long. The Civil War produced a reversal of the College's vocational influence, from which it was extremely slow to recover. In a society united by an opposition to monopolies, the price of survival was to tolerate interlopers, in the hope that conditions of restrictive practice would eventually return. But as the restoration history of the College shows, it became almost impossible to suppress the fertile developments in popular medicine which had occurred during the two decades of derestriction.

In addition the intellectual reputation of the College was in the balance. The Fellows were regarded as the guardians of Galenic medicine, which was subjected to increasingly damaging criticism from the Paracelsians. Indeed, William Harvey, himself a prominent Fellow, unwittingly abetted the critics of Galen by his physiological researches, which provoked a reappraisal of ancient ideas about man's physical nature. The speed with which attitudes changed can be assessed from the mechanistic physiology which Thomas Hobbes had evolved by 1650. This incorporated the ideas of Harvey into a system which represented a complete reaction against the outlook of the Galenists. Despite these adverse conditions, the task of retrenchment was accomplished extremely successfully by Harvey and his colleagues. Vocationally, expectations were wisely kept low and the preservation of institutional integrity was recognised as an accomplishment in itself. On intellectual matters, the Fellows were strikingly successful in capturing an up-to-date image, although it proved difficult to implement a compromise with Paracelsian medicine.

208. C. Goodall, *An Historicall Account of the College's proceedings Against Empiricks . . . to the Murther of King Charles the first* (London, 1684).

There can be no doubt that at the outset of the Civil War the majority of the Fellows, particularly in the older generation, would have harboured royalist sympathies. The Royal Physicians, who were *ex officio* Fellows of the College, attended the king and queen in the provinces. The most eminent Royal Physician, William Harvey, was appointed Warden of Merton College during the royalist occupation of Oxford. After the fall of Oxford he retired to live quietly with his family in the home counties. The restrained behaviour of the royalist Fellows spared the College political embarrassment and facilitated its passive submission to the *de facto* rulers. It must have been a cause of regret to the royalist physicians that the College felt obliged to exclude such an able physician as Walter Charleton. The refusal to admit him to a fellowship must have been occasioned by his obdurate adherence to the royal party; had this not been publicly announced on the title pages of his many books, he might have been spared.[209] Fortunately, few concessions of this kind were called for; politically the College played a completely passive role. When the Royal Physician Alexander Frazier was expelled on the technical grounds of long absence without permission, he was replaced by another royalist, Charles Scarburgh, and it was agreed that Frazier might be restored upon his return from abroad.[210]

The increasing parliamentarian party in the College behaved with the same restraint as the royalists, also in the interests of institutional unity. New Fellows and executive members were elected without obvious reference to their political or religious views.

From the very beginning of the Civil War, an extremely cautious attitude was adopted to the activities of practitioners under the jurisdiction of the College. Offences were conveniently overlooked, particularly when committed by practitioners with puritan or parliamentarian connections. Only token accusations against empirics were made and very few convictions occurred. Unlicensed practitioners settled in London, practised, and were promoted to important offices without objection from the College. When Dr. William Currer, a prominent iatrochemist was summoned before the Fellows for illegally practising in London, he was gently advised (*Monetur amice*) that he should abide by the statutes.[211] There is no indication that he or others responded to this advice. The College also endured without complaint the arrogant behaviour of apothecaries and surgeons, and Culpeper's unauthorised translations of *Pharmacopoeia Londinensis* and *De Rachitide*, both of which had been compiled by committees of Fellows. A good indicator of the changing conditions is the College's relationship with Peter Chamberlen. Before the civil wars, it had successfully undermined

209. Annals, 6 July & 2 November 1649, 3 May & 16 July 1655. Clark (50), i, pp.281–2; Webster (316), pp.393–8. The political divisions within the College will be considered in a forthcoming paper by Lindsay Sharp of Queen's College Oxford.

210. Annals, 25 June 1650.

211. Annals, 2 April 1652.

Chamberlen's plans to incorporate midwives under his own supervision. After spending some time on entrepreneurial activities in the low countries Chamberlen returned to England as an eloquent partisan of radical puritanism; his re-emergence on the English scene was announced by a scheme for a system of public baths. Although this was overtly opposed by the College, parliament duly granted a patent to Chamberlen. This is indicative of the minor role played by the College on matters of public health. Decisions about the medical services of the army and navy, hospitals, and poor relief were made largely without reference to the London College.

In the absence of legal sanctions, it was necessary for the College to introduce positive inducements to membership. The number of Fellows was tending to fall below the statutory limit, affecting both the income and morale of the College. Hence some of the more arbitrary requirements were gradually relaxed. It was decided that incorporation at Oxford or Cambridge would no longer be a condition of candidature for British physicians with foreign MDs. The number of candidates was raised from six to twelve. These modifications were incorporated into the revised statutes which were completed on 3 May 1647.[212] But on questions of internal management and ceremonies, the 1647 statutes were even more rigid and oligarchically orientated than the *statuta vetera*. The medical texts prescribed for examination were precisely the same Galenic and Hippocratic works which had been specified a century before. Sample questions indicate that physicians were expected to be skilled in phlebotomy, purgation, cauterisation, etc., the very practices which were coming under violent attack. Latin was maintained as the medium of communication for all basic activities, including the medical lectures.

Perhaps the most important of the innovations was the less restrictive attitude to licentiates, who were to be granted permission to practise, even if foreign or medically unqualified, relatively unlearned or inexperienced, if judged of sound abilities and character. Such liberality was expressly designed to avoid the accusation of monopoly (ne Collegium nostrum monopolii accusetur). A final, slight gesture to popular medicine was the introduction of the category of Honorary Fellow, the first elected being Henry Pierrepoint, Marquis of Dorchester, a celebrated amateur physician, who combined an interest in chemistry with a position of political influence. Such additions to the College were valuable for earning goodwill and securing much-needed injections of funds.[213]

The result of these modifications was relatively slight. The College was able to maintain its appeal to the class of physicians from which it had traditionally recruited. Few licentiates came forward, perhaps owing

212. Clark (50), i, pp.277–81.

213. 'Statuta Collegii Medicorum Londinensium', 1647, Clark (50), i, pp.393–417. For Pierrepoint, see *DNB*; Munk (195), i, pp.282–92.

to the small annual fee, but more probably because there was no legal inducement to join; many possible applicants would have had little sympathy for the medical views of the Fellows.

Only towards the end of the Republic was there any thought of taking measures against empirics and non-licensed practitioners. This later concern may have been prompted by intelligence about the rival medical College proposed by Rand and his associates. More importantly, many candidates came forward to complain that empirics were unrepentantly and audaciously undermining established practices (de Agyrtarum insolentia, audaciaque praeter solitam praxin conquerebantur). Dr. Edward Greaves delivered an impressive speech on this subject on behalf of the aggrieved candidates. A large committee was established to report on the matter.[214] But despite protracted discussions and arguments about the correct course of action, no solution was found to this problem and only sporadic action was taken against empirics, although menacing speeches by the candidates continued. Almost all cases of concerted action were against the lowest class of empirics.[215] The graduate Paracelsian and Helmontian physicians were rarely mentioned and never fined. Intellectual rather than legal means were required to meet the threat of such competition.

With the emergence of a coherent and aggressive Paracelsian movement during the Commonwealth, the College of Physicians was forced to define its attitude to chemical therapy. Hitherto, as witnessed by the first edition of the *Pharmacopoeia Londinensis* (1618), Fellows with Paracelsian sympathies were able to encourage the use of a number of chemical remedies, without arousing controversy or hostility. This trend towards a peaceful compromise was not acceptable to the Paracelsians outside the College. The chemical remedies in the *Pharmacopoeia* were ridiculed as perfunctory gestures towards the new medicine which could not be understood or applied without a complete abandonment of Galenic beliefs. College chemistry was 'pseudo-chymistry' or 'misochymistry'; its defects and disjointed nature were exposed by the Culpeper translation of the *Pharmacopoeia*. The minor amendments which were made in the 1650 edition in no way undermined these criticisms; indeed, under the watchful eye of Baldwin Hamey, chemical therapy was kept well in the background.[216]

Rather than embark on a general defence of Galenic medicine, with the attendant risk of appearing authoritarian and unsympathetic towards experimental philosophy, the College shrewdly emphasised its positive role in furthering the empirically sound elements of Paracelsian

214. Annals, 13 & 31 March 1656.

215. Annals, 4 & 25 April, 2 May 1656.

216. George Thomson, *Misochymias* (London, 1671), p.4. Noah Biggs (25), p.14. Clark (50), i, p.230, comments on the *Pharmacopoeia Londinensis*: 'The earlier revisions apparently lagged behind the advance of knowledge, and it seems difficult to praise them except in so far as they were the products of good intentions.'

medicine. The College claimed to take an open-minded approach to all methods of therapy; proven remedies were acceptable whatever their source. There was even an attempt to regain the advantage by fostering the view that the Paracelsians were peddling a collection of useless or potentially dangerous and untested drugs. The final proof offered of the genuine commitment of the College to chemical therapy was the employment of a professional chemist to build up a college laboratory or 'chymicall repository'.

Laboratories were not an entirely new idea in the world of organised medicine. Collections of chemical apparatus were commonly assembled by individuals investigating alchemy, or by distillers for commercial purposes. As early as 1623 the Apothecaries had seen the commercial advantage of a laboratory; in 1641 their President offered £800 for the erection of a laboratory at Blackfriars.[217]

Certain Fellows of the College of Physicians may have been motivated by dissatisfaction with the quality of chemicals supplied by apothecaries when they agreed in 1648 to the President's suggestion that the College should establish a chemical laboratory. However, that some members had reservations about this development is indicated by Ralph Palmer's 'Life of Baldwin Hamey', a biography of one of the most influential Fellows: 'Chemistry now began to come into vogue, which Dr. Hamey could not well be reconciled to, from his Galennical Principles . . . it seem'd to him as a Stroke of Quackery, and perhaps was first us'd in that way; incourag'd by the Vanities of Paracelsus'.[218] In view of the rise of the Paracelsians the laboratory proved fortuitously to be a blessing. The college chemist, William Johnson, was soon granted a room, although there were long delays before he was provided with apparatus. None the less he was forced to give an undertaking that he would bring preparations before the College for monthly inspections.[219] Shortly after the inception of this scheme Robert Child reported optimistically that the College had established a laboratory 'in which all chymical medecins may the better bee prepared, every doctor taking his turne to attend it'.[220]

Johnson's credentials made him an ideal apologist for the College when the tide of provocative and antagonistic literature produced during the Commonwealth could no longer be tolerated. Johnson's publications were nicely designed to imitate the popular iatrochemical works emanating from French and his associates. A critical examination indicates that Johnson achieved his end with the minimum of effort and the maximum of publicity directed against the critics. His first literary exercise was the re-issue of a collection of translations of short works by Paracelsus and his disciples Fioravanti and Quercetanus, published

217. Barrett (*op. cit.* n.20), pp.58–9.
218. Royal College of Physicians, MS 249, fol. 54.
219. Annals, 26 June & 24 October 1648; 23 January & 2 April 1651.
220. Ephemerides 1648 & 1649.

originally by the pioneer Elizabethan Paracelsian John Hester in 1596.[221] Direct acknowledgment of Hester was made only in the second preface, the first being signed 'J.H. W.J.'. Johnson's contribution was extensive prefatory matter drawing attention to the chemical activities of the College. It was announced that a 'Chymical Artificer' had been appointed to supply the London public with chemical remedies; in other words, Johnson's Amen Corner laboratory was to supply any of the remedies mentioned in the book. These claims suggest that Johnson hoped to exercise an independence in medical matters, acting more as an authorised Paracelsian *physician,* than as a dispensing chemist. The College Annals on the other hand are quite explicit about what his duties were expected to be; the Fellows intended him to operate in the humble and routine capacity of laboratory assistant to the physicians.

Most of Johnson's preface consisted of separate vitriolic attacks against the two major critics of the College. The first, 'Short Animadversions upon the Book lately Published by one who stiles himself Noah Biggs, Helmonta Psittacum' defended the College from accusations of exclusiveness and neglect of chemical therapy. Biggs was accused of being an uncritical admirer of van Helmont. In the second Johnson turned to 'Friend Culpeper'; numerous points from the preface to his English translation of the London *Pharmacopoeia* were quoted and refuted. Culpeper's background as an apothecary's assistant was emphasised in order to underline how little qualified he was to speak as a medical authority.

Johnson's second publication, *Lexicon chymicum,* was presented as an original work.[222] This elementary dictionary of Paracelsian terminology retained its popularity into the later seventeenth century. However an examination of its contents indicates that Johnson had abstracted his material verbatim from the distinguished Paracelsian *Lexicon* of Martin Ruland.[223] Even the title was closely modelled on that of this earlier work. The most obvious departures from Ruland were: less scrupulous adherence to alphabetical order; the omission of many important terms; and the abbreviation of long definitions. Johnson's greatest problems were caused by Ruland's having interspersed texts in German. These were omitted, or where an entire subject was discussed in German, a page reference to Ruland's *Lexicon* was given. In the numerous cases where Ruland gave only the Latin term and its German

221. *Three Exact Pieces of Leonard Phioravante Knight* (London, 1652); Sudhoff (274), Nos. 239, 371, 505.

222. *Lexicon chymicum cum obscuriorum verborum, et rerum hermeticarum, tum phrasium Paracelsicarum, in scriptis ejus: et aliorum chymicorum, passim occurentium planam explicationem continens* (London, 1652); other editions 1652/3, 1657, 1660. Sudhoff (274), Nos. 371, 372, 380, 391.

223. *Lexicon alchemiae sive dictionarium alchemisticum, cum obscuriorum verborum, & rerum hermeticarum tum Theophrast Paracelsicarum phrasium, planam explicationem continens* (Frankfurt, 1612); Sudhoff (274), No. 291.

synonym, Johnson gave either the Latin term alone, or omitted the entry. Consequently this dictionary cannot be taken as evidence of Johnson's familiarity with Paracelsian medicine, or of his abilities as an expositor. French's modest 'Chemical Dictionary' appended to his *New Light of Alchemy* was similar to Johnson's work. Indeed the latter may have designed his book to compete with French's dictionary.

After these nondescript works by Johnson, neither the Fellows nor their acolytes made further direct excursions into Paracelsian literature. The official laboratory was briefly mentioned in Charleton's account of the College published in 1657, where it was claimed 'that plenty of choice Chymical remedies, [are] daily confected in the Elaboratory belonging to the College, by the directions and prescriptions of the Fellows'.[224] In the official records of the College, however, Johnson and his laboratory quickly sink into obscurity. Whatever the merits of its chemical preoccupations, the College was not successful in convincing critics that it had absorbed sufficient benefit from the Paracelsian teachings. The chemical remedies of the London *Pharmacopoeia*, Johnson's apologias, the laboratory, and the chemical interests of Fellows were dismissed as 'this new way of Mimical Chymistry', designed to build up an immunity against the new medicine.[225] Starkey and his associates believed that a failure to embrace Paracelsus and van Helmont with less than total commitment, signified a negative attitude to the new science which was motivated by vocational conservatism and personal greed. It was not possible for the converted to bring their old wealth into the kingdom of heaven. Complete emancipation from the past was obligatory before a regenerated system of medicine could be evolved. Accordingly *ad hoc* adoption of Paracelsian tenets or individual remedies was unconvincing to the puritan medical reformers. Compromise was as alien to them in the medical context as it was in religious life. Therefore they were impelled to attack compromise with, perhaps, even greater ferocity than that used for totally reactionary opinion. To be exposed to the light and turn from it, was an even greater sin than to live in perpetual darkness. Just as the Presbyterians rather than the Anglicans were regarded as the immediate obstruction to religious reformation, so the College of Physicians was cast in the role of chief enemy to medical reform. In view of the overriding importance of vocational and medical issues, any well-intentioned scientific endeavours among the Fellows appeared to be insignificant or irrelevant. Detached from this situation, the intellectual historian tends to make an entirely different assessment. Even if a vocationally backward attitude is acknowledged to have existed among the Fellows, their intellectual activities may be found to be extremely important for the later development of experimental science.

224. Charleton (46), p.42.
225. Starkey (268), pp.244–5.

(x) Solomon's House

The period of the Republic was a crucial testing time for the College. It was essential to discover some means of maintaining the corporate spirit of the Fellows at a time of spectacular decline in their vocational influence. Adroit political behaviour saved the College from the most immediate threats—a notable contrast to the university colleges. It was also realised that any attempt to reassert the College's vocational authority would have been counterproductive. But the College was in a much stronger position on intellectual matters. The Fellows were not obliged to respond in only a completely passive and guilt-laden manner to the insults of the Paracelsians and Helmontians. The first protective measure was a failure; the poorly-conceived attempt to represent the College as a patron of Paracelsian medicine must have appeared disingenuous to critics, and as a dangerous adventure to many Fellows. However there were other methods of avoiding being stigmatised as the unthinking guardian of authoritarian and ineffective Galenic medicine. It was possible for the College to identify with other expressions of experimental science. For instance by cultivating the experimental philosophies of Bacon and Harvey, the College could take up a position on scientific matters more *avant-garde* than that of the Paracelsians, but without placing cherished medical traditions at risk. It was this policy which set the seal on the survival and even success of the College in the unfavourable atmosphere of the Republic. Hence Walter Charleton was able to portray the Fellows as the legitimate heirs of Bacon, declaring that: 'In the Colledge of Physicians in London . . . you may behold Solomon's House in reality.'[226] Charleton's survey in 1657 of the formidable scientific achievements of the College shows how effectively the defensive position was prepared. Thus on intellectual grounds at least the College could command an unassailable height of esteem.

William Harvey played a crucial role in this reorientation from humanistic Galenism to experimental natural philosophy. As the Lumleian lecturer of the College since 1615 Harvey had established critical standards of commentary on many aspects of anatomy and physiology; the discovery of circulation vindicated this approach. His work exemplified the merits of non-doctrinaire experimental philosophy, combining detailed knowledge of classical authors with dissection, comparative anatomy and vivisection. His model investigation of one organ system created a precedent which could be readily applied to other areas. Perhaps equally important, Harvey's biological philosophy was open-minded and undogmatic, allowing many points of contact with the Helmontians and Paracelsians, while exposing points of divergence with the increas-

226. Charleton (46), p.34. Charleton's description of the College is considered fully in Webster (316). Similar sentiments were expressed in Sprat's *History of the Royal Society* (1667), p.130, and in poetic form by John Collop, a London physician, in *Poesis Rediviva* (London, 1656).

ingly popular iatromechanism.[227] Thus Harvey displayed a philosophical attitude which was unlikely to lead to an uncritical acceptance of any of the new systems developed during the seventeenth century. Indeed Harvey's intellectual stature was sufficient to ensure a relatively calm acceptance of his ideas in England. The revolutionary theory of circulation was accepted by the College without incident. Harvey's medical and vocational influence increased steadily. There were very few critics of Harvey in England and they are not of great importance compared with the younger generation of physicians who enthusiastically supported the new experimental physiology. This group became Harvey's disciples and collaborators in his later work on embryology. In his celebrated journey through Italy Harvey was accompanied by George Ent, who subsequently became one of his closest friends. Having returned home Ent composed one of the first defences of circulation by an Englishman, and became a prominent Fellow of the College during the Republic, acting as its major contact with Harvey.[228] Harvey's influence was not confined to London. During his brief period at Merton College Oxford, he influenced many young scholars who played an active part in science in London and Oxford during the 1650s. At Cambridge Harvey's friend Francis Glisson occupied the Regius chair of physic from 1635. Glisson's activities produced a continuous stream of students sympathetic to the new physiology. As a result of these trends, when the medical faculties revived after the Civil War an entirely new approach to medical science was in evidence. Accordingly the physicians who filtered into the College of Physicians during the Republic tended to reflect the interests and bias of Harvey.[229] No conflict was allowed to develop over adherence to the time-honoured therapeutic techniques of Galenism; the new sciences of comparative anatomy and experimental physiology were cultivated without direct reference to their medical implications. Traditional medical lore sustained vocational life, while the new science was an appealing intellectual diversion. It was realised that the new physiology would inevitably influence medicine, but its immediate findings gave no grounds for a wholesale assault on Galenic theory.

Members of the College embarked upon many research projects, which often had direct reference to Harvey's techniques and concepts. Significantly, much of this work was undertaken at Amen Corner, often in conjunction with the lectures and public meetings at the Col-

227. For Harvey see particularly Walter Pagel, *William Harvey's Biological Ideas* (Basel and New York, 1967). See also Pagel, 'Harvey and Glisson on Irritability with a Note on van Helmont', *Bull. Hist. Med.*, 1967, *41* : 497–514; Pagel and Winder, 'Harvey and the "modern" concept of disease', *Bull. Hist. Med.*, 1968, *42* : 496–509.

228. George Ent, *Apologia pro circulatione sanguinis* (London, 1641); revised edition 1685. Ent's work made reference to Paracelsian chemical theories.

229. Of the list of nine candidates recorded in the preface to the 1650 edition of the *Pharmacopoeia Londinensis*, four (Charles Scarburgh, Thomas Wharton, Christopher Merrett and Samuel Collins) were disciples of Harvey.

lege. This collaborative enterprise was reflected in certain major works published between 1650 and 1660. After Ent's *Apologia pro circulatione sanguinis* (1641) and similar continental works, further direct defences of Harvey were unnecessary. After a period of literary inactivity during the Civil War, the Fellows embarked on a revision of the *Pharmacopoeia Londinensis.*

In 1648 a small committee was established to revise the Jacobean pharmacopoeia.[230] Owing to the influence of de Mayerne, the first edition of 1618 had contained a significant proportion of chemical preparations. The 1650 preface forestalled alarm by assuring the reader that the introduction of 'subsidiary' or 'auxiliary' chemical medicines involved no threat to traditional practices. Furthermore most of the chemical preparations were themselves derived from Dioscorides. Of the innovations, some were from Paracelsian sources, others from anti-Paracelsian writers with chemical interests. The committee concerned with the 1650 revision lacked any convinced advocate of chemical therapy. Indeed Baldwin Hamey, one of its members, had a deep aversion to Paracelsianism. Thus the revised *Pharmacopoeia* had twelve fewer chemical preparations than the 1627 issue (130 compared with 142), and about the same number as the 1618 edition and 1638 issue. Munk's comment on the work of this committee is apposite : 'There is little in the body of the work, or in the address to the reader, or the epilogue, but the usual quaintness of Hamey's style to call for special comment.'[231]

The most notable communal activity of the Fellows during these years was the investigation of rickets, begun by a committee of nine in about 1645. For some years they collected data, exchanged information and held meetings at Amen Corner, before entrusting the composition of a treatise to three of their members. Ultimately, Glisson, who was concerned with theoretical aspects of the problem, so impressed the others that he was entrusted with the composition of the whole work, which enjoyed great success, in both Latin and English versions.[232] From a historical point of view, it is important, as both the first descriptive monograph on rickets and the first pathological work to employ explanations in terms of the circulation of blood. The study bore a strong imprint of Glisson's theories, which were soon to be expressed in an even more important work, *Anatomia Hepatis* (1654). Glisson's monograph on the liver, besides containing an extremely accurate anatomical survey, reassessed the physiology of the abdominal viscera in terms of circulation, and of Glisson's own theory of irritability, which was to become

230. *Pharmacopoeia Londinensis: Collegarum hodie viventium studiis ac symbolis ornatior* (London, 1650); *Pharmacopoeia Londinensis of 1618 Reproduced in Facsimile with a Historical Introduction by George Urdang* (Madison, Wis., 1944). See also Debus (71), pp.152–6 for a discussion of the first edition.

231. Munk (195), iii, p.378; Clark (50), i, pp.281, 287.

232. *Tractatus de rachitide, seu morbo puerili, quo vulgo The Rickets dicatur* (London, 1650).

the central feature of his later writings. *Anatomia Hepatis* was dedicated to the College of Physicians and Cambridge University. On internal and circumstantial evidence, Glisson's text emerges as the culmination of a long period of dissection and discussion at the College. Particular credit was given to his colleagues Ent and Wharton in the frequent textual references to experiments performed with London colleagues. *Anatomia Hepatis* gave considerable prominence to the lymphatic system, which had taken the place of circulation as a subject of European medical controversy. Glisson was primarily concerned with physiological questions, but most other authors concentrated on the priority dispute between Bartholin and Rudbeck in Scandinavia. Glisson complicated this issue by introducing a claim to the independent discovery of the lymph ducts for a candidate of the College of Physicians, George Joyliffe, who lectured on this subject to the College in 1653, at the height of the priority controversy.[233]

Complementary to Glisson's work on the liver was Thomas Wharton's systematic study of the glands, which was also conceived during discussions at the College's anatomical lectures.[234] Wharton's project was begun in 1652 at the instigation of the President. The preface acknowledged the collaboration of colleagues, Glisson and Ent obviously having played a particularly active part.

The published works of Glisson and Wharton, and the edition of Harvey's final work, *De Generatione* (1651) which Ent supervised, furnish ample proof of the acceleration of momentum in anatomical and physiological studies at the College during Harvey's later years. This view is supported by evidence about other research projects, begun during the Republic at the College of Physicians, but reflected in later publications often associated with the Royal Society. Glisson's pupil Charles Scarburgh, probably with the assistance of Wren and Charleton, was analysing the action of muscles according to the principles of mechanics. Taking their clue from a little-known German dissertation, a geometrical model of muscular action was developed which assumed constancy in muscle volume, so contradicting both the ancient and Cartesian explanations which relied on muscle expansion. The correctness of the College's work was later shown by the plethysmograph experiment of another Fellow Jonathan Goddard, at the Royal Society, while William Croune and others evolved an iatrochemical explanation for muscular action.[235] This work and much other physiological speculation at the College of Physicians was probably faithfully reflected in

233. *Anatomia Hepatis,* Chapter XLV; this claim was revived by Timothy Clarke, *Phil. Trans.* No. 35, 1668, pp.672–82; Munk (195), i, p.280. For details of the Scandinavian controversy, W. Kock, 'Anatomical Science and Education in the Seventeenth Century', *Analecta Medico-Historica,* 1968, *3*: 281–92.

234. *Adenographia, seu descriptio glandularum totius corporis* (London, 1656). Dedicated to Hamey, Glisson, John Bathurst and Ent.

235. Charleton (46), p.37. For commentaries on this subject, see Webster (316), pp.400–1.

Charleton's *Oeconomia animalis* (1659), which became one of the most popular textbooks of physiology of the latter part of the century.[236]

Some of the scientific activities of the College were not so sustained or productive. These usually were also more remote from Harvey's work on human anatomy and physiology. In the earlier history of the College, occasional references were made to a physic garden, but the College neither established a garden nor achieved any reputation for expertise in botany. In 1649, when the Oxford Botanic Garden was well-established and many private gardens had achieved celebrity, it was reported that George Bate was offering to endow a garden, at the residence of either Tradescant or the Earl of Arundel.[237] This garden was not established and the idea was never effectively revived. However there were, perhaps in connection with the revision of the pharmacopoeia, some minor figures attached to the College who were eager to promote a more positive interest in botany. The first expression of this enthusiasm was *Phytologia Britannica* (1650), a handlist of English plants produced by William How, an Oxford MA, who was associated with the College.[238] How was a man of wide interests which ranged from mathematics to alchemy and natural history; he established a garden which became the nucleus of the famous Chelsea Physic Garden of the Society of Apothecaries. *Phytologia Britannica* was published anonymously; its title pages gave great prominence to the imprimatur of the President and Censors of the College; it had every appearance of being an official publication. However the quality of this work was extremely poor, even when compared with the herbals of the apothecaries Johnson and Parkinson. There was an obvious need for a revised edition, which was undertaken by a small group of physicians and botanists headed by Christopher Merrett, the College Librarian. Although this catalogue was extended to include animals, fossils, minerals, etc., the quality improved only slightly. It was certainly no competitor to the rival 'Phytologia', begun by the Cambridge academic John Ray in about 1659, after his eminently successful catalogue of Cambridge plants.[239] There was a similarly disappointing conclusion to the work on comparative anatomy undertaken during these years, perhaps at the instigation of George Ent; he had worked with both of the pioneers in this subject, Harvey and the Italian Marcus Aurelius Severino. But the dissections at the College and at the Royal Society, although often mentioned, led to no consequential publications. As with botany, the major advances were made during the later part of

236. Charleton also produced an abbreviated English edition, *The Natural History of Life, Nutrition and Voluntary Motion* (London, 1659).

237. Ephemerides 1649.

238. Annals, 6 December 1650.

239. Merrett, *Pinax rerum naturalium Britannicarum* (London, 1667); Ray, *Catalogus plantarum circa Cantabrigiam nascentium* (Cambridge, 1660); *idem, Catalogus plantarum Angliae* (London, 1670). Ray's English flora contained much information on the medical uses of listed species.

the century by a few determined outside investigators, such as Ray, Grew, Willis and Malpighi.

The successful collaborative researches undertaken by the members of the College of Physicians were extremely important in re-establishing the corporate spirit of their institution. It was perhaps a desire to encourage these fertile developments and bolster the morale of his medical colleagues, which prompted Harvey to endow the College with premises suitable for these activities. This important gesture was made with Harvey's characteristic modesty. The College responded promptly and graciously to his anonymous offer to endow 'a library and a repository for simples and rarities'.[240] The 'Musaeum Harveianum' was opened in February 1654.[241] This name for his institution is not previously mentioned in the records of the College. Its choice is probably not without significance. The celebrated Danish physician Olaus Worm had established a large collection of rarities relating to medicine, natural history and antiquities, and this collection was augmented by materials sent from all parts of Europe by Worm's correspondents. There were many indirect associations linking Harvey with Worm.[242] In England an analogous development occurred at the house of John Tradescant in South Lambeth; the College had already considered this as the site for its botanical garden, which would have been based on the rich collection of exotic plants collected on Tradescant's American voyage. Equally notable was the Tradescant Museum, a collection ranging from *objets d'art* to medical specimens.[243] Even before the Tradescant catalogue was published, the museum was widely visited, arousing the curiosity and envy of Elias Ashmole, who was ultimately to gain possession of this collection. At the end of the century the museum became the nucleus of the Museum Ashmoleanum at Oxford. Harvey probably recognised that an institution of this kind could serve as a focus for the wide-ranging enquiries of the Fellows. Thus, by establishing a museum as well as a library, the College might provide a repository for its collections and also encourage discussions of research. Harvey's friends would have applauded this idea; quite possibly he collaborated in the planning of the museum along these lines.

At the official opening of the Museum, according to Aubrey 'a noble

240. Annals, 4 July 1651; Munk (195), iii, pp.323–4; Clark (50), i, pp.285–6, 298–9; Keynes (175), pp.397–406. Clark's assertion that 'Harvey did not intend to promote any new kind of organisation for research' (p.300), takes an unduly pessimistic view of Harvey's bequest.

241. Annals, 2 February 1653/4.

242. Thomas Bartholin, Worm's son-in-law and enthusiastic disciple of Harvey, was the most important link: E. Gotfredsen, 'The Reception of Harvey's Doctrine in Denmark', *Acta Medica Scandinavica,* Supplement (Copenhagen, 1956). Axel Garboe, *Thomas Bartholin* (Copenhagen, 1949: Acta Hist. Scient. Nat. et Med. ed. Univ. Hauniensis vol. 5).

243. John Tradescant the younger, *Musaeum Tradescantianum; or a collection of rarities* (London, 1656); M. Allen, *The Tradescants, their Plants, Garden and Museum* (London, 1964). Ashmole's *Diary,* ed. Josten (*op. cit.* above, p.129, n.97) makes many references to this collection.

building of Roman Architecture (of Rustique work, with Corinthian pillasters)', Harvey's scientific protégés dominated the proceedings. Ent gave the major address; Glisson was elected to the Anatomical Lectureship, and Merrett was nominated as the first Librarian. As reward for his munificence Harvey was elected President of the College.[244] The statutes of the museum were worked out in minute detail by a committee, which again was dominated by Harvey's friends. It was explicitly ordered that the library was to include books relating to the sciences in general, as well as to medicine. Only chemistry was conspicuously absent from this catalogue, which included besides medicine, geometry, geography, cosmography, astronomy, music, optics, zoology, physics, mechanics and accounts of voyages of exploration.[245] Merrett's catalogue of the Harveian Museum and Library indicates the liberal scope of the collections, which were approaching the range of the Musaeum Tradescantianum. Merrett was also translating and compiling a lengthy commentary for an Italian work on glassmaking.[246] Evidence relating to the museum and its curator shows that the outward-looking course advocated by the statutes was diligently pursued.

During these years there was a rapid accumulation of material from diverse sources. The only discordant note recorded was over Harvey's request for the Museum to display pathological specimens obtained by the Helmontian George Thomson. This episode indicates Harvey's disinterested scientific attitude, which could not be shared by his younger colleagues who were at that time engaged in fierce controversy with the Helmontians. It would have been inappropriate to give publicity to the Helmontians in the Harveian Museum. Hence yet another cause for the embitterment of relationships between the College and Helmontians emerged, the repercussions of which went on into the restoration.[247]

An additional spur to scientific activity was provided by another bequest by Harvey. This was the annual Harveian oration, which was designed to encourage Fellows to 'search and study out the secrets of Nature by way of Experiment'.[248] Relatively little is known about these lectures, but the one delivered by Scarburgh in 1662 shows much

244. Annals, 30 September 1654; Keynes (175), p.400.

245. Annals, 26 June 1654 – 29 June 1656. The Rules were printed at the beginning of Christopher Merrett's *Catalogus librorum, instrumentorum Chirurgicorum, rerum curiosarum, Exoticarumque Coll. Med. Lond. quae habentur in Musaeo Harveano* (London, 1660). Rule 17 ordered 'Praeter libros medicos, illos potissimum in Musaeo huic commodos atque idoneos judicamus, qui vel Geometriam, vel Geographiam, vel Cosmographicam, vel Astronomiam, vel Musicen, vel Opticen, vel Historia Animalium, vel Physicen, vel Mechanicam tractant, vel ad remotiores terrarum regiones itineraria complectuntur.' For a translation of the Rules, Keynes (175), pp.401–2.

246. *The Art of Glass* (London, 1662). The author of the Italian text was Antonio Neri; Sir Charles Dodds, 'Christopher Merrett, FRCP, First Harveian Librarian', *Proc. Roy. Soc. Med.*, 1954, *47*: 1053–6.

247. Webster (316).

248. Munk (195), iii, p.361; Keynes (175), p.404.

sympathy for the ideals expressed by Harvey. In an historical account of scientific studies in the College, Scarburgh concentrated on its achievements in anatomy and physiology, which were attributed primarily to the influence of Harvey. Other formative influences on the general scientific outlook of the Fellows singled out for mention were the works of Gilbert, Bacon and Digby. In so doing Scarburgh was making a fair assessment of the outlook of the College during the Republic.[249]

The members of the College of Physicians were effective exponents of experimental philosophy, but they developed a characteristic outlook which differed markedly from that of their rivals, the Paracelsian practitioners. The viewpoint adopted by each of these two groups was very much influenced by their respective social positions, as well as by their political and religious alliances. The Fellows exhibited virtually no response to the social crisis which accompanied the Civil War, although medicine was directly relevant to many problems. As much as possible they preserved the vocational role for their medical élite which had been defined under the Tudors. While awaiting the passing of the storm, they reorganised their statutes, revised the *Pharmacopoeia* and made every effort to preserve their corporate identity. Harvey as already indicated paid considerable attention to the enhancement of corporate aspects of the College. He enjoined the Fellows to 'continue mutual love and affection' and to remember that 'Concordia res parvae crescunt, discordia magnae dilabuntur'.[250] The profession of physician continued to be reasonably lucrative, supported by a social élite which represented a rapidly diminishing segment of the London population. For this inward-looking group of practitioners, there was no incentive to abandon traditional practices or professional affiliations, which had served the educational and intellectual requirements of generations of physicians. These traditions were part of a system which had slowly perfected itself during the humanistic revival in medicine. New ideas were absorbed, but not to the extent of significantly disturbing the equilibrium of Galenic medicine. Compromise with Paracelsian or Helmontian medicine could only be countenanced at a superficial level. A greater degree of acquiescence to new doctrines would have brought ideologically dangerous associations. Thus neither the new edition of the *Pharmacopoeia* nor the literary activities of William Johnson gives any real impression of significant response to Paracelsian medicine. The only important penetration of iatrochemical ideas came in the sphere of physiology, where chemistry provided a convenient basis for the description of physiological mechanisms. Thus Glisson, Ent, and Willis displayed a degree of familiarity with iatrochemical writings which

249. L. M. Payne, 'Sir Charles Scarburgh's Harveian Oration', *Journal of the History of Medicine*, 1957, *12*: 158–64.

250. Inaugural address at the establishment of the Harveian Orations, Munk (195), iii, p.361; Keynes (175), p.404.

would not be anticipated from their vocational affiliations. Ent's *Apologia* and Glisson's *Anatomia Hepatis* introduced iatrochemical ideas in as uncontroversial a manner as possible. But such findings became extremely difficult to integrate with humoral theory. Glisson's explanation of rickets for example suggested that the new physiology had an important medical dimension. His work was paralleled at Oxford by that of Thomas Willis, whose synthesis of Harveian physiology and iatrochemistry was first announced in his work on fevers published in 1659.[251]

The work of Glisson and Willis had little appeal for the Paracelsians. Attention to fine anatomical detail was regarded as attention not paid to the fundamental questions of medicine. A negative attitude to Paracelsus was taken as a sign of reactionary social and intellectual attitudes. From the point of view of the Puritan Revolution, the intellectual priorities of the College resulted in an insensitivity to the severe social problems of the time and a lack of interest in proposals to establish more adequate medical services for the community. However from the different perspective of the historian of science this social conservatism was responsible for directing effort into fundamental anatomical and physiological research, reinforcing Harvey's influence, and laying the foundations for modern medicine. This was achieved without attacking Galen; the new physiology of Harvey seemed to be a logical continuation of the work begun by the humanist scholars of the Renaissance. Accordingly the College of Physicians accomplished the feat of promoting experimental science while acting as faithful guardian to a system of classical medicine.

251. For further discussion of this subject see A. B. Davis, *Circulation Physiology and Medical Chemistry in England 1650–1680* (Lawrence, Kansas, 1973).

V

Dominion Over Nature

'For man by the fall fell at the same time from his state of innocency and from his dominion over creation. Both of these losses however can even in this life be in some part repaired; the former by religion and faith, the latter by arts and sciences. For creation was not by the curse made altogether and for ever a rebel, but in virtue of that charter, 'In the sweat of thy face shalt thou eat bread', it is now by various labours (not certainly by disputations or idle magical ceremonies), subdued to the supplying of man with bread; that is, to the uses of human life.'

Francis Bacon, *Novum Organum,* Bk.II, aphorism 52.

'But the new world of the sciences and the new geographical world do not agree in the old being more refined than the new. On the contrary, it is certain that the augmentations to the arts show themselves greatly superior to those we have, so as not only to bend nature gently, but to conquer and subdue, even to shake to her foundations. For it almost always happens that what is easy to discover is infirm in performance, since the roots of things where the strength resides are covered deeply. But if to any one given to the love and worship of contemplation, this frequent and honourable mention of works sounds somewhat harsh and offensive, let him be assured that he thwarts his own wishes. For in nature works are not only benefits to life, but pledges of truth. The rule of religion that a man should justify his faith by works applies also in natural philosophy; knowledge should be proved by its works. For truth is rather revealed and established by the evidence of works rather than by disputation, or even sense. Hence the human intellect and social conditions are enriched by one and the same means.'

Francis Bacon, *Cogitata et Visa, Works,* iii, p.612.

(i) Dominion Over Nature

Puritan attitudes to technology and agriculture were developed in the context of speculation about the primitive condition of man. In the Garden of Eden Adam willingly submitted to the discipline of work and his labour was pleasant. Because of this obedience he was given complete control over his environment, until the Fall. Then he and his descendants were punished by being condemned to irksome toil. Genesis and *Paradise Lost* described this transformation in identical terms: 'In the sweat of thy face shalt thou eat bread, till thou return unto the ground.' Man's disobedience caused God to 'change his pleasure into labour, and his ease into industry'.[1] But even after this fateful episode God had permitted man to turn the situation to advantage. Through penitent labour degenerate man was allowed to evolve an ordered civilisation in which the human condition was ameliorated to a certain degree. Furthermore the human intellect perceived a distant goal of purity and bliss. This image of the New Eden was particularly clear at certain stages in the history of civilisation and it acted as an incentive to attempt to transcend the degenerate condition.

The Puritan Revolution was one of these periods of utopian insight and endeavour. The practical arts were God's gift to His undeserving children. It was a constant source of amazement and consolation

> 'Why plowing, building, ruling and the rest,
> Or most of those arts, whence our lives are blest
> By cursed Cains race invented be.'[2]

With the protestant emphasis on an ascetic and active approach to vocational and communal life, the arts were 'not to be despised, and a vertue to be praised'. Persistent application to the practical arts was regarded as an ideal test of obedience.[3] Because man was 'shut out of Paradice into the subburbs of this world', he might only return to grace through a relentless search for purity, both in personal life and in nature. To struggle with the environment was to attempt to restore nature to its primitive purity. Thus life was a continuous course of 'chymistry', in which it was ordained 'that we should labour to get our bread, and other necessary things for this present life, as Natures Labourers, not lazily, but in the sweat of our browes, that by this means, by laying the Cross upon us which we should bear with patience, it might stir up our industry in this LAND of LABOUR to attain the fruits of Terrene and Coelestiall Wisdome.'[4] Such sentiments reflect the emergence of a social ethic which placed considerable emphasis on unremitting toil and which accorded high esteem to the manual arts. This ethical viewpoint is characteristic of the followers of Bacon and Paracelsus discussed below. As an inducement to active participation in commercial and industrial life, the same social ethic has been regarded by Weber and others as a major source for the rise of capitalism in areas of protestant, and especially Calvinist or puritan influence.

1. Genesis 3:19; Milton, *Paradise Lost,* x, lines 205–6; Pettus (209), p.153.
2. Donne, *Progress of the Soul,* II, lines 514–16.
3. Calvin (43), pp.151–2.
4. Pinnel (216), p.96. Capitals as in the original. Similar terms were used by John Elliston: 'And herein lieth the Mystery, or central science of the high Philosophical Work in this Spagyrick Art, which consummates the Cure not only for the Body, but also for the Soul.' Preface to *Signatura Rerum* (31), sig.A4r.

Adam was a source of inspiration for the experimental philosophers, who were encouraged to value 'harmless industry (it seems one of the pleasures of Paradise)'; to serve the community, and freely to communicate scientific information.[5] Increasingly scientific activity was influenced by utilitarian criteria. Increasingly the unproductive, scholastic disputes were judged to be subversive to the active Christian life. Adoption of the idea of the sanctity of manual labour encouraged a more direct involvement with nature, in the quest for productive knowledge and service to the community. The final reward for such exertions might be man's return from the suburbs into paradise. The restoration of dominion over nature became one of the major aspirations of the Great Instauration.

The academic scholar and the gloved physician became subjects for censure. Colliers and craftsmen were held up as models of virtue by Bacon and the Paracelsians, who believed that the divorce of scholars from craftsmen had been a serious disadvantage to western society. However, industrial developments and the acceleration of economic development since the Reformation could be seen as indications of a reawakening. The pioneer experimental philosophers believed that unification of effort could lead to even more substantial achievements. Although the arts were generally thought to reflect God's beneficence to fallen man, they were often traced back to the more perfect age; indeed it was sometimes stated that 'all lawfull and profitable Arts, were known and practised of Adam'.[6] Adam was usually described as a gardener and naturalist. However mining and metalworking were also thought to have been among his highest attainments, and he was even credited with abilities in transmutation and other chemical processes. Considerable importance was attached to metallurgy, and it was regarded as a discredit to the English nation that its mineral resources had been poorly exploited. Adam was supposed to have known gold, bdellium and onyx; these were immediately useful, but they were also symbolic of his wider attainments in applied chemistry: 'God placed him in Paradise, and commanded him to dig or till the Earth: As also a Refiner; otherwise, why should it be made known to him, that the River Pison did encompass the Land of Havilah where Gold was, if Adam were not to wash and refine it from the less valuable Earth?'[7] By exegetical ingenuity, Adam could be transformed from a simple gardener into a proficient metallurgist.

Speculative reconstructions of the lives of Adam's progeny amplified the picture of ancient technology and agriculture. Most of the patriarchs were thought to have played some part in the development of the crafts. For instance Tubal-Cain, son of Lamech, was 'instructor of every arti-

5. Pettus (209), p.27.
6. Gibbens (115), p.204. For a discussion of this subject, see Williams (334), pp.144–8.
7. Pettus (209), sig.B2r. Genesis 2:11–12.

ficer in brass and iron'. This ancient period was thought to have been marked by the development of the whole range of refining and alloying techniques.[8] The secrets of medicine and transmutation had diffused to the Egyptians, before being fully restored to the Jewish race by Moses. In response to those who claimed supernatural powers for Moses, it was emphasised that his knowledge was based on 'the laudable Sciences of Arithmetick, Politicks, natural and lawful Magick . . . the Art of Medicine, and knowledge of natural and artificial things'.[9] From Moses this sacred wisdom was imparted to Bezaleel and Aholiab, who were supposed to have possessed 'all manner of workmanship', as well as knowledge of the general principles of natural philosophy. They were familiar with gold, silver and brass work, the cutting of stones, wood carving, embroidery, weaving and probably dyeing, in fact 'any manner of cunning work'. Accordingly Bezaleel and Aholiab became models for the Christian virtuoso. For example Descartes at first seemed to Henry More to possess the virtues of Bezaleel and Aholiab, but on later reflection More felt that weaknesses in Cartesian metaphysics rendered this comparison inappropriate. Descartes was not, after all, the proponent of a truly Christian philosophy.[10] Ultimately divine wisdom was vested in Solomon, whose empire and wealth were established on technological and scientific foundations. The *Song of Solomon* presented an optimistic account of the potentialities of fallen man. Indeed, the Fall was almost a blessing in disguise, leading to a more resilient intellect and greater maturity of judgement. By persistently resisting temptation and continually reconsecrating himself to divine ends, Solomon was rewarded with dominion over all things.

The sparkling image of the agricultural and technological proficiency of the ancient Hebrew culture was contrasted with the subsequent backwardness of the Roman Empire and catholic Christendom. These institutions had buried knowledge in the cells of monks and friars, or allowed it to be concealed by adepts. Artisans and miners were increasingly impeded by their traditions and mysteries, until they were reduced to a bare subsistence. The sign of reawakening came with a handful of prophets led by Paracelsus, who were gifted with an 'insatiable desire for the knowledge of the secrets of nature'. A dedication like theirs to experimental science was regarded as the only way to restore true knowledge. Following the example of Paracelsus, various authors had systematically studied mining and metalworking. Germany was held up as an example to the rest of Europe as the pioneer of technological and religious reformation.[11]

It is apparent from the above comments that it was not merely dis-

8. Webster, *Metallographia* (327), p.2; Genesis 4:22; 41:42.

9. Webster (327), p.8.

10. Exodus 35:30–5; More, *Conjectura Cabbalistica* (190), p.104. Webster (327), pp.2–3; Hartlib (144), pp.9–18.

11. Webster (327), pp.15, 17–19.

interested historical curiosity which inspired such widespread interest in the technological attainments of Jewish antiquity. Writers were concerned to give a vivid impression of the great power sacrificed at the Fall, in order to galvanise their contemporaries into an effort to restore the primitive condition. John Beale's letters to Hartlib frequently cited the biblical precedent. He recalled the 'devine Wisdome exemplified & executed by Moses' which could 'effect strange alterations in the World'. Solomon had been able to augment his wealth by similar powers. Daniel had recovered and reformed this knowledge, and predicted that a future golden age of knowledge was to come. Hence the reformers of the seventeenth century were prompted to ask: 'What Magique . . . doe wee find in all or any of his enterprizes, or what methode of Wisdome, or of knowledge, or of power, or of acquiring wealth, which is still allowable to the progress & industry of Gods deare people?' Beale was optimistic that 'powerful mysteries' would be placed in the hands of those who adopted a regime of holy discipline and who were pledged to live free from controversy:

> 'And as Man is thus by Light restord to the dominion over his own house, soe, by Magnalias that are brought to light, Hee is restored to a dominion over all the beasts of the field, over the birds of the ayre & over the fishes of the Sea. Here you must adde the discovery of, or dominion over all the Workes of God; the conversion of Stones into Metalls & backe againe; of poisons into powerful Medicines, of bushes, thornes & thickets into Wine & oyle, & of all the Elements to take such guise as Man by divine Wisdome commands. . . . And let all these Naturall, Artificiall & Spiritual Wonders bee allwayes recorded to the prayse of the Most High.'[12]

This ecstatic vision of the scientific gifts of the elect was the development of a view found in the *Instauratio Magna* of Bacon, the philosophical reformer who most influenced Beale. Although Bacon was averse to drawing scientific principles from the scriptures, he fully accepted that they, like the classical fables, conveyed moral precepts which were important for the natural philosopher. Bacon thought it noteworthy that the most ancient biblical records were careful to 'honour the remembrance of the inventor both of music and works in metal'. This was thought to reflect the susceptibilities of Moses, who was himself skilled in these arts. Bacon's greatest curiosity was reserved for 'Salomon the king, as out of a branch of his wisdom extraordinarily petitioned and granted from God, is said to have written a natural history of all that is green from the cedar to the moss, . . . and also of all that liveth and moveth' (I Kings 4:33). As a reward Solomon was granted power over nature and a 'mighty empire in Gold'. Above all Bacon

12. Letters from Beale to Hartlib, 15 September 1657 & 26 March 1659, HP LI.

admired Solomon's modesty and dedication, pronouncing that 'The Glory of God is to conceal a thing: the glory of the King to search it out' (Proverbs 25:2). Solomon's work in compiling natural histories was regarded as an example to all future ages, of conscientious scientific enterprise.[13] It is consistent with this view that Solomon, to whom God gave 'knowledge of holy things, made him rich in his travails, and multiplied the fruits of his labours' (Wisdom of Solomon 10:10), became the inspiration for *New Atlantis*. The head of this utopian state, named Salomona, was credited with many of the moral attributes and interests of Solomon. Accordingly he founded an ideal scientific institution, appropriately naming it 'Solomon's House', after his Jewish predecessor. Among its cherished possessions were the natural histories of Solomon, which western scholars believed had not survived from antiquity.

The above illustrations underline the strength of the protestant belief that the fall of man was not irreversible; spiritual salvation would be accompanied by the renewal of his dominion over nature. This would repeat the experience of Solomon and complete the prophecy of Daniel. Support for this view was derived from the *Corpus Hermeticum*, a source influenced by the biblical texts quoted above, but generally accorded greater antiquity by sixteenth-century authorities. The hermetic writer, supposedly the Egyptian prophet Hermes Trismegistus, strongly emphasised the power of any of the elect to operate as a magus, controlling nature by spiritual powers. The hermetic texts attracted a considerable following during the Renaissance, inspiring dreams of knowledge and power for the adept which underlined the potentialities of science, but ran counter to the basic moral values of Andreae, or Bacon and his followers. Hence although the superficial literary influence of the hermetic texts was pervasive the hermetic philosophy was treated with considerable reserve by the experimental philosophers. By contrast the scriptures prescribed a form of science which was compatible with the protestant ethic. Bacon's ideas about the Fall, the residual wisdom of Jewish antiquity and the moral conditions for restoration, were completely in keeping with the dominant Calvinist tradition in England. His 'experimental philosophy' represented a striking reaction against the hermetic worldview, involving a 'scientific ideal of co-operative, diligent research . . . opposed to esoteric philosophies thriving on allusion, ecstasy, intuition, mystery . . . inspired by Moses [Moschus], Zoroaster, Hermes, Plato, Plotinus, Proclus, and pseudo-Dionysius.'[14] Bacon's attitude undoubtedly represented an over-reaction against metaphysical speculation, but he was concerned to prevent the demanding regimen of experimental philosophy from becoming contaminated by the seduc-

13. *Valerius Terminus,* Bacon *Works,* iii, pp.219–20. See also, *Instauratio Magna, Works,* i, p.124; *Novum Organum, Works,* i, p.222; *Cogitata et Visa, Works,* iii, p.610.

14. Rossi (250), p.56. Corrected quotation.

tive attractions of hermeticism. Thus the idea of the return of man's dominion over nature was basically biblical in inspiration. The hermeticist interpretation of this concept was only accepted by the English Baconians to a limited degree.

Scriptural sources were also relevant to such specific theoretical issues as the theory of matter. At many points it was relevant to speculate about the origins and nature of elements, their degree of permanence and their capacity for growth and transmutation. The dominant Aristotelian theory of elements was assailed by rival theories which were more consistent with biblical cosmogony. Although the Paracelsian theory of matter, which attained such widespread influence in the seventeenth century, is generally described in terms of the three principles, salt, sulphur and mercury, it defies such simple exposition. Paracelsus believed that his three principles were more fundamental than the four elements of Aristotle, but they too rested on a complex ontology. The problem of fundamental importance was the nature of the prime matter. Here Paracelsus drew insight from the opening of the fourth gospel; the foundation of the world was the Word (Fiat) and the Word became Flesh. With the materialisation of the Word, God created water as the matrix or seed of all other creatures. At one level water was an incorporeal spiritual entity, at another the material substratum for the basic chemical principles.[15] By this means the Paracelsian cosmogony could be firmly related to the text 'the Spirit of God moved upon the face of the waters' (Genesis 1:2). From the prime matrix emerged salt, sulphur and mercury, the *tria prima,* which were the source of the four Aristotelian elements, or all species of the mineral, plant and animal kingdoms. At this stage it is not necessary to give a detailed review of this theory of matter, except to emphasise that each of the three principles differed from the common chemical of that name. Finally the conceptual differences between the Aristotelian-four and Paracelsian-three element theories are so considerable that it is not possible to regard them as simply related.[16] Even the adoption of *three* principles was related to the trinitarian basis of the 'Triune' word Fiat. The Godhead had a threefold nature which was reflected in his Word, which in turn marked the beginning of heaven, earth and all creatures.[17] This trinitarian relationship of the three-principle theory was also emphasised in Jacob Boehme's *Signatura Rerum*, which was translated by John Elliston in 1651.

Such speculations about the ultimate nature and origins of matter were not divorced from practical chemistry. For instance, van Helmont modified the Paracelsian theory to derive all entities from a single pri-

15. W. Pagel, *Paracelsus* (Basel, 1955), pp.95–8.

16. For detailed discussion of Paracelsus's theory of matter, see Pagel, *op. cit.; idem,* 'The Prime Matter of Paracelsus', *Ambix* 1961, *11*: 112–35. K. Goldammer, 'Bemerkungen zur Structur des Kosmos und des Materie bei Paracelsus', in H. H. Eulner *et al.* (eds.), *Medizin-geschichte in unserer Zeit* (Stuttgart, 1971), pp.121–44.

17. Pinnel (216), pp.31–3.

mary principle, which he identified as water. This viewpoint could be related to the creation story, in which the basic divisions of the cosmos were described in terms of dividing the waters (Genesis 1:2-9). Furthermore God said: 'Let the waters bring forth abundantly the moving creature that hath life, and fowl that may fly above the earth in the open firmament of heaven.' (Genesis 1:20). Van Helmont illustrated this principle by his celebrated quantitative willow-tree experiment, which appeared to prove decisively that plants were derived solely from water. Robert Boyle was among the many experimentalists who repeated this trial; at a more practical level, it provided the incentive for a wide range of water-culture experiments which were fundamental to the investigation of plant nutrition and the principles of crop fertilisation.[18]

One of the most important aspects of the theory of matter related to the processes of chemical change. There was general opposition to the scholastic view that the types of substance were generated in the earth at the moment of creation. Following Paracelsus, the major English writers Jorden, Webster and Pettus, opposed the view that the species of minerals were commixtures of the four Aristotelian elements. They adopted a more hylozoic theory, stressing the unity of the organic and mineral kingdoms. Minerals were thought to have a genesis and growth analogous to that of higher organisms. In elaborating this view, most writers followed the Paracelsian view that all generation was from 'seeds' bearing the specific characteristics of each chemical substance. The seminal forms lay dormant in the earth until the appropriate conditions for their growth appeared. Jorden proposed that 'there is a Seminarie Spirit of all minerals in the bowels of the earth, which meeting with convenient matter, and diuvant causes, is not idle, but doth proceed to produce minerals, according to the nature of it, and the matter which it meets withal.' Similarly Webster believed that 'in Vegetables there is a seminal spirit, vapour, or steam, that doth transmute and assimilate the juice of every Plant into this or that individual: . . . and in stones there is a petrifying quality, vapour or steam, that doth turn the matter aggregated, into the nature of this or that stone.'[19] From the moment of creation God 'hath plac'd Metals and Minerals in the Mountains, Valleys and Veins of the Earth, and causeth them to grow there.'[20] Such views could aptly be supported by close similarities between the veins of minerals, and fronds of plants; the earth appeared to be a vast organic form, which was constantly in a state of flux and generation. Consequently it could readily be believed that subterranean waters were 'circulating' in the manner of body fluids, that the minerals in exhausted mines would regenerate given suitable conditions, or that given suitable circumstances minerals could be transformed into higher

18. Partington (205), ii, pp.223–4; Webster (314).
19. Jorden (166), pp.84–5; Webster (327), p.46.
20. Pettus, *Fleta Minor* (London, 1676), preface. This work is a translation of Lazarus Ercker, *Was einem Probirer zu Wissen von nothen ist.*

species. Indeed, perhaps all minerals were naturally evolving towards the state of gold. Instances of minerals in a 'liquid' condition were supposed to provide evidence for transitional states. It was believed that by investigating the properties of mineral waters and conditions in mines, the process of generation could be understood and eventually repeated in the laboratory: 'These diversities of metals being come to pass by accidental causes, is the cause that Art (being Natures Ape by imitation) hath endeavoured to perform that wherein Nature was hindered.'[21] The laboratories of Solomon's House investigated such processes of imitation, with the aim of discovering methods of stimulating nature into greater productivity. Gradually the emphasis shifted from the straightforward exploration and exploitation of natural resources, towards research into methods of artificial production. Hence nature was not only a valuable treasury of natural products but also both stimulus and guide to the creation of useful materials by human ingenuity. Any worker who 'shall refuse no pains and difficulties to get experience, by the industrie of his handie work, he shall (if the grace of the most high favour be infused into him) bring forth far greater things out of the open bosome of Nature, than they seem to promise at first sight.'[22]

Just as the early colonial adventurers dreamed of discovering rich hoards of gold, so many of the natural philosophers were hypnotised by the quest for the philosopher's stone. Thus science could rapidly lead to a Faustian degeneration of the intellect and a self-imposed isolation from society into pretentious and secretive brotherhoods like the Rosicrucians. The principle of transmutation was almost universally accepted by seventeenth-century chemists, but although this problem was used as a means to attract interest in chemistry, the moral temper of experimental natural philosophy precluded excessive concentration on the transmutation of base metals into gold. In *Macaria,* the traveller's offer to demonstrate transmutation is greeted with enthusiasm. Plattes used this device to capture interest for his scheme for a state laboratory, which was primarily intended to produce chemical medicines and yield improvements in chemical technology and agriculture. Transmutation was regarded as a subsidiary long-term objective. This view is substantiated by Plattes's other writings. In his metallurgical work *A Discovery of Subterraneal Treasure* (1639), one short section of three pages was taken up with transmutation, while the remainder of the text was devoted to refining and assaying. More surprisingly, his 'Caveat

21. Gerard Malynes, *Lex mercatoria* (186), p.256. This section of Malynes's work was reprinted as an appendix to Hartlib's *Chymical Addresses* (144).

22. Plattes (218), pp.40–3; Hartlib (144), p.85. French gave a similar admonition to those seeking after transmutation; they should 'inquire into the Nature of Mines, and Metalls, as also of Vegetables, . . . thus Art is not placed in fortune, or casuall invention, but in a reall Science . . . without the knowledge of naturall things, especially in the Minerall Kingdome, thou shalt be like a blind man that walketh by use.' *New Light of Alchymie* (108), pp.119–20.

for Alchymists' was primarily concerned with underlining the responsibility of all aspiring adepts to seek 'perfection in the knowledge of nature, especially in minerals, that by his own speculation and practice, without help of books, he can write a rational discourse of either animals, vegetables, or minerals, in such a solid way, that no man can contradict it, without shame upon fair tryal, the question being rightly stated.'[23] Bacon, Jorden, French, Webster, Pettus and Boyle joined Plattes in admitting the possibility of transmutation into gold, but the part which this played in their writings was very limited. They were much more concerned with evolving fruitful methods and in accumulating a reliable body of information about the natural world. It was recognised that the technological application of scientific knowledge offered a means to national economic prosperity. From a moral point of view this was regarded as a much safer route to utopia, than that of investing all energies in the search for transmutation into gold.

In Eden all human needs had been satisfied by pleasant and diverting labours. In later ages dominion over nature would not be granted so readily. The magus or Rosicrucian tended to be mesmerised by dreams of personal grandeur; he adopted unproductive methods and was inclined to dissipate his energies in spiritual and literary virtuosity. By contrast the experimental philosopher was confident that his dedication to social service, open communication of useful knowledge and adoption of rigorous empirical procedures, were consistent with his Christian moral code.

The followers of Bacon aimed at becoming 'servants' or 'ministers' of nature. By collaborating with enlightened craftsmen they hoped to prepare the ground for a technological revolution. During the mounting economic crisis between 1620 and 1650 such a prospect may have appeared absurdly utopian, but it was taken seriously by a significant body of intellectuals and craftsmen. Given their views about providence and the millennium such ambitious goals appeared to be attainable and realistic.

Baconian science became an integral part of plans for economic development. Gerard Malynes excused the insertion of a section on the generation of metals into his economics treatise because he held 'it not amisse for a man to have knowledge in most or in all things: for by this study of Alcumie, men may attain to many good experiments of distillations Chimicall, Fire-works, and other excellent observations in Nature.' Perhaps one positive result of this interest was his claim to be able to manufacture alum at one-sixth of the price charged by the state monopoly.[24]

23. Plattes, 'Caveat', in Hartlib (144), pp.85–6.

24. Malynes (186), p.180; Price (228), pp.83–4. Bacon adopted a similar attitude to alchemy, claiming that the search for gold had 'brought to light a great number of good and fruitful experiments, as well for the disclosing of nature, as for the use of mans life.' Bacon *De Augmentis* (13), p.21; *Novum Organum,* Bacon *Works,* i, pp.173–4.

Jorden and especially Plattes and Webster were depressed by the obvious neglect and backwardness of mining and metalworking in England compared with Germany. They were confident that England was rich in mineral resources, but exploration and exploitation had been neglected, owing to the inadequacies of the practitioners, the inefficiency of industrial organisation and the failure to take advantage of technological improvements. Plattes claimed to have been since childhood 'a strict observer of the great losse that came to this country, partly through ignorance, and partly through negligence, in raysing that benefit out of the superficiall, and subterraneall Treasure of the Earth'.[25] His experience of mining and agriculture was similar; both called out for rationalisation and innovation. Plattes adopted an empiricist approach to knowledge; with 'strong love to knowledge, [I] addicted my self so strongly to true experiments, judging no knowledge perfect till it was thereby confirmed'. Having established sound experimental procedures he believed that it would be possible 'to turne Plowe-men into Philosophers; and make them to excell their predecessors, even as a learned Physician excelleth an Empiricke'. Improvements in agriculture and mining were seen as the only economically sound solution to the problem of the distressed poor.[26] Recognition of the economic implications of experimental science was apparent in Plattes's first publications in 1639, and again in *Macaria* composed two years later. *Macaria* was designed to interest the members of the Long Parliament in scientific planning.

Plattes was not the only writer to stress the economic relevance of science. Webster attributed the general economic superiority of the Dutch to their extreme diligence 'in all manual performances, while the English are supine and idle'. Thus it was common to find that raw materials which were mined in England, such as black lead, were controlled by the Dutch. He generalised:

> 'The Common Disease or Condition of the English Nation that we are accustomed too much to dote upon foreign commodities, and imported Wares; which makes them negligent in looking into, or improving their own native commodities, and such things as their own Country yields.'[27]

In Webster's view science could lead to economic self-sufficiency, greater self-esteem and higher international status. His educational tract *Academiarum Examen* (1654) pointed out that the prevailing form of higher education failed to equip the élite for an economically active role. He therefore joined other educational reformers in proposing radical reform of the scholastic curriculum; the universities could then

25. Plattes (218), sig.B1v–2r.

26. Plattes (217), p.6, sig. a1v. For a similar point of view see Blith (27), sig. a1r–2r.

27. Webster (327), pp.24–5.

produce scholars who would be able to apply their knowledge of medicine, chemistry or mechanics to everyday problems. Pettus believed that knowledge about gold 'The Cordiall of all humane Commerce' was an essential part of education. In order to appreciate this subject, a general knowledge was required of metallurgy and mineralogy, which in turn would be 'noble invitations to the Study of Geography, Hydrography and other Sciences, thereby to learn the Wonders of the Land and Deeps; insinuating also to us the richest Minerals, Plants, and Precious Stones'. Then would follow study of streams, rivers and finally the sea; whence 'the Art of Navigation is known and improv'd, and Merchandizing thereby encouraged.'[28]

The puritan intellectuals realised that the English were not only a long way short of regaining dominion over nature, but that they were also considerably more backward than European neighbours in their command of agriculture and technology. In addition, they knew that the prevalent social attitudes and educational institutions of the élite were not favourable to any redress of this balance. Nevertheless biblical sources provided an insight into a much higher plane of economic and social life. With the models of Eden and the New Jerusalem in mind the activists framed programmes for the development of applied science. In this utopian endeavour they were guided by the *Instauratio Magna* of Francis Bacon.

(ii) Literate Experience

Francis Bacon developed a coherent system of natural philosophy which was consistent with the social ethic of protestantism. It was also framed with reference to the millennial expectation of man's dominion over nature. Hence it is not surprising that Bacon's philosophy was assimilated into the general religious worldview of the Puritans. Indeed his writings came to attain almost scriptural authority. The Puritans were particularly impressed by Bacon's insistence on reference to utilitarian functions. More than any other exponent of the new philosophy, Bacon paid attention to the sociology of knowledge. His writings were framed with conscious reference to ideological obstacles preventing the transformation of intellectual values. If his labours were manifestly unsuccessful in solving specific scientific problems, or in detecting the fertile developments in the physical sciences made by his contemporaries, no figure was more influential in stimulating his countrymen's active participation in experimental science and in drawing the natural philosopher and the craftsman into the centre of the social scene.

Technology impinged on Bacon's thought at many levels. The mechanical arts were used as a model for the reform of natural philosophy and all other sciences. Specific technological case-histories were used to demonstrate the manner in which intelligent application could

28. Pettus (209), pp.41–2.

lead to economic progress and intellectual advancement. The productivity of the mechanical arts was contrasted with the sterile metaphysical debates of scholastic natural philosophy. Bacon was confident that his radical reform of natural philosophy would lead to an even greater acceleration of technology until both were in a position to influence all human affairs. With the promise of such tangible and wide-ranging rewards, it was hoped that such great enthusiasm for experimental science would be generated, that the élite would abandon their disdain for manual labour, and submit to full-hearted collaboration with the widest social spectrum of artisan practitioners. By this great communal effort the foundations could be laid for the general social and intellectual regeneration of the Great Instauration.[29]

The inductive method and natural history formed the twin pillars of Bacon's system, each being treated with equal and proprietary interest. If anything, induction was accorded greater prominence during the early phases of composition of the *Instauratio Magna,* while natural history came to predominate towards the end of Bacon's work. Technology played a decisive part in both of these facets of his natural philosophy.

Induction was framed as a means to circumvent, on the one hand, unproductive scholastic logic, and on the other, sceptical negativism. It is a commonplace that Bacon's inductive logic states many of the elements of sound procedure in experimental science. Bacon himself insisted that the exhaustive search for certain causes should not be distracted by attempts to obtain premature rewards. In the terms of one of his favourite metaphors: experiments of light should take precedence over experiments of fruit. Such priorities could be supported by scriptural authority. On the first day the Creator gave light alone; only on the second day were the first fruits brought forth. The myth of Atalanta was also relevant; in turning aside to pick up the golden apple, the course was interrupted and victory irretrievably sacrificed.[30] Bacon concluded that 'the very beholding of the light is itself more excellent and a fairer thing than all the uses of it'. Hence the contemplation of things and incisive attempts to understand their operations, would grant a liberation from error which was more worthy than 'all the fruit of inventions' (in seipsa magis digna est, quam universus inventorum fructus).[31]

Such statements have been taken as unambiguous pronouncements about the independence of scientific enquiry; Bacon seemed to be arguing that the quality of scientific judgement would be necessarily impaired by reference to utilitarian values. Such a view of Bacon's methodology can only be defended by taking aphorisms from *Novum Organum* out

29. For general discussions of Bacon stressing the utilitarian aspect, see R. F. Jones (163), pp.41–61; W. E. Houghton (153); B. Farrington, *Francis Bacon Philosopher of Industrial Science* (London, 1951).

30. *Instauratio Magna,* Bacon *Works,* i, pp.128–9. *Novum Organum,* 1, 70, 117 & 121, *Works,* i, pp.179–81, 212–13, 215–16.

31. *Novum Organum,* 1, 129, Bacon *Works,* i, pp.221–3.

of context and ignoring related passages which appear to assert the opposite conclusion. Thus Bacon could claim, that in the study of the works of creation 'Truth and utility are here the very same things' (ipsissimae res); or that works themselves were of greater value as pledges of truth than as contributions to the comforts of life; or again that social amelioration and enrichment of the intellect were undertaken by one and the same means.[32]

Either Bacon was genuinely inconsistent, or alternatively the two apparently opposite sets of values are reconcilable. I suspect that the inconsistency would not have been at all apparent to Bacon himself. Only with the increasing separation of science and technology at a much later date did his position seem to be ambiguous and self-contradictory. The difficulty is overcome by reference to the religious maxim applied by Bacon himself. In religion the perfect inner light of personal revelation was the highest ideal, but it was also essential to test and prove this faith by works. Similarly, in science, perfect knowledge of the inner workings of nature was the ultimate goal, but this knowledge could best be attained through the investigation of the arts which related to everyday life. The value of knowledge in this area would be proved by its capacity to yield socially beneficial rewards. Hence, by establishing the mechanical arts as the most satisfactory territory for scientific enquiry, it was possible for Bacon to claim that truth and utility were the very same things. He was not lapsing into naive utilitarianism in claiming that the basic rule for natural philosophers was 'that all knowledge is to be limited by religion, and to be referred to use and action', or alternatively 'Now the true and lawful goal of the sciences is none other than this : that human life be endowed with new discoveries and powers'. By the judicious application of the inductive method of 'literate experience' it was anticipated that innovation would become systematic and productive; the new rational foundation would overcome the reliance of the arts on sporadic and random improvements.[33] When governed by the above principles the experimenter would never lose sight of practical applicability, while maintaining a scrupulous vigilance against premature utilitarian exploitation.

Bacon's attitude to the mechanical arts was not uncritical. The procedures of *Novum Organum* were designed to test commonly held superstitions or asserted cases of magical phenomena. As a community, mechanics were often backward and secretive, but they had nevertheless achieved considerable successes. Such figures as Agricola, Palissy and Stevin were willing to bridge the gulf between the scholar and the craftsman; they had exhibited the enormous potentialities of literate technology. On the other hand neither the scholastic philosophers nor

32. *Cogitata et Visa,* Bacon *Works,* i, p.612 (see above, p.324). *Novum Organum,* 1, 81, 124, *Works,* i, pp.88, 127–8.

33. *Valerius Terminus,* Bacon *Works,* iii, p.218; *Redargutio philosophiarum, Works,* iii, p.573. *Novum Organum,* 1, 81, 110, *Works,* i, pp.188, 208–9.

their critics could satisfy Bacon that they were sufficiently aware of the need to relate natural philosophy to its natural roots in experience. Indeed he claimed that the sciences became increasingly ossified as they were passed from master to pupil in scholastic education. By contrast the mechanical arts had sprung into life and were 'continually thriving and growing, as having in them a breath of life; at first rude, then convenient, afterwards adorned, and at all times advancing'. The accelerating development of technology was primarily attributable to the rapid accumulation of small improvements, the method being essentially collaborative, empirical and 'democratic'. By contrast, the scholastic 'dictatorships' were most productive at their inauguration; thereafter under the orthodoxy of the schools there had been a rapid intellectual decline.[34] The inductive method was thoroughly consistent with the democratic methods of the mechanic—a 'subdued and perpetual intercourse with the thing itself'; this was the only infallible means to a sound understanding of nature. In the accumulation of scientific knowledge the virtuosity of dictators, or fidelity of schools, would be at a discount; by following the rules of induction 'but little is left for the powers of wit'. Consequently Baconianism represented a 'real and legitimate union between the empiric and rational faculties', creating a unity of outlook which would be mirrored in the social sphere by full intellectual sympathy between the scholar and the craftsman.[35]

Bacon had various reasons for preferring scientific investigations to concentrate on subjects already treated by the craftsman. Owing to the mechanics' enterprise, knowledge of materials and techniques was already well advanced, particularly in such areas as metallurgy and horticulture. Thus a solid foundation had been laid for more sustained experimental investigations. Nature would be forced to reveal her full potentialities when 'forced out of her natural state, and squeezed and moulded' in the workshops of craftsmen. In this she was like Proteus, who was induced to reveal his true shape only when straightened and held fast. Similarly it was necessary to submit nature to the trials and vexations of art.[36] As a lawyer Bacon naturally applied familiar professional terminology to the activities of the craftsman. By 'interrogation' applied with extreme determination and cunning, nature would be 'tortured' into revealing her secrets; she would then submit to voluntary 'subjugation'. However the scientific 'trial' necessitated a degree of sensitivity analogous to religious feeling, and an intuitive respect for nature of the kind already familiar to the physician or member of a mining guild. Hence *Novum*

34. *Cogitata et Visa,* Bacon *Works,* iii, p.616; *Instauratio Magna, Works,* i, pp.127–8. *Novum Organum,* I, 74, *Works,* i, pp.183–4. *De Augmentis, Works,* iii, pp.289–90.

35. *Instauratio Magna,* Bacon *Works,* i, p.131; *Novum Organum,* I, 61, 122, *Works,* i, pp.172–3, 216–17. For a full discussion of this point with reference to Gilbert, see Zilsel (350).

36. *Novum Organum,* I, 98, Bacon *Works,* i, p.298. *De Augmentis, Works,* iii, p.333.

Organum opened with the phrase, *Homo, naturae minister et interpres;* man was the minister and servant of nature, bound to his vocation by spiritual bonds. In order to succeed it was necessary to proceed with humility and complete dedication to empirical methods—'Nature to be commanded must be obeyed'.[37] Using an analogy drawn from the gospels, it was emphasised that a complete reorientation of intellectual values was required, in accordance with the maxim that only those offering childlike submission would be eligible for salvation. Natural philosophers must become 'children again and infants, not scorn to take ABC thereof in hand, and in finding and searching out the interpretation thereof, let them spare no labour', even to the point of death.[38]

By the rigorous application of the rules and experimental methods of *Novum Organum* it was hoped to ascertain the conditions necessary and sufficient for the production of natural phenomena. Then it would be possible to imitate nature at will and unleash a variety of operations useful to man. The seriousness of this utilitarian purpose is confirmed by the direction taken by Bacon's interests following his provisional statement of the inductive philosophy. Even in *Novum Organum,* it was apparent that inductive study of particular problems was to be accompanied by the systematic collection of observations and experiments; thus natural history would gradually encompass all facets of nature. Both inductive science and natural history were deserving of urgent attention. The failure of past generations to record their arts and sciences had been lamentably short-sighted. Equally, Bacon's own generation was indicted for its failure to accumulate reliable scientific and technological information. Indigence, idleness, or preference for the gossip of the streets, had critically reduced the quality of the intelligence available to experimental philosophers desiring to embark on an inductive study. On all subjects information was scattered, unreliable and qualitative. More ambitious investigations were precluded until serious attention was given to natural history: 'Good hopes may therefore be conceived of natural philosophy, when natural history, which is the basis and foundation of it, has been drawn upon a better plan, but not till then.'[39]

Natural history came to dominate Bacon's outlook during his later years. *Historia naturalis* was always regarded as a fundamental unit of the *Instauratio Magna,* its role being outlined briefly in both the *Distributio Operis* and *Novum Organum* published in 1620. *Novum Organum* was left incomplete with only two of its eight books written.

37. *Novum Organum,* I, 1, Bacon *Works,* i, p.157. *Instauratio Magna, Works,* i, p.144.

38. *Novum Organum,* I, 3, 129, Bacon *Works,* i, pp.157, 222. *Historia Ventorum, Works,* ii, p.15.

39. *Instauratio Magna,* Bacon *Works,* i, p.126. *Novum Organum,* I, 98, *Works,* i, pp.194–6. For a discussion of Bacon's views on natural history, see J. Spedding in *Works,* i, pp.369–90.

In the final part of book two, the 'auxilia intellectus' were passed over rapidly, as a prelude to the final section 'Parasceve ad Historiam Naturalium et Experimentalem', a plan for the construction of natural histories which concluded with a 'Catalogus Historiarum Particularium'. Therefore *Novum Organum* terminated with a clear emphasis on natural history. Bacon's next publications confirmed and explained the reasons for this bias. The preface to the *Historia Ventorum* announced that the new logical instrument could attain nothing without assistance from natural history, whereas the latter could unaided 'much advance instauration, or renewing of sciences'. In the enlarged version of the *Advancement of Learning*, a greatly expanded section on *historia naturalis* was included, which was derived from the 'Parasceve'.[40]

Thereafter Bacon's energies were devoted to the compilation of natural histories of winds, life and death, density and rarity, as well as various fragments which were either lost, or included in the posthumous *Sylva Sylvarum*. Finally the description of Solomon's House in *New Atlantis* demonstrated how the inductive natural histories could be related to utilitarian functions.

The mechanical arts were as relevant to natural histories as to the philosophy of induction. In the 'Parasceve' a basic dichotomy was recognised between the natural world and the arts. First priority was accorded to the natural history of trade; this was 'the most useful since it exhibits bodies in motion, and leads more directly to practice'.[41] Furthermore

> 'the use of History Mechanical is of all others the most radical and fundamental towards natural Philosophy; such natural philosophy as shall not vanish in the fume of subtile, sublime, or delectable speculation, but such as shall be operative to the endowment and benefit of man's life: for it will not only minister and suggest for the present many ingenious practices in all trades, by connection and transferring of the observations of one art to the use of another, when the experiences of several mysteries shall fall under the consideration of one man's mind; but further it will give a more true and real illumination concerning the causes and axioms than is hitherto attained.'[42]

Thus, as in *Novum Organum,* the identity of truth and utility was an essential premise for the conduct of natural history. Primary emphasis was to be on the arts directly involved in manipulating natural materials —agriculture, cookery, chemistry, dyeing; the investigation of glass, enamel, sugar, gunpowder, fireworks, paper, etc. Next came the arts

40. *Historia Ventorum,* Bacon *Works,* v, pp.133–4; *De Augmentis, Works,* iii, pp.330–4.
41. *Parasceve,* Bacon *Works,* i, pp.388–9.
42. *De Augmentis,* Bacon *Works,* iii, pp.332–3.

concerned with working prepared materials with instruments—weaving, carpentry, architecture, milling and clock-making. It was Bacon's 'firm intention to cause streams of every species of mechanical experiment to flow from all quarters into the ocean of philosophy'. He was as optimistic about the scientific potentialities of the histories as about their obvious capacity to rationalise and improve the arts. Whatever the balance of these advantages, it was anticipated that considerable energies would be invested in compiling histories of trade. Reference to the one hundred and thirty topics listed in 'Catalogus historiarum particularium' confirms this impression. The first forty were concerned with the history of natural objects, coinciding with the subject matter of the well-known Renaissance natural histories. Apart from two final topics, the remainder were histories of man, ranging from anatomy, physiology and medicine to a central core of about forty histories of trade. These were comprehensive enough to include such specific subjects as osier work and gardening (112 & 116). Under each heading the scope was specified in detail. For instance, the hundredth history included ironworking, lapidary art, brick, tile, lead and glassmaking, pottery, cements and incrustations, and finally woodworking.[43]

The shift of emphasis from inductive logic to natural history, and finally towards histories of trade involved increasing reference to collaborative enterprise and free communication between different social groups. Consequently Bacon's attention was increasingly directed to the organisation and patronage of science. The preface to *Novum Organum* ended with an invitation to James I to imitate Solomon by promoting the compilation of a Natural and Experimental History, serviceable for raising a superstructure of sound natural philosophy. This request was reinforced by one of Bacon's favourite biblical citations: 'It is the glory of God to conceal a thing: but the honour of kings to search out a matter' (Proverbs 25 : 2).[44] Bacon usually cited this passage to support the idea of there being a general obligation to participate in experimental science. Here it was applied to induce royal patronage for a venture which would bring esteem, wealth, and empire to the English nation. From the point of view of Bacon's personal reputation, this request could not have been made at a more unfortunate time, but he remained convinced that the promoters of the *Instauratio Magna* deserved to be furnished with a substantial institutional establishment.

Tentative thoughts about such a foundation were entered in private memoranda during July 1608. Its aims were to be the compilation of first a history of marvels, and secondly a history of the observations and experiments of all mechanical arts. Natural history of marvels never played more than a subsidiary role, but its presence illustrates the influence of della Porta's *Magia Naturalis,* a work which provided the chief inspiration and quarry for *Sylva Slyvarum.* Histories of trade were

43. Bacon *Works,* i, pp.405–11.
44. *Ibid.,* pp.132–3.

subject to greater attention, a list of queries being drafted relating to a college designed for the purpose. The list began :

> 'Gyving pensions to 4 for search to compile the 2 Histories ut supra. Foundac. of a college for Inventors. 2 Galeries with statuas for Inventors past and spaces for Inventors to come. And a Library and an Inginary.'[45]

This entry provides a synoptic view of the scheme which ultimately matured into the Solomon's House of *New Atlantis*. As advocated in *Novum Organum* research was to be conducted under royal patronage, in conscious imitation of Solomon. The declared function of Solomon's House, 'the Knowledge of Causes and Secrett Motions of Things; And the Enlarging of the bounds of Humane Empire, to the Effecting of all Things possible' provides an apt epitome of Bacon's natural philosophy, re-echoing yet again the functional unity of truth and utility. Even more than the conquest and colonisation of new territories, the empire of man over nature was regarded as a noble ideal.[46] Solomon's House provided a model of the working relationship between inductive research and cumulative natural history. Not surprisingly operational emphasis was on the mechanical arts. Indeed, within the space of a few pages Bacon made references to a large percentage of the topics listed in his 'Catalogus historiarum particularium'. For instance mines and artificial caves were used by the workers of Solomon's House for the collection of ores and experiments concerning their properties. New 'artificial' metals were produced by amalgamation, specimens being tested underground for durability or transmutability. The products of this work could then be made available for use in technology or medicine. The officers of the House were involved in experimental work, in composing natural histories, in compiling a new philosophy, or in dispensing benefits to the public.

New Atlantis ended abruptly after the description of Solomon's House; like the majority of Bacon's writings it was bequeathed to posterity as a fragment. Indeed at the time of Bacon's death the whole *Instauratio Magna* was in the form of a series of fragments. It was thought more necessary to provide an outline of the whole edifice, than to pursue one section to completion. On each topic he was content to terminate his labours after stating fundamental doctrines. But Bacon's work was sufficiently complete to provide guidance on such basic issues as experimental method, or on the conduct of natural histories, and on the organisation of scientific enquiry. During the Puritan Revolution there was no shortage of labourers to take up the philosophy of the *Instauratio Magna*. Puritan intellectuals initiated an attempt to apply Baconian principles to the widest sphere of human activity.

45. Bacon, *Letters & Life* (263), iv, pp.25, 66.
46. *New Atlantis*, Bacon *Works*, iii, p.156; *Cogitata et Visa*, *Works*, iii, p.612.

(iii) The Burden of Perpetual Patents

The myth of Atalanta stated a dilemma which was crucial both to Bacon's personal career and to the life of the whole English nation. For individual intellectual attainment, or general exploitation of scientific knowledge, it was essential to persevere with long-term objectives, resisting the temptation to fall prey to any promise of immediate rewards. Nevertheless Bacon's dramatic personal decline and the gathering economic crisis of the 1620s suggest that it was extremely difficult to transcend the imperfections of Jacobean social life to attain the moral integrity and economic policies needed to accomplish the return of dominion over nature. In both experimental science and industrial organisation, the foundations were laid for spectacular advancement, but like Atalanta the English projectors were led astray by seductive counter-attractions.

During his erratic public career Bacon displayed traces of that breadth of vision which characterised his natural philosophy. He reached towards religious reconciliation, political union, organised colonisation of Ireland and America, rationalisation of the exchequer, and the codification of case and statute law. However, Bacon's pre-occupation with immediate contingencies stifled the development of his political programme. Furthermore he himself became rapidly engulfed in the seething cauldron of court life, in which rapacious competition for immediate rewards appeared to offer the only guarantee for survival. Thus Bacon's general programme attracted only negligible attention or support; the personal success of the great architect depended entirely on his ability to administer to the recurrent crises in the royal finances. Tragically, his short-term solutions invariably conflicted with requirements for general economic growth, and thereby they were incompatible with the lofty goals of the *Instauratio Magna*.

This conflict is well-illustrated by his dilemma over patents. The patent system had evolved during the reign of Elizabeth as a means to attract the importation of foreign crafts and to stimulate native ingenuity. The protection of the crown was given to patentees on condition that new techniques were developed and diffused to native workmen. This system had been a considerable asset to industries in the late sixteenth century. Bacon must have been aware of the potentialities of patents to stimulate ingenuity and scientific enquiry providing that they were correctly administered. He stated unambiguously that rewards were deserved by 'any man [who] out of his own industry or endeavour finds anything beneficial for the commonwealth, or brings in any new invention'. Subsequently he was intimately involved with the machinery devised by James I to ensure the efficient operation of the patent law. Bacon was appointed to the Commissioners for Suits, the permanent body instituted to investigate each request; he was one of its two most prominent members. Moreover, as Attorney-General and subsequently as Lord

Keeper, he was familiar with every patent under consideration in the years before 1620, the period of the most spectacular proliferation of patent grants.[47] It is apparent that Bacon was involved in a system granting patents according to criteria quite different from those originally envisaged. Patents intruded into all aspects of national life; they affected toothpicks and Welsh butter, inns and ale-houses. Monopolists were not obliged to import new crafts, to introduce genuine inventions, to stimulate the diffusion of expertise, or to improve industrial organisation for the public advantage. Quite the contrary, patents were intended to assist predatory courtiers to appropriate sections of the economy, with guaranteed profits and security from competition, regardless of the social consequences. The price that Bacon gave for the tolerance of court favourites was his connivance at economic abuses of this kind. He himself received a proportion of Alienations profits and Star Chamber fines, among other gratuities. Such compensations were very considerable, enabling Bacon to live in ostentatious style, but they were contemptible compared with the gains of such figures as Buckingham. Manipulation could be defended in terms of the prerogative powers of the monarch, or potential benefit to the privy purse, but monopolies proved ultimately to be both financially unrewarding and politically disastrous.[48] Monopoly became a watchword in the agitation against the delinquency of the early Stuarts and their advisers. Individually the economic influence of monopolies was often slight, although the cumulative effect was significant. In certain cases, such as the notorious Cockayne project, the introduction of monopoly produced a devastating setback to the nation's major export. Howell reported from Hamburg that it had caused 'both Dutch and Germans to turn necessity to a virtue, and made them far more ingenious to find ways, not only to dye but to make cloth, which hath much impaired our markets ever since'. According to his impression British exports had been reduced by two-thirds, a figure which is generally supported by modern estimates.[49] From the technological point of view one of the worst features of the Jacobean patent system was its disregard for invention; obsolete methods were perpetuated and such genuine inventions as Lee's stocking frame, or the innovations introduced by Hugh Plat were refused grants. Meanwhile the predatory search for income extended to glass, soap, silver and gold thread, and fen drainage,

47. Price (228), pp.25–6. Between 1561 and 1603, 55 patents were granted, compared with 108 granted by James I: E. W. Hulme, 'The History of the Patent System under Prerogative and Common Law', *Law Quarterly Review*, 1896, *12*: 141–54; 1900, *16*: 44–56.

48. The older literature on Bacon includes protracted debates over his role in monopolies. S. R. Gardiner, *History of England 1603–1642*, iv, pp.1–55, followed Bacon's editors by adopting an apologetic tone. For more realistic appraisals, see Price (228); G. Unwin, *Industrial Organisation in the Sixteenth and Seventeenth Centuries* (Oxford, 1904), pp.172–92; Menna Prestwich, *Cranfield, Politics and Profit under the Early Stuarts* (Oxford, 1966), pp.267–85; Clark (49), pp.104–9.

49. Howell (156), p.300.

occasionally stimulating innovation, but always causing social discontent. This was exacerbated by more general economic decline, poor harvests, rising prices, decline in cloth exports, increasing population. The period between 1620 and 1640 was marked by fluctuations, uncertainty and deflation. European markets were adversely affected by the Thirty Years War; harvests were particularly bad; epidemics reduced morale. Unemployment and depressed wages created hardship and famine for the working population of agricultural workers, wool operatives and the by now sizeable body of employees in the newer industries.[50] Faced with such depressing conditions at home, many were tempted to seek security in the New Jerusalem across the Atlantic. Stagnation, corruption and repression in England formed a striking contrast to Bacon's Island of Bensalem, where all families 'doe flourish and prosper ever after in an extraordinary manner . . . You shall understand that there is not under the Heavens, so chaste a Nation, as this of Bensalem; Not so free from all Pollution, or foulenesse. It is the Virgin of the World'.[51] In his final years, Bacon retreated into the ideal world of *New Atlantis,* where he could create a utopian state which was becoming increasingly remote from the realities of English life.

Despite the generally dismal condition of England under the early Stuarts, the spirit of innovation generated in the Elizabethan era was not extinguished. Indeed the foundations continued to be laid for the mercantilist prosperity of the later part of the century. Economic conditions under the Stuarts merely delayed the fruition of this endeavour. Intellectuals and craftsmen were actively collaborating on many scientific and technical problems; the pervasive quest for economic applications proved to be no handicap to the development of more abstract aspects of mathematics and science. Indeed it could be claimed that Bacon's natural philosophy was not so much an isolated and prophetic statement, as a formal and coherent expression of the dominant viewpoint in the Jacobean scientific movement. Although Bacon had only limited contacts with leading scientific practitioners, his outlook was considerably influenced by the scientific enterprise of the period.

Bacon's close concern with patents would have ensured familiarity with a wide range of inventions, inventors and projectors, from whom he would have gained an impression of the potentialities of science. This varied experience found expression at many points in his description of Solomon's House. Patents were overwhelmingly concerned with mining.[52] Solomon's House was introduced by an optimistic description of mines sunk to six hundred fathoms, ten times the depth of the most ambitious

50. For general discussion of these trends, see B. E. Supple, *Commercial Crisis and Change in England 1600–1642* (Cambridge, 1959); C. Wilson, *England's Apprenticeship 1603–1763* (London, 1965), pp.89–140.

51. Bacon, *New Atlantis, Works,* iii, p.152.

52. Nef (198), i, p.254. 75 per cent of the patents granted between 1561 and 1688 were directly (43 per cent), or indirectly (32 per cent), concerned with mining.

shafts sunk and inadequately drained by Bacon's contemporaries. There are many indications that these grandiose dreams of mines, mills, distillations and new metals were symptomatic of Bacon's serious involvement with chemistry and technological projects. He made preliminary enquiries for a natural history of metals. According to Bushell he was the leading proponent of the use of adits for draining mines. Bushell also claimed that his own success in mining silver in Cardiganshire was due to the exploitation of Bacon's methods. Bacon took out leases for mining in Wales and was involved with the successful wireworks at Tintern, the seat of much minor mechanical and metallurgical innovation by German technicians. He was consequently familiar with the techniques of the production of osmond iron, the drawing of wire by water power and the operation of slitting mills. Finally, he recognised that ignorance of refining techniques involved the loss of valuable silver found in lead deposits. Since the Dutch were importing and refining this ore, Bacon advocated the suppression of lead exports, pending the successful development of refining in England. The information we possess about Bacon's various involvements with metallurgy is sufficient to indicate the intimate relationship between experimental science, technological innovation, and industrial and economic policy. Bacon was in a position to view science from all these perspectives and to appreciate the subtle interrelationship of the various factors affecting its development.[53]

Most of the inventors were humble specialists who were seeking rewards for minor improvements to their trade. They designed new ploughs, draining machines, or furnaces; they introduced new preparations for varnishing, dyeing, or protecting the hulls of ships from worms. Their combined efforts gave Bacon an impression of a fertile spirit of innovation among the craftsmen engaged in the nation's nascent industries. A few of the practitioners had remarkably wide interests and uncontainable zest for innovation. David Ramsay was given licence 'to multiply and make Salt Peter in an open Field, in fower Acres of Ground, sufficient to serve all Our Dominions; To raise Water from low Pitts by Fire; To make any sort of Mills to goe on standing waters by continual motion, without the help of Wind, Waite or Horse.' Besides his interests in saltpetre, perpetual motion and possibly a kind of steam engine, Ramsay also claimed to have invented a new method of making tapestry, improvements in sailing, new drainage and metalworking techniques, a method of increasing soil fertility and finally a process for bleaching yellow wax.

53. Partington (205), ii, pp.389–414; 'Inquisitions touching the Compounding of Metals', 'Articles of Questions touching Minerals', Bacon *Works,* iii, pp.793–817. The latter differs from 'Articles of Enquiry touching Metals and Minerals', appended to the 1661 edn. of *Sylva Sylvarum.* See also *Histoire Naturelle de Mre. F. Bacon* (Paris, 1631), pp.34–40. A spurious speech supposed to have been prepared for the parliament of 1621, 'Speech touching the recovering of drowned mineral works' was printed by Bushell in *Abridgment of the Lord Chancellor Bacon's . . . Mineral Prosecutions* (London, 1659), sig.A3r–4v. H. G. Nicholls, *Iron Making in the Forest of Dean* (London, 1866), pp.29–30; Rees (238), pp.174, 215, 453–61, 497. Price (228), pp.55–9.

Unfortunately the inventor left no further evidence about his prodigious achievements![54] Many innovations were no doubt confined to the imagination, but preserved records indicate the seriousness, patient determination, technical competence and even unexpected virtuosity among the inventors. Edward Jorden's patent for smelting tin, iron, lead and copper with pitcoal, peat and turf, was backed by a sound knowledge of chemistry.[55] Equally, evidence from divers sources relates to the work of the two immigrant practitioners, Salomon de Caus and Cornelius Drebbel. It has been perceptively suggested that their curious repertoire of inventions provided the inspiration for Bacon's description of Solomon's House.[56] Bacon was also undoubtedly influenced by a wider circle, including such projectors as David Ramsay and Thomas Bushell, and by the general community of the mechanics. De Caus replaced Simon Sturtevant as the builder of the elaborate waterworks at Hatfield House. His celebrity rested on fountains and ingenious devices designed to simulate musical instruments, using jets of water or steam. Similarly Drebbel designed a Neptune's fountain in which Neptune, tritons and nymphs emerged from a cave and progressed in a horse-drawn chariot until out of sight behind a jet of water. The construction of articulated 'automata' is an echo of the scarab constructed by John Dee. Talents were not entirely absorbed in providing entertainments in domestic architecture for aristocratic patrons. Almost every author of such aesthetic diversions was involved in some serious economic enterprise. Sturtevant was given the first patent to smelt ores using coal; de Caus was a drainage engineer and pioneer (along with Ramsay and the Marquis of Worcester) of experiments in the use of steam power. Drebbel was involved in one of the fen-draining partnerships, but his chief success was the establishment of a dyeworks. The development occurred in the wake of the ill-fated Cockayne project, which exposed the inadequacy of the English dyeworks. From fireworks, Drebbel developed the torpedo used on the Duke of Buckingham's La Rochelle expedition, while his famous submarine was thought to have important military and engineering applications.[57] The combination of dilettante curiosity and economic awareness was also displayed by Edward Somerset, Marquis of Worcester, who employed the Dutch mechanic Caspar Kalthoff on a wide range of activities at the Vauxhall ordnance factory during the reign of Charles I.

54. *Specification of Patent, No. 50,* 21 January 1630/1; Rymer, *Foedera,* xix, pp.239–41.

55. *Specification of Patent, No. 61, 1632. A Discourse of Naturall Bathes and Mineral Waters* (London, 1631); Dud Dudley, *Mettallum Martis* (London, 1665), p.3.

56. Rosalie L. Colie, 'Cornelius Drebbel and Salomon de Caus: Two Jacobean Models for Salomon's House', *Huntington Library Quarterly,* 1954/5, *18*: 245–60.

57. L. Stone, 'The Building of Hatfield House', *Archaeological Journal,* 1956, *112*: 100–28; F. M. Jaeger, *Cornelis Drebbel en zijne Tijdgenooten* (Gröningen, 1922); Dudley, *op. cit.,* p.3; Nef (198), i, pp.248–52; Price (228), pp.180–92. Thomas Bushell claimed to have displayed to Charles I waterworks like those of de Caus and Drebbel, *Mineral Overtures,* 1659, p.6.

When the extensive premises were confiscated by parliament, the inventory listed not only the expected forges and casting works, but also two 'model rooms' containing water drainage engines, perpetual motion machines, fountains and improved wagons.[58]

Much of this inventive effort was dissipated owing to absence of capital support or sufficiently sustained research. For instance the numerous rival patentees who claimed to use coal for the smelting of iron ore made extravagant claims but little metal. Nevertheless coal became more extensively used; it was successfully introduced into the glass and brewing industries in the early seventeenth century. With the discovery of coking coal, coke partly replaced wood in brewing, while the technique of sealing crucibles enabled coal to replace wood in glassmaking.[59] Technical proficiency and the application of German expertise also facilitated the successful silvermining projects in Cardiganshire of Sir Hugh Myddelton and Thomas Bushell. In another ambitious venture, Myddelton's New River Company, fresh water was carried from Hertfordshire for piping to London houses. The accurate surveying of Edward Wright was vital to the success of this scheme. Myddelton attracted the backing of speculators, including James I.[60] Drebbel was the proponent of a similar project. Even greater capital resources were required for the fen-draining projects which came to fruition during Charles I's reign. A preliminary exercise was undertaken in the northern fens, where the drainage works were undertaken by Thomas Lovell and William Engelbert.[61] The greatest returns were to be expected from schemes to drain the Great Level in the southern fens. Pioneers hoped to undertake this work for the large sum of £150,000, an indication of the scale of this enterprise. Associated with the undertakers were Henry Briggs and Drebbel, who were probably engaged to supervise surveying and drainage engineering respectively. This group was overtaken by rivals who were employing Cornelius Vermuyden as their drainage expert. The success of his 'little Army of Artificers, venting, contriving, and acting outlandish devises' is well-known.[62]

Perhaps the most conscious attempts to apply science and mathe-

58. *Century of Inventions* (London, 1663; composed c.1655); H. Dircks, *The Life, Times and Scientific Labours of The Second Marquis of Worcester* (London, 1865); C. ffoulkes, *The Gunfounders of England* (London, 1937), pp.52–3, 114; W. H. Thorpe, 'The Marquis of Worcester and Vauxhall', Newcomen Society *Transactions,* 1932–3, *13*: 75–88.

59. Nef. (198), i, pp.215–20; E. W. Hulme, 'English Glass-Making in the Sixteenth and Seventeenth Centuries', *The Antiquary*, 1894, *30*: 210–14; 1895, *31*: 68–72, 102–6, 134–8. W. A. Thorpe, *English Glass* (London, 1961), pp.114–34; *VCH Surrey,* ii, pp.299–302.

60. J. W. Gough, *The Superlative Prodigall. A Life of Thomas Bushell* (Bristol, 1932); *idem, Sir Hugh Myddelton* (Oxford, 1964); Rees (238), pp.453–64.

61. H. C. Darby, *The Draining of the Fens* (Cambridge, 1940), p.45; John Norden, *The Surveiors Dialogue* (London, 1610), p.149.

62. Vermuyden had successfully drained Hatfield Chase, financed primarily by Dutch speculators. Darby, *op. cit.*, p.42; J. Korthals-Altes, *Sir Cornelius Vermuyden* (London, 1925); L. E. Harris, *Vermuyden and the Fens* (London, 1953).

matics to economic ends before 1640 occurred in the areas of navigation and surveying. Already during the reign of Elizabeth, John Dee had given an exhaustive exposition of the potentialities of mathematics. His text provided a definitive guide to the emergent class of mathematical practitioners, who had attained a firmly established position in the capital by 1600. As contrivers and manufacturers of instruments ranging from telescopes to calculating devices they emerged from apprenticeship into European dominance during the first part of the seventeenth century.[63] On the basis of certain common mathematical principles a whole range of astronomical, navigational and surveying instruments was contrived, gradually perfected, and simplified for popular use. The progress of instrument-making was an ideal confirmation of Bacon's judgements about the growing proficiency of the mechanical arts. In the sophisticated work of the physical astronomers, and the simple routines of the landmeter, instruments were being applied in the manner advocated by Bacon, to transcend the limitations of the senses and to compile an accurate body of information about the terrestrial and celestial environment. In surveying, the new decimal chains of Rathborne and Gunter passed quickly into general use, while in astronomy Horrox and his associates devised Keplerian telescopes and micrometers, which were used for the first proficient observation of a transit of Venus in 1639.

The rise of practical mathematics is strikingly confirmed by extensive publishing activity in the area; textbooks were produced for all branches of the art. Initially practitioners depended heavily on translations of Spanish and Dutch navigational texts and charts. An increasing degree of originality was indicated by Edward Wright's *Certain Errors in Navigation* (1599), which reflected the growing concern with oceanic navigation, taking account of compass variation and convergence of the meridians. The first part of the seventeenth century saw the rapid rise of ephemerides and mathematical tables. Mathematical navigation was then greatly advanced by trigonometry and logarithms, which made their impact between 1614 and 1620. In order to popularise these fundamental developments Gunter evolved 'Gunter's scale', a durable calculating instrument which enabled the humble practitioner to manipulate logarithms according to simple rules. 1616 was a particularly important year; it was marked by the edition of Napier's preliminary work on logarithms prepared by Wright and Briggs, as well as by Rathborne's exhaustive textbook of surveying.[64] At this point it was declared that

63. John Dee, preface to Henry Billingsley (ed.), *The Elements of Geometrie of the most auncient Philosopher Euclide of Megara* (London, 1570). For full discussion of the mathematical practitioners, see Taylor (278); D. W. Waters, *The Art of Navigation in England in Elizabethan and Early Stuart Times* (London, 1958); F. R. Maddison, *Medieval Scientific Instruments and the Development of Navigational Instruments in the XVth and XVIth Centuries* (Coimbra, 1969). See Figure 2, p.489 below.

64. *A Description of the Admirable Table of Logarithms* (London, 1616); Aaron Rathborne, *The Surveyor* (London, 1616).

'if any be desirous so to enrich his understanding with Mathematicall knowledge, he shall find the works both of ancient and moderne writers so plentifully, as that there were never better or neer helpes for the attaining thereof, then are at this present, as may well be proved by those excellent workes and Inventions, that have lately beene published, namely the admirable Table of Logarithmes'.[65]

The ramifications of practical mathematics were considerable. By systematising accounts and introducing double-entry book-keeping, personal and commercial accounts were regularised and separated; tables were evolved to facilitate estimates relating to numerous commodities, and for calculation of rates of interest. Mathematical practitioners were concerned on estates with surveying, drainage, estimation of the value of timber and construction of impressive buildings, gardens and waterworks. The advancing ambitions of surveyors were indicated in John Norden's *Surveyors Dialogue* (1607); Norden's own energies were devoted to a comprehensive topographical survey, county by county, a project which is mainly remembered for his county maps and similar ones prepared by Speed. The mathematicians extended their work to the colonial territories of Ireland and America. The mathematician Thomas Harriot demonstrated the manner in which an American voyage could be productively recorded in terms of charts, maps and regional surveys.[66] English navigators collected magnetic data, hoping that the study of compass variation would hasten the solution of the longitude problem. Then the work on the declination and inclination of the compass was an indispensable background to the theoretical work of William Gilbert. The longitude problem was constantly debated, but was not solved during the seventeenth century. These rich developments support Taylor's view that 'English geography entered upon a distinctly mathematical phase' in the seventeenth century.[67]

Mathematics came to have universal application. Telescopes were applied to the study of lunar geography; the micrometer was used to measure celestial phenomena. The estate owner and the merchant obtained an accurate estimate of their property and wealth by applying mathematical methods. Such estimates called for tables of interest, rates of exchange, etc., but also for more elaborate treatises, combining the provision of useful data with economic analysis and a consideration of national policy. Rational examination of the national economy was particularly stimulated by the worsening economic depression. Policy makers came to recognise the relevance of accurate economic data and quantitative economic theories. There was an increasingly close rapport between mathematicians, geographers and merchants.

In considering the defects of natural history, Bacon declared, 'Nil

65. George Gilden, *A Prognostication* (London, 1616), sig.B2r–v.

66. A. C. Littleton & B. S. Yamey (eds.), *Studies in the History of Accountancy* (London, 1956), pp.185–237, 288–312. Taylor (279); A. W. Richeson, *English Land Measuring to 1800* (Cambridge, Mass., 1966).

67. Taylor (279), p.68.

debitis modis exquisitum, nil verificatum, nil numeratum, nil appensum, nil dimensum in naturali historia reperitur.' This point was re-emphasised in the *Parasceve,* where Bacon made a plea for quantification in natural history, including by implication the histories of trade:

> 'We moreover recommend that all natural bodies and qualities be, as far as is possible, reduced to number, weight, measure, and precise definition; for we are planning actual results and not mere theory; and it is a proper combination of physics and mathematics that generates practice.'[68]

Gerard Malynes approached economics in the general spirit of Bacon's aphorism; he founded his comprehensive treatise on the principle that all commercial transactions were 'distributed by Number, Weight and Measure'; this biblical tenet was utilised by both Bacon and his later disciple William Petty. The same text assumed fundamental importance in the writings of Malynes as well as in those of Petty, and it provided an exemplary biblical foundation for the new science of Political Arithmetic. Like the Baconians, Malynes declared his intention of writing the law of merchants 'in plaine and compendious writing, by undoubted principles, familiar examples, and demonstrative reasons, without affectation of curious words'. The first qualifications for the merchant were arithmetic, knowledge of weights and measures, geometry, cosmography, mathematics and geography, both of lands and seas.[69] Malynes's textbook included an elaborate quantitative survey of all aspects of the economy, with digressions on various topics, including bee-keeping, the generation of minerals, and the usefulness of copper farthings. Malynes was also involved in a vigorous debate about England's economic decline. There was particular concern about the export of bullion and specie, which was regarded as the root cause of the shortage of money and decay of trade. According to Malynes, this drift was caused by the recent manipulation of European currencies, which had resulted in the undervaluation of English coin. Therefore the remedy lay in the revision of rates of exchange. A rival interpretation was proffered by Thomas Mun, who suggested that loss of bullion was a reflection of the adverse flow of trade. Accordingly the solution rested in precise estimation of the trade balance, the more effective exploitation of natural resources, the encouragement of local industries, and the prohibition of imports of certain manufactured items and export of raw materials. Many of Mun's ideas were reflected by economic proposals of the later part of the century, in particular those which urged the importance in national policy of regulating the balance of trade.[70]

68. Bacon, *Novum Organum,* 1, 98; *Works,* i, pp.202–3. *Parasceve, Works,* i, p.400.

69. Gerard Malynes (186), Preface, pp.6–7. See Wisdom of Solomon, 11:20.

70. Thomas Mun, *Englands Treasure by Foreign Trade* (London, 1664; composed c.1622–3). For detailed discussion of the debates between Malynes, Mun and Misselden, see B. E. Supple, *Commercial Crisis and Change in England*

In order to realise the potentialities of the mathematical sciences it was necessary to diffuse knowledge to the widest possible audience. The appreciation of mathematics was not helped by the conservative habits of seamen, or the scholastic education of the élite. It was hoped that the crown or the merchant companies, primary beneficiaries of the economic applications of mathematics, would take responsibility for promoting the work of the mathematical practitioners. However, the response was disappointing. Mathematical teachers and writers continued to lack state support and there was no adequate institutional basis for the education of craftsmen or merchants who might benefit from the mathematical arts. An institution comparable with the *Casa de Contratación* at Seville would have been suitable for this purpose. But by the standards of Spain and Portugal, state enterprise was noticeably deficient in England. During the reign of James I Prince Henry earned celebrity for his patronage of mathematicians and artisans, but his example was not followed systematically. The Privy Council supervised translation of *Spiegel der Zeeaert* (*The Marriners Mirrour,* 1588), while in 1634 Henry Bond was employed to teach mathematics at the Chatham dockyard.

Further patronage was left to the merchant companies, which were increasingly obliged to pay attention to navigation as their ships undertook longer voyages. In the later sixteenth century they established substantial fleets in the Baltic and Mediterranean, while in the first part of the next century, regular traffic was initiated with the East Indies, North America and West Indies.[71] The Muscovy Company, a pioneer of long-distance trade, employed some of the best navigators in the later sixteenth century; its patronage assisted the popular writers Robert Recorde, and Richard Eden the translator of the *Arte de Navegar* (*The Art of Navigation,* 1561). The East India Company was less conspicuous as a patron. It purchased a copy of Hakluyt's *Principal Voyages* for the edification of members of its Indian depot and grudgingly provided employment for Edward Wright for a few years before his death. By contrast many individual navigators and aristocratic patrons maintained an intimate association with mathematicians, some of whom became members of their households or were tempted to take part in voyages of exploration. Dee, Harriot, Bavin and Wright benefited by this type of patronage.

Private teachers in London were the most effective promoters of the skill of practical mathematics. They often taught mathematics as a sideline to either instrument-making or instrument and book selling. A

1600–1642 (275), Chapter IX. See also C. H. Wilson, 'Treasure and Trade Balances', *Economic History Review*, Second Series, 1949–50, *2:* 152–61; Clark (49), pp.126–7.

71. R. Davis, *The Rise of the English Shipping Industry in the Seventeenth and Eighteenth Centuries* (London, 1962).

teaching role probably originated from attempts to publicise their wares by offering elementary instruction to purchasers. Such a system protected their proprietary rights, whereas provision of complete details in instruction manuals would have assisted competitors. There was also some recognition of the value of public lectureships. In the later sixteenth century a group of wealthy patrons established a mathematical lectureship in London for Thomas Hood. A more permanent endowment was provided by Sir Thomas Gresham, himself an economist and advocate of new methods of accountancy. Gresham College was inaugurated in 1597, and its professors of geometry and astronomy paid particular attention to applied mathematics. Owing to the enthusiasm and competence of such professors as Briggs, Gunter and Gellibrand, Gresham developed into the natural focus for London mathematical practitioners and amateurs. The leading private mathematical teacher, William Oughtred, maintained strong associations with the Gresham circle, and a continual flow of young university students, including John Bainbridge, John Greaves, Wallis, Ward, Wilkins and Wood, benefited from London mathematical teaching. Inevitably these experiences opened vistas of a new approach to education and professional life; comparisons were made which operated to the disadvantage of the scholastic curriculum of universities. In a sharp censure of Aristotelianism, William Watts, addressing 'venerable Artists and younger Students in Divinity' at Cambridge, declared that 'it's not to be doubted, but that the careful reading of our Books of Voyages would more elucidate the History of Nature, and more conduce to the improvement of Philosophy, than any thing that hath beene lately thought upon'.[72] Watts was one of many minor authors pressing for the educated classes to enter into more active participation in economic affairs. Of this group, Watts was a clergyman-mathematician, Malynes a merchant, Pettus a mining expert, and Webster an iatrochemist. Increasingly this group reflected the views of Bacon and by 1640 its members tended to fall into line with the Baconian programme as a whole.

The multiplicity of developments summarised above vindicated the belief that a technological utopia was within the reach of the English nation. But it was equally apparent that the smooth operation of science and its fruitful application to social amelioration depended on individual moral attitudes and national economic policy. Internal policies and events in Europe conspired to undermine economic development; the crisis deepened and there was mounting social discontent. Instead of stimulating ingenuity and innovation, the monopoly system suppressed initiative in the quest for easily won profits. Thus science existed in a state of inhibition. The years before 1640 were marked by uncertain

72. Appendix to Gellibrand, *Appendix concerning Longitude* (London, 1633), sig.S2r. See also, Thomas Hood, *A Copie of the Speache: made by the Mathematicall Lecturer* (London, 1588); F. R. Johnson, 'Thomas Hood's Inaugural Lecture', *JHI*, 1942, *3*: 94–106.

rewards, irregular patronage and failure to establish institutional foundations. John Pell circulated his *Idea of Mathematics* in the 1630s with the hope that the kingdom was not entirely 'destitute of learned Nobility and Gentry' willing to support his plan for a mathematical intelligence centre. Bishop Williams regretted that none could be found to support 'so fundamentall universaly usefull and eminent science as Mathematics'.[73] Similarly, when Kynaston's academy, designed to support the founder and six professors, failed soon after its inception, Fuller remarked that it was 'begun in a bad time, when the world swarmed with proleing Projectors and necessitous Courtiers, contriving all waies to get moneys'. Chamberlain in noting the obvious economic disadvantages of monopolies, exclaimed that 'the world doth even grone under the burthen of these perpetuall patents'. After a strenuous effort, the parliament of 1621 failed to correct the deficiencies of the monopoly system, leaving the final blow to the Long Parliament, which in November 1640 swept the entire edifice aside.[74]

Despite various pernicious aspects, the policies of the early Stuarts were not sufficient completely to inhibit the economic momentum created under Elizabeth. The all-important woollen industry declined sharply, but a nucleus for future prosperity was provided by a whole range of embryonic new industries, concerned with manufacturing iron, glass, salt, alum and saltpetre; increasingly industries made use of coal which replaced timber as the staple fuel for certain purposes. These developments were sufficiently impressive to be described by Nef as 'An Early Industrial Revolution'. He pointed out as a microcosmic expression of the fertile spirit of innovation, the use at the end of the sixteenth century of 'boring rods for finding out the nature of underground strata, and railed ways with large horse-drawn wagons for carrying coal . . . devised by the ingenuity of some inventors who remain anonymous, apparently in southern Nottinghamshire, where at about the same time, in 1589, William Lee gave the world his celebrated stocking-knitting frame'.[75]

Many of the families involved in the process of economic diversification provided recruits for the new science. The mine-owning Willughby family of Nottinghamshire produced the mathematician and naturalist Francis Willughby, the patron of John Ray; John Evelyn's family held the important saltpetre monopoly; Robert Boyle's father, the first Earl of Cork, was concerned with the development of ironworking in Ireland; the father of William Brouncker was joint founder of the Distillers' Company; Christopher Merrett's father was involved in the tobacco-growing project in the West Midlands. Hartlib's family were

73. Pell, *Idea of Mathematics,* 1651 edn., pp.41–2; Aubrey, i, p.129. Christopher Hill (149), Introduction, draws attention to the prevailing pessimism of the period between 1614 and 1640.

74. N. E. McClure (ed.), *The Letters of John Chamberlain,* 2 vols. (Philadelphia, 1939), ii, p.311. Price (228), pp.35–46.

75. Nef (198), pp.165–89. *Idem,* 'The Progress of Technology and the Growth of Industry in Great Britain', *Economic History Review,* 1934, *5*: 3–24; pp.17–18.

involved with dyeing and Eastland trade. At a more modest level Petty was son of a Romsey weaver and dyer. The family of the alchemist William Backhouse were active in Myddelton's New River project. William Harvey's family were engaged in East India and Levant trade. William Harvey himself was mentioned along with his merchant brothers, in 1638, as a dedicatee of *The Merchants Map of Commerce* by Lewis Roberts. These examples show that involvement in the new trades was not confined to any one social or political group.

The above evidence indicates the great extent of the awareness of the economic implications of science during the first decades of the seventeenth century. By 1640 there was also a high degree of individual participation in the quest for innovation. Projectors and patents were common, but subscription to the more ambitious Baconian goal of utopian scientific and economic planning was noticeably lacking. Indeed Bacon himself failed to behave in a manner consistent with the objectives which he preached. Thus despite his lofty statements of intention the treasures of science were left for later generations to claim.

(iv) The Riches and Abundance of the World

The revival of parliamentary authority renewed interest in economic planning. A new group of theorists emerged, who formulated social and economic policies for the puritan faction. Not all of their ideas were new. Indeed many had received sporadic expression in the earlier part of the century. But the writers of the Puritan Revolution incorporated these proposals into a more coherent programme, which embraced a broader range of issues, and they gave high priority to policies designed to ameliorate the condition of the lower classes. Accordingly they took up popular grievances, supported the Long Parliament's attack on the monopoly system, and framed alternative policies which would guarantee national prosperity without causing harm to any section of society. Consistently with the mood of the times the economic writings tended to take on an optimistic and utopian flavour. The new writers came to terms with the changing economic situation and sought to turn the conditions to advantage. They believed that the decline of traditional textiles could be compensated for by the development of the new draperies; it was realised that future prosperity required economic diversification and the ability to manufacture at competitive prices. Above all the theorists shared the Baconian view that local conditions and natural resources placed no limitation on economic development. Providence guaranteed that ample rewards would be forthcoming, provided that problems were approached in a resourceful and scientific manner.

The new phase of economic speculation began in 1638. It was initiated by the publication in 1638 of Roberts's *Map of Commerce,* a work which established continuity with the earlier period. Roberts's book was in some ways a complement to Malynes's *Consuetudo,* providing a substantial guide to the economic resources of every continent. Also in 1638 Hartlib published *An Idea of Mathematics written by Mr. John Pell to Samuel Hartlib.* This set the tone for the brief but ambitious reform tracts produced during the next few years. In 1639 Plattes issued *A Discovery of Infinite Treasure,* which contained a series of proposals for agricultural reform. Shortly afterwards he produced a briefer companion volume on mining and metallurgy, *A Discovery of Subterraneal Treasure.* The establishment of the Long Parliament provoked a further burst of economic writings. Plattes organised his proposals into a utopian tract, *A Description of the Famous Kingdom of Macaria* (1641). *Englands Safety in Trades Encrease* (1641) by Henry Robinson was the most detailed exposition of the new economic theory; much the same ground was covered by Lewis Roberts in *The Treasure of Traffike* (1641). More limited aspects of economic planning were considered in brief tracts by William Goffe and Sir Thomas Roe.[76]

This collection of short works represents a refreshing and incisive contribution to economic theory. The writers themselves collaborated to a certain degree; all (with the possible exception of Goffe) were associated with Samuel Hartlib. Apart from Roe they were active supporters of the parliamentary party. They were expert and experienced in their area: Robinson and Roberts were cosmopolitan merchants; Pell was a well-known mathematician; Plattes had spent many years working in agriculture and mining. Roberts is probably typical of the group. He was a member of John Goodwin's congregation at St. Stephen's Coleman Street, an officer in the Honourable Artillery Company, and engaged in East India trade.

These authors drew a contrast between the natural wealth of the earth and its current unexploited condition. Failure to realise this potential was blamed on man's own neglect:

> 'The earth, though notwithstanding it yeeldeth thus naturally the richest and most precious commodities of all others, and is properly the fountaine and mother of all the riches and abundance of the world, partly as is said before, bred within its bowels, and partly nourished upon the surface thereof, yet is it observable, and found true by daily experience in many countries, that the true search and inquisition thereof, in these our dayes, is by many too much neglected and omitted.'[77]

Plattes complained that because of inefficient agricultural methods, 'the barrenness both by little and little increase, and the fertilitie decrease every yeare more and more'. This agricultural decline brought

76. William Goffe, *How to advance trade of the Nation and Employ the Poor* (1641), *Harleian Miscellany,* iv, pp.385–9. Sir Thomas Roe, *His speech in Parliament: wherein he sheweth the cause of decay of coin and trade* (London, 1641).

77. Lewis Roberts, *The Treasure of Traffike, Or A Discourse of Foreign Trade* (London, 1641).

economic hardship which in turn, according to Plattes, had sown the seeds of civil strife. He believed that this position was unnecessary since 'Nature is no niggard, but giveth riches to all that are industrious'.[78] Similarly Robinson wrote that:

> 'England may have the advantage of all the World besides, by reason of her situation surrounded by the Sea, her Inhabitants populous for Manufactures, skilfull in Navigation, and unparalleld for safeties, her superfluitie of sundry commodities to furnish most Nations that stand in need of them, and lastly her Fishing, than which nothing is so peculiar to her, a treasure equall to that of both Indies in the richnesse.'[79]

The reformers called for dedicated industry, assisted by legislation designed to remove restrictions and encourage the flow of trade. Robinson and Roberts strongly subscribed to Mun's view that national wealth depended primarily on status in international trade. Parliament was asked to support measures designed to promote the expansion of trade. For the benefit of merchants they sought improved credit facilities, customs duty reforms, a more rational company organisation and freedom from restrictive impositions. Both writers advocated wider use of bills of exchange, reduced interest rates, and a national bank. It was recognised that improvement of roads, bridges, river navigation and postal services would greatly facilitate inland trade. Robinson proposed that parliament should undertake utopian planning, which would involve the creation of new industrial centres situated with regard to local resources and communications. Robinson joined Plattes in calling for agricultural improvement, wishing to set 'wits and hands a worke for improving of the soile'.

There was general agreement that an aggressive attitude to foreign trade deserved high priority. The reformers sought to imitate and ultimately surpass the Dutch to become the 'sole soverayne of the sea'. In this context they appealed for the encouragement of the fishing industry and of colonisation as a means to stimulate growth of the merchant fleets. Reformed tariffs would be framed with regard to their influence on the volume of trade rather than to immediate financial returns. Robinson became the pioneer English advocate of entrepôt trade.

Although neither Roberts nor Robinson made explicit reference to technological innovation, many of their proposals (e.g. improved river navigation, a restored coinage, extraction of salt from sea water) might have involved an important technical ingredient. Robinson's associate Samuel Hartlib was an extremely active advocate of innovation almost from the time of his arrival in England. In planning his first journey

78. Plattes, *Infinite Treasure* (217), sig.C3v, p.78.
79. Robinson, *Englands Safety* (246), pp.3–4.

to the continent, Hartlib's colleague, John Dury, expressed his intention to collect books and documents relating to 'the Preservation and Encrease of wealth by trades and mechanicall Industries, either by sea or Land; either in Peace or Warre'.[80] Subsequently Hartlib's correspondence assembled intelligence on all aspects of 'useful learning'. John Pell was particularly concerned with the development of mathematics. Between 1630 and 1634 he originated an ambitious plan for a Baconian natural history of mathematics. He proposed to establish a mathematical 'public library' which would prepare abstracts and research reports as well as collecting books and instruments. It would keep up with recent developments by maintaining a correspondency and by compiling a register of mathematical teachers and practitioners. Besides being an employment exchange for mathematicians, the agency would protect the public by issuing testimonials 'after examination to all sorts of practisers, as Pilots, Masters, Landmeters, Accomptants, &c. of their speculative ability and practical dexterity, that those that have occasion to use such men, be not abused by unable undertakers, to their exceeding damage'.[81] Pell's proposals probably reflect the growing social importance of the mathematical practitioners. Although their immediate impact was slight, many of Pell's ideas were later repeated in a slightly different context in Hartlib's Office of Address. The *Idea of Mathematics* became extremely well known. It was widely circulated abroad by Hartlib and Haak; it was reprinted as an appendix to *The Reformed School* (1651), and later by the Royal Society.

During the 1630s Hartlib was closely involved with the work of mathematical practitioners and inventors. He expected that significant practical achievements would result from the work of the Gresham professors Briggs and Gellibrand, whose work he frequently mentioned.[82] He was also acquainted with Dury's uncle, David Ramsay, who was one of the most active inventors of the years before 1640. Hartlib also took up the cause of the Moravian exile Johann Christoph de Berg who patented 'many Inventions, as well mathematicall as mechanicke engynes and instruments not hitherto knowne or used in any of our Domynions'.[83] Hartlib publicised de Berg's work and probably arranged for him to enter into an association with Kynaston.[84] Thereafter Hartlib interested Pym in the Moravian's abilities as a mine-drainage expert. Pym obviously had high expectations of de Berg and he enthusiastically solicited de

80. Turnbull, *Samuel Hartlib* (284), pp.10–12, 'The Purpose and Platforme of my Journey into Germany', 1631.

81. Pell, *Idea of Mathematics,* quoted from the 1651 edn. (89), p.38. For the editions, see Webster (320), pp.15–16 & *passim.* See also the edition by P. J. Wallis, 'An early mathematical manifesto—John Pell's Idea of Mathematics', *Durham Research Review,* No. 18, April 1967: 139–48.

82. Ephemerides 1635. Hartlib greatly admired Gellibrand, of whom he reported 'these 2 hundred years not the like published as Gellebrand hase done de Magnete'. *Ibid.*

83. *Specification of Patent, No. 92A,* 1636.

84. Agreement between de Berg & Kynaston, HP LXIV 19 & Ephemerides 1634.

Berg's assistance with drainage operations at coal mines near Coventry. This kind of service was undoubtedly important in cementing Hartlib's friendship with a number of important puritan politicians who proved to be invaluable allies at a later date.[85]

Hartlib and Joachim Hübner hoped that Comenius's Universal College might devote some attention to the mechanical arts. At one stage Hübner was confident that Comenius would deliver the Verulamian instauration of knowledge, and turn his back on the inane speculations of scholastic physics, metaphysics and astronomy to elaborate a philosophical system which would generate progress in the area of mechanical arts.[86] But to their disappointment his interest in technology was limited to dabbling in perpetual motion. When in 1639 Gabriel Plattes emerged out of obscurity to publish his tracts on agriculture and mining, Hartlib realised that this author could complement the work of Comenius.[87] Whereas Comenius was concerned with general intellectual reform, Plattes could demonstrate the relevance of science and technological innovation to the utopian social programme. Plattes was not only concerned with 'raysing that benefit out of the superficiall, and subterraneall Treasures of the Earth' by diffusing information about agricultural and metallurgical practices; he was also aware of the relevance of this work to a lasting solution of the outstanding social problems of poverty and unemployment. He believed that the poor would be assisted more by their own, productive labour than by charity. Because of his own limited education, general empiricist disposition and desire to reach a wide audience, Plattes's writings were extremely well-organised, simple and direct. He hoped that by taking account of his advice the common people would at negligible cost become able to improve their land, detect and assay ores, and even become expert in the use of chemical indicators and controls for crop diseases.

Despite the utopian guise of *Macaria* its reform proposals were obviously directed at the English situation. Plattes's attitude to social and economic policy was consistent with the proposals of his fellow pamphleteers Roberts and Robinson. Adopting the utopian genre enabled Plattes to describe extremely idealistic constitutional changes which would facilitate economic development; thereby a state would be created in which 'the people doe live in great plenty, prosperitie, health, peace, and happinesse'.[88] General supervision of reform was to be vested in five Councils of Parliament, which would be concerned with Husbandry, Fishing, Trade by Land, Trade by Sea, and New Plantations. It may be presumed that Plattes intended these councils to implement policies of the kinds advocated by Robinson and Roberts. Indeed the division of responsibility between the councils of *Macaria* was remi-

85. Letters from Pym to Hartlib, HP XXXI 3.
86. Letter from Hübner to Hartlib, 1 December 1636, *MGP* II, pp.70–2.
87. Plattes, *A discovery of Infinite Treasure,* 1639 (217); *A Discovery of Subterraneall Treasure,* 1639 (218).
88. Plattes, *Macaria* (219), p.2.

niscent of the proposals made in *Englands Safety in Trades Encrease.* For instance the Council of Husbandry was designed to supervise systematic 'improving of lands, and Making High-wayes faire, and bridges over Rivers; by which means the whole Kingdome is become like to a fruitfull Garden'. These subjects were included in Robinson's fourteenth proposal.[89]

While Roberts and Robinson placed their emphasis on finance and the regulation of trade, Plattes stressed improvement and innovation. His national laboratory or 'Colledge of experience' was intended, like Solomon's House, to collect 'any experiment for the health or wealth of men'. It was anticipated that parliament would sanction the publication of works beneficial to the public, such as his own new book of husbandry and trade which was given the provisional title 'Treasure House of Nature Unlocked'. Plattes hoped that the laboratory of the College would make further progress towards understanding and controlling 'transmutation of sublunary bodies', a subject which had already been briefly discussed in *A Discovery of Subterraneal Treasure.*[90] In an oblique manner Plattes was drawing attention to his own previous writings and offering preliminary intimations about more substantial work in progress. His premature death prevented the completion of further tracts, but the fragments subsequently published by Hartlib indicate continuing preoccupation with metallurgy and the improvement of husbandry.

The approach to science defined in *Macaria* became firmly established among the puritan intellectuals. They took up the philosophy of Bacon, emphasising still further his commitment to histories of trade. Thus their attitudes towards science were framed with reference to their general economic and social programmes. Although many features of puritan social and economic policy were delineated without direct reference to science or technology, these factors were never far from sight. Workhouses were designed to solve the problem of the able-bodied poor; they would also assist the diffusion of new industries and techniques. Enclosure provoked popular antagonism, but it could be defended as a necessary preparation for scientific agriculture. Finally, more general economic policies were increasingly framed with reference to the collection and analysis of data. Thus we find the emergence of an embryonic scientific economics which had many points of contact with the new science.

(v) The Employment of the Poor

Every proponent of the idea of a technological utopia must have been aware that the economic changes of the seventeenth century were tending to swell the numbers of the poor. Crippling poverty became as en-

89. *Ibid.*, p.4; Robinson (246), pp.42–5.
90. Plattes, *Macaria* (219), pp.5, 11; *A Discovery of Subterraneall Treasure* (218), pp.40–3.

demic and unwelcome as the diseases which accompanied it. Accordingly many of the puritan reformers regarded the solution of the problem of poverty as a first priority; innovations were regularly judged by their relevance to this issue. It was also essential to show that industrial and agricultural progress need not be accompanied by dispossession and redundancy.

Before 1640 legislation and impressive private philanthropy had failed to stem the growing tide of pauperism. But whether motivated by a sense of Christian charity, or by fear of popular unrest, philanthropy provides an impressive feature of social life between 1600 and 1640.[91] When alms or hospitals were insufficient, inducements were given to the surplus population to emigrate to the colonies. With the Civil War poor relief was strained and the plight of the poor deteriorated still further. It is not yet possible to make a final assessment of the poor law policy of the parliamentarian authorities, but it is evident that the plight of the poor attracted eloquent apologists, whose efforts found expression to a limited degree at both national and local levels. Most of the action proposed was of a traditional kind. For instance, engrossers, forestallers, maltsters, badgers and alehouse-keepers came under attack from authors who were disturbed by the shortage and high price of grain.[92] In 1647 the parliament established a London Corporation for the Poor, which was eventually granted an income of £1,000 per annum and two houses to be used for rehabilitation. It was hoped that this model would be imitated throughout the country. The proceeds of the tax on coal were partly devoted to the poor and there is evidence that many local agencies were active in raising funds and initiating schemes to set the poor to work. Miss James believed that the emphasis of poor relief rapidly shifted from benevolence to the destitute poor, to the suppression of vagrancy. Recently Cooper has revised this view to conclude that the 'Commonwealth's intentions were at least as good as those of the Privy Council before 1640; in some places the results were better'.[93]

Whatever the success of palliative measures, these efforts failed to satisfy the active pamphleteers who pressed for a national policy of relief firmly based on vocational training and integrated with other aspects of social policy. Their enthusiasm for the expansion of agriculture and trade enabled them to envisage a permanent solution to the problem of poverty; all classes were expected to share in the anticipated commercial prosperity of the nation. Genuine humanitarian

91. W. K. Jordan (167), Chapter 7. E. M. Leonard, *Early History of English Poor Relief* (Cambridge, 1900).

92. For a typical list of proposals, see John Cook, *Unum Necessarium,* 1648 (57); a valuable and balanced account of poor law under the Commonwealth is given by Aylmer (12), pp.308–11, and by J. P. Cooper, 'Social and Economic Policies under the Commonwealth', in Aylmer (11), pp.121–42. See also James (158), Chapter VI.

93. Cooper, *op. cit.,* pp.126–9; James (158), p.299.

convictions provided a continuing motivation for the poor relief proposals, but the reformers were also encouraged by the possibility of turning a national burden into an economic asset. It was also more commensurate with the puritan social and utopian ideal, that all members of society should be engaged in productive labour, rather than that one section be endowed with great wealth and an obligation to support their less fortunate brethren.

Plattes argued that the improvement of land rather than the provision of almshouses offered the only satisfactory method of supporting the population. Likewise Robinson proposed a national system of workhouses, which would educate the poor and furnish them with adequate means to further their vocations and 'increase the Manufacture and Handicraft workmanship of the Nation'.[94] Miss James was absolutely wrong in detecting a fundamentally unsympathetic attitude to poverty among these puritan writers. From the writings of Plattes and Robinson at the outset of the Puritan Revolution, the tone was predominantly sympathetic. More conservative writers pressed parliament to restore traditional poor law measures, while the innovators manifested a genuine desire that the poor should be allowed to share fully in the profits of commerce and industry. Their plans were designed to protect the poor from exploitation. It was realised that simple scientific improvements could do much to secure the independence of artisans and agricultural workers. The reformers' proposals ranged from the severely practical schemes for workhouses of Hartlib, to utopian sketches for ideal communities. Hartlib developed Robinson's brief comments about poor relief into a detailed scheme for a system of workhouses for 'the imployment of the poore, the suppressing of idle Counterfeits; and the education of all poore Children'. Hartlib's workhouses were not akin to the repressive institutions of Victorian England; they were vocational training centres which would have been adapted to the requirements of each locality. Hartlib proposed that flax and hemp grown in each area should be purchased by central funds, housed in a 'Magazin' and distributed to poor workers, who were to be trained in the techniques of the new draperies by skilled artisans. Poor children were to be taught to read and write in part of each day, while they would also 'doe some work to help relieve them'.[95] The new draperies were regarded by Robinson as one of the main causes for the greatness of the Dutch. The growth and utilisation of flax and hemp would solve the problem of rural and urban poverty. Thereby it would set 'multitudes of poore people a worke, who thereby maintaine their wives and families in good order, which otherwise might bee burdensome, and perhaps

94. Plattes, *Discovery of Infinite Treasure* (217), Preface; Robinson, *Englands Safety in Trades Encrease* (246), pp.43–4; *idem*, *Certain Proposals* (248), pp.23–5. Cook (57) hoped that 'one fruit of this War will be I hope, to teach men good Husbandry': p.29.

95. Hartlib, *The Parliaments Reformation*, 1646 (135).

starve'.[96] These proposals were taken up enthusiastically and it is probable that the poor-relief pressure group influenced the decision to establish the London Corporation for the Poor. Industrial training schemes would have enjoyed the support of merchants like Robinson, who recognised the productive potential of the unemployed masses. To their disappointment the Corporation made only token efforts at introducing rehabilitation schemes, so precipitating renewed pamphleteering by Hartlib and his colleagues.[97]

Undeterred by the lethargic response to their ideas, the reformers went on to evolve even more ambitious training schemes and plans for community development. Hartlib's ideas on vocational training and education of poor children were further elaborated in Petty's *Advice,* which proposed a system of *Ergastula literaria* or literary workhouses for all children above the age of seven. Besides providing valuable physical exercise and inducing respect for manual labour, these workhouses would enable poor children to earn sufficient income to support them during the sophisticated education which was described in detail by Petty. This instruction was to terminate with training in mathematical instrument-making and other fine works of craftsmanship and applied art. At a more advanced level it was proposed to establish a *Gymnasium Mechanicum,* a fellowship of skilled artisans who would represent the highest level of attainment in each mechanical art. These artisans would be furnished with rent-free accommodation, and they would collaborate with colleagues and outsiders willing to assist the resident experts. Accordingly 'all Trades will miraculously prosper'. The college would compile histories of trade; and 'Active and Philosophicall heads' would be encouraged to further the 'Interpretation of Nature'. Upon reflection a critic wrote that Petty's scheme was too ambitious, estimating that it would need between two and three thousand pounds for its implementation. He thought that histories of trades could be produced by a voluntary 'Society and Corporation for the Advancement of Arts and Manufactures', formed under the supervision of a 'Chief Workman' chosen by national competition.[98]

An equally ambitious and probably related proposal for assisting skilled artisans emerged from discussions between Dury and Worsley. The former recognised that the royal ordnance complex at Vauxhall offered an ideal basis for a 'College For Inventions and Advancement of all Mechanical Arts and Industries'. Hartlib designated this institution as one of the eleven constituent colleges of his proposed University

96. Robinson, *Englands Safety* (246), pp.18–19.

97. Some of the most important of the poor relief tracts are Hartlib, *Londons Charitie* (1649); *idem, London Charity enlarged* (1650); Rice Bush, *The Poor Mans Friend* (London, 1649); Hugh Peter, *Good Work for a Good Magistrate* (London, 1651); Balthazar Gerbier, *A New Years Result* (London, 1652).

98. Petty, *Advice* (210), pp.4, 7. Anon., 'A Remonstrance of the feasibility of the Designes described by W.P.', HP. LIII 36. A system of colleges for vocational education was proposed by Snell (262), but with very limited educational standards.

of London. As already mentioned, Vauxhall had been the base for the activities of the Marquis of Worcester and his technicians before the Civil War. The parliamentary survey of September 1645 found the house, gardens and metalworking plant to be in reasonable condition. The buildings included, besides the large melting house with seven furnaces, equipment for working various metals, and two rooms containing an extensive series of models which were the work of Worcester, Caspar Kalthoff and William Joulden.[99] There was considerable delay over the disposal of Vauxhall and other crown properties. When the Act was introduced on 16 July 1649, it declared that the sale would not 'extend to the House called . . . Vauxhall, nor to the Grounds, Houses, Buildings, Models, Utensils, or other necessaries for practical Inventions therein contained, . . . but they shall remain and continue for the use of the Commonwealth, to be employed and disposed of by the Parliament, as they shall think fit.' Henry Robinson, as Comptroller for the Sale of Crown Lands, may have been instrumental in determining this outcome. Hartlib reported with satisfaction that 'As for Vauxhall, there is a proviso put into the act, that it shall not be sold'.[100] In an interesting memorandum composed to guide the authorities, Dury emphasised the importance of preventing dispersal of the Vauxhall plant, which could be readily employed by the state to advance the mechanical arts.[101]

'A Memorandum for Setting Faux-hall apart for Publick Uses

1. To keepe all manner of Ingenuities, rare Models and Engines which may bee useful for the Common-wealth.
2. To make Experiments and trials of profitable Inventions, which curious Artists ofttimes canot offer to the knowledge of skilful men and to public Use for want of a place of Adresse to meet with them, and of other necessarie conveniencies to show a proofe of their skill, wherof in Fauxhall is great store.
3. To bee a place of Resort wherunto Artists and Ingeniers from abroad and at home may repaire to meet with one another to conferre together and improve many ways their abilities, and hold forth profitable Inventions for the use of the Commonwealth.

The Reasons

1. The late king did designe that place for such an Use and that wee should be lesse mindful of the Public than hee did seeme to bee, will bee a disparagement unto us.

99. See above, pp.347–8.

100. Firth & Rait, ii, pp.190, 692; *CJ*, vi, p.261; *CSPD 1651/2*, pp.406, 413; *1652/3*, p.198; *1653/4*, p.355. Letter from Hartlib to Boyle, 24 July 1649, Boyle *Works*, vi, p.78.

101. Undated letter; no names are mentioned, but it is clearly from Dury to Worsley: BL vii. J. J. O'Brien, 'Commonwealth Schemes for the Advancement of Learning', *British Journal of Educational Studies*, 1968, *16*: 16–41, wrongly attributes this proposal to Worsley.

2. The conveniences of forges, furnaces, mills, and all manner of tooles for making of Models and Experiments being there already will bee a great losse to the Common-wealth if they should bee destroyed, and if the House bee alienated into some privat hand this will fall out.
3. In other Common-wealths as in Switzerland and the Low-Countries and the free Imperial Cities of Germany, there are places designed for all manner of Ingenuities, which they call *kunst-kameren* that is the chambers of Artifices.
4. It will encourage Artistes of all sorts at home and abroad to looke towards us, to esteeme of us, and to repaire to us, as men of Public Spirits and Lovers of Ingenuities, which will not only bee a credit to the Parliament, but an occasion of much profit. For to have a magazin of all manner of Inventions, and a ready way to encrease the same and trie the usefulnes thereof, is a treasurie of infinit and unknow'n Value in a Common-wealth which by setting this place apart for Public Use may bee gained.'

Vauxhall College represented the opposite end of the educational spectrum from Hartlib's workhouses, which were to be concerned primarily with basic literacy and elementary technical instruction. At Vauxhall, which was perhaps the intended location for Petty's *Gymnasium Mechanicum,* skilled artisans would be free to pursue scientific work and promote technological innovation. State protection, public service and freedom from entrepreneurial exploitation were features taken over from the College of Experience proposed by Plattes in *Macaria.* Letters composed by the Hartlib circle at this time indicate that the scheme was promoted by Boyle, Dury, Worsley and the influential Independent MP John Trenchard. Among the inventors who were expected to participate were William Wheeler, David Ramsay, Cressy Dymock, Kalthoff and Petty. Their current pre-occupations included the development of drainage wheels, furnaces and agricultural machinery, which were designed to facilitate schemes for the improvement of ore-refining, fen-drainage and agriculture. Worsley exclaimed that 'if Kalthoff and Petty might be joined together, they might doe wonders'.[102]

Dury's Vauxhall model probably influenced Petty's ideas on the reform of Gresham College. This institution had in the past played an important practical role, but it had declined during the 1630s. Petty felt that it could once again become an important stimulus to economic improvement. He proposed to replace the chairs of Divinity, Civil Law and Rhetoric with chairs in magnetism, optics, industrial chemistry and inventions. At this time Hartlib was seeking a means 'how Mr. Petty may be set apart or encouraged for the advancement of experimental

102. See the above letter and the one to which it was a reply, dated 18/28 May 1649. BL VII.

and mechanical knowledge in Gresham college at London'. Petty was appointed professor of music at Gresham, but the more ambitious schemes for Gresham and Vauxhall were not implemented.[103] Many appointments were made at Gresham during the Puritan Revolution but none of the professors showed interest in the kind of reconstruction advocated by Petty. Indeed after securing his appointment Petty seems to have taken little interest in Gresham College, owing to his pre-occupation with affairs in Oxford and then in Ireland.

The Vauxhall project continued to be discussed. John Trenchard obtained ownership of the property, probably on behalf of his colleagues in the Hartlib circle. Eventually it was proposed that the house should be returned to the Marquis of Worcester, who intended 'to bestow the use of that house upon Gasper Calehof and his son . . . for he intends to make it a college of artisans'. Hartlib hoped that it would be possible to employ Dymock at this establishment.[104] Otherwise, Hartlib and his associates devoted their main energies to the creation of an Office of Address, which was intended to assume responsibility for the patronage of experimental philosophy and technology.

Although no permanent state-regulated institution devoted to Baconian science and technological innovation was established, the various projects are an indicator of the enthusiasm for institutionalisation among the Baconians during this period. The projects of Hartlib and Dury find a parallel at the universities in John Wilkins's mathematico-chemico-mechanical school at Oxford. A particularly bizarre expression of the trend was Thomas Bushell's opportunistic proposal to establish Solomon's House either in London or at Wells. Recognising that advocacy of the Baconian philosophy was a means to win patrons and secure political rehabilitation, Bushell first proposed to establish in Lambeth Marsh a 'foundation or building, which is designed for the execution of my Lord Verulam's New Atlantis'. His primary aim was to persuade prospectors to bring their specimens to Lambeth for free assaying, a service which would have provided Bushell with useful information about current geological exploration![105] Bushell's fertile imagination evolved the phantasy that he was Bacon's chosen disciple, ordained to vindicate his master's knowledge of mining. Bushell next proposed to establish 'Solomon's House in all its dimensions' in the city of Wells. Again the discovery of 'Mineral Treasures' was to be his immediate task, but perhaps in conscious satirical imitation of the puritan tracts, Bushell asserted that the House would persuade debtors and criminals to 'walk hand in hand with you towards Christ's paradise, the Saints

103. Letter from Hartlib to Boyle, 24 July 1649, Boyle *Works*, vi, p.78. Ward (305), p.218. *Petty Papers*, ii, p.172. For Petty's proposals for Gresham, see Appendix VII below.

104. Letter from Hartlib to Boyle, 8 May 1654, Boyle *Works*, vi, p.88. Dircks, *Life . . . of the Second Marquis of Worcester*, pp.262–8.

105. Letter from Hartlib to Boyle, 8 May 1654, Boyle *Works*, vi, p.88; Bushell, *Abridgment* (London, 1659), pp.6–9; J. W. Gough, *op. cit.*, p.98.

New Jerusalem'. His agency would also feed the poor, increase trade, augment customs receipts and discover new arts for the 'universal good and honour of this Nation'. Bushell sought to attract publicity to his ideas by erecting statues to leading philosophers and issuing medallions to subscribers.[106] Bushell was undoubtedly a gifted projector, who opportunistically appreciated that Baconianism was the key to puritan sensibilities; but his reiterated assertions of dedication to the public good were insufficient to conceal the dominant motive of self-interest.

Science and technology had some part to play in the proposals for planned communities. These extremely diverse and usually impracticable schemes paid some attention to education and vocational training, but economic prosperity was sought primarily through the efficient distribution of labour. However social planners became increasingly aware that innovation and technical accomplishment were considerable assets to their communities. On the basis of biblical texts, Hugh Peter argued that the magistrate was obliged to support the advancement of learning, the improvement of nature, the advancement of the arts, and increase in trade.[107] His specific proposals were an amalgam of Robinson's economic theories and Baconian natural philosophy. In agreement with the supporters of a national technical institution, Peter advocated rewards for inventors and agricultural innovators. He believed that each town should devote a proportion of its income to the improvement of the environment, by such means as drainage schemes or the manuring of pastures.[108]

Peter's ideas were given more systematic expression by Winstanley, whose social theories assumed that his communes would undertake the more effective exploitation of nature. All benefits would be applied to the improvement of society as a whole, rather than passing to individual engrossers.[109] Providing there were adequate safeguards, it was permissible to proceed with innovation. Each craftsman would be taught by a skilled overseer, 'that young people may learn the inward knowledge of the things which are, and find out the secrets of Nature'. Like the children in Hartlib's workhouses, or Petty's Literary Workhouses, those of Winstanley's community were forbidden to concentrate on scholastic subjects; they would at an early stage be 'set to such Trade, Arts and Sciences, as their bodies and wits are capable of'.[110] Active involvement with the mechanical arts and with experimental philosophy was regarded as socially and spiritually desirable. It was incumbent upon each citizen to search after hidden knowledge and to 'arise to search it out'. Accordingly Winstanley exhibited a kind of intuitive Baconianism, championing the 'actor' against the 'contemplator', as a contributor to

106. Bushell, *Minerall Overtures* (London, 1659), pp.8–16; Gough, pp.116–21.
107. Hugh Peter, *Good Work for a Good Magistrate,* 1651 (208), p.73.
108. *Ibid.,* pp.74–81.
109. Winstanley, *Law of Freedom,* 1652 (336), p.23. For his acknowledgment to Peter, see p.11.
110. *Ibid.,* pp.43, 68–9, 70–1.

fruitful learning. His designation of the various spheres of knowledge worthy of further investigation closely paralleled the Baconian programme for histories of trade. Thus the inhabitants of Winstanley's communes were expected to share in the benefits of experimental philosophy in the same manner as the citizens of *New Atlantis* or *Macaria*.[111]

An entirely different approach to solving the problem of poverty was shown in the ramshackle schemes of Peter Chamberlen. Although a physician and inventor, he was primarily interested in promoting large-scale poor relief on a financially profitable basis. The intellectual outlook of the participants, and their capacity to generate improvements were of lesser concern. Chamberlen believed that application of the joint-stock principle could set 200,000 poor to work. In addition to providing for their subsistence, the fund would support schools and hospitals. The labours of the poor were expected eventually to make a profit for the subscribers. This profit would be further increased by the engines and inventions of the artisans. Economic benefits would also flow from an academy associated with the project, which was expected to attract talented foreign scholars.[112] The joint-stock principle was approached in a more sensitive manner in the 'society of mutual love' of Peter Cornelius Plockhoy van Zurick-zee. Cornelius, like members of the Hartlib circle, was impressed by the primitive simplicity of the Anabaptist communes in Transylvania and Hungary. The Anabaptist virtues of pacifism, industry and brotherly love were combined by Cornelius with more sophisticated educational and intellectual attitudes. He proposed that his society besides embracing classical languages and cultural subjects, should derive the maximum benefit from science and technology. Cornelius initially hoped to influence the social policies of the Protectorate. After the death of Cromwell, he reverted to a more modest proposal for a colony, which enjoyed a transitory existence in America under Dutch auspices before being suppressed by English colonists. The Hartlib circle had come to similar conclusions, abandoning their long-cherished programme for social reform to seek instead a patron willing to support 'a real Macaria', possibly in the Bermudas.[113]

Both the plans for utopian communities and the optimistic social programmes which were heralded by Plattes's *Macaria*, showed a common awareness of the capacity of science and technology to smooth

111. *Ibid.*, pp.56–7, 69–71. Winstanley divided the arts into five major groups, dependent on the type of material worked. The agricultural arts were listed in one category, and the arts relating to the cultivation of trees and woodworking under another. Winstanley and Plockhoy were imitated by William Covel, who described his utopian community in more detail, but with less impressive insight. Man was enjoined to compare the beauty of creation with the vanity of human society. In an attempt to improve the latter, the precedent of nature should be followed: *A Declaration Unto the Parliament* (London, 1659).

112. Chamberlen, *The Poore Mans Advocate* (44), pp.3–4, 7, 38.

113. Plockhoy, *A Way Propounded to make the poor of these and other Nations happy* (London, 1659); Schenk (255), pp.144–8; Worthington *Diary*, i, pp.156, 211–12.

the way towards a harmonious society. By stressing the rewards of technical proficiency and the 'improvement of nature', the poor could be stimulated to increased effort in the search for the fruits of nature. Thus the lower classes were not only encouraged to seek economic independence; they were also accorded a high degree of human dignity.

Baconian ideas became an important element in humanitarian proposals for poor relief and in Winstanley's plan for the organisation of his communes. The state was no longer obliged to regard the poor as a great social burden, a drain on private charity and public resources, tempting Puritans to link charities with punishment for vagrancy. Given suitable incentives and a favourable social climate, the poor would share in the general economic prosperity. In addition their combined labours would provide an impetus to the compilation of Baconian histories of trade. This kind of collaborative research assumed a central importance in Winstanley's commune. Although the direct practical influence of the utopian literature and general social programmes was limited, these imaginative designs enabled reformers to visualise the social role of science and to evolve a scientific ideology suited to various types of planned society.

(vi) The Advancement of Arts and Ingenuities

One legacy of *Macaria* was a flood of proposals for general social reform; designs for utopian communities became one of the hallmarks of the Puritan Revolution. An equally important and related manifestation of the puritan social ethic was the emergence of groups of intellectuals dedicated to the Baconian ideal of the national patronage of science and technology within the framework of wider social and economic planning. Success in this area demanded both an ability to generate support among influential politicians, and a sensitive appreciation of fruitful developments in experimental science. Extreme political instability and the proliferation of new scientific systems made the fulfilment of these conditions difficult. Nevertheless the puritan natural philosophers displayed considerable resilience; they achieved positions of appreciable influence without sacrificing their commitment to productive scientific enquiry. This degree of success was rendered possible by the close identity of interests between experimental philosophers and puritan politicians over a wide range of issues. Particularly fertile interaction took place over economic policy; the advocates of economic diversification appreciated the value of Baconian science, whereas the Baconians realised that economic diversification offered the best conditions for the development of their scientific work. There was accordingly a mutually beneficial relationship between these two spheres of interest. Hence it is not surprising that the philosophers whose formative years fell during the Puritan Revolution formed cordial relationships with merchants and tradesmen; they also took an interest in economic speculation. This group of merchants and Baconians was therefore well-equipped to make a decisive contribution towards the foundation of scientific economics.

This unity of endeavour was already apparent before 1642, in the writings of the group which embraced the technician Plattes, the mathematician Pell and the merchants Robinson and Roberts. Their associates, Dury, Hartlib, Culpeper and Nicholas Stoughton, ensured that technology was to the forefront in the social programme framed during the early years of the Long Parliament. The momentum created in 1641 was sustained for the rest of the Puritan Revolution. Within the group organised by Hartlib a continuous succession of young intellectuals was familiarised with the work of artisan inventors and introduced to political patrons.

A general framework for activity was provided by the schemes outlined in *Macaria*. Hartlib pressed forward with the work of the College of Experience without state patronage, in the hope that his more ambitious schemes would ultimately be implemented. Particularly after the death of Plattes it became necessary to induce other inventors to enter into the spirit of reformation and public service. It was not easy to evolve an ethical code which would encourage the active participation of inventors whose social attitudes had been formed during the period of monopolies. After the extreme reaction against monopolies in 1640, it was gradually admitted that some degree of regulation was necessary. Consequently, corporate privileges and a few individual patents were granted, so restoring certain of the practices of the Stuart industrial organisation. However, in important respects the corporations were in a weaker position and individual patents were not allowed to proliferate. Reformers wished to promote an ordered economy, which would ensure efficiency and guarantee adequate rewards, but prevent degeneration into uncontrolled monopolies. Plattes urged the state to remunerate inventors, as an inducement for them to utilise their knowledge for the public good. In 1645 Culpeper stated principles which were consistent with the spirit 'to advance the publicke aime that is amongst us'. He proposed that practitioners should voluntarily resign their rights of exploitation into the hands of a trust which would ensure that inventions were used 'wholly and solely for the benefits of some such publique worke or workes as (by certaine persons thereto appointed) from time to time shall be thought fitt to be undertaken and noe other use whatsoever'. As recompense, either the inventor or the trust were to be allowed to sponsor projects based on the invention.[114] This idea quickly matured into a plan for a national agency to supervise technological innovation, which became fundamental to the Office of Address proposals of Hartlib.

Even before the Office of Address was announced, the members of the

114. Letter from Culpeper to Hartlib, 5 November 1645, HP XIII.

Hartlib circle entered into negotiations with promising individuals whose efforts seemed relevant to the public interest. Their patronage of two Huguenot innovators and William Wheeler illustrates the laborious and uncertain nature of early attempts to apply technology to the service of the Commonwealth. The Huguenots Peter Pruvost and Hugh l'Amy, provided a link with the colonisation projects of earlier decades. In 1629 a plan was introduced to settle French protestants in Virginia, with the aim of exploiting their native skills in vine and olive growing and the manufacture of silk and salt. This project matured into an elaborate proposal to create a 'Carolina' colony with Hugh l'Amy as Receiver General of Rents. Despite prolonged deliberation, the Carolina colony was not established, but l'Amy and his disciple Pruvost remained active propagandists for plantations.[115]

The Huguenots reappeared before the public eye in 1645, when Hartlib was confident that a parliamentary committee would be established to examine their proposals which had been translated and redrafted by Dury. But regardless of vigorous preparatory work, parliament appears not to have formed the anticipated committee. Pruvost disclosed his plans only in the most general terms. His main public service was to be the reduction of unemployment: 'For now multitudes of People that are without Rule in a manner desperat & wilde under noe government shall bee reduced to certain employments & brought under inspectors, who may bee directed how to teach them & order their wayes in their callings to the attainment of knowledge & the exercises of temperance of Righteousnes & Godlinesse'. This approach coincided with Hartlib's proposals for workhouses and even more closely with various schemes for settlements. Pruvost was insistent that state sponsorship of an American colony was preferable to a patent to protect specific inventions. He was totally averse to establishing any 'kind of monopoly in trade'. Previously the petitioners had promised profits to the king and various courtiers; now they offered to solve the problem of unemployment and generate profits for the state. From the rather inscrutable proposals it is clear that the Huguenots intended to reveal methods of husbandry and fishing practised on the continent. Pruvost and l'Amy appear to have been skilled in the techniques of intensive agriculture, fisheries and the salting and drying of fish.[116] On all of these topics, the English were most anxious to benefit from continental expertise. Pruvost visited England to press his claims, but it is clear that considerable suspicion was encountered; there was also

115. *Cal. State Papers Colonial 1574–1660,* pp.108, 115, 129.

116. The main collection of papers relating to Pruvost and l'Amy is HP LIII 14; see also LIII 31, 32 & XXV 8. Many of the drafts exist in multiple copies or variant forms. The main document framed by Dury and probably intended for publication is 'The Proposals of Mr. Pruvost with a discourse thereupon' dated 30 November 1645. There are five copies of 'A Summarie of the Propositions to be tendred to the Parliament by the French Protestants mentioned by Mr. Hartlib in his petition to the House of Commons'.

much debate over the exact terms of any formal agreement. The relevant documents were widely circulated and Dury reported that Westrowe had called a meeting of nine or ten gentlemen who had expressed sympathy with the scheme, providing that benefit to the state could be guaranteed. Culpeper introduced the scheme to Hugh Peter, himself an experienced colonist.[117] There was some discussion about the terms of the patent sought by the projectors, but the basic difficulty arose over their land-tenure proposals. Culpeper was disturbed that these left too 'little liberty for a man to dispose of his owne', savouring of the authoritarianism of the previous age. Despite the exemplary aims of the projectors Culpeper demanded that Pruvost

> 'will quitte that resolution of takinge mens estates & disposinge of them without theire consente. A state never yet acted suche a thing since the worlde began, & I am confident this Parliament (after soe many pressures & noe satisfactory accounte) will not thinke themselves in case to doe it, & in truthe, if soe much good be like to be effected, to every particular man in his owne private concernements, every body will see that there will be noe neede of constrainment—An inseparable companion of most former monopolies'.[118]

Support for the Huguenots had placed Culpeper in an ambiguous position; while he favoured state intervention on their behalf to promote economic diversification, their intention to introduce state management of natural resources provoked anxieties about the repressive powers of central authority. In this test case Culpeper would rather sacrifice reform than risk incursions against personal freedom. To the regret of Culpeper Pruvost soon left England—'I feare wee have loste Provoste & doe very much grieve for it'.[119] However his proposals continued to circulate in the Hartlib circle and were soon to re-emerge under a new and more influential sponsor.

Even with such sympathetic characters as the Huguenots, difficulty was encountered in framing proposals acceptable to the projectors, their puritan sponsors and to the parliamentary authorities. Much greater problems beset negotiations with inventors lacking puritan commitments. Many younger practitioners were willing to subscribe to the ideal of public service, but older inventors like William Wheeler guarded their work with jealous secrecy. Like the Huguenots, Wheeler had been involved with Sir William Boswell, who had financed Wheeler's operations in the Netherlands. The inventor dabbled in a wide range of subjects, but his main energies were devoted to the perfection of a snail wheel (*slercrat*) drainage mill, a machine potentially of great

117. Letter from Dury to Hartlib, 25 August 1646, HP III. Letter from Culpeper to Hartlib, 20 September 1647, HP XIII.

118. Letter from Culpeper to Hartlib, 13 October 1647, HP XIII.

119. Letter from Culpeper to Hartlib, 10 November 1647, HP XIII.

economic importance. Apparently, after demonstrating his device, Wheeler was granted a patent by the States General in 1639, followed by an English patent in 1642—the very last granted by Charles I. At this point Wheeler's reputation was high. When his principle was copied at Leyden, the Englishman obtained substantial indemnification in return for his assistance in improving the wheels replenishing a canal. The claim that his invention approached a perpetual motion created additional interest in this wheel.[120] Wheeler was the subject of intensive discussion among Hartlib's correspondents, at first with a view to attracting him into full collaboration. Soon they became disenchanted. When Worsley visited the low countries, he enquired after Wheeler's mills, but no examples were discovered or reported. Furthermore Wheeler had deserted Boswell without paying his debts, and could not be traced. Nevertheless Boswell was confident that the invention was 'very good, and behoovefull to the country if used', attributing its failure to the conservatism of the Dutch. Worsley echoed this sentiment: 'although they have printed a paper to shew the use and excellency of it, and prooved it Mathematically in Diagrams, By the statick Art against the Fabriques that opposed it, and have shewed, how that even they also have added to it . . . yet they can sell none; neither do the country care for contracting for them'.[121]

The inventor proved insensitive to all offers of assistance which were conditional on devotion to public service, defending his work against critics and offering his services to new patrons until his death in 1653. Various members of the Hartlib circle withdrew gratuities granted to him; Culpeper realised that fruitful collaboration required a less mercenary attitude from the inventors. It was necessary for them to recognise that their gifts were God-given and should therefore be used for the benefit of all. One solution, which would satisfy the interests both of the public and the inventor, was for parliament to 'appointe a committee for the examining & rewardinge of Ingenuities & purchasinge them for publique use'. Culpeper thought that this committee should become the trustees for an Office of Address, which seemed to be the appropriate vehicle for ensuring the maximum participation of technologists in the work of the commonwealth. Until that relationship was established 'the Divine will hinder the worlde, of a great parte of the happines which it might injoy'.[122]

120. Doorman (81), pp.42–3, 144, 177. *Specification of Patent No. 127*, June 1642. Wheeler's invention was described in *Bewys van der Hoedanigheyt en Werking der geoctroyeerde waterschepraden geinventeert bij Jker Willem Wheler* (Amsterdam, 1642). See also D. Seaborne Davis (70), pp.93–5. Wheeler's pamphlet is translated in B. Woodcroft (ed.), *Supplement to the Series of Letters Patent*, vol. I (London, 1858).

121. Letter from Worsley to Hartlib, 4/14 February 1647/8, HP XXXVI 8. Elsewhere Worsley claimed that Wheeler's mill was better than 'any other can bee, if there come no Perpetual Motion': letter to Dury, 18/28 May 1648, BL VII.

122. Letters from Culpeper to Hartlib, 16 June 1647 & 15 May 1648, HP XIII. Most of Culpeper's letters written in 1647 were concerned with Wheeler. See also

Although denied the support of inventors like Wheeler, the puritan intellectuals persisted with their technological endeavour. Gradually Plattes's role was assumed by Benjamin Worsley, whose project to manufacture saltpetre occasioned considerable comment during 1646. Furthermore, as Culpeper noted, Worsley had taken up the ideas of Pruvost which he found to be consistent with his new propositions on saltpetre. Dury was convinced that these schemes could not 'be demanded and advanced excepte the intereste as well as the authority of a State be ingaged in it'. An appropriate mechanism would be 'the extensiones of that colledge you [Hartlib] have in your mind' which might 'free minds from necessary worthy cares & set them upon such universall objects as leade moste to Gods Glory, in our nayghbors good'. The result would be the discovery of a 'sea of ingenuities', and an increase of the fruits of the earth, by which men would return to dominion over nature and reconciliation with God.[123] With such an inspiring aim in mind it was essential to enter into close association, to 'stirre up one another, to press forward, to that marke that is set before us'.[124]

'Examining & rewarding of Ingenuities & purchasing them for publique use' was adopted as one of the main functions of the Office of Address. Pell's mathematical agency and the College of Experience of *Macaria* were two of the principal scientific elements which were incorporated into the Office of Address proposals which were announced to the public in the decade between 1647 and 1657. Culpeper in particular recognised that public patronage and free communication of technological intelligence were such striking departures from traditional practices that determined opposition was likely from the monopolists and the Presbyterians. Consequently Dury's initial description of the Office took considerable care to explain that the institution was compatible with the generally acknowledged parliamentarian religious and social doctrines. Universal applause would have been gained by the promise to increase employment in all 'Vulgar Trades', uprooting vagrancy 'even as weeds are to be rooted up and cast out of a fruitful garden'. The introduction of a repressive tone into Dury's tract perhaps lessened the impact of the more unorthodox and liberal measures enunciated by Hartlib. From the outset the Office of Address was conceived in two parts; an Address for Accommodations concerned with 'Outward Things' and an Address for Communications dealing with 'Inward Things'. The two parts were to maintain a fruitful intercourse, but remain independent in administration, even to the extent of being located in different towns. The obvious location for the Office

---

Wheeler's apologetic tracts, *Mr. William Wheelers Case from his own relation* (London, 1644); *A List of Some Chief Workes which Mr. William Wheeler Offereth to undertake* (Amsterdam, 1651).

123. Letter from Culpeper to Hartlib, n.d. [1646], HP XIII.

124. Letter from Culpeper to Hartlib, 10 January 1645/6, HP XIII.

of Communications was London, while at first Dury favoured Oxford for the Office for Accommodations.[125]

The Address for Communications 'for the Relief of Human Necessities' had an entirely economic function. By compiling up-to-date registers concerning employment, trade and estates, the Office could provide a valuable service for employers, employees, merchants and those engaged in estate transactions. Hartlib recognised that the registers could be applied to 'all things which either may be any way offered by one man to any or to all'. The registers would be of two types, information being distributed according to its degree of permanence. A basis for operation would be provided by Permanent Registers containing geographical, demographical, statistical and economic data, relating to all trading nations, and also for each region of Britain. This collection of reference material would take over the functions of Roberts's *Map of Commerce,* a work which was circulated among the Hartlib group at this time. Permanent data of this kind would provide the basis of registers relating to four main aspects of economic life—the employment of the poor, commercial transactions, artisans and professions, and 'Ingenuities, and Matters commendable for Wit, Worth and Rarity'. This last register would catalogue information about books, manuscripts, inventions, mathematical instruments, or collections of rarities, which might prove of value to the public. Accordingly, following Hartlib's plan, the Permanent Registers had a strongly scientific bias, while the Temporary Registers included much technical information. It could therefore be legitimately claimed that a major function of the Office was 'an Orderly and effectual Correspondencie and Agencie . . . for the Advancement of Universall Learning, and all manner of Arts and Ingenuities'.[126]

In its basic form the Office had already proved its worth in the Parisian *Bureau d'adresse* of Théophraste Renaudot. There was immediate enthusiasm for establishing such agencies in London, although the various competing proprietors concentrated on the distribution of routine commercial information, rather than the wider charitable and intellectual functions advocated by Hartlib.

The Office for Accommodations was entrusted to the capable hands of Henry Robinson, while Hartlib concentrated on the Office for Communications. As first outlined by Dury the Communications Office was reminiscent of the Universal College of Comenius. There was little

125. Dury, *Considerations tending to the Happy Accomplishment of Englands Reformation,* 1647 (86), pp.42–3, 53.

126. Hartlib, *A Further Discoverie of the Office of Publick Addresse,* 1648 (136), pp.2–4. A manuscript, 'Q. and desiderata of O. of Addresse' by Hartlib confirms the intention to compile detailed 'Histories of Manufactures' containing a description of all relevant operations, instruments and tools: HP LIII 21. Samuel Lambe (178), p.8, admired the Dutch for rewarding 'profitable and delightful Arts and Mysteries' from a public stock.

specific reference to science, apart from passing praise for Bacon's *De Augmentis Scientiarum* and a call for 'the most profitable Inventions' to be deployed by the state for the public good.[127] By contrast the detailed proposals which eventually won state approval had a strongly scientific and technological bias. The evolution of this 'Agency for the Advancement of Universal Learning' has already been described.[128]

John Wilkins was suggested as a suitable head or 'president of the standing council of universal learning'.[129] The choice of a leading university figure appears somewhat anomalous in view of the harsh criticisms of academics voiced by the advocates of the Office of Address. On the other hand Wilkins's support would have been invaluable in the period after Cromwell's death. Also Wilkins was not an altogether alien figure. The spirit of his natural philosophy as expressed in *Mathematical Magick,* and the thirst for invention displayed by Wilkins's protégés at the Oxford Experimental Philosophy Club, indicate genuine points of contact with the Baconianism of the Office of Address. Wilkins predicted that the study of mechanics would yield 'real benefit' in 'Drayning, Mines, Cole-pits &c'. In terms reminiscent of Bacon, he commended the mechanical arts because of their power to 'overcome, and advance nature'. Accordingly they were not 'to be esteemed less noble, because more practical, since our best and most divine knowledg is intended for action, and those may justly be counted barren studies, which do not conduce to practice as their proper end.'[130] *Mathematical Magick* was a resourceful attempt to discuss the various types of mechanical contrivance in terms of elementary mechanical principles. There is little trace of his own work as an inventor at this stage; rather Wilkins drew upon well-established texts on mechanics and the Theatres of Machines of such authors as Ramelli, Zoncha and Besson. Occasional reference was made to the exploits of Cornelius Drebbel, whose perpetual motion device and submarine were discussed in detail. Perpetual motion formed the climax of Wilkins's book; one by one the various types of alleged perpetual motions were scrutinised and eliminated. Closest attention was devoted to the spiral waterwheel of the type built by Wheeler, which was recognised as a highly efficient and economically significant invention. Although Wilkins realised that this was not a true perpetual motion, inventions of this type were encouraged, because 'our searching after it may discover so many other excellent subtleties, as shall abundantly recompense the labour of our enquiry'.[131] It will be recalled that Bacon had given a similar justification for alchemy.

127. *Considerations* (86), p.47.
128. See above, pp.66–77. See also Appendix VIII, below.
129. Letter from Hartlib to Boyle, 16 December 1658, Boyle *Works,* vi, p.115.
130. Wilkins, *Mathematicall Magick* (331), sig.A4v, p.31.
131. *Ibid.,* p.293.

After experience of such treatises as *Mathematical Magick* contemporary observers like Aubrey could detect no abrupt discontinuity in approach to science between Wilkins and the Baconians associated with Hartlib. Aubrey believed that a utilitarian and experimental attitude united a broad group of intellectuals which included Boyle, Petty, Potter, Wilkins and Wren. They experimented with chemical medicines; they produced a wide range of useful mechanical inventions, including perpetual motion devices, ploughs, double-writing instruments, agricultural engines, mathematical and optical instruments. When John Lydall of Trinity College Oxford entered into correspondence with Aubrey, it was very much in the spirit of Hartlib's intelligencers : 'I shall bee very happy & willing to preserve continuall intelligence with so truly sincere and ingenious friend . . . I desire you to write what new discovery or experiment you shall chance to make or meet with.'[132] These undoubted similarities of interest contrast with a divergence of attitude between the various groups of Baconians over the social function of their knowledge. Hartlib anticipated that innovation would be applied by the state to solving the problems of poverty and unemployment, while more orthodox virtuosi were influenced by the traditional motives of self-interest and gentlemanly curiosity.

Because of their concern with public service and social policy, Hartlib's associates were obliged to pay attention to wider issues of economic policy. Benjamin Worsley's scientific outlook became particularly strongly influenced by general economic objectives. His ability to initiate fruitful experimental enquiry and frame national economic policies made him appear as the natural heir to the Lord Chancellor as an advocate of the utopian goals of science. Whatever the limitations of his scientific accomplishment, his example constituted an incentive for other young puritan intellectuals to enter into public service.

Worsley first attracted public attention by his attempt to translate a simple scientific principle into economic practice. As described above, the chemists believed that metals, minerals and salts were generated in the earth whenever conditions were suitable. They were somewhat optimistic about the possibilities of such processes, and their explanations of chemical change were false. However it is true that chemical changes which produce salts naturally occur in soil mixtures owing to the influence of bacteria, which perform the functions of the 'semina' of the Paracelsians. Hence in principle the generation of saltpetre could be undertaken on an industrial scale. Much advice was available on the subject. Ercker gave instructions for the continuous production of saltpetre by this method. Jorden believed that rich earth would breed saltpetre when exposed to sunlight. Vegetation was thought to be nourished by the saltpetre which had been generated in the soil. Thus nitrous

132. Letter from John Lydall to John Aubrey, 18 September 1649, Bodleian, Aubrey MS 12, fol. 304r. For the inventions of Wilkins and his associates, see above, pp.163–72. See also Frank (105).

water was an effective fertiliser bringing 'all plants to perfection farre sooner then any other dung'.[133]

During the Civil War saltpetre was in very great demand for gunpowder manufacture and metallurgical works; chemists believed that if produced economically it might also become an important fertiliser. Such extension of use was precluded by expensive and inefficient methods of production. For most purposes the trade depended on the unpopular breed of saltpetre men who excavated cellars, outhouses and chicken runs in search of the black nitrous earth, which was mixed with lime and ashes, and then leached for its salts. Finally the impure solution was boiled and partially purified, a process which consumed large quantities of wood or coal. This unsatisfactory method was partly circumvented after 1639 by various East India Company merchants who imported saltpetre from India. But their supply was variable in both quantity and quality, while reliance on such imports was recognised as politically and economically undesirable.[134] Failure to organise adequate supplies of saltpetre, the cause of mild concern before 1640, became a major burden to both parties during the Civil War. Saltpetre men and importers assumed a factitious importance. Parliament gave considerable attention to the complex ordinances controlling saltpetre digging, in order to limit the unpopularity and inconvenience of the searches. In 1631 little interest had been aroused by David Ramsay's claim that a small saltpetre farm could supply sufficient salt for the whole nation. There was a more positive response in 1646 when Worsley introduced a similar scheme supported by scientific reasoning and backed by influential merchants. The foundation for Worsley's project was 'De Nitro Theses quaedam', a brief tract containing a synopsis of current chemical theory about saltpetre, and miscellaneous experimental evidence, perhaps drawn from Plattes and Ramsay. Worsley's views on the chemical nature of saltpetre were Paracelsian; the salt was regarded as a product of fixed and inflammable elements, which were separated in combustion and then reunited in the process of generation. He believed that saltpetre was normally formed in the surface layers of earth, where it was a fundamental nutriment for plants, from which it passed to the bodies of animals. Saltpetre was a good fertiliser; reciprocally, materials which were effective fertilisers were thought to be rich in saltpetre. Accordingly seeds which had been steeped in saltpetre solution produced more vigorous seedlings. Worsley thought that saltpetre could be generated in mounds containing mixtures of suitable

133. G. Agricola, *De Re Metallica,* trans. H. C. & L. H. Hoover (London, 1912), pp.561–4; J. Pettus [Ercker], *Fleta Minor* (London, 1683), pp.338–40; Edward Jorden, *A Discourse of Naturall Bathes* (London, 1632), p.48. Webster, *Metallo graphia* (327), pp.43–6, repeats Jorden; J. R. Glauber, *Prosperitas Germaniae* (Amsterdam, 1656), Bk. III.

134. Nef (198), i, pp.185–6; *VCH Surrey*, ii, pp.299–302. For typical ordinances see *LJ*, viii, pp.147–8, 7 Feb. 1646; Firth & Rait, i, pp.320–1 & *passim.* See also Aylmer (12), p.39.

material, providing that the aetherial constituents of saltpetre were at the bottom and the more fixed elements above. When impregnated with dung possessing the semina of saltpetre, the aetherial and fixed elements would be brought together and fused into saltpetre within three to four weeks.[135]

Providing that a supply of raw materials could be guaranteed, Worsley's method appeared to offer few difficulties. His scientific thesis was backed by a popular petition drawing attention to unsatisfactory aspects of current methods of saltpetre production. The new process would avoid infringing the liberties of the subject, employ the poor, improve the land and increase yields for the poor husbandman. Such was the anticipated efficiency of Worsley's process that for every ton purchased, an additional sixty pounds was offered free. At a more practical level, Worsley and his sponsors requested parliamentary permission to manufacture saltpetre throughout England, using turf, firs and ferns cut from royal forests. In return they offered to supply saltpetre, as well as fertiliser produced from the refuse.[136] The new method quickly won supporters. A certificate was obtained from a committee of London aldermen, which added authority to the draft proposals presented to parliament. Worsley's petition was granted, 'considering the great Use and Necessity of Salt-petre' and the 'certain Experiments' supporting the new method. Parliament appreciated that Worsley's method would release the citizens from an irritating burden and offer a means to employ 'divers Poor in this Kingdom'.[137]

In the long term the saltpetre project slightly damaged Worsley's reputation, but at first it greatly enhanced his public celebrity and contributed to increase expectations about the economic potentialities of experimental science. The saltpetre enterprise was supported wholeheartedly by the Hartlib circle and it may well have provided one of the main incentives for Boyle's interest in experimental chemistry. References to Worsley's project mark the beginning of Boyle's scientific correspondence. Boyle was promptly informed by Lady Ranelagh about the passage of the 'Saltpetre Act'. He expressed his congratulations to Worsley : 'I must confesse to you, that, in my wishes for the prosperity of your pious powder-plot, my private interests would needs mingle with more public considerations, I having been lately so vexed by those undermining two-legged moles, we call saltpetre-men.'[138] Boyle's subse-

135. 'De Nitro Theses quaedam', HP XXXIX 1. This copy is inscribed by Hartlib 'Mr. Worsleys Salt-Peter.' It is followed by a collection of letters about saltpetre composed between 1652 and 1654.

136. 'Certain Propositions in the behalfe of the Kingdome. Concerning Salt-Peter' & 'An *Acte* for a new way of making Salt-Peter', HP LXXII 15. For similar documents see HP LIII 26.

137. Certificate of Committee of Aldermen, 7 March/7 April 1646 & 'The Humble Petition of Benjamin Worsley', *LJ,* viii, pp.573–4, 21 November 1646.

138. Letter from Boyle to Worsley, [November 1646], Boyle *Works,* vi, p.40. In a letter to Boyle, 5 April 1659, Hartlib criticised Worsley's refusal to comment on saltpetre, a subject which he had formerly been 'so hot upon . . . both for

quent investigations on plant nutrition and the generation of salts may have been instigated by Worsley's work. In the *Sceptical Chymist* and other writings he continued to accept the theory that 'the seminal principle of nitre, latent in the earth, does, by degrees, transform the neighbouring matter into a nitrous body'. Thus in principle it was possible to establish 'a perpetual mine of salt petre'.[139] Similar views were expressed in the 'History of the Making of salt-Peter' by Thomas Henshaw, which was selected for inclusion in Sprat's *History of the Royal Society.*

The saltpetre project of Worsley was quickly incorporated into a wider economic programme, which was also influenced by the colonisation proposals made by Pruvost. Worsley's general statement of policy was headed 'Proffits Humbly presented to this Kingdome'. This opened with sections on the production and uses of saltpetre. Besides its obvious incorporation in gunpowder manufacture, Worsley proposed to experiment with the use of saltpetre for manuring, for preserving fish, for counteracting crop diseases and for improving the quality of wool. Worsley pointed out that by such simple expedients imports would be reduced, home production increased; and thereby bullion would be saved, commodities made cheaper, customs receipts increased, agriculture improved and the poor employed. Instead of explaining his intentions about saltpetre in detail, Worsley turned to more general economic questions, since many of his development proposals rested on wider issues. Recognising the dominance of the Dutch in maritime trade, Worsley suggested that their example should be emulated by developing 'Our own shipping, from our owne Plantations'. Like other contemporary economic writers he attached great importance to the enlargement of dominions and expansion of shipping. Agricultural and technological innovation was not irrelevant; it was to be undertaken whenever appropriate. But its application was dependent on the implementation of more general policies. Worsley predicted that by applying these

---

writing and acting'. Boyle *Works*, vi, pp.116–17. Petty's comments on this issue were even more acid. See also various letters from Culpeper to Hartlib February–December 1646, HP XIII. Dr. T. C. Barnard kindly informs me that Worsley revived the saltpetre project while serving as Surveyor General in Ireland. In this context see Boyle *Works,* vi, pp.80–1.

139. *Sceptical Chymist* (1661), Boyle *Works,* i, p.566. In the *Usefulnesse* (32), Boyle quoted the same evidence to prove that 'Metalline Bodies were not all made at the beginning of the World, but have some of them a Power, though slowly to propagate their Nature when they meet with a disposed Matter.' Bk. I, pp.77–8; Bk. II, part 2, pp.4–6. Ephemerides 1655 reports Boyle's interest in Starkey's experiment 'to make out of a certain quantity of saltpeter twice or 4 times as much or more' within 4 months. Boyle's views on the agricultural uses and generation of saltpetre were given fully in the appendix to *Usefulnesse,* 'How Experiments may become useful to Humane Life', pp.4–13. For Henshaw, see Sprat (266), pp.260–83. For a later echo of such projects, see R. P. Multhauf, 'The French Crash Program for Saltpeter Production 1776–94', *Technology and Culture,* 1971, *12*: 163–81.

policies the nation would achieve an unparalleled position of wealth and honour. Parliament would then be able to complete the task of reconstruction, by undertaking law reform, propagation of the gospel, educational expansion and the 'Advancement of Learning by men appointed and maintained to keep an Universall Correspondency, by erecting of Treasure Houses for the Collection of the History of Nature, for experiments both Chymicall and Mechanicall & by increasing of choice and public Libraries'. Ultimately he looked forward to the millennial conversion of the Jews and reconciliation of the churches.[140]

Worsley effectively demonstrated how a co-ordinated programme of innovation and economic reform could be used to guide the nation towards a utopian goal. After reading these propositions Culpeper declared his sympathy for Worsley's ultimate aim for glorification of God 'throughout the whole worlde, . . . not the family, Country, Nation, but whole mankind'.[141] 'Proffits Humbly' probably assumed considerable importance as a statement of general policy in the discussions of the 'Invisible College' which Worsley and Boyle organised in 1646. It is apparent from the comments of Boyle that the members of this College were equally concerned with immediate utilitarian improvements and ultimate utopian aims. For instance after announcing that he was teaching his labourers about husbandry and composing an essay on this subject, Boyle promised to transmit to Worsley 'any thoughts or experiments of mine, that I shall judge conducible to the furtherance of your great design,' which would lead to the composition of a *de usu partium* for the whole world. When describing the College to Marcombes, husbandry was suggested as an ideal pursuit for a member; to Tallents he stressed the universalist intention : 'they take the whole body of mankind for their care.' Finally, in answer to Hartlib's enquiries, he reaffirmed the utopian nature of the Invisible College.[142]

Once Hartlib was introduced to the Invisible College, he sought its integration within his wider circle of correspondents. Boyle, Worsley and Boate were drawn into participation with the Office of Address. Thenceforth the Hartlib circle embarked on an exceedingly wide range of technological and economic activities. Many others besides Boyle were attracted to study 'natural philosophy, the mechanics, and husbandry, according to the principles of our new philosophical college, that values no knowledge, but as it hath a tendency to use'.[143] Experimental philo-

140. 'Proffits humbly presented to this Kingdome', HP XV(II) 23. The full text is given in Appendix V below.

141. Letter from Culpeper to Hartlib, n.d. [1646], HP XIII.

142. Letters from Worsley to Boyle, [November 1646]; Boyle to Marcombes, 22 October 1646; Boyle to Tallents, 20 February 1646/7; Boyle to Hartlib, 8 May 1647. Boyle *Works,* i, pp.xxxiv–xxxv, xl; vol. vi, pp.40–1. For the history and membership of the Invisible College, see above, pp.57–67.

143. Letter from Boyle to Marcombes, 22 October 1646, Boyle *Works*, i, pp. xxxiv–xxxv.

sophy was not valued only for its immediate utilitarian application. Boyle and his colleagues also believed that problems having economic relevance could readily yield productive scientific knowledge and an appreciation of the manifestations of providence. Increase in understanding and return of dominion over nature were expected to proceed in harmony.[144] Following Bacon, it was emphasised that the distinction between luciferous and fructiferous knowledge should not obscure the underlying unity of experimental science and technology:

> 'For though that famous Distinction, introduc'd by the Lord Verulam, whereby Experiments are sorted into *Luciferous* and *Fructiferous,* may be (if rightly understood) of commendable Use; yet it would much mislead those that should so understand it, as if Fructiferous Experiments did so meerly advantage our interests, as not to promote our Knowledg; or the Experiments called Luciferous, did so barely enrich our Understandings, as to be no other waies useful. For though some Experiments may be fitly call'd Luciferous, and others Fructiferous . . . there are few Fructiferous Experiments, which may not readily become Luciferous to the attentive Considerer of them . . . And on the other side those Experiments, whose more obvious use is to detect to us the Nature or Causes of things, may be . . . exceedingly Fructiferous. For since as I have formerly observ'd, man's Power over the Creatures consists in his Knowledg of them; whatever does increase his Knowledg, does proportionately increase his Power.'[145]

Worsley was equally insistent that dedication to economic objectives need not prejudice success in experimental science:

> 'For humane knowledge I honour only that which is immediately deduced from, or built upon Reall & certayne Experiments; & those so many, as to make an infallible universall; seeing according to the Schooles science is not of particulars. All men therefore sedulous in Experiments, I honour alike, whether they be physicall or naturall, medicinall, Astronomicall, Opticall or any way mechanicall or Chymicall; all Knowledge carefully grounded upon these, beeing not only certaine, or Reall, but Usefull.'[146]

This point of view was also taken up in the early writings of William Petty. His *Advice to Samuel Hartlib* (1648) propounded a system of practical education and research adapted to 'the general good and comfort of all mankind'. In reaction against the rationalistic natural philosophy of Descartes and More he asserted that science must progress

144. Boyle, *Usefulnesse* (32), Bk. I, pp.1–2, 19–20.
145. *Ibid.*, Bk. II, part 2, pp.44–5. A similar view is found in Wilkins, *Mathematicall Magick,* Bk. I, Chapter II.
146. Letter from Worsley to Hartlib, 27 July 1648, HP XLII 15.

by an inductive method which would establish principles explaining all phenomena 'equally well, & that soe easily, as that a meane capacity may be able to foretell the effects of nature by them before they happen, and consequently produce great Noble pieces of art, tending to the happiness of Mankind'.[147] Once this methodological standpoint was adopted, neither scholastic nor Cartesian natural philosophy could rival the attractions of Bacon's natural histories. The Baconians became confident enough to assert with Glauber that university learning was sterile and a distraction from 'that knowledge of Nature, which I . . . now possess; neither doth it ever repent me, that I have put my hands to the Coals, and have by the help of them penetrated into the knowledge of the Secrets of Nature'.[148]

From the above quotations, it is apparent that the English experimental philosophers increasingly adopted the philosophy of Bacon. Their ultimate priorities and objectives were guided by the *Instauratio Magna,* while both in concept and language Bacon provided a framework for their philosophy. On specific issues Paracelsus, van Helmont and Glauber exercised considerable influence, but without disturbing the fundamental Baconian orientation. Thus with calculated fidelity the philosophers of the Puritan Revolution perpetuated the ideals of Bacon, repeating his anti-scholasticism, dedication to experimental philosophy, and inclination to give priority to natural history and histories of trade in the quest for the achievement of dominion over nature. A large number of practitioners were recruited to support this programme; and in spite of their failure to create substantial institutional foundations, their unity of outlook and dedication to public service guaranteed extremely fruitful collaboration.

Although the immediate social influence of the puritan Baconians has been acknowledged, they have been judged harshly by historians of science. Violent assaults on scholasticism are not thought to have been matched by sustained or serious interest in the experimental philosophy which was championed so vehemently in the reform literature. Entanglement with social and religious doctrines has been regarded as an impediment which prevented the Puritans from transcending their pious slogans and vulgarisations to enter into active participation in experimental science. Indeed the Invisible College, Office of Address or plans for specialist colleges for mechanics might have been well-intentioned but only ephemeral fancies, inconsequential manifestations of the passing swell of utopian schemes generated during the optimistic phase of the Puritan Revolution. However, the evidence cited above provides evidence of serious intention; projects were interrelated and drafted after extensive discussions among the practitioners, whose uninterrupted

147. 'Mr. Petty's letter in answer to Mr. More', 1648/9, HP VII 123; Webster (319), p.367.

148. Johann Rudolph Glauber, *Prosperitas Germaniae,* quoted from *Works,* trans. C. Packe (1689), p.307.

efforts to promote Baconianism extended through the two decades of parliamentary supremacy. In view of the failure of the puritan natural philosophers to establish their own scientific institutions, it is crucial to assess the significance of their informal efforts to relate experimental science to current social needs. It is only possible to counter claims that the scientific work and impact on society of the Puritans were insignificant, by elucidating specific case histories illustrating the degree to which they were successful in promoting their objectives. For present purposes discussion will be limited to five representative examples.

First, attention will again be drawn to chemistry, a subject often mentioned in two previous chapters, to illustrate the great enthusiasm for a subject which had achieved a new vitality, fitting it to play an integral role in the advancement of a Baconian programme.

Secondly, an account of the debate over coinage rationalisation will demonstrate the concern with technological innovation and the application of mathematical principles in an area of central concern to the state.

Thirdly, consideration of activities in Ireland will illustrate the work of the natural philosophers employed in the civil service. The conquest of Ireland provided an ideal opportunity for the Baconians to elaborate a regional natural history. This exercise in collaborative research revealed certain personal antagonisms, but it also led to an important extension of perspective.

Fourthly, reference will be made to attempts to relate the Baconian programme to wider social and economic policies which carried natural philosophers into the centre of political debate, where they had an opportunity to influence the general economic policies of the Commonwealth and Protectorate.

Fifthly, attention will be paid to husbandry as the area in which the Baconians made their most sustained attempt both to promote innovation and lay the foundations for a consistent, scientific approach to agriculture.

(vii) Chemistry: the Key to Nature

Some of Bacon's harshest comments were reserved for the chemists and alchemists. In his view chemistry had the greatest potential importance for industry, agriculture and medicine, but the chemists had completely failed to establish their art on a sound, scientific basis. Even Paracelsus, despite his appeals for emancipation from ancient authority and for a reliance on the Light of Nature, had misled his followers with writings which were characterised by 'noisy trumpeting, the cunning of their obscurity, their religious affiliations, and other specious allures', which turned out not to be 'sources of true knowledge, but empty delusions'. Nevertheless Bacon also adopted an unexpectedly sympathetic attitude to Petrus Severinus, the main contemporary exponent of Paracelsianism, and furthermore he admitted that the chemists 'by their activity and persistence, have done much to advance and help mankind, by bringing to light a great number of not unimportant discoveries for the benefit of man's life and estate'. Bacon appealed to the chemists to conduct their experimental work in a more systematic manner; then they would transcend their sporadic discoveries to gain true mastery over nature.[149]

Quite independently the continental Paracelsians were beginning to react against the introverted and secretive attitudes of traditional alchemy. Bacon's opinions were echoed in Andreae's condemnation of the delusions of the alchemists and Rosicrucians. Andreae's friend Joachim Jungius undertook a sophisticated eclectic synthesis of chemical theories, which aimed at relating Paracelsian views to current empirical knowledge.[150] At a more popular level the well-ordered exposition of theory and the adequate descriptions of large numbers of chemical preparations in the textbooks of Croll, Quercetanus and Beguin served to increase the influence of Paracelsus and provide a fresh impetus to experimental chemistry. Through these handbooks an audience was introduced to the controlled manipulation of a wide range of substances; and the preparation of mineral acids and salts in particular became the foundation for a new school of practical chemistry. The writings of Jorden and Plattes shortly after Bacon's death illustrate the degree of proficiency attained in the chemical techniques required for the preparation and testing of the salts of iron, copper, antimony and mercury. In a complementary area, Drebbel, although primarily an engineer, was successful in his work on dyes and explosives.[151]

The industrial and medical aspects of the new chemistry were intimately related; they had many techniques in common and both were concerned with processes involving metals and metallic compounds. The physician Edward Jorden studied medicinal springs, but his writings betray an equal interest in mining and metallurgy. Plattes was a mining expert; but his proposed College of Experience was expected to benefit medicine as much as metallurgy. Clodius's Chemical College possessed five furnaces which were employed to produce 'diverse choice chemical experiments, for the advancement both of health and wealth.'[152] The preparation of medicines gave insight into the properties of commercial products, while industrial by-products could be useful in medicine. In the search for an effective cure for ulcers, Hartlib was advised to

149. Bacon, *Temporis Partibus Masculus, Works,* iii, pp.533, 538; *Redargutio Philosophiarum, Works,* iii, pp.575–6; *Cogitata et Visa, Works,* iii, pp.605–6.

150. J. V. Andreae, *Christianopolis* (146), Chapters XLIV & XLV. E. Wohlwill, *Joachim Jungius und die Erneuerung atomistischer Lehren im 17. Jahrhundert* (Hamburg, 1887); H. Kangro, *Joachim Jungius' Experimente und Gedanken zur Begründung der Chemie als Wissenschaft* (Wiesbaden, 1968).

151. For Paracelsianism in the early seventeenth century, see Partington (205); Debus (71); Sudhoff (274).

152. Letter from Hartlib to Boyle, 28 February 1653/4, Boyle *Works,* vi, p.81. For Clodius and his College, see above, pp.302–4.

obtain a 'most precious medicine', the volatilised compound produced during the manufacture of brass from copper and lapis calaminaris at a Lambeth foundry.[153] At one stage in his career Dury took up chemistry with a view to solving his financial difficulties. At first he inclined to practise as a distiller, until Worsley warned him that his training scarcely fitted him for such a demanding 'mechanick trade'. By way of compromise it was suggested that he would be wise to specialise in expensive cordials, which might be prepared from French wine and herbs, distilled in a glass alembic over boiling water. Worsley himself had considered retiring to the country to earn a comfortable living by preparing herbal cordials and perfumes.[154] This episode illustrates the spectacular rise of experimental chemistry among the educated classes, who provided the enthusiastic audience for the large volume of iatrochemical literature published between 1650 and 1660.

An additional stimulus was given to this movement by the writings of van Helmont and Glauber. The rise of 'Helmontian' medicine has already been discussed. Glauber shared many of van Helmont's views, but his character was much more than that of a pragmatic industrial chemist; his famous laboratory was concerned equally with medicine and industry. His voluminous publications had the aim of improving chemical techniques and promoting the development of chemical therapy and industrial chemistry. His first book *Furni Novi Philosophici* (1646) was immediately successful; new sections were added in 1648, 1649 and 1650 and the first complete edition appeared in 1651. During the 1650s he produced *Operis Mineralis* (1651), *Miraculum mundi* (1653), *Pharmacopöa Spagyrica* (1654) and *Dess Teutschlands Wolfahrt oder Prosperitas Germaniae* (1656) as well as many minor tracts. *Prosperitas Germaniae* brought together many of his earlier ideas, with a view to encouraging the economic recovery of Germany after the devastation of the Thirty Years War. Glauber described improved furnaces and methods for refining metals, gave instructions for producing chemical medicines and also detailed advice on the manufacture of saltpetre.[155] His furnaces were perhaps the predominant interest of chemists between 1646 and 1660. Not surprisingly many of Glauber's ideas were incorporated in plans to make chemical technology a basis for the prosperity of England. Worsley's saltpetre project afforded a dramatic if inconclusive inauguration of this programme.

153. Letter from Hartlib to Boyle, [June 1658], Boyle *Works*, vi, p. 111. The same substance was recommended by Merrett and Harvey: A. Neri, *The Art of Glass*, trans. Merrett (London, 1662), p.300.

154. Letter from Worsley to Hartlib, 22 June 1649, HP XXVI 33. Many other letters relate to this project, as well as two brief sets of instructions by Worsley, 'Of Distilling' and 'Of the distilling or drawing of spirits, some Animadversions': *ibid.*

155. For further information on Glauber, see Partington (205), ii, pp.341–61; K. F. Gugel, *Johann Rudolph Glauber 1604–1670 Leben und Werk* (Würzburg, 1955). John Winthrop Jr.'s library contained 23 volumes by Glauber: Wilkinson (333), pp.157–61.

Immediately after the appearance of the first part of *Furni Novi Philosophici* the English Baconians sought fuller acquaintance with Glauber and his work. Showing characteristic initiative, Worsley made a prolonged visit to the low countries in order to visit Glauber's laboratory and to gather other technical and commercial intelligence. Through Hartlib's friend Johann Morian other English visitors like William Rand were introduced to Glauber and practical chemistry. Immediately the first part of *Furni Novi Philosophici* was published, Culpeper requested a 'transcript of soe much of his booke to be printed heerafter as concernes the oven'. He also wished to find out more about Glauber's methods of brewing and boiling in wooden vessels, an invention which Culpeper accredited to Sir Hugh Plat. Appelius reported that Morian was acting as Glauber's agent and had without difficulty secured the author's permission for translation, since Glauber's main desire was to ensure the maximum dissemination of the chemical techniques which he had hitherto taught privately.[156] At once a translator was appointed, but his work gave little satisfaction to Culpeper, who proceeded to correct the translation, at one stage attempting to enlist the assistance of Petty. The work was nearing completion in the autumn of 1647, but publication of further parts of Glauber's book caused delay. Nevertheless, Culpeper's prompt start and access to manuscripts probably assisted John French, who published an English translation of the whole shortly after the appearance of the first complete version in Amsterdam. A manuscript translation of Ercker's book was also being circulated at this time, although no English translation was published until 1683.[157]

Glauber's works were an important factor in the rehabilitation of chemistry as an exact and empirical science. During the 1650s it was translated from a position of relative neglect and low esteem to one of central concern among English natural philosophers. Distillation techniques and furnace construction became central pre-occupations; itinerant chemistry teachers acquainted with furnace practice were in considerable demand. In London Webster learned chemistry from Hunniades; in the University of Oxford Staehl established successful chemistry classes, while Küffeler was considering a similar venture at Cambridge or Durham. Increasingly the experts banded together to establish chemical laboratories employing skilled laboratory attendants. Laboratories sprang up in connection with the universities, the College of Physicians, and Hartlib's Agency, as well as many other private groups in London. Culpeper attempted to obtain original examples of Glauber's furnaces, in order to repeat his experiments and guarantee the accuracy of the translation of *Furni Novi Philosophici*. One of Boyle's first refer-

156. Letter from Culpeper to Hartlib, 1 October 1646, HP XIII. Letter from Appelius to Hartlib, 16/26 August 1647, HP XLV 1.

157. Ephemerides 1650. For the first published translation, see Sir John Pettus, *Fleta Minor* (London, 1683).

ences to scientific matters expresses acute disappointment when a 'great earthen furnace' obtained from abroad arrived 'crumbled into as many pieces, as we into sects'.[158] At Cambridge John Ray's circle was sponsoring the production of Glauber's iron retorts, while Henry Power's chemical notebooks record numerous experiments using the new furnaces. Robert Child introduced Starkey to Hartlib as an inventor of furnaces, whose abilities equalled those of Glauber himself. The spontaneous and dramatic rise of experimental chemistry provided the opponents of scholastic learning with one of their most valuable weapons. As a subject lying entirely outside the scholastic curriculum, chemistry was used to underline the sacrifice of fruitful knowledge ensuing from the failure to reform education. Thus chemistry was fundamental to the puritan educational programme of John Webster, while in a similar context John Hall declared that chemistry 'hath snatcht the keyes of Nature from the other sects of Philosophy, by her multiplied experiences'.[159] It is difficult for the modern reader to appreciate the intensity of the enthusiasm for chemistry felt among this generation. His belief that chemical experiments were the key to the innermost secrets of nature, inspired the practitioner to approach this labour with religious dedication. In this spirit Boyle declared that:

> '*Vulcan* has so transported and bewitched me, that as the delights I taste in it make me fancy my laboratory a kind of *Elysium*, so as if the threshold of it possessed the quality the poets ascribed to that *Lethe*, their fictions made men taste of before their entrance into those seats of bliss, I there forget my standish and my books, and almost all things, but the unchangeable resolution I have made of continuing till death.'[160]

During the Republic the chemists embarked on an ambitious range of projects; they attempted to improve techniques in established industries, and to apply chemistry in new directions. The ultimate goal of undertaking transmutations of all kinds—the 'key, clearly and perfectly to know, how to open, ferment, putrify, corrupt and destroy . . . mineral, or metal'—was never forgotten.[161] A representative chemical practitioner, whose interests were widely shared, was Johann Sibertus Küffeler, who worked from the Stratford-le-Bow dyeworks founded by his father-in-law Drebbel in about 1607 and continued after Drebbel's death by various members of the Küffeler family. The Küffeler papers indicate

158. Letter from Culpeper to Hartlib, 7 September 1647, HP XIII. Letter from Boyle to Lady Ranelagh, 6 March 1646/7, Boyle *Works,* i, pp.xxxvi–xxxvii. See also *Works,* vi, p.86.

159. C. E. Raven, *John Ray* (235), p.47; Turnbull (291), pp.224–5; Hall (127), p.27.

160. Letter from Boyle to Lady Ranelagh, 31 August 1649, Boyle *Works,* vi, pp.49–50.

161. Letter from Worsley to Hartlib, quoted in a letter from Hartlib to Boyle, 28 February 1653/4, Boyle *Works,* vi, p.79.

familiarity with a wide range of dyeing techniques, ranging from a black dye using an iron sulphate mordant to a series of red and blue dyes. Drebbel's most successful innovation was Bow dye, apparently produced from cochineal using a tin (or pewter) mordant. The secret of Bow dye was kept closely by Abraham who intended to reveal it to his brother Johann Sibertus on his deathbed. He died before this intention could be fulfilled, although the secret was discovered in some other way. J. S. Küffeler continued this interest in dyes. In 1647 it was reported that he was operating a dyeworks at Arnhem, as a neighbour of Glauber, while in 1657 Hartlib passed on to him an Italian technique for watering tabbies and mohairs, recently obtained from an informant in Tours.[162]

William Petty's interest in dyeing is evident from the *Advice* (1648). At this time he was investigating the techniques of manufacturing and dyeing pintado, a type of calico imported from the East Indies. He believed that the technique of dyeing the coats of horses, practised in Poland, might assist with his work on pintado. His information on dyeing was ultimately condensed into a succinct but thorough 'History of the Common Practices of Dying' which was read to the Royal Society in 1662 and reprinted in Sprat's *History of the Royal Society*.[163] Bow dye was regarded by Boyle as an ideal example of the beneficial consequences of scientific activity. He believed that the invention had resulted in considerable gains to tradesmen both in England and elsewhere. Drebbel was not merely a technician; the inventor was not 'bred a dyer nor other tradesman' and was not even aware of the traditional methods of dyeing scarlet; on the contrary he was an educated 'Mechanicien, and a Chymist'. Boyle was confident that further innovations of this kind would be effected by chemists. One result would be the substitution of native woad for imported indigo. He was also actively interested in inks and varnishes, whereas his friend John Beale wrote a long manuscript treatise on the purple dyes of the ancients.[164]

162. Letters from Hartlib to Boyle, 20 June 1657 & 27 April 1658, Boyle *Works*, vi, pp.93, 102–3; Partington (205), ii, p.324; F. M. Jaeger, *Cornelis Drebbel* (Gröningen, 1922), pp.88–94, 136–7. Although the secret of Bow dye was usually ascribed to Drebbel, Evelyn on one occasion attributed it to 'the Noble Hunniades' (*Numismata* (1697), p.280). There was probably jealousy between Küffeler and Hunniades, explaining the former's remark that Hunniades was 'a very idiot laborant and one that knew nothing at all': Ephemerides 1656. Evelyn mentioned Drebbel as the dye's inventor in his *Diary* (97), iii, pp.446–7. Letter of Appelius to Hartlib, 16/26 August 1647, HP XLV I.

163. Ephemerides 1648; Sprat (266), pp.284–306; Birch (26), i, pp.41, 50, 82–4, 109.

164. Boyle, *Usefulnesse* (32), Appendices, *How Experimental Philosophy . . .*, pp.31–41; *The Goods of Mankind . . .*, pp.22–3. *On Colours*, Boyle *Works*, iii, p.139. Beale, 'Purple of the Ancients . . . together with Civile & Scholasticall Disquisitions', HP LI. For continuing interest in this subject see A. J. Turner, '*Purpura anglicana:* A Bibliographical Note', *Jnl. Soc. Bibliography of Nat. Hist.*, 1970, 5: 361.

Küffeler's work diversified in many directions. Appelius thought that few could match his knowledge of metallurgy. His introduction of glass stoppers for bottles was thought by Boyle to have various applications.[165] Undoubtedly of more importance was his self-regulating oven, a device which could be applied for medium-temperature experiments, incubating eggs, or baking bread.[166] A portable version could be used for supporting armies in the field. But Küffeler's celebrity was primarily due to his 'firework', an explosive device, derived from Drebbel's torpedo which had probably been evolved to destroy French ships during the Duke of Buckingham's expedition to the Ile de Rhé in 1628. The torpedo invention probably influenced Küffeler's decision to follow the example of Drebbel and his brother Abraham by settling in England. Having 'perfected a dreadfull Engine for the speedie and effectuall destroying of Shipping in a Moment' in 1653, during the Dutch War, he presented his proposals to the Council of State. Thenceforth Küffeler's invention was recommended to the Protector by Hartlib and other prominent supporters. Alarmed by the potentialities of this weapon Hartlib believed 'the dreadfull effect of this invention to be such as would enable any one nation that should be first master of it to give the law to other nations'. Accordingly he pressed the Protector to secure English control of the invention in order to prevent it from falling into the hands of the enemies of religion. After various minor delays, a ship was appointed for a trial and the torpedo was demonstrated at Deptford on 4 August 1658, the effect being 'exceedingly beyond expectation and did a far greater execution than what the petitioner had promised'. Cromwell was so impressed that he ordered a reward of £10,000 for Küffeler, but no payment was made owing to the death of the Protector. Thereafter the inventor pressed Richard Cromwell and Charles II to develop the torpedo but without response. The dramatic demonstration at Deptford made an immediate impact; the invention is widely discussed in the letters of such figures as Boyle, Beale, Worsley, Oldenburg and Winthrop. Repercussions continued into the restoration, resulting in a visit to the inventor by Pepys, who 'doubted not the matter of fact, it being tried in Cromwell's time, but the safety of carrying them in ships'. From the various accounts it is apparent that the time fuse was kindled before the torpedo was propelled towards its target. After travelling across the intervening water, the torpedo would penetrate the ship at any point of the hull, making an explosion which would cause sinking within two minutes. There was considerable debate over the precise nature of the explosive mixture used by Küffeler. It may have been *aurum fulminans*, since Appelius reported that Küffeler 'had lately been trying his Aurum fulminans', with the

165. Boyle *Works*, vi, p.109. *Usefulnesse* (32), Bk. II, pp.163–4. Glauber also used glass stoppers.

166. Jaeger, *op. cit.*, pp.84–7; Evelyn, *Diary* (97), iii, pp.446–7. B. Monconys, *Journal des Voyages* (Lyons, 1666), part 2, p.40.

result that he had 'lost almost his whole hand & life'.[167] Draft agreements outlining the conditions under which Küffeler was willing to impart his secrets to private individuals, indicate that the greatest demand was for his scarlet dye, the self-regulating oven and his services as a teacher of practical chemistry.[168]

Küffeler appears to have derived most of his ideas from Drebbel and reports of his own innovations seem to have been exaggerated. Nevertheless his virtuosity and ability to exploit inventions having considerable commercial or military possibilities made a deep impression upon his contemporaries. He was a leading member of an extensive community of technicians and chemists whose resourceful ingenuity provided valuable information for such figures as Evelyn, Petty and Boyle. The notability of such figures as Küffeler significantly enhanced the image of Baconian science. The degree to which the approach of the technical chemists was valued is indicated by Petty's declaration that in philosophical matters 'I shall preferre Cornelius Drebbel before him [Descartes] though he understood no Latin as one that hath done more though said less'.[169]

The chemists studied mining and metallurgy with renewed vigour, hoping to encourage more effective exploitation of England's neglected mineral legacy. From their personal experience in the West Midlands, Derbyshire, and Northern Counties, Jorden, Plattes, Pettus and Webster argued that the nation possessed substantial deposits of tin, copper, lead, iron, lapis calaminaris, antimony and alum. Coal was mined in considerable quantities; tin, lead and iron were exploited to a limited degree; but apart from sporadic attempts by a few resourceful individuals, other substances were neglected. But the successes before 1640 of Bulmer and Bushell in exploiting copper and silver respectively were indicative of the rewards open to efficient promoters. After 1646 Glauber's works renewed interest in attempts to find solutions to some of the technical problems of mineralogy and metallurgy. It was asserted that expansion in this area would yield a remedy for the bullion shortage, a source of metals for recoinage, a direct and indirect stimulus to trade, and a solution to the problem of unemployment.

Alchemists and prophets optimistically hoped that divine intervention, inner illumination or textual investigations would reveal the secret of the Philosopher's Stone, so facilitating the multiplication of gold and other

167. Letters from Hartlib to Boyle, 13 May, 25 May, 10 August 1658, Boyle *Works*, vi, pp.108, 109, 113. Jaeger, *op. cit.*, pp. 76–8. Pepys, *Diary*, ed. Latham & Matthews, iii, pp.45–6. *CSPD 1661/2*, p.327. Monconys, *op. cit.*, part 2, p.40. Pepys, *Tangier Papers* (London, 1935), p.44. Oldenburg *Correspondence*, i, pp.180, 181, 191. Turnbull (292), pp.42–3. 'To his Highnesse Richard Lord Protector . . . The Humble Petition of Dr. John Sibertus Küffeler', HP LIII 5; various testimonials about Küffeler are preserved in HP LIII 41. Letter from Appelius to Hartlib, 27 Sept. 1647, HP XLV 1.

168. HP XXVII 13 & 49.

169. 'Mr. Petty's letter in Answer to Mr. More', HP VII 123, & Webster (319), p.368.

precious materials. The Republic coincided with an eruption of interest in transmutation, which infected both scholars and mechanics, whether of Anglican or puritan persuasion. The search for the Philosopher's Stone inevitably tempted chemists to make excessive claims, or to indulge in imaginative phantasies. George Starkey attempted to increase the authority of his writings by the claim that he was the agent for an adept whom he called Eirenaeus Philalethes. Starkey published a series of Philalethes tracts, asserting that he had been initiated into the mysteries known to his master. This elaborate fiction convinced not only contemporaries but also certain modern historians that the adept existed and various attempts have been made to identify him, thus to a certain extent vindicating Starkey's method of publicising his activities.[170] Predictions about transmutation became numerous, confident and specific. For instance considerable interest was provoked by Mary Rand's speculation that 'making of Gold shal be vulgarly knowne A.1661'.[171]

Although such claims were treated seriously, it would be wrong to assume that puritan energies were much dissipated in the pursuit of the Philosopher's Stone. Indeed, puritan chemists tended to adopt the attitude of Bacon and Plattes, denigrating speculative and literary alchemy, while advocating concentration on experimental problems having utilitarian relevance. But it was not possible or desirable to avoid all concern with 'Transmutation', a concept which embraced a wide variety of chemical changes. Conversion of base metals into gold was merely one aspect of transmutation, and control over this phenomenon was thought to be wholly consistent with the return of man's dominion over nature. Thus curiosity about transmutation was entirely compatible with an active participation in experimental chemistry. This conclusion was aptly expressed by Beale:

> 'I cannot tell whether the philosophers stone will become soe speedily vulgar, as Mary Rante hath prophesyed, but I see many juste grounds of appreciating gold, & of raysing vulgar things to bee more truely excellent, than gold or any Jewells . . . Is it not high time for all that can believe so much as is nowe become obvious & in a manner exposed to their natural eyes, to unite together & joyne

170. Starkey's Philalethes writings were compiled into *The Marrow of Alchemy* (London, 1654/5). For Starkey as an alchemist and the dispute over Philalethes see G. H. Turnbull (291); R. S. Wilkinson, 'George Starkey, Physician and Alchemist', *Ambix,* 1963, *11*: 121–52; *idem,* 'The Problem of the Identity of Eirenaeus Philalethes', *Ambix,* 1964, *12,* 24–43; *idem,* Letter to the Editor in *Ambix,* 1972, *19*: 204–8.

171. Letter from Oldenburg to Boyle, 10 September 1658, Oldenburg *Correspondence,* i, p.178; letter from Hartlib to Boyle, 5 April 1659, Boyle *Works,* vi, p.116. Mary Rand's prediction was made in *Clavis Apocalyptica,* listed in Pierre Borel, *Bibliotheca Chimica* (Paris, 1654), p.25. For similar views, see Starkey, *Marrow;* Eirenaeus Philaletha Cosmopolita, *Secrets Reveal'd* (London, 1669; composed 1645); 'Prognostication what shall happen to Physicians, surgeons . . . alchemists & miners . . .' in Hartlib, *Chymical Addresses* (144), Appendix. See also Hill (151), pp.119–20.

their strength & counsayles into the execution, performance & practise of the best things & for the best ends?'[172]

Most chemists were persuaded to concentrate on more readily attainable, and socially relevant goals. Once the military hostilities ceased the mining and metallurgical projects of the 1630s were resumed, very often by the former projectors, who were obliged to accommodate themselves to the new situation. As already noted Thomas Bushell dramatically reorientated himself into conformity with the puritan social ethic, seeking to advance his entrepreneurial mining activities under the guise of utopian philanthropy. Most practitioners were happy to adopt a more modest course, pursuing limited objectives, but in a more consciously scientific spirit than previously. Their work was assisted by the increasing acquaintance with foreign authors. Having translated Glauber, French announced in 1652 that Ercker was about to be published in English and that plans had been made to translate Agricola, although the cost of woodcuts was causing delay.[173] French's translations were related to his practical activities; Hartlib reported of him that he had 'beene in trials for many years together and knows all the places for minerals in England'. Similarly Webster, after his initiation in chemistry with Hunniades, concentrated on the preparation of his *Metallographia,* a work which drew together ideas on the origin, nature and properties of metals. It formed a more chemically biased complement to the technical treatises of Ercker and Agricola; Webster's information was drawn from an extremely wide range of sources, including some quite obscure Paracelsian authors. Webster also displayed first-hand knowledge of technical processes used in mining in the Northern Counties, paralleling French's familiarity with the Yorkshire mineral springs.[174] Christopher Merrett accumulated some useful information about the distribution of minerals and metallurgical techniques, while working on his survey of the natural products of Britain. In 1649 Merrett also began preparing a lavishly annotated version of Neri's important little work on glass. Gerard Boate's natural history of Ireland gave more prominence to mining and metallurgy than to any other topic.[175] These authors were probably in contact with Robert Child, who was undertaking similar

172. Letter from Beale to Hartlib, 22 March 1658/9, HP LI.

173. Ephemerides 1652. The Ercker translation was delayed until 1683 and Agricola's book was not published in English until the present century. Plattes's *Discovery of Subterraneall Treasure* was reissued in 1653.

174. Ephemerides 1648. Webster, *Metallographia, or An History of Metals* (London, 1671). Ferguson (98), ii, pp.530–1. From the text it is clear that Webster's work was largely completed by 1660.

175. Merrett, *Pinax rerum naturalium Britannicarum* (London, 1667); *The Art of Glass* (London, 1662). Gerard Boate, *Irelands Naturall History* (30), 1652, pp.122–41. Merrett and colleagues at the College of Physicians subscribed to a testimonial supporting the mining ventures of Thomas Bushell in 1652: J. W. Gough, *The Superlative Prodigall* (Bristol, 1932), p.93. Edward Jorden's *Discourse of Naturall Bathes* (1631) opened with a letter of recommendation from leading members of the College of Physicians.

exploratory work in New England. In 1645 he reported to Hartlib that 'the country abounds with minerals, esp. Iron stone' which, along with other mineralogical specimens, had been despatched to London for investigation by Leonard Buckner and Merrett.[176]

The above evidence suggests the chemists were becoming completely conversant with the technical and scientific literature on mining and metallurgy. Furthermore this growing expertise was supported by experimental work, by preliminary attempts to survey natural resources, and by the compilation of information relevant to the histories of the metallurgical arts. This effort was of course intended to lead to industrial improvement. At this point the scientist met a number of obstacles which could not be overcome by literature surveys or scientific work. It was necessary to override legal barriers and vested interests; it was not easy to gain entrepreneurial support, or skilled labour for projects in the remote areas where mining might be profitable. In the unsettled conditions of this period, it was rarely possible to bring together at any one moment the complete combination of factors necessary for the establishment of a successful mining venture. Thus the frequently inconclusive and frustrating attempts to promote mining projects supply an unhappy contrast with the successful scientific foundation work which had been undertaken. Nevertheless, even when the immediate practical results were disappointing, the enterprises of this period influenced developments which were to bear fruit after the restoration.

The work of Glauber and other chemists was relevant to many industrial processes. In certain industries, the work of innovation was already underway; it has been perceptively noted that 'Glassmaking was one of the first trades to benefit by this mood of critical investigation' of the Baconians.[177] There is every indication that the lessons learned from the furnaces of the small-scale, cosmopolitan and London-based glass industry were applied in the more demanding field of metallurgy.

The manner in which grandiose schemes could be turned to practical benefit, and made to generate productive exchanges of ideas, is indicated by the mining projects initiated after the Civil War. Playing his usual active role, Worsley attempted to establish a partnership to promote mining projects. Hartlib introduced him to William Hamilton, the Scottish chemist and Fellow of All Souls College, who was interested in promoting mines in Scotland. The experienced innovators Dud Dudley and David Ramsay 'who travelled afoote all the Kingdom of Scotland ever affirmed that Scotland would proove another Indies if mines and caves were improved as easily as they might by them and their associates. I say much more by Glauber's skill and knowledges.'[178] Glauber's techniques were seen as the key to the more efficient treatment of ores.

176. Letter from Child to Hartlib, 24 December 1645; quoted from Turnbull (290), pp.50–3.
177. W. A. Thorpe, *English Glass,* 3rd edn. (London, 1961), p.144.
178. Ephemerides 1648.

Hence during his visit to the low countries Worsley was supplied with information about British mineral deposits to guide his enquiries into furnace techniques at the laboratories of Glauber and Morian. Dury sent information from his uncle Ramsay about the state of both English and Scottish mines. The best prospects in England appeared to be the antimony, silver-bearing lead, and iron ore deposits near Durham, while Scotland was thought to possess mines as rich as any in the world, likely to yield gold, silver, antimony, tin and lead. Furthermore Ramsay claimed to possess a patent to authorise his exploitation of the Scottish deposits. He now required financial backing and technical assistance from Worsley, who was asked to learn methods of separating silver from lead, gold from copper and above all, processes for the removal of impurities of arsenic, sulphur and antimony from all ores. Ramsay felt that these problems could be solved by pre-treatment of ores or by more refined furnaces. Worsley completed his 'Mineral Experiments' in the Netherlands, and he claimed to have evolved 'furnaces which might bee conducible to this way of refining'.[179]

By improving ventilation, introducing chimneys of different lengths, and dividing the interior into compartments, Glauber's various furnaces were able to perform a considerable variety of operations under controlled conditions and at higher temperatures than had hitherto been attained in more conventional small furnaces. Other refinements enabled Glauber to perform separations and distillations in closed containers, or in earthenware distillation vessels separated from the fuel source. The English chemists anticipated that Glauber's furnaces would lead to revolutionary improvements in their methods of refining ores. Boyle regarded the improvement of furnace techniques as the first of his 'better wayes of doing many things in Chymistry'. He advised that it was necessary to follow Drebbel's example by applying the principles of mechanics to the design of chemical equipment. Thereby the chemist would achieve 'the Saving of Fuel, or to the making the utmost use of Heat afforded by the Fuel they do employ, or as to the intending Heat to the height, or as to the regulating Heat at pleasure'. Boyle suggested the more economical use of heat by having one fire heat a number of vessels, or various ovens of a complex furnace. He recognised that Glauber's chimney was of fundamental importance for the elimination of fumes and for improving ventilation to obtain high temperatures without the aid of bellows. Drebbel had been able to melt Venetian chalk in his furnaces, a feat which Boyle had not yet achieved in 1663, although he was confident that silver or gold might be cupelled in small furnaces without bellows. Boyle stressed that the efficiency of furnaces could be still further improved by the use of new fuels which might 'give a greater, or a more durable Heat; or to be lesse offensive by their smoak or smells; or else by discovering some cheap way of doing, without fire,

179. Undated letters from Dury to Worsley, [1649] and 17 August 1649, HP I 2.

what was wont to be done by it.' There was already considerable interest in ovens heated by dung or fermenting liquids, which might be used for such purposes as hatching eggs. Even more important were attempts to find substitutes for wood and charcoal, which were increasingly expensive commodities. Coal was cheap, but noxious, rendering it unsuitable for many processes, although Boyle reported its successful use in manufacturing aqua fortis. The utility of coal could be greatly increased by 'charring' to produce coke. This operation, performed in pots, greatly increased the price of fuel, but it was found that coke was more suitable for furnaces, being reduced 'into coherent Masses, of a convenient bignesse and shape, and more dry and apt to kindle.' Coke was also economical in use and it produced a more intense heat. Improved coking methods would ensure its complete superiority over coal. Boyle reported that at least one acquaintance was coking without pots, thereby supporting the continuous operation of furnaces which were used for producing chemical medicines, at one quarter of the normal expense.[180]

Boyle's comments on furnace design and fuels show the degree to which scientific and economic considerations were interconnected. The improvement of furnace operation was recognised as having equal relevance for chemistry and industry. The problems which he mentioned were by no means new, but the arrival of improved chemical techniques encouraged the translation of laboratory methods into industrial practice.

Within industry itself conspicuous efforts had been made to improve furnaces and introduce new fuels since the later sixteenth century. Blast furnaces employing water power to drive bellows had opened up an 'entirely new phase in smelting to set the stage for the first industrial revolution, and to change the course of the iron industry in Britain to a more productive purpose by the indirect and double process involved in the blast furnace and the forge'.[181] Blast furnaces considerably improved output over the traditional bloomeries; this made possible permanent industrial sites, at which fuel consumption was increased, and ever-increasing pressure placed on local charcoal and timber resources. It has been estimated that about 2,000 cubic feet of solid wood were required to produce one ton of bar iron at the iron foundries of the 1620s.[182] The expanding and voracious iron industry is thought to have been one of the important factors contributing to the 'timber famine' which was frequently mentioned as a social grievance in the seventeenth century. Whether timber shortage was more than a local phenomenon or not, or even if it was a misfounded scare, timber conservation became a leading theme among the social reformers in the mid-seventeenth

180. Boyle, *Usefulnesse* (32), Bk. II, pp.160–2, 166–7.

181. Rees (238), p.179. See also H. R. Schubert, *History of the British Iron and Steel Industry from c. 450 B.C. to A.D.1775* (London, 1957), p.157.

182. G. Hammersley, 'The Charcoal Iron Industry and its Fuel 1540–1750', *Economic History Review*, 1973, *26*: 593–613; p.605.

century.[183] Attempts at timber conservation, shortage and high prices created an incentive for the use of alternative fuels.

In many boiling processes the substitution of coal for other fuels presented no problems, but the disadvantages mentioned by Boyle prevented the use of coal at first for brewing, baking, glassmaking and iron smelting. Gradually the technical problems were solved; the numerous patents taken out for coal utilisation processes reflect the strong interest in this question. In glass-making the use of sealed earthenware pots protected the chemicals from contamination; brewers were the first to exploit coke extensively. Coal could be used in calcining and smelting many ores. But iron smelting, the most important process of all, proved to be unamenable to coal. Some coal was used in fineries and chaferies, but no substitute was found for charcoal in the blast furnace. The solution of this problem was a golden fleece hunted assiduously by the pre-Civil War patentees, led by the notorious Dud Dudley. Despite their protestations there is no evidence that more than feeble success was achieved by any of the innovators, whether using coal or coke, reverbatory or direct heating methods.[184] It is generally assumed that, with the collapse of the patent system, the momentum of experiment fell off until well after the restoration; and that later results were at first indifferent, before success was finally achieved at the end of the century by Abraham Darby at Coalbrookdale. It will be seen that this is a wholly false impression.

In view of the striking growth of interest in fuels and furnaces during the interregnum, it is important to determine whether there was any positive attempt to apply the new expertise to the unsolved problems of iron smelting. Dud Dudley certainly continued his own experiments, and was aware of competition from other innovators, during the Republic. The work of improvement continued despite the lack of patent protection, and the severe dislocation and slow recovery of the mining and metallurgical industries.

The Forest of Dean ironworks may be taken as an example of an industrial enterprise which was severely affected by the Civil War, and which was subsequently revived as a highly successful pioneer experiment in state management. Furthermore, there is clear evidence of attempts to promote new industrial methods.

183. The timber famine has been emphasised by Nef and most other writers; see also A. & N. Clow, 'The Timber Famine and the Development of Technology', *Annals of Science,* 1956, *12*: 85–102. G. Hammersley, *op. cit.,* believes that the extent of this shortage has been exaggerated.

184. Nef (198), i, pp.215–20, 245–52. Dud Dudley, *Mettallum Martis: or, Iron Made with Pit-coale* (London, 1665). T. S. Ashton, 'The Discoveries of the Darbys of Coalbrookdale', Newcomen Soc. *Transactions,* 1924–5, *5*: 9–14; R. A. Mott, 'Dud Dudley and the Early Coal-Iron Industry', Newcomen Soc. *Transactions,* 1947, *27*: 247–51; H. R. Schubert, 'The Truth about Dud Dudley', *Jnl. Iron & Steel Inst.,* 1958, *166*: 184–5. For a recent revision, see G. R. Morton & M. D. G. Wanklyn, 'Dud Dudley—a New Appraisal', *Jnl. of West Midlands Regional Studies,* 1967, *1*: 48–65.

The development of the Forest of Dean ironworks repeated a pattern found in many other locations. James I had considered establishing his own ironworks, but this plan was abandoned in favour of private grants. Various projectors were involved from 1612 onwards, until in 1640 the leases passed to Sir John Winter. By this stage there were just over ten furnaces and about the same number of forges, but many would have been in a poor state of repair. Production had been purposely held back in an attempt to preserve timber; at one time only two furnaces and four forges were permitted to operate simultaneously. From a detailed inventory of 1635, and subsequent excavations, it is clear that the furnaces were of the conventional square-outline type, but they appear to have been taller than furnaces elsewhere, with the result that they were capable of a higher weekly output of iron. In the period before 1640 these furnaces produced between two and three tons per twenty-four hours.[185]

During the Civil War the works continued under new ownership, but they were not operated at capacity. The Council of State was undecided whether to revive the industry under private ownership, or destroy the furnaces in the interests of timber preservation. At first the latter consideration was dominant. Various orders were made to control the cutting of timber, until finally it was decided to demolish the ironworks altogether.[186] However the increased demand for great shot and ordnance owing to the Dutch War brought about a modification of this policy. In 1653 Major John Wade, who had previously been appointed as a 'Preservator', was invested with the responsibility of re-establishing the Dean ironworks, while having due regard for the preservation of timber.[187] Since the state was already responsible for forest management, similar control of the ironworks provided an opportunity to co-ordinate the supply of naval timber and iron required for shipbuilding and armaments. Under the entrepreneurs ironworks had developed at the expense of timber; the nationalisation of the industry created a fresh opportunity to restore this balance and there is every indication that Wade was sympathetic to this policy. He conscientiously attempted to revive the ironworks and prevent plunder of timber, although insufficient resources were provided for him fully to achieve either objective. Wade frequently expressed frustration at the inability of the authorities to prevent the loss of timber and at times he had difficulty in obtaining sufficient funds for financing development and paying workmen. However

185. H. R. Schubert, *History of the British Iron Industry,* pp.185–7; *idem,* 'The King's Ironworks in the Forest of Dean 1612–1674', *Jnl. of the Iron and Steel Institute,* 1953, *173*: 153–65; H. G. Nicholls, *Iron Making in . . . The Forest of Dean* (London, 1866); R. Jenkins, 'Iron making in the Forest of Dean', Newcomen Soc. *Transactions,* 1925/6, *6*: 42–65. These sources have been largely superseded by G. F. Hammersley's encyclopaedic 'The History of the Iron Industry in the Forest of Dean Region 1562–1660' (Unpublished Ph.D. dissertation, University of London, 1972).

186. Hammersley, 'Iron Industry', pp.217–26.

187. *CSPD 1653/4,* p.107, 27 August 1653.

the ironworks quickly became operational; initially a furnace was erected at Parkend and subsequent developments there included the erection of forges and casting works. Wade aimed at producing fifteen tons of shot a week. The furnace was traditional in form, but its greater height (28 feet) resulted in improved performance. Wade claimed in addition that the furnace was one of the best-watered in the nation, with the result that an effective blast could be produced. Production was continuous between February 1654 and January 1660, the account books showing that a sustained output of three tons per twenty-four hours was attained.[188] Wade's works supplied the navy with shot, nails and castings, while private buyers were found for pig, bar iron and chimney backs. From a commercial point of view, Wade's ironworks were a remarkable success. As Hammersley concludes: 'one furnace and one forge made 3,750 tons of pig iron, 700 tons of shot and over 720 tons of bar iron and possibly some forgings in six and a half years, producing a gross income of approximately £41,000 and a total profit of about £12,000.' This represented a clear profit of £1,250 per annum and a return of 26 per cent on cost.[189] The creation of the state ironworks in the Forest of Dean would have been approved by the puritan economic theorists. Largely owing to the abilities of John Wade, this integrated organisation of woodland and industrial components was a major success.

To what extent was there an interest in technological innovation at the enterprising Forest of Dean ironworks? For instance, the exploitation of local coal deposits for smelting the ore might have been economically advantageous and it would have contributed to the preservation of timber. Although timber shortage was not a serious problem for Wade, there seems to have been some interest in the more widespread use of coal in the West Midlands during the Republic. The Forest of Dean, with its iron ore and coal deposits in close proximity, was an excellent location for an experiment on the use of coal for iron smelting. The leading representative of the independent operators was Dud Dudley, who has left a highly unsympathetic account of his competitors. In the Mendips, the other experienced projector, Thomas Bushell, and his German assistant, fought unsuccessful battles with local miners in an attempt to establish control of copper mining. Petty and Hartlib noted that Bushell, like Dudley, was experimenting 'melting of iron with sea-coale'.[190] But all such efforts were probably unsuccessful, resulting in a sense of frustration which was expressed as bitter animosity towards all rivals. Dudley gave a highly distorted but informative account of the establishment of an ironworks in the Forest of Dean. This was described as a private venture of Cromwell, Wildman and other army officers. After

188. Schubert, 'The Kings Ironworks . . .', pp.154–62. Nicholls, *op. cit.*, pp.41–3. There are numerous references to the affairs of Wade's ironworks in *CSPD 1654–8*. For full details see Hammersley, 'Iron Industry', pp.206–40.

189. Hammersley, 'Iron Industry', pp.237, 393–407.

190. Dudley, *Mettallum Martis*, pp.21–7. Gough, *The Superlative Prodigall*, pp.107–13. Ephemerides 1649.

securing patents for Jeremy Buck, they established 'at vast charge' furnaces in the Forest of Dean. Then they indulged in expensive

> 'Invention and Experiments, which was done in spacious Wind-Furnaces, and also in Potts of Glass-house Clay, and failing afterwards, got unto them an Ingenious Glass-Maker, Master Edward Dagney an Italian then living in Bristow, who after had made many Potts, for that purpose went with them into the Forrest of Dean, and built for the said Captain Buck and his Partners, a new Furnace, and made therein many and sundry Experiments and Tryals for the making of Iron with Pit-cole and Sea-cole etc.'[191]

A further expert involved in these experiments was Captain John Copley, whose failure was also greatly relished by Dudley. This state-sanctioned enterprise would certainly have been followed with interest by Wade, whose successful venture was pointedly ignored by Dudley. In publicising what he thought of as failure, Dudley unwittingly provided the historian with valuable evidence about an experimental aspect of the Forest of Dean ironworks. It is impossible to know from present evidence whether the attempts to introduce coal were successful. Perhaps they were little more effective than the methods employed earlier. Indeed they may have been abandoned shortly after Wade's ironworks entered into production. But the specific details given by Dudley indicate that a serious attempt was made to apply experience gained in other metallurgical fields, to iron smelting. Buck's patent was granted in 1651, for a method which initially employed the reverbatory principle, in the form of a 'Wind-Furnace'. This was probably an imitation of the furnaces which had been successfully introduced in Germany for copper smelting.[192] Buck's work was known to Robert Child, who was seriously worried about the wastage of wood in iron smelting; he commended 'some Ingenious men, who lately have got a Patent for making Iron with Sea-coal'.[193] The alternative method was copied directly from the glass-works, with earthenware pots supplied by Edward Dagnia, a member of the celebrated Italian family of glass-makers. In the early years of the seventeenth century the English glass-workers began to place the constituents of glass inside sealed earthenware pots which could then be heated in a coal furnace. The Dagnia family would have been among the first practitioners of this method. An analogous technique was applied by Buck and Dagnia at the ironworks, but apparently in some cases the heat was insufficient to melt the ore, and in others the pots fractured. How-

191. Dudley, *op. cit.*, p.38 [sic; p.22].

192. 'An Act concerning the new Inventions of Melting down Iron, and other metals, with Stone Coals, . . . without Charking thereof', Firth & Rait, ii, pp.509–10, 2 April 1651. R. Jenkins, 'The Reverbatory Furnace with Coal Fuel, 1612–1712', Newcomen Soc. *Transactions,* 1933–4, *14*: 67–81. Rees (238), pp.393–6.

193. Robert Child, quoted from Hartlib, *His Legacy* (142), p.49.

ever it is known that this method was applied successfully in steelmaking at a later late.[194]

Dudley admitted that the Forest of Dean experiments were undertaken at considerable care and expense. At one stage Dudley himself was called in to inspect the inventions. He noted that both soldiers and medical men were involved in the work. The physician George Starkey might have been attracted by this venture, since he made a brief visit to Bristol in 1656, where it was reported that he had discovered a mine of a metal like antimony and was returning to London to patent 'an invention for a continual blast'.[195] John Copley, another participant, was working with John Benson, a former associate of Dudley; Benson was described by Hartlib as a great admirer of Glauber. They were in active competition with Bushell:

> 'Cap. Copley is getting a patent with Benson for melting downe of oare with sea-coale, which wil be a mighty saving of the wood to the whole nation. Thomas Bushel to whom he had revealed this whole skil went about to circumvent him in it.'[196]

Intrinsically Copley was the most likely to succeed, since he operated with a blast furnace, using coke mixed with the ore. Dudley was called in to assist with the improvement of Copley's bellows.[197]

James I had considered becoming the proprietor of the Forest of Dean ironworks. However considerations of short-term financial advantage caused him to abandon control of this project, with the result that a commercially viable industry was established at the cost of a slow destruction of the forest. This policy operated to the detriment of both national security and the iron industry. The establishment of the state ironworks was one of the more imaginative and constructive policies of the Republic. From our point of view it represents an interesting attempt to balance conflicting interests by policy and perhaps by technological innovation. With the exploitation of local coal for smelting, the iron industry could develop without prejudicing the valuable forest trees. By modifications of furnace design, experiments with coal and coke, direct and indirect heating, the officially nominated practitioners attempted a longer-term solution to the fuel problem. A numerous personnel was involved, perhaps including administrators, soldiers, physicians, mechanics, and chemists familiar with the works of Glauber. Per-

194. E. W. Hulme, 'English Glass Making in the Sixteenth and Seventeenth Centuries', *The Antiquary,* 1895, *31*: 102–6. Thorpe, *English Glass,* pp.114, 124.

195. Ephemerides 1656.

196. Ephemerides 1654.

197. Copley's coke was to be produced by a partnership of Joseph Wellington, Edmund Warcarp and John Grosvenor: Rees (238), pp.294–5. By coincidence the former owner of the Forest of Dean ironworks, Sir John Winter, was also experimenting with producing coke, at Greenwich. A patent was obtained for his method in 1661. See Evelyn, *Diary* (97), iii, pp.180–1, August 1656. Winter too may have been hoping to use coke for smelting iron.

haps even Boyle at Stalbridge in Dorset knew about this enterprise. The economic importance of the episode was limited. After the restoration Wade resigned; the ironworks operated for a time, but they were then demolished in the interests of timber conservation. Before the demolition, the furnaces were probably visited by a member of the Royal Society. From his description, it is apparent that the traditional square furnace had been abandoned in favour of a circular outline, creating an interior similar to the modern egg-shape.[198] Thus an important step forward was made at about this time, possibly at the very works operated by Wade. The attempt to introduce coal was probably not successful, but the experiments were more wide-ranging and systematic after 1640 than in the previous period. The experience accumulated during the interregnum was probably helpful to later innovators such as Frederick de Blewston who introduced a reverbatory furnace for iron smelting in Staffordshire in 1677. In this case-history the Republic recognised the need for experiment; support and even a rarely granted patent were given to the innovators, who were confident that their new skills in experimental chemistry could solve one of the most intractable of industrial problems.

This example of managerial competence and technical ingenuity was not without parallels. For instance John Winthrop Jr. and Robert Child were confident that New England would yield rich deposits of minerals. They approached this enterprise in a thoroughly scientific manner, and they both possessed libraries specialising in metallurgical and chemical literature. There seemed to be various alternative natural resources suitable for exploitation, but their greatest efforts were devoted to the development of iron foundries. Their project moved forward, and in 1641 Winthrop visited England to gather capital and skilled workmen for the ironworks. Hugh Peter and Emmanuel Downing were among the pious backers of this enterprise. The ironworks made some progress, particularly after the appointment of Richard Leader, Hartlib's friend, as the director of operations. In 1645 Child reported that he had discovered ten or twelve types of iron ore, which were being sent back to London for analysis. He commented: 'I doubt not (by the grace of God) but we shall prosper in Iron works, and make plenty of iron speedily.'[199] This proved to be an accurate prediction; the iron foundries at Saugus and Lynn became the established base for the New England iron industry. As Hartlib's notes indicate, Leader proved to be a keen proponent of innovation. Although the iron foundries developed along traditional lines, their initiation was very much due to the puritan Baconianism of Winthrop and Child.[200]

198. Henry Powle, 'An Account of the Iron-Works in the Forest of Dean', *Phil. Trans.*, No. 137, 1678, *12*: 923–5. See also R. Plot, *The Natural History of Staffordshire* (Oxford, 1686), p.128.

199. Letter from Child to Hartlib, 24 December 1645, quoted from Turnbull (290), p.52.

200. Kittredge (176), pp.6–13; Morison (192), pp.269–88; Robert C. Black III,

(viii) The Honour and Great Advantage of the Commonwealth

Because of their interest in precious metals, chemists and metallurgists were often concerned with problems of currency. By such methods as increasing the output of the Mines Royal, or by attempting transmutation, projectors sought to increase the flow of gold and silver to the Mint. Even copper and tin mining ventures were undertaken in the expectation that these metals would be used for coins of low denomination. On the basis of Thomas Bushell's success with mining silver in Cardiganshire, a mint was established at Aberystwyth, which produced a small but regular supply of coins until the work was interrupted by the Civil War. Apart from this pilot project little success was encountered in establishing mints supplied with native bullion. Nevertheless, chemists retained their interest in the technology of coining and in economic problems relating to the Mint.

The problem of 'scarcity' of money remained. As Vaughan later complained : 'the want of money makes the life of the citizens penurious and barbarous.' The overall national economic crisis was accompanied by depleted bullion stocks, owing to an accelerated export of precious metals, and clipping of coin. Among the lower classes shortage of small change and farthings was a serious cause of complaint. Although the reformers believed that the full restoration of prosperity rested on agricultural, industrial and commercial development, they also claimed that it was essential for the state to restore the Mint and if possible prevent the further deterioration of currency by culling and clipping. In an entirely different context, for the sake of the dignity of the Republic, it was desirable to replace the royalist currency by an aesthetically impressive issue of commonwealth coinage. The Mint was also responsible for the production of official seals and medals. The importance of the currency problem is indicated by the protracted debate over the Mint which lasted throughout the Commonwealth and Protectorate. Traditional economic questions were relevant to decision-making, but a dominating role was assumed by the problem of technological innovation, owing to the emergence of an ambitious proposal to mechanise minting operations. Once a decision had been reached on this issue, the state was faced with the even more radical proposal of currency decimalisation. In a more direct manner than in the case of the nationalised ironworks, the attempt to re-establish the Mint introduced questions of scientific analysis and technological innovation.

The Younger John Winthrop (New York & London, 1966), *passim;* G. H. Haynes, 'The Tale of Tantiusques, An Early Mining Venture in Massachusetts', *Proceedings of the American Antiquarian Soc.*, New Series, 1901, *14*: 471–97. E. N. Hartley, *Ironworks on the Saugus* (Norman, Oklahoma, 1957).

The currency available in 1649 had been produced almost entirely by the traditional method of hammering. Discs of a required weight were stamped out from thin bars of silver. The discs were then marked by hammering between two dies. This technique could not produce a deep or precise image, with the result that most of the hammered coinage is of an extremely unimpressive quality. Furthermore, the discs varied in weight and the imprint was seldom centred perfectly. Thus there was every inducement to cull out heavy coins, or clip unmarked edges. With crude designs it was quite possible to impinge even further inside the margin. The excess silver could be used as bullion, or alternatively, it could be easily counterfeited into further inferior coinage.

For the new regime it was a great challenge to produce a coinage which would not be susceptible to such deterioration and would thereby serve to strengthen confidence in the national currency. At first mint affairs appear to have been conducted in a traditional manner. A more active policy began in 1649, with a radical overhaul of the mint staff.[201] Although the Master of the Mint appointed in 1649 was the Helmontian physician Aaron Gurdan, once installed he showed no propensity for experiment, and co-operated fully with the Moneyers' Company. His lack of efficiency and professional knowledge of mint affairs caused concern to all parties. The Mint was controlled by a large and fluctuating committee, the dominant member of which was Sir James Harrington, while at later stages an active role was also assumed by Lambert, Jones, Wolseley and Strickland. Under Harrington's vigorous leadership this Committee quickly embarked on investigations of the true par of English and foreign coins, mint ratios, export of bullion, tin and copper farthings, and mint organisation, as well as the technology of coining. Expert witnesses such as the aged Sir Ralph Maddison or the opportunistic Thomas Violet provided the Committee with a considerable body of evidence. Violet rapidly assumed a highly partisan position, attempting to direct decisions along lines congenial to the Moneyers' and Goldsmiths Companies.

The Council of State lost no time in authorising the first issue of commonwealth coinage, which was produced by the moneyers by hammering in the autumn of 1649.[202] Although this type of coinage continued to be issued during the Commonwealth and Protectorate, its distressingly poor quality and design caused the Committee to consider alternative methods of production.

In February 1650 the Committee openly declared its intention 'to consider how the moneys of the Commonwealth may be better made'.[203] Perhaps realising the inferiority of the workmanship of the dies, the poor

201. Aylmer (12), p.41.

202. *CSPD 1649/50,* pp.106–8, 201–2, 206, 284, 394, 396, 402–4, 429–30, 437–8, April–December 1649. Firth & Rait, ii, pp.191–2, 281–2, 17 July and 16 November 1649. Henfrey (147), pp.29–31.

203. *CSPD 1649/50,* p.503, 2 February 1650.

quality of the coin produced by the workmen employed by the moneyers, and the susceptibility of this product to clipping, the Committee had already begun negotiations with Pierre Blondeau, who had been invited over from France by the Council of State in the autumn of 1649 to 'see what use may be made of him and his skills'.[204] Blondeau came with a strong recommendation from an English agent (probably René Augier), who described him as 'one of the ablest of his age in the art' of coining in gold, silver and copper. Indeed certain techniques could be performed only by him. His merits had been recognised by Richelieu, from whom he had received protection until 1642. Then owing to persecution by the French moneyers he decided to offer his services to the Commonwealth. Upon arriving in England he attracted the support and co-operation of reformers such as Hartlib, but at the cost of again arousing the enmity of the local moneyers.

For almost a century before 1640 there had been various trials of strength between the innovators and the moneyers in both England and France, in which advocates of machined coinage had never won more than pyrrhic victories. Immediately Blondeau arrived in England the parliamentary Committee came under strong pressure to resist innovation. But the outcome on this occasion was to be different. Building on long experience Blondeau had achieved conspicuous competence in coin technology. Also the intrinsic and serious defects of hammered coinage were coming to be universally admitted. Finally, the parliamentary Committee felt no particular regard for the vested interests of the moneyers, and was in sympathy with the mood of innovation among the Baconians.

The ultimate source for the techniques of machined coinage was the instruments developed to produce medals during the Renaissance.[205] Machines had been developed for drawing out and stamping sheets of metal into perfect discs of uniform thickness. The blanks were then placed between two dies in a screw press or *balancier,* which was capable of achieving the necessary relief in one blow. This technique was sporadically applied to coinage in Italy, France and England in the later sixteenth century, when inscriptions or milling round the edge were introduced to prevent clipping or forgery. After a series of conflicts machined coinage was established in France in 1645. The Frenchman Nicholas Briot (c.1579-1646) was allowed to experiment with machined coinage at the mints of Charles I in London and Edinburgh, but opposi-

204. *CSPD 1649/50,* pp.295, 305, 503–5, 30 August, 11 September 1649 and 2 February 1650.

205. W. J. Hocking, 'Simon's Dies in the Royal Mint Museum, with some notes on the early history of coinage by machinery', *Numismatic Chronicle*, 4th Series, 1909, *9*: 56–118. Sir John Craig, 'British Coins and Coinage', *Jnl. Royal Soc. of Arts,* 1949/50, *98*: 959–86. For the general history and detailed description of the coinage produced during this period, see Craig, *The Mint* (Cambridge, 1953); R. Ruding, *Annals of the Coinage of Great Britain*, 3 vols. (London, 1840); H. A. Grüber, *Handbook of the Coins of Great Britain in the British Museum* (London, 1899).

tion from the moneyers prevented the widespread application of his methods.[206] By the time of the Commonwealth, Briot's machines had fallen into disuse, but advocates of mechanised methods were still vociferous. Parliament purchased Briot's mills, tools and presses; it also possessed William Engelbert's machine for minting pence and half-pence, while in 1649 the coining 'engine' of one Estcourt was examined by a parliamentary committee.[207]

Blondeau showed great initiative in representing his case in broadsheets, published tracts and unpublished memoranda submitted to the Mint Committee. He painted an alarming picture of the weakness of English coinage and indicated how the basic defects could be remedied by his particular mechanised method of producing coins.[208] Immediately the moneyers replied to Blondeau's criticisms, he hit back with unrestrained attacks on the mint officials and vested interests attempting to obstruct his petitions.

It was pointed out that coin worth £100 at face value, by weight was worth only £70-£80. In addition heavy coins were culled and exported, to the benefit of the goldsmiths, but to the detriment of the poor. Those coins remaining in circulation were 'the counterfeited, clipped or lightest'.[209] Blondeau urged that the only solution was coining according to a rigorous standard, which would ensure equality of the weights of coins and introduce markings to prevent clipping. Blondeau's method of coining in a large *balancier*, requiring intensive labour and extensive premises, would greatly decrease the likelihood of forgery, whereas hammered coins could be produced by implements of pocket size which might be used at a simple charcoal brazier. The ultimate insurance against forgers and clippers was the marking of edges. Blondeau was familiar with the old technique of surrounding the coin in the press with a jointed collar (*virole brisée*) engraved with appropriate lettering. However this was not the method which he intended to employ, but a 'new way, known only to myself, of marking the coins on the edge, the old way spoiling many stamps and engines,

206. H. Farquhar, 'Nicholas Briot and the Civil War', *Numismatic Chronicle,* 4th Series, 1914, *14*: 169–232; F. Mazerolle, 'Nicholas Briot Tailleur Générale des Monnaies', *Revue Belge de Numismatique,* 1904: 191–203, 295–314.

207. Farquhar, *op. cit.,* p.193. Petition from Plattes to the Mint Committee claiming ownership of Engelbert's engine, HP LXXI 4. *CSPD 1649/50,* p.318; *1650,* p.83.

208. See particularly *The Humble Representation of Peter Blondeau* [1651]; *An Answer to several objections* [1651]; *A Most Humble Memorandum From Peter Blondeau* [1653]; all three also printed in Violet (298), with replies to Blondeau. 'The French Minters Second Propositions', 26 Feb. 1649/50, *CSPD 1650,* pp.14–15, and Henfrey (147), pp.227–8. *To the Parliament of the Commonwealth of England,* folio broadsheet, June 1650; 'Propositions of Blondeau to the Mint Committee' [1651], in *CSPD 1651,* pp.174–5, 1 May 1651. *A Most Humble Remonstrance of Peter Blondeau* [1653]. Copies of *The Humble Representation, An Answer* and *A Most Humble Remonstrance* are found in HP VIII 20, XXVI 48, XXXIX 2f.

209. Blondeau, *The Humble Representation,* pp.4–5. Blondeau's analysis is confirmed by Horsefield (152), and Letwin (180), pp.64–7.

and being impracticable on thin money'.[210] Despite Blondeau's repeated insistence that his technique was novel, it was believed by critics (and even by Henfrey) that he used the *virole brisée*. However, subsequent close examination of his coins by Hocking has proved that he used a thin strip of steel bearing the inscription in incuse letters, which was placed inside a steel collar surrounding the blank. After the blank was struck in the screw press, the steel strip was removed from the coin using a wooden peg.[211] The simplicity of this principle accounts for Blondeau's confidence that enemies would not be able to discover his secret. Superficial inspection of his mills and presses would have suggested the use of techniques currently applied in France. Indeed the methods he used for drawing out metal, stamping blanks, or for rounding and milling edges between parallel steel bars bearing engraved indentations, followed the French example.[212]

Blondeau's final and crucial asset was the collaboration of the official mint engraver and brilliant medallist Thomas Simon. The engraver would have been attracted to the mechanised methods, since they must have permitted his artistic abilities far greater opportunity for expression. The ample evidence about Blondeau's technical competence would have inclined Simon to enter into partnership with the Frenchman, even at the risk of unpopularity with colleagues at the London Mint. The two partners placed specific proposals before the Mint Committee, estimating their costs and requesting £1,000 for machinery and £400 for buildings.[213] After hearing the views of various parties, the Committee quickly reached a decision in favour of Blondeau:

> 'Resolved upon the Questions that the Patterns of Coyne offered by the Frenchman, with Letters upon the Edges, is a better fashion of the money of England: And is for the honor and great advantage of the Commonwealth: Provided the said Coyne be made at a moderate charge.'[214]

As in commonwealth affairs in general, it proved much easier to take a decision than to achieve the desired end. Detecting that their arguments against mechanisation on grounds of expense, inefficiency, or damage to the interests of poor workmen, had produced little effect,

210. 'Propositions of Blondeau to the Mint Committee', *CSPD 1651*, pp.174–5, 1 May 1651. Similar claims were made elsewhere in Blondeau's writings. At the outset of his petitioning he stated 'I can do it in another manner, which is my particular invention, and no man but I can do it, whereof I made several trials, and the pieces I have exhibited are of my making that way': *CSPD 1650*, p.14, 26 Feb. 1650. See also *A Most Humble Memorandum* [1653], p.6.

211. Hocking, *op. cit.*, pp.89–91.

212. Craig, 'British Coins', p.961; Hocking, *op. cit.*, p.92.

213. 'Propositions of Blondeau to the Mint Committee', 1 May 1651, *CSPD 1651*, p.174. For Simon, see G. Vertue, *Medals, Coins and Great Seals and other Works of Thomas Simon* (London, 1730); H. Farquhar, 'Thomas Simon, "One of Our Chief Gravers"', *Numismatic Chronicle*, 5th Series, 1932, *12*: 274–310.

214. *CSPD 1651*, p.175, 1 May 1651. Blondeau, *A Most Humble Memorandum*, p.9.

the moneyers themselves became advocates of machine-struck coinage. With the assistance of David Ramage, Briot's former assistant, the Moneyers' Company rapidly drew up proposals to make mill money 'as fair, beautiful and cheap as any Frenchman in the world'.[215] Faced with this new situation Harrington authorised a trial between the two parties, who were set to produce pattern pieces with the motto 'Truth and Peace 1651', and engraved edges. In order to assist the moneyers, Simon was instructed to supply them with certain instruments, whereas previously Ramage had been ordered to place all of Briot's equipment in Simon's care.[216]

After a grant of six weeks' extension for the moneyers, the test pieces were produced in the summer of 1651. Each side scorned the products of its rival, but the survival of many of the original pieces has enabled modern specialists to make an impartial estimate. Ramage produced relatively few coins and there is general agreement that his work was greatly inferior to the engraving of Simon, or the coining of Blondeau. Indeed Henfrey claims that the Blondeau-Simon test pieces were superior to any coins previously produced in England.[217]

This trial produced no immediately conclusive outcome. The moneyers, with the assistance of Violet, continued to assert the superiority of Ramage's work. They expressed a willingness to produce machined coins, but warned the state that this would involve considerable expense and delay. They also predicted that counterfeiting would be easier as a result of mechanisation because, they claimed, machine-struck coins could be made by small, silent presses. Consequently the moneyers placed estimates for machined coinage, in the knowledge that all delay operated in favour of the continued production of coins by the established practitioners, using traditional methods.[218] In addition it was suggested that Blondeau should be prosecuted for producing coin outside the Mint; finally, even the mint officers and especially Gurdan were criticised for failure to take decisive action.

Frustrated by the loss of momentum within the Mint Committee and the Council of State, Blondeau published tracts outlining his views on the economic crisis and also providing a brief history of his dealings with the parliamentary Committee and the moneyers. He too criticised Gurdan, but his most bitter comments were reserved for the ignorant 'Irish locksmith' Ramage who, he alleged, was not only a mediocre craftsman, but also disloyal to parliament. Throughout Blondeau, like Simon, emphasised his loyalty to the Republic, while attacking the opportunism and political unreliability of Violet and his associates.[219]

215. *CSPD 1651*, p.174, 7 May 1651; Violet (298), pp.22–3.

216. *CSPD 1651*, pp.174–7, 253, 8 May & 14 June 1651.

217. Henfrey (147), pp.67–71, for a full description of the test pieces. Simon claimed to have produced 300 coins for this test: *CSPD 1654*, pp.131–2.

218. 'Propositions of the Moneyers', 21 October 1651, *CSPD 1651*, pp.487–8.

219. For the tracts produced by Blondeau between the autumn of 1651 and 1653, see note 208 above. Two of these tracts with replies on behalf of the

Increasingly Blondeau's negotiations with the Mint Committee concentrated on the precise terms for a contract, rather than the principle of machined coinage. This latter point at least seems to have been settled by 1653.[220]

The debate between Blondeau and the moneyers lasted into the Protectorate. Once Cromwell was firmly established, steps were taken to make effective use of Blondeau's abilities. At first it was planned that he should establish an Irish mint. He was paid for a journey to Ireland and provision was made for the construction of machinery there. However, regardless of continuing anxieties about the state of Irish currency, nothing seems to have been accomplished.[221] But Blondeau was granted a state pension and it was agreed that he and Simon should be employed to coin bullion captured from the Spaniards in 1656.

A report made by Lambert and Wolseley confirmed and amplified the decision made by Harrington in 1651. It was accepted that machined coins would avoid the inconvenience of the great variation in size found in hammered coinage. Blondeau's coins could neither be clipped, nor readily counterfeited. Furthermore they would be most handsome, without involving excessive cost. Objections had been heard from officers of the Mint, but the only gesture made towards their position was that Blondeau was to be required to undertake a trial of his methods in Ireland. In the event, this condition was not enforced and the trial was conducted in London. It was proposed that Blondeau should be given charge over the English Mint if the trials were successful. A house was to be provided for Blondeau's work and the engraver ordered to prepare dies with appropriate inscriptions and devices. One side of the coins was to bear the Protector's effigy, while the other was to display his arms.[222]

For the trial it was decided to coin £2,000. In order to protect Blondeau from vindictive critics at the Mint, various alternative sites were considered for the machine-coining. Eventually the 'kitchen, larder, cellars, coach house etc.' of Drury House were placed at his disposal, care being taken to protect his works from damage.

In November 1656 Simon's designs were approved and inscriptions selected for the surfaces and edges, while in February 1657 Blondeau was paid £200 for 'the Charge of Coyning of 2000l. according to his

---

moneyers were reprinted in T. Violet, *The Answer of the Corporation of Moniers* (London, 1653).

220. *CSPD 1651*, pp.488–9; *CSPD 1651/2*, pp.152–3, 156–7.

221. *CSPD 1655*, p.215, 26 June 1655. Henfrey (147), pp.84–9. At this time the proposals of James Standish on the Irish mint were under consideration (Henfrey, p.84). William Potter sent proposals for the use of native metals for Irish coinage to Hartlib: 'Advertisements about Coyne', 13 Dec. 1658, HP LIII 30

222. *CSPD 1656/7*, p.49, July 1656.

New Invention'.[223] In this operation seven types of coin were produced (fifty-shilling piece, broad, half-broad, crown, half-crown, shilling and sixpence). The series of coins produced by Blondeau and Simon has been judged 'undoubtedly [to] excell in a high degree all previous examples of English numismatic art. By means of the power and precision of Blondeau's machinery, the bold and striking outlines of Cromwell's portrait on Simon's dies were faithfully reproduced in comparatively high relief'.[224]

The superiority of the Cromwellian coinage is attributable to both technical and artistic qualities. By using Blondeau's presses, Simon was able to achieve a quality in coinage comparable with that of the medals of the Renaissance. The high-relief bust of Cromwell was modelled in full detail, standing out prominently against a polished table or background. The surface was varied by frosting on the bust, heraldic crosses, and inscription. Blondeau improved this effect even further by using finely polished blanks of perfect circularity, protected against clipping by milled edges or inscriptions. Thus the trial vindicated Blondeau's original claims that machine-struck coinage could serve the economic objective better than traditional hammered coinage while also assisting the dignity of the state by its superior aesthetic qualities.

Having completed the trial, preparations were made to produce a national coinage at Drury House. After passing through various committees, Blondeau's request for £1,440 to build machinery weighing 30,000lb was granted. The necessary funds were allowed and assistants appointed in the winter of 1657/8.[225] The manufacture of crowns, half-crowns, shillings and sixpences bearing Cromwell's bust probably began during the summer of 1658, perhaps only a month before the Protector's death in September. Although a high quality was maintained, the work was discontinued after Cromwell's death. Nevertheless the experience gained by this experiment in mechanised coinage was not wasted. With the restoration of Charles II the moneyers took the initiative and resumed the minting of hammered coins. The resultant dramatic decline of standards was apparent to Henry Slingsby, the new Master of the Mint, who was described by Pepys as a great friend of Blondeau. It was 'strange to see how good they are in the stamp and bad in the money, for lack of skill to make them. But he says Blondeau will shortly come over and then we shall have it better, and the best in the world.' The hammered coinage was so unsatisfactory compared with the Cromwellian coinage, that Blondeau was recalled from exile to resume his partnership with Simon. Thereafter hammered coinage was permanently abandoned and, after a brief period of reinstatement, Ram-

223. *CSPD 1656/7*, pp.48, 106, 156–7, 286–7. The Order of Council, 27 November 1656, is attached to Wood's decimalisation proposals in HP XXVII 20.

224. Hocking, *op. cit.*, pp.96–7; Henfrey (147), p.112.

225. *CSPD 1657/8*, pp.30, 37, 52, 63, 168–9, 226, 301.

age was ejected from his post as Superintendent of Mills. Thus Blondeau's hard-won victory over the moneyers during the Protectorate was finally confirmed, and the coinage of Charles II was produced according to the high technical standards established during the Cromwellian period. Aesthetic standards are less easy to assess. Certainly the Cromwellian coins continued to attract admiration. Indeed Pepys's celebrated remarks indicate that Simon's standards were difficult to match.

> 'There dined with us today Mr. Slingsby of the Mint, who showed us all the new pieces, both gold and silver . . . , that are made for the King by Blondeau's way, and compared them with those made for Oliver—the pictures of the latter made by Symons, and of the King by one Rotyr [John Roettier], . . . He extolls these of Rotyrs above the others; and endeed, I think they are the better, because the sweeter of the two; but upon my word, those of the Protectors are more like in my mind than the King's—but both very well worth seeing. The Crownes of Cromwell's are now sold it seems for 25s and 30s a-piece.'[226]

The decision to embark on extensive recoinage, and the acceptance of the standardisation of procedures according to the proposals of Blondeau were accompanied by the discussion of a wide range of issues relating to currency. It was necessary to decide which metals to use for each denomination, the degree of use of alloys, and the values of coin to be issued. It was also necessary to respond to the extensive public agitation for a national issue of farthings. Mostly the debate followed well-worn paths, but an essentially new dimension was added by the proposal for currency decimalisation. The introduction of a more rational currency system, in line with similar reforms of weights and measures, would have brought to economic life the advantages of one of the latest trends in mathematics. This innovation was probably seen as a useful complement to Blondeau's technologically advanced methods at the Mint. Since the introduction of mechanised methods involved the production of a series of new dies by Thomas Simon, this appeared to be an ideal moment to carry the reform a stage further, by adopting decimalisation. Not surprisingly this idea found expression among the mathematicians recruited to the Cromwellian civil service.[227] Decimalisation was not a completely new idea, but plans for its widespread application had been relatively few. For the ultimate source of the Cromwellian proposals, it is necessary to refer back to an analogous situation during the early period of the stabilisation of the United Netherlands;

226. Pepys, *Diary*, ed. Latham & Matthews, ii, pp.38–9, iv, p.70, 19 Feb. 1661 and 9 March 1663. See also H. Farquhar, 'Thomas Simon . . .', pp.292–4.

227. For a brief discussion of this subject see my 'Decimalisation under Cromwell', *Nature*, 1971, *229*: 463. Published to mark Britain's decimalisation of currency on 15 February 1971.

thereafter, the fuller exploitation of the decimal principle was delayed until the eve of the French Revolution.

The first significant decimalisation proposals came from the fertile and inventive mind of Simon Stevin. His advice on public affairs was frequently sought during the early years of the United Netherlands. One of his early writings, *Die Thiende* (1585), illustrated the widespread mathematical and practical implications of the decimal treatment of fractions. This apparently simple device, of reducing fractions to the computational method already applied to integers, had received only sporadic application previously: astronomical usage had determined the predominant sexagesimal treatment of fractions.[228]

Stevin devoted equal attention to the theoretical and practical aspects of this question. His book was composed in Flemish; it was addressed primarily to mathematical practitioners and contained a lengthy appendix explaining the practical application of his idea to surveying, the measurement of textiles, liquid and solid measure, astronomy, weights of precious metals, and money. The preface suggested that surveyors had already found decimal scales useful, and the subsequent history of decimalisation underlines the closeness of the association between practitioners and theorists. It would be interesting to know the degree to which Stevin's ideas on decimalisation were stimulated by intuitive craft experience.

In a final and particularly prophetic paragraph of *Die Thiende* Stevin appealed for the decimalisation of weight, measure and money, and with respect to the latter he advised that 'principally the new coins, might be valued and reckoned upon certain primes, seconds, thirds, etc.' This advice, to the States General of the United Netherlands, was to be repeated in similar terms more than fifty years later, by the economic advisers to the Protectorate.[229]

Die Thiende became widely known, mainly owing to Stevin's French translation of his tract. Soon the decimal arithmetic had many advocates and some rival claimants to independent discovery, but no author developed the idea so clearly or with such regard to practical implications, as Stevin.

The value of decimalisation was recognised in England by practical mathematicians and theorists; *Die Thiende* was faithfully translated into English with minor additions by the gunner Robert Norton, who was the son of the poet Thomas Norton and the nephew of Archbishop Cranmer.[230] While Robert Norton was the author of mathematical

228. D. J. Struik (ed.), *The Principal Works of Simon Stevin*, vol. 2a (Amsterdam, 1958), pp.373–455. G. Sarton, 'The first explanation of decimal fractions and measures', *Isis*, 1935, *23*: 153–244. F. Cajori, *A History of Mathematical Notations*, 2 vols. (Chicago, 1928), i, pp.314–26.

229. Struik, *op. cit.*, p.453.

230. Robert Norton, *Disme: The Art of Tenths* (London, 1608); Taylor (278), p.189. Struik reprints Norton's translation, but reads the title as 'Dime' and gives Norton's first name as 'Richard'.

works, his father had been the translator of protestant theological treatises, including Calvin's *Institutes*. Decimal fractions would have been further popularised by Norton's brief appendix to Recorde's popular introduction to arithmetic.[231]

Norton's translation was in all probability the inspiration for Henry Lyte's *The Art of Tenths, or Decimal Arithmetic*, which was in circulation as a manuscript for about ten years before publication.[232] This brief and rare book is usually described as a translation of Stevin; but it should be regarded as an original work, consisting of an introduction to decimal computation which contains a summary of Stevin's treatment of fractions, followed by a series of exercises illustrating the value of the decimal principle for calculations in various spheres of commercial mathematics. Like Stevin, Lyte appreciated that decimal arithmetic would be assisted by the introduction of decimal instruments. Evidence that such instruments were already in production is provided by the advertisement included in Lyte's book, for decimally divided yard and two-foot rulers which could be obtained from John Thomson, a prominent London instrument maker.[233]

Lyte's book was an indication of a general receptivity to Stevin's ideas among the English mathematical practitioners, particularly the surveyors. Aaron Rathborne's decimalised perch chain, 198 inches long, divided into 10 'primes' and 100 'seconds', adopted a nomenclature for its units which was directly taken from Stevin. At about the same time Edmund Gunter introduced his celebrated rod chain, divided into 100 'centesmes', every tenth link being marked by a brass ring. Gunter's calculations were decimal, and where appropriate his instrumental scales were decimal; he remarked that customary duodecimal divisions of the foot 'doth breed much trouble both in Arithmetick and the use of instruments'. As indicated below, this author made a further contribution to decimalisation by undertaking the application of base-ten logarithms to trigonometry.[234]

Lyte gave instructions for a yard ruler which would be divided decimally; a second scale would give the square measure for each division. A similar approach was adopted for monetary calculations. Tables were provided for the conversion of duodecimal currency into decimals (perhaps the first decimal conversion tables), and examples were given to indicate the ease of decimal accountancy. Without engaging in radical proposals for the decimalisation of weights, measures and

231. *Recordes Arithmetick*, 1615 edn., appendix, 'The Art and Application of Decimall Arithmeticke'.

232. Henry Lyte, *The Art of Tenths* (London 1619), Preface, sig. ¶5r. Lyte was the son of Henry Lyte, translator of R. Dodoens's *Cruyde boeck* (1563), as *A Niewe Herball* (London, 1578). See H. C. Maxwell Lyte, 'The Lytes of Lytescary', *Proc. Somerset Arch. & Nat. Hist. Soc.*, 1892, *38* : 57–8.

233. Lyte, *The Art of Tenths*, sig. ¶4v.

234. Aaron Rathborne, *The Surveyor in Foure Books* (London, 1616); Edmund Gunter, *Description and Use of the Sector* (London, 1623). See A. W. Richeson (244), pp.104–9, 113, 141.

money, various practical mathematicians followed Lyte's example by providing interconversion tables, which allowed a wide range of calculations to be undertaken in decimal terms.[235]

The important implications of Stevin's ideas became particularly apparent after Napier's invention of logarithms. Napier, in close collaboration with Henry Briggs, appreciated the advantage of logarithms calculated to the base ten. The first tables of base-ten logarithms, from one to one thousand, were by Briggs calculated to fourteen places of decimals using a recognisably modern notation.[236]

Briggs, as a teacher of mathematics at Gresham College, lost no opportunity of using his lectures to popularise logarithms and point to their practical applications. His friend Edward Wright, the writer on navigation, promptly translated *Mirifici Logarithmorum canonis descriptio* (1614) for the benefit of mariners. This was published posthumously, edited by Briggs and dedicated to the East India Company. In his preface Briggs pointed out the relevance of logarithms to navigation and astronomy, through their application to trigonometrical tables. As an illustration of their commercial application he provided an example of a calculation of compound interest using logarithms.[237]

Commercial arithmetic of this kind rapidly became a standard part of works on logarithms; simple rules were given for conversion between decimal tables and duodecimal currency. Examples were supplied of the application of logarithms to a wide range of investment transactions, to illustrate the ease with which complex calculations could be performed without loss of accuracy.

Decimalisation had an important part to play in the development of trigonometrical tables. In 1620 Gunter applied base-ten logarithms to tables of sines and tangents; Briggs recognised a further implication, criticising the traditional sexagesimal 360° division of the circle and proposing that it would be more satisfactory to divide the circle into 100 parts. As a compromise, his trigonometrical tables divided the degree centesimally, a practice which had already been anticipated by Stevin.[238]

Although Briggs believed that this change was widely desired, his decimal division of the circle had little lasting influence, with the result that there was constant need for interconversion between sexagesimal readings and decimal calculations. The authoritative trigonometrical tables continued to be constructed according to the traditional division

235. Lyte, *The Art of Tenths,* pp.20–1, 24ff. See also William Barton, *Arithmeticke Abreviated* (London, 1634); William Leybourne, *Arithmetick, Vulgar Decimal & Instrumental* (London, 1657).

236. Briggs, *Logarithmorum chilias prima* (London, 1617). See J. W. L. Glaisher, 'Logarithms', *Encyclopaedia Britannica,* 9th edn., xiv, pp.773–5.

237. Napier (196), sig. A6r–8r.

238. Briggs, *Arithmetica Logarithmica* (London, 1624), Chapter XVII, pp.41–5. Expanded in Briggs, *Logarithmical Arithmetike* (London, 1631), Chapter VII, pp.8–16. *Idem, Trigonometria Britannica,* ed. H. Gellibrand (Gouda, 1633), pp.1, 49.

of the circle. None the less Briggs's idea attracted occasional commendations. Wallis remarked that sexagesimal division was not altogether convenient or desirable, being the result of tenacious custom and thoughtless imitation of the ancients.[239]

The influence of Briggs is evident in the writings of Wallis's friend, the mathematical teacher William Oughtred (1574-1660), whose rectory at Aldbury was visited by numerous young mathematicians during the first half of the seventeenth century. Oughtred's fame was greatly enhanced by *Clavis mathematica* (1631), one of the most concise, modern and effective textbooks of the period, which gave an enormous impetus to mathematical studies in England.[240] The Puritan Revolution marked the climax of Oughtred's influence. His textbook was revised, translated and augmented. In 1647 the second augmented edition was produced in both Latin and English forms. In 1648 the Latin edition was reissued, and a third even more expanded edition appeared in 1652. The responsibility for the preparation of Oughtred's work was undertaken by his grateful disciples, most of whom were associated with Oxford. The *Clavis* opened with an introduction to decimal arithmetic; Oughtred commented in passing that 'this decimall Logistica or accounting is for Astronomical calculations much easier and neater than the Sexagenarie common in use'. He also praised his friend Briggs for decimalising the canons of sines. Oughtred's *Trigonometria* (1657) was one of the few books to follow Briggs's centesimal division of the degree. In the second and subsequent editions of the *Clavis* Oughtred gave rules for sexagesimal-decimal interconversion and instructions for the use of logarithms; he also included a brief treatise 'of anatocisme, or compound Usury'.[241] Considering the decimal bias of the *Clavis,* it is not surprising that the idea of decimal currency took root among his pupils. Jonas Moore recollected that he could acquire no knowledge of mathematics until 'at last by a most happy accident I had Mr. Oughtred's Clavis Mathematicae bestowed upon me'. Moore's *Arithmetic* followed the *Clavis* by opening with an introduction to decimal arithmetic; it then urged that decimalisation should be adopted more widely: 'it were yet worthy the name of Reformation to cause the fractions of mony and weight to be altered: And as concerning the case in measure, Surveyors and Land-meters, who use the decimall chaine, and those who use a decimall foot, yard or scale can best certifie upon experience.'[242] Like Briggs and Oughtred, Moore planned to construct astronomical tables on the decimal principle.

239. Wallis, *De Algebra Tractatus,* quoted from *Opera Omnia* (London, 1693), ii, p.37.

240. For editions of the *Clavis,* see Madan (184), Nos. 2203, 2772; P. J. Wallis, in *The Bibliotheck,* 1964, *5*: 147–8.

241. Oughtred (203), pp.2, 169–72.

242. Moore, *Arithmetick* (London, 1650), Preface and p.14. Moore's abilities at mathematics are acknowledged in the preface to the 1647 English edition of Oughtred's *Clavis.*

A particularly rigorous exponent of decimalisation was Robert Wood, who had been an undergraduate at Merton College Oxford. Henry Briggs, the first Savilian professor of geometry, had died shortly before Wood entered Merton. After taking his MA in 1649, Wood was appointed by the parliamentarian Visitors as Fellow of Lincoln College Oxford. As he explained in a letter to Hartlib, his mathematical education had been undertaken at Aldbury 'under that admirable and deservedly famous Mathematician, old Mr. Oughtred'.[243] His work in preparing the 1647 English translation of the *Clavis* was acknowledged by Oughtred in its Preface. In 1651 Oughtred entrusted the preparation of the 1652 Oxford edition of the *Clavis* to Wood and the Savilian professors Wallis and Ward. Although there is little direct information about Wood's activities at this time, later evidence indicates that he was on good terms with his fellow Oxford mathematicians. Aubrey mentions Wood as one of Petty's particular friends; this was perhaps a significant factor in directing him towards participation in economic affairs and public service.[244]

Wood directed his energies to a variety of economic problems. His first and most complete economic writing was 'Ten to One', the proposal for decimal currency, which was probably written in the winter of 1655/6. Its author was no doubt hoping to influence the outcome of the discussions which led to the new coinage of 1658. Because periodically it was necessary to consider renewing national coinage, decimalisation was more practicable in this area than in the more stable, but more localised traditions of measurement and weights. Although too sophisticated to solve any of the numerous elementary problems relating to recoinage, Wood's proposal is of the greatest interest as the first fully developed defence of decimal coinage. Furthermore it shows an appreciation of the virtue of establishing the monetary system on the soundest rational basis.

Wood's pamphlet, which is reproduced in Appendix IV below, is one of the more rigorous, concise and direct examples of the economic writings of this period, a benefit undoubtedly deriving from the mathematical background of the author. In general outlook Wood operated within the context of the tradition established by Robinson and his friends in 1641. 'Ten to One' was addressed to Cromwell and his economic advisers: it argued that general economic advantages would follow if a monetary system was adopted which was completely in line with decimal arithmetic. Since integers and fractions were decimal, pounds should likewise be divided decimally. It was inconsistent to adopt decimal calculation for monetary integers (pounds), while maintaining monetary values as shillings, pence and farthings: 20th, 240th

243. Letter from Wood to Hartlib, 1 July 1657, HP XXXIII 1.

244. Letter from Oughtred to Wood, 19 April 1651, Aubrey, ii, pp.113–14; see also p.141. Wood was not specifically mentioned as the translator in the 1647 English *Clavis*, but he was in the preface to Halley's new edition of 1694.

and 960th divisions of a pound. Accountancy under such a system 'causeth distraction of the mind' whereas it should be a 'delightfull recreation'. The duodecimal system inevitably introduced errors into accountancy. Wood's solution was to introduce decimal coins of three types, the Tenth, the Hund (or Hundredth) and the Thous (or Thousandth), the first being equivalent to two shillings, the second being about two pence, and the third about a farthing.

Certain difficulties were raised by Wood's plan. First, he accepted that the new decimal coinage might operate alongside the conventional non-decimal coinage. Secondly, although farthings were widely used at this time, Wood had no settled opinions about the smallest unit. He hinted that the thousandth might be altogether abolished, a proposal which would not have been acceptable since no half-penny unit was to be substituted. No doubt Wood anticipated that private farthing tokens, already widely produced, would remain in circulation. The half-penny was avoided out of a desire for mathematical consistency. For the same reason he expunged his own proposal for a half-Hund piece (a two-hundredth part of a pound), ten of which would equal the shilling. Had he not done so, he might have avoided another awkward feature of his proposal, which left no unit between two pence and a farthing. The absence of the farthing would have made the position even worse. This situation has been avoided in the modern decimal system by the adoption of the half new penny, the non-decimal element tentatively considered by Wood.

'Ten to One' shows that Wood was fully aware of the practical problems which would be incurred by the introduction of decimalisation; he appreciated that it was most difficult to construct a monetary system according to a rigorous rational principle. His ultimate solution was a compromise; it preserved a strictly decimal system, alongside the old duodecimal currency which he hoped would gradually become redundant. Wood discounted the criticism that a new coinage system was inadmissible because of public resistance to change, or because of the difficulty of teaching the lower classes to use the sophisticated new system. Wood averred that the intrinsic rationality of decimalisation would ensure easy comprehension by all classes. But regardless of this he believed that the public could adjust to any monetary system and he pointed out that there had already been a smooth transfer from testons and groats to the current coinage. Once the commercial convenience of the new currency was recognised, Wood believed that non-decimal habits would be abandoned. This opinion would appear to have been justified in view of the recent success of decimal arithmetic, which had gained widespread popularity among mathematicians and artisans alike.

If Wood's proposal had been adopted accountancy would have been saved from troublesome interconversions rendered necessary by the prevailing practice of calculating interest decimally. Elementary arithmetics gave considerable space both to methods of conversion, and techniques of calculating compound interest, annuities, etc. The use of logarithms to speed such operations was increasingly common. Wood described logarithms as 'the most rare and absolute invention for the despatch of Arithmetical Operations that are or perhaps ever will be discovered'. Since most logarithmic tables were calculated to the base of ten, they could readily be used in decimal currency calculation.

While 'Ten to One' skilfully argued the advantages of decimalisation and elaborated a simple procedure for its introduction, it is clear from Wood's tone that he was not confident of success. Hence he included an uncontroversial suggestion, that the two-shilling piece might be introduced immediately, to replace the non-decimal half-crown. Ironically Wood's incidental remark that the new currency should portray the Protector was the only one of his proposals to be realised in the new coinage, and this outcome was obviously not due primarily to Wood. The modest request for a two-shilling piece was not acted upon, until the florin was introduced in 1849.

Wood was more successful in the second objective of 'Ten to One', which was to create public support for decimalisation. Realising that there would be antagonism to his proposal, his first action was to gather from the comments of a monetary theorist the main objections, and to answer them point by point.

Wood's critic (probably William Potter) was totally sceptical about the need for decimal currency, or indeed decimalised weights and measures. He believed that the introduction of decimal coins alongside the old coinage would lead to unnecessary complications. Accordingly if decimal coins were introduced, it would be necessary to embark on a complete recoinage. In view of the smooth operation of the duodecimal system and the various systems of weights and measures, he could see no reason for reform. Even the introduction of two-shilling pieces seemed to be unnecessary in view of the existence of shillings.

Wood defended the parallel system on the grounds that 'variety of Coynes are looked upon as advantageous both to the buyer and seller'. The poor understood the already complex English system, or the even more varied coinage in Ireland. The gradual introduction of the decimal coins would give ample time for familiarisation with the new system, during which the public would appreciate the value of a more rational and straightforward method of computation. He insisted that 'no hurt it can do, so that it may do some good, and might perhaps make way for the introduction of such a Decimalisation as no Cavaleere or Leveller would have any occasion to complaine of, in weights and measures, now (as I heare) under publick consideration'.[245]

245. Potter, 'Objections Against Ye Discourse of Decimal Coins'; Wood, 'An Answer to the objections against the Discourse of Decimal Coynes', HP XXVII 20. Letter from Wood to Hartlib, 8 April 1657, HP XXXIII 1.

Having clarified his views on decimalisation Wood sought to take advantage of the success of Blondeau, further to promote reform. He commented to Hartlib that 'I am glad that Monsieur Blondeau's ingenious designe for coyning goes on so well to prevent abuses of Clipping &c. and should not be sory if my proposals for decimall mony (which I conceive may prove of some advantage to the publicke) might take effect with his; the new pieces of 2s value or the tenth of a pound would be capable of inscriptions on the edge and very convenient for payment.'[246]

'Ten to One' and appended documents were sent to Hartlib on 1/11 March 1655/6, with the intention that they would be circulated among the officials concerned in the recoinage debate. As indicated above Hartlib was already following the discussions about recoinage, and he had ready access to a wide range of relevant officials, from the Council of State to the Master of the Mint. Nothing is known about the official response to decimalisation proposals, but the letters from Wood to Hartlib indicate that there was a generally favourable reception. 'Ten to One' might even have been instrumental in securing Wood's preferment from Oxford to the Irish civil service.

At the outset of his work in Ireland Wood wrote requesting a copy of 'Ten to One' for use there. Margaret, Lady Broghill had passed a copy to her husband Roger Boyle, Lord Broghill, an influential member of the Irish and Scottish Councils. Broghill's sister, Lady Ranelagh, had also read the proposal but was convinced that it would be difficult to introduce. Wood's enthusiasm for decimal coinage gradually waned, but nevertheless he announced his intention of developing a scheme for decimal weights and measures. It would be interesting to know whether he was by this time aware of Stevin's anticipation of these ideas. Wood may have found some consolation in the favourable reaction to his ideas among the mathematicians, both in Ireland and at Oxford. Decimalisation was accepted by his old associate Petty and by Miles Symner, the professor of mathematics at Trinity College Dublin. A similar response was elicited from 'our Mathematical professors and others' at Oxford, a group consisting predominantly of Oughtred's pupils Ward and Wallis, and probably Wilkins and Wren, who are mentioned in other contexts in letters written during this period.[247]

It is not surprising that Wood's ideas were more acceptable to mathematicians than to politicians, since at this time decimalisation was more important as a rational principle than as a solution to immediate monetary problems. Significantly it was again mathematicians who introduced decimalisation into the heated debate preceding the recoinage of 1696. It is perhaps a reflection of Wood's influence that two of the three later proponents of decimalisation were among his supporters

246. Letter from Wood to Hartlib, 6 January 1657, HP XXXIII 1.

247. Letters from Wood to Hartlib, 8 April 1657, 1 August 1657, HP XXXIII 1.

during the Protectorate.[248] Again, at this later time, decimalisation was overshadowed by more pressing economic questions. As in the case of sexagesimal notation in astronomy, the traditional monetary units held such a tenacious grip on the public mind at all levels, that it was to be centuries before a government could be persuaded to implement Wood's proposals.

(ix) The Frame of a Whole State

Bacon's later writings show that the compilation of natural histories came to assume for him an overwhelming importance. This need not have distinguished him from the naturalists of antiquity, the Renaissance encyclopaedists, or indeed the increasingly proficient botanists and zoologists of his own day. Descriptive lists of animals, plants and minerals were becoming impressively comprehensive, while regions ranging from English counties to American colonies were subjected to cartographical, geographical and historical scrutiny. But Bacon believed that conventional natural history required reform before it could make its optimum contribution to natural philosophy. He considered that too much energy had been devoted to superficial description; despite voluminous writings, nothing of consequence was contributed to the 'Instaurations of Philosophy'. A more systematic approach was advocated: labour should be organised to undertake minute investigation of all processes of generation and change; it was equally important for the observer to expand his horizons to embrace astronomy, meteorology and the systematic study of mountains, rivers, tides, sands and woods. The natural history of marvels (*magnalia*) or wonders of nature was another neglected area, for by tracing out 'the footings of nature in her wilful wandrings; . . . so afterward you may be able at your pleasure, to lead or force her to the same place and pastures again'. However the greatest rewards could be expected from investigation of the mechanical arts, a hitherto almost completely neglected course but one which 'to the raising of Natural Philosophy is of all other the most radical and fundamental'. From the understanding of the mechanical arts would emerge:

> 'Such Natural Philosophy, I understand, as doth not vanish into the fumes of subtile and sublime speculations, but such, as shall be effectually operative to the support and assistance of the incommodities of mans life: For it will not only help for the present, by connecting and transferring the observations of one Art, into the use of others, . . . but farther, it will give a more clear illumination,

248. J. K. Horsefield (152), pp.292, 325, lists two tracts on decimalisation during this period. One was anonymous, the other by Sir Christopher Wren. A slightly ambiguous remark by Petty might suggest that he too was favourable to the idea of decimalisation: *Petty Papers,* ii, p.271.

than hitherto hath shined forth, for the searching out of the causes of things, and the deducing of Axioms.'[249]

Accordingly Bacon shifted the emphasis of natural history towards the manual arts, believing that the meticulous study of 'small and mean things' would provide the key to fundamental explanations of natural phenomena. From this standpoint, it was only a short step to the investigation of economic and social aspects of the manual arts and the development of natural history into a general scientific study of society. Bacon occasionally apprehended this possibility; as at the point when he stated that the inductive method was applicable to all sciences, including medicine, ethics, and politics.[250] With respect to medicine specific directions were given for the compilation of case histories of diseases, the study of pathological anatomy, *anatomia comparata,* and vivisection studies. On wider issues Bacon's directives were less precise, but they were nevertheless sufficiently suggestive for Petty to declare that 'the *Advancement of Learning,* hath made a judicious *Parallel* in many particulars, between the *Body Natural,* and *Body Politick,* and between the Arts of preserving both in Health and Strength: And it is as reasonable that as Anatomy is the best foundation of one, so also of the other; and that to practice upon the Politick, without knowing the *Symmetry, Fabrick,* and *Proportion* of it, is as *casual* as the practice of Old-women and Empyricks'.[251] Equally important for the redirection of effort was the insistence that 'nothing duly investigated, nothing verified, nothing counted, weighed, or measured is to be found in natural history: and what in observation is loose and vague, is in information deceptive and treacherous'.[252]

Bacon was not able to make a substantial contribution to natural history or to the histories of trade, but his writings provided useful materials and unequivocal advice for his successors on the direction of the great collaborative enterprise for the instauration of philosophy. The priorities outlined by Bacon were ideally suited to the social ethic of the Puritans. Distrust of natural history for its own sake, concentration on the mechanical arts, appeal to collaborative effort, the promise of social amelioration, and the dream of great national power, were factors which contributed to the influence of Baconian natural history among the puritan reformers. The Puritans tended therefore to drift away from descriptive natural history, and to concentrate on agriculture, industry, trade and social analysis. Such a bias acted to the detriment of certain problems in the physical sciences to which natural

249. Bacon, *De Augmentis* (13), p.54; see also pp.49–55. *Novum Organum,* I, 98. See above, pp.335–42. For an excellent general discussion of histories of trade, see Houghton (153).

250. *Novum Organum,* I, 127.

251. Petty, *The Political Anatomy of Ireland* (213), author's preface.

252. *Novum Organum,* I, 98. For a similar statement, see *Parasceve,* Bacon *Works,* i, p.400.

philosophers had traditionally attached considerable importance. But Bacon believed that this reorientation was desirable and he would have applauded the extension of his methods into the fields of regional and economic geography. The increasing influence of his particular form of natural history was perhaps reflected in the popularity of *De Augmentis Scientiarum, Sylva Sylvarum* and *Historia vitae et mortis,* during the Puritan Revolution. This interest extended to a wide public, commonly finding its echo in the exhortation to 'put into practice the Lord Verulam's Designations' to improve nature or encourage the arts, made by such preachers as Dury or Peter. At a more specific level, it has already been mentioned that Baconian natural history provided the general framework for Winstanley's plans for the distribution of labour in his communes, for Petty's design for the compilation of histories of trade, and for Hartlib's programme for the Office of Address.[253] Furthermore it was hoped that through the creation of collegiate organisations of the type advocated by Bacon, the study of natural history would be officially sanctioned by the state.

Hartlib's *Further Discovery of the Office of Address,* which appeared in 1648, was of the greatest importance in drawing together Baconian natural history and systematic commercial abstracts of the kind advocated by Lewis Roberts.[254] 'Mutual Help' was the basic principle upon which Hartlib's plan was founded. Hartlib hoped to establish a central agency which would maintain numerous registers of information relating to such areas as trade, property conveyancing, and employment. Thereby all involved in these activities would have access to comprehensive, accurate and up-to-date intelligence, with the result that their efficiency would be greatly increased. The services were particularly important for the unemployed poor, but Hartlib's ultimate aim was to increase the momentum of the commercial life of the whole nation.

Registers of a most complex nature were required if the Office was to exercise its widest function, 'to set every body in a way by some direction and Addresse, how to come speedily to have his lawfull desires accomplished, of what kind soever they may be'.[255] Hartlib's basic registers were designed to provide economic and geographical information. Therewith the public would 'know the scituation of any of the Provinces, Shires, Counties, Cities, Towns, Villages, Castles, Ports; and such like places'. In a manner reminiscent of Roberts's *Map of Commerce,* these registers were to be amplified with economic information about each locality. But the success of the registers depended on their ability to comprehend the constantly changing daily needs of the population. It was recognised that this necessitated the compilation of detailed demographical and statistical information, relating to all classes and professions. The poor were to be listed, with special details about

253. See above, pp.373–6.
254. *A Further Discoverie of the Office of Publick Addresse,* 1648 (136).
255. *Ibid.,* p.6.

those who had failed to receive public or private charity. The sick poor would be the object of special reports describing their condition, which would then be circulated among physicians able to diagnose and suggest suitable treatment for their illnesses. Records of these case histories, if preserved by the Office, would have provided a valuable basis for a natural history of diseases of the kind recommended by Bacon. Elaborate commercial statistics would be maintained, including details of real estate transactions, monetary affairs, weights and measures, agricultural commodities, raw materials relating to industry, medicines, drinks, as well as 'All living Creatures in the Earth, Aire and Waters, Beasts, Fowls, and Fishes'. The 'Register of Persons' would provide lists of professions, trades, servants, and many incidental personal affairs. Strangers, whether scholars, or tradesmen, rich or poor, would be included in the various registers. Finally the 'Register of Ingenuities' would collect scientific information, which again would be relevant to histories of trade.[256] In conclusion it was foreseen that the compilation of these registers would greatly contribute to the understanding of the mechanism of the state, and provide an indispensable basis for a scientific approach to social policy.

> 'He that can look upon the frame of a whole state, and see the constitution of all the parts thereof, and doth know what strength is in every part, or what the weaknesse thereof is, and whence it doth proceed; and can, as in a perfect modell of a Coelestiall Globe, observe all the motions of the Spheres thereof; or as in a Watch, see how all the wheels turn and worke one upon another for such and such an ends, he only can fundamentally know what may and ought to be designed; or can be effected in that State for the increase of the Glory, and the settlement of the Felicity thereof with Power according to Righteousnesse.'[257]

In the *Further Discovery* Hartlib provided both a general context and many specific proposals for a 'Political Anatomy'. Not only was the concept of natural history extended to embrace geographical, economic and social phenomena, but Hartlib also appreciated that it was necessary to organise this material on a regional basis. Thus implicit factors in Bacon's interpretation of natural history were rendered explicit in the *Further Discovery*. The natural history aspect of the Baconian programme had an immediately widespread appeal. Among the first to amplify Hartlib's ideas was William Petty, whose *Advice* was presented as a contribution to the Office of Address design. He described the Office as the 'great instrument of this Designe . . . whereby the wants and desires of all may be made knowne unto all'.[258] Once it is

256. *Ibid.*, pp.8–26.
257. *Ibid.*, p.26.
258. Petty, *The Advice of W.P.*, 1648 (210), pp.1–3.

realised that the *Advice* was intended as a sequel to the *Further Discovery,* Petty's schemes for technical and medical education, as well as his plans for the compilation of a history of trades, emerge as a complement to the functions of the Office of Address. At this stage Petty's immediate enthusiasm was for histories of trade, but involvement with the Office of Address was probably partly responsible for stimulating his interest in the wider concept of political anatomy. Over the next few years both Petty and other members of the Hartlib circle were to pursue this idea further, until it eventually matured into Petty's brilliant conception of 'Political Arithmetic'.

History of trades remained a basic pre-occupation. Education in Petty's Literary Workhouse was designed to produce intellects which would be responsive to 'the advancement of Reall Learning'. After the completion of their basic education, Petty recommended his students to follow either Pell's systematic survey of the mathematical arts, or his own projected work entitled *Vellus Aureum, sive Facultatum Lucriferarum Descriptio Magna,* which was an introduction to all means of gaining subsistence. In particular he recommended that the 'History of Arts or Manufactures might first be undertaken as the most pleasant and profitable of all the rest'. He urged an intensive practical study of each art; these would be recorded in detail, with coloured illustrations of all relevant tools and machines.[259] With characteristic practical insight, Petty gave detailed instructions for the study of trades, with warnings about possible causes of error and indications of the most fruitful sources of enquiry. His aim was to inculcate a comprehensive scientific understanding of techniques, with the result that the information, when collected and analysed, would suggest innovations which might readily be applied in local circumstances. As in the Office of Address, all books on the subject were to be collected and excerpted, but Petty repeatedly advised his students to examine the arts 'per Autopsiam, and Re-experiment the Experiments contained in them'. This labour would guarantee full insight into the mysteries of trades, to the intellectual satisfaction of the intelligentsia and the enlightenment of mechanics. The emancipation of trades from traditional restrictions and the employment of all classes along more productive lines would boost trade and manufactures to make England 'potent and rich' like the Netherlands. Having outlined the methodology of histories of trade, Petty's *Advice* ended by referring the reader to Bacon's *De Augmentis,* where he would find a division of natural history into 'History of Nature free', and 'History of Trades', that is, 'of Nature vexed and disturbed'. Furthermore Bacon's *Catalogus historiarum particularum* provided an 'exact and judicious' list of histories for future investigation.[260]

By contrast with Bacon, Petty possessed a sound first-hand knowledge of trades. As the son of a clothier he had direct experience of cloth

259. *Ibid.,* p.18.
260. *Ibid.,* pp.3, 18–26.

working and dyeing. In addition, a natural curiosity in boyhood had led to an interest in the work of smiths, coachmakers, carpenters, joiners, etc.[261] Once associated with Hartlib he compiled a general scheme for a history of trades which was passed on to Boyle, with a comment that one history was virtually complete. The outcome is not reported, but Petty's papers contain lists of histories as well as notes on various trades, which were probably all composed at about this time.[262]

The early catalogues of histories resemble the classifications of trades given by Bacon or Winstanley. One consists of an ordered list of natural products, with appended information on trades and products which were related. Thus under 'Iron' Petty listed four types of smith; smelting, casting and forging at ironworks; two types of ironmonger, three grades of cutler; grinders; makers of cross bows, edge tools, fish hooks, shaping irons, hooks and eyes, needles, screws, weights, drills for surgical instruments, nails, tweezers, saws, files, rasps, axes, hammers, springs, augers, pots, kettles and wire. In a second 'History of Arts illiberal & mechanique', the trades were listed according to antiquity, succession, dependence, dignity, etc. Eight categories were distinguished: 1. Useful and purely mechanical. 2. Mean and less honourable. 3. Servile. 4. Rustical. 5. Female. 6. Polite and more Liberal. 7. Curious. 8. Exotic. Long lists were given for each category, ending with inventions for flying, and a book of tools and models shown in perspective and exactly proportioned.[263] In addition Petty made collections of observations on paper making, printing inks, ship design and cloth making. The latter was the most extensive, and may have been the history which was virtually complete in 1647.[264]

Petty's ceaseless quest for novelty and his crowding professional commitments prevented the completion of the histories on which such substantial progress had been made by 1647. Inventions relating to brewing, distillation, perfumery, agricultural mechanisation, textile dyeing, printing, optical instruments and mechanics competed for attention in his thoughts. Petty believed that by organising the poor to exploit new inventions the foundations would be laid for collaborative histories of trades. Thus the workhouses planned by Hartlib could take on the functions of the *Gymnasium mechanicum;* they could both solve a serious social problem, and fulfil a positive intellectual role. Although Petty became pre-occupied with other problems he remained interested in the history of trade and he communicated this interest to others, furnishing Robert Wood with various papers relating to the subject in 1657. When Beale revived Petty's scheme for a College of Artificers,

261. Aubrey, ii, p.139.

262. Letter from Hartlib to Boyle, 16 November 1647, Boyle *Works,* vi, pp.76–7. *Petty Papers,* i, pp.205–7. BM Sloane MS 2903, fols. 1–65. Mr. Lindsay Sharp informs me that this document, perhaps deriving from William Petty's work, was possibly written by Abraham Hill.

263. *Ibid.,* fols. 59r–60v; 63r–65v.

264. *Ibid.,* fols. 13r, 26r–38v, 55r–57r; 61r–62r.

Wood noted that it would be an ideal preliminary for 'History of Trades (at least some of them) I mean after the manner of natural Historie, which would in my opinion [be] the most desirable work I can thincke upon'.[265]

Active and systematic interest in trades became a hallmark of the Baconians. By 1645 Child was regularly sending specimens of New England minerals and seeds to Merrett and Leonard Buckner in London. Upon arriving in England Child collaborated on many subjects with Merrett, whom he commended to Hartlib for his 'mechanical endeavours and industries'. Child was pleased about the completion of How's *Phytologia Britannica* (1650) and he pressed for Merrett to undertake its correction, and extension to cover all subjects. In 1649 Merrett was already projecting a translation of Neri's *De Arte Vitraria,* a work which eventually was regarded by Boyle as a model history of trade. Child also recommended that the College of Physicians should embark on 'the History of all incurable diseases . . . accurately recorded from year to year'.[266]

Boyle's work on the history of trades was published in the final part of the *Usefulness*. Because of his widespread experience of collaboration with London artificers and involvement in scientific issues relating to trade Boyle was well qualified to write on this particular aspect of the usefulness of experimental philosophy. He aimed to 'carry Philosophical materials from the shops to the Schooles and divulge the experiments of Artificers, both to the improvement of trades themselves and to the great enriching of Artes and Nature'. A whole section was devoted to the proposition 'that the Goods of Mankind may be much encreased by the Naturalists Insight into Trades'. Following Bacon, it was emphasised that trades, even though practised by illiterate mechanics, were to be reckoned among the more noble parts of any history of nature. Rather than attempting comprehensive histories of particular trades, Boyle preferred to give a large number of specific examples of the manner in which industrial problems had been solved by innovation. He drew extensively upon the work of the 1650s, often recording inventions discussed many years before by Hartlib. For instance, Thomas Duckett's chemical method of tanning was mentioned often by Hartlib before its appearance in Boyle's essay.[267]

Interest in histories of trade spread rapidly from Hartlib's circle to the virtuosi. Wilkins's proposed mathematico-chemico-mechanical school at Oxford was probably intended to assist with the history of mech-

265. Ephemerides 1647 and 1648. Letters from Wood to Hartlib, 8 April and 10 June 1657, HP XXXIII 1.

266. Letters of Robert Child, HP XV v; Ephemerides 1649 & 1650. For a summary, see Turnbull (290); Boyle, *Usefulnesse* (32), Bk. II, part 2, sig. *4v. Merrett's annotated translation of Neri was published in 1662 and his *Pinax rerum Britannicarum* in 1667.

267. Boyle, *Usefulnesse* (32), Bk. II, part 2, pp.18–19. Ephemerides 1654, 1656, 1660.

anical arts. John Evelyn found the utilitarian ideal congenial, and he confessed that he 'had an inclination to the imployment upon a public account'. His thoughts wandered over a wide range of subjects as he searched for suitable topics for his first histories. Although superficially Evelyn appears to share the aspirations of his puritan correspondents, closer examination betrays a significant difference in approach. Evelyn's mind unerringly flew to the gentlemanly diversions of the virtuosi; the first area which he outlined was etching, painting in oil, painting in miniature, annealing in glass, enamelling, and marbling. Furthermore, running against the basic principle among the puritan reformers of free communication, he decided not to publish this history, since he wished to protect established craftsmen and prevent debasing 'much of their esteem by prostituting them to the vulgar'. This work was no sooner begun, when Evelyn discovered that he had a 'rural genius'. He quickly produced a translation, *The French Gardener: instructing how to cultivate all sorts of Fruit trees and Herbs for the Garden* (1658). After this apprenticeship, he sent Hartlib a plan for an extensive history of 'ornaments of gardens'. This evolved into the ambitious project for an *Elysium Britannicum,* which was to be a comprehensive history of formal gardens. This project attracted much interest at meetings of the Royal Society.[268]

Hartlib's primary energies were increasingly devoted to the accumulation of materials relating to husbandry. His great success in drawing together the work of numerous agricultural and horticultural investigators will be discussed below. However, despite the impressive nature of this collaborative enterprise, the final results were tentative and fragmentary. This experience would have indicated the magnitude of the task facing the compilers of any major history of trade. Hence a general history of trade would have seemed to be a remote prospect, a labour which could only be effectively undertaken by a large, dedicated and well-organised group of scholars and craftsmen. However the task became of more manageable proportions if the natural history was confined to a discrete geographical region, perhaps an English county, or one of the colonial territories. There are signs that natural history was pursued on this regional basis, both in England and in the colonies.

Regional bias was not an altogether new tendency. The antiquaries of the earlier part of the century showed a sensitive appreciation of local conditions in their chorographical writings. In the case of such authors as Henry Burton or Richard Carew, their works were organised on a county basis. However these were a long way from the systematic county natural histories which were attempted by Plot, Aubrey and their associates in the later part of the century. The roots of this move-

268. Letters from Evelyn to Boyle 9 May 1657, 9 August 1659, Boyle *Works,* vi, pp.287–8; letter from Evelyn to Lady Sunderland, 4 August 1690, Evelyn (96), iii, pp.317–18. For Evelyn's later work, see Denny (79). The suggestion to translate the *Jardinier Français* was originally made by Arnold Boate; see letter from Hartlib to Boyle, 8 May 1654, Boyle *Works*, vi, p.85.

ment may be traced to such enterprises as Beale's sketch of an agricultural history of Herefordshire, which will be discussed below, or to Gerard Boate's natural history of Ireland.

Ireland was an ideal location for a pilot attempt at a comprehensive natural history. It was conveniently near, not too large, or too highly developed; its past attractions for planters had been considerable and the collapse of the rebellion opened up new opportunities for plantation. Furthermore many Baconians had become associated with the Irish army or civil service and were anxious to demonstrate their worth by promoting planned exploitation of the province. Accordingly Ireland became to the Puritans a more immediate source of attraction than even the American colonies.[269]

For once Baconian aspirations and political necessity coincided. It was imperative for the Republic rapidly to achieve an Irish settlement, since the military reduction lasting from 1649 to February 1653 had produced severe civil dislocation and had generated mounting arrears of salaries which could be most adequately satisfied by grants of forfeited lands. There was also a longer-term arrangement whereby war loans raised among Adventurers in London would be repaid in Irish land. Accordingly Ireland was looked to as a land of promise; military and civilian creditors anticipated ample rewards and the state prayed that the resources of forfeited lands were sufficient to meet its obligations. In order to retain the goodwill of the army, the Republic was obliged to make immediate preparations for the repayment of debts. A first necessity was the assessment of Irish lands, a formidable task which soon involved the administration in a surveying operation more complex and detailed than had ever been previously undertaken in the history of civilisation. The authorities were faced with a technical problem, which, if not approached with initiative, could place the stability of the Republic at risk. This responsibility was quickly transferred to parliament's Baconian advisers; it provided one of the most exacting tests of their ability to translate political anatomy and Baconian natural history into practical terms.

Even before the cessation of military activities the ground had been prepared for further scientific work, by the natural history of Ireland undertaken by the brothers Gerard and Arnold Boate. After a promising start in 1645 this work was destined to be devastatingly interrupted by the vicissitudes of human life. The natural history was initiated by Gerard Boate, the London medical practitioner, whose interest in Ireland was probably prompted by his brother's reports from the province. Then upon leaving Ireland in 1644 Arnold provided

269. Especially relevant to the following section are T. C. Barnard (18), Chapter VI; F. V. Emery, 'Irish Geography in the Seventeenth Century', *Irish Geography*, 1954–8, *3*: 263–76; Y. M. Goblet, *La transformation de la Géographie Politique de l'Irlande au XVIIe siècle dans les cartes et essais anthropogéographiques de Sir William Petty*, 2 vols. (Paris, 1930).

Gerard with information gained during eight years of travelling and medical service in that country. Subsequently Gerard received information from Irish gentlemen such as Sir William Parsons and his son, Richard Parsons, before eventually settling in Ireland himself in late 1649. Only the first part of the natural history was completed by the time of his death a few months later.[270] But this part was of sufficient general interest to merit the publication by Hartlib in 1652 of a text edited by Arnold; this was furnished with a long letter of dedication composed by Dury, but signed by Hartlib. Dury's dedication to Cromwell and the Lord-Deputy, Fleetwood, was an inspiring piece of religious writing, albeit displaying only limited relationship to the text.

Dury declared that he knew 'nothing more usefull, than to have the knowledg of the Natural History of each Nation advanced & perfected'; as a prelude, in this case, to the replanting of Ireland by Adventurers, exiled Bohemians or other protestant refugees. The *History* would also prepare the way for the efficient exploitation of natural resources, and the expansion of trade.[271]

Boate's *Natural History,* despite its modest format and unpretentious approach, represented a major development in economic geography. Abandoning the chorographical tradition stemming from Camden, with its attendant absorption in antiquities, ecclesiastical foundations, archival sources, and local history, Boate provided a regional description strongly orientated towards economic affairs. The author furnished the settler with a brief documentary account of the region; he avoided exaggerated claims, and his work was not embellished with accounts of local marvels, or colourful digressions. Considerable information had been gathered and it was organised with little more elaboration than the digests of useful information contained in almanacs. Despite Boate's academic background and previous authorship of a Latin philosophical work, he abstained from interspersing his text with citations from classical authors; even references to modern authorities like Bacon were rare. By contrast, the 'natural history' composed by the royalist clergyman Childrey was a miscellaneous collection of travellers' tales, designed to entertain the rich and over-awe the poor with its pseudo-erudition.[272] Boate's economical style precluded explicit reference to sources of influence. Nevertheless it is clear that his work was conceived within a Baconian context; he was also probably indebted to the economists Roberts and Malynes. Of the regional surveys, he would have valued the new natural history of Brazil by two of his fellow countrymen.[273]

270. Boate, *Irelands Naturall History* (30), sig. A6r–8r, 'To the Reader', by Arnold Boate.

271. *Ibid.*, sig. A3r.

272. Joshua Childrey, *Britannia Baconiana: Or, the Natural Rarities of England, Scotland & Wales* (London, 1661).

273. Willem Piso and Georg Marcgraf, *Historia naturalis Brasiliae, in qua non tantum plantae et animalia, sed in indigenarum morbi, ingenia et mores describuntur* (Leyden, 1648).

Also relevant, as with Petty, was the medical education which he had received in the Netherlands. Anatomy, which had revealed the structure of the human body, could be applied to anatomise nature; the chemistry of chemical therapy was also the chemistry of mining and metallurgy. Finally, Boate's association with Hartlib and the Invisible College would have confirmed his adherence to the aims of the Office of Address, which was intended to sponsor a comprehensive political anatomy. Goblet is probably correct in believing that the scientific and utilitarian character of Boate's work persuaded Hartlib to undertake its publication.[274]

Boate provided only the briefest account of Irish topography and he did not include maps or illustrations of any kind (pp.1-10). The rest of the book consisted of twenty-three brief chapters (pp.10-186), which summarised information on each aspect of economic geography, beginning with ports and ending with diseases. While the coastline was poorly described, great attention was devoted to ports. Rivers were treated as means of communication or as fisheries. In this context, subsequent surveys suggest that Boate was correct in asserting the importance of the fresh-water fisheries. The description of general terrain, and comments about the distribution of mountains and bogs were brief, but fine details were given about local manuring and marling techniques, or about practices used for the draining of bogs. Although Ireland was richly wooded, it was admitted that quite severe impoverishment of timber resources had been caused by the English settlers.

As advertised in the title, the *Natural History* worked systematically through the natural resources, 'its Metalls, Mineralls, Freestone, Marble, Sea-coal, Turf, and other Things that are taken out of the Ground', before treating the climate, health and disease. Prospects for mining silver and lead were assessed with caution and with unusually specific reference to informants (pp.141-7). Glass works were also described briefly (pp.160-2). In accordance with their greater economic importance, iron ore mines and ironworks were described in considerable detail. Indeed this was the most detailed section of the book (pp.122-41), probably reflecting the deep general interest in mining and metallurgy, which has already been noted above with respect to England. Boate described the types of ore, and mines, their distribution, profits, transport facilities and relationship with furnaces. The latter were described in particular detail (pp.138-9); furnace design followed the traditional square pattern, with charcoal as the sole source of fuel.

It is apparent from this summary that the first part of the *Natural History* was basically a survey of the natural resources of Ireland. Three further parts were planned, dealing with plants, other living creatures and finally the 'Natives of Ireland, and their old Fashions, Lawes and

274. Goblet, *op. cit.*, i, p.153. For an estimate of this 'première étude de géographie physique moderne du pays', see *ibid.*, pp.147–53; Emery, *op. cit.*, pp.264–6. Taylor (279), pp.132–3.

customes'.[275] It may be safely assumed that the sections on plants and animals would have been approached in a predominantly utilitarian spirit, whereas the anthropological study of the natives would have been intended as a prelude to their 'improvement'.

In the preface to the *Natural History* Arnold Boate hinted that, although he was resident in Paris, he would continue his brother's work. Towards this end he contributed two additions to the second edition of Hartlib's *Legacy* (1652). The first was an 'Appendix', which consisted of extracts of his letters on husbandry. The second was a twenty-five page section bearing a separate title-page: *An Interrogatory Relating more particularly to the Husbandry and Natural History of Ireland.* This consisted of an alphabetical list of queries relating to Ireland, commonly known as the 'Alphabet'. The *Interrogatory* was frequently detached and circulated separately. The general principle of using an 'interrogatory' to gather information on scientific problems was known to Bacon, but Boate appears to have been the first author in England to publish such a questionnaire. Queries relating to all aspects of Irish natural history were included. Further information was sought on topics already treated by Gerard Boate, such as minerals, types of earth, alum, coal, and the distribution of bloomeries and glasshouses. But the largest number of questions related to plants, animals and agriculture. Information was requested about the distribution of numerous birds, including such subsequent rarities as the osprey. Even more attention was devoted to fresh-water and salt-water fish, reflecting the significance of fishing in the Irish economy. The distribution and state of regeneration of the main types of forest was a further popular topic. Finally Boate inquired about the introduction and commercial use of fruit trees, vegetables, and such plants as flax and hemp. He hoped that his Irish informants would provide information which would allow comparisons with the state of horticulture and agriculture elsewhere in Europe. Because of the great public interest in his work, Arnold Boate was tempted to return to Ireland, but died en route from France in late 1653.

Reporting this loss Hartlib lamented that it would be extremely difficult to find a substitute for Arnold Boate. Nevertheless he appreciated that there were various able Baconians in Ireland qualified to shoulder the burden of completing the natural history. Boyle and Child in particular were 'solemnly' called upon to take up the task. Accordingly copies of the *Interrogatory* were dispatched to Boyle, with the recommendation that they should all be 'judiciously answered'. Hartlib optimistically reported a few months later that 'divers' replies to the *Interrogatory* had been obtained. For Boyle's benefit, he also summarised recently acquired information about certain species of animals and plants which were either characteristic of Ireland, or unexpectedly rare.[276]

275. Boate (30), sig. A6r.

276. Letters from Hartlib to Boyle, 28 February and 8 May 1654, Boyle

Hartlib's nominee for the organisation of further work on the natural history was his friend Robert Child, who had arrived in Ireland in May 1651.[277] Child was extremely well prepared for this work. Indeed he had already shown commitment to the idea of regional surveys during his first visit to Massachusetts, some time before 1640. A contemporary witness described the broad-ranging nature of Child's work: 'At his first coming to New England he . . . fals upon a dilligent survey of the whole Countrey, and painefully travells on foot from Plantation to Plantation; takes notice of the Havens, situation, strength, Churches, Townes, number of Inhabitants'.[278] This revealing comment shows that Child was not merely concerned with natural resources, or even economic intelligence, but that, at this early stage, his work had extended into the field of social statistics. In other words, Child's investigations in Massachusetts were an anticipation of developments which occurred in the Irish history more than a decade later.

We know little about Child's findings in New England, although some relevant information was included in the 'Large Letter' which formed the bulk of the first edition of Hartlib's *Legacy*. Immediately Child arrived in Ireland he settled into his normal routine of collecting botanical specimens and encouraging innovation in agriculture and horticulture. He studied each aspect of Irish agriculture as a prelude to suggesting improvements suitable for each locality. In view of the prevailing backwardness, he recommended the settlement in Ireland of Dutch experts in modern agricultural methods.[279]

The importance of the natural history project was immediately evident to Child. His copy of Boate's book was circulated among his neighbours, who had acquired a great enthusiasm for agricultural improvement. In view of their immediate concern with draining and fertilising, the recent books by Boate and Walter Blith were especially welcome. However Child commented that Boate's general survey of natural resources and communications in the first part of the *Natural History* was not particularly relevant to the agricultural community. Accordingly the completion of the second part, on plants, was a matter of urgency. He therefore began to gather 'stubble' for the *Interrogatory,* to be transmitted to Arnold Boate.[280]

No sooner had Child taken on primary responsibility for the *Natural History* in the early months of 1654 when he too died. Thus between

---

Works, vi, pp.81, 84–5. Five copies of the interrogatory were sent with the second of these letters, and a further fifteen on 15 May 1654: *Works,* vi, p.89.

277. For general description of Child's years in Ireland, see Turnbull (290) and Kittredge (176), pp.119–24.

278. Letters from Child to Hartlib, 1 August and 13 November 1651, [February] and 11 March 1652, HP xv v. Turnbull (290), pp. 30–4.

279. E. Winslow, *New Englands Salamander* (London, 1647), pp.7–8.

280. Letters from Child to Hartlib, 2 February, 8 April, 7 July and 28 October 1653, HP xv v. Turnbull (290), pp.36–7.

1650 and 1654 Hartlib lost three valuable colleagues and with them all hopes of prompt completion of the history.

The letters of Child and Arnold Boate published in the various editions of the *Legacy* were not particularly pertinent to the Irish work, since they were selected primarily for their relevance to general agricultural questions. Many scattered notes in Hartlib's papers probably derive from Child, but they were insufficient to support publication of the second part of *Irelands Natural History*. Enquiries were made about Child's papers, but nothing was discovered apart from already-known information about clover, flax and woad.[281]

After the death of Child, work on Boate's natural history tended to be more sporadic, but the enthusiasm for husbandry remained, and observations continued to be made with reference to the *Interrogatory*. Particularly important in this context is the partnership between Miles Symner and Robert Wood. Immediately upon his arrival in Ireland Wood began to experiment with 'clover husbandry'; thereafter his interests extended to other aspects of natural history. Wood reported progress in his work on the *Interrogatory* in various letters to Hartlib, specifically mentioning his observations on butter, cheese and the causes of loughs. Sheets of answers were circulated to Lady Ranelagh as well as to Hartlib.[282] For the most part Wood was content to assist his more experienced colleague Symner, who intended to

> 'correct diverse faults in the Natural History of Ireland which you published, both which his long experience and travels in this country have enabled him to do. We expect accurate Mapps of Ireland from Dr. Petty's surveyes; those of Speed, all others taken out of them being extremely defective in many particulars and grosly faulty.'[283]

Minor observations were passed to Hartlib and Lady Ranelagh, but nothing consequential was produced. Although Symner was enthusiastic, his other duties prevented serious attention to the natural history. This marked the last serious effort of the Hartlib circle to complete a natural history of Ireland. Despite an excellent start, an impressive body of active participants and general popular interest, no further sections were prepared for publication. This apparent failure, amid such favourable circumstances, might be construed as a reflection of the intrinsic defects of the Baconian enterprise. It might be thought that the goals of the Baconians were too remote and too badly defined to stimulate sustained scientific enquiry, so that the energies of Gerard and Arnold Boate, Child, Boyle, Wood, Symner, Morgan and their many anonymous helpers, were not applied to any wholly practicable ends.

281. Letter from Hartlib to Boyle, 8 May 1654, Boyle *Works*, vi, p.85.

282. Letters from Wood to Hartlib, 13 May & 10 June, 24 June and 27 July 1657, HP XXXIII 1.

283. Letter from Wood to Hartlib, 27 May 1657, HP XXXIII 1. For three sheets of replies by Symner to the *Interrogatory*, see HP LXII 45.

However, closer examination indicates that the Irish natural history left a significant legacy. Rather than the project being abandoned, the emphasis was shifted to a fundamental and more pressing aspect of the natural history, which had been too briefly considered by Gerard Boate —the problem of the precise topographical survey of the province. Accurate maps were unobtainable at the time of Boate's work, but the above comment by Wood indicates that the position had changed by 1657. Not only had maps been produced, but these maps were of a kind particularly relevant to the socio-economic aims of the natural history of Ireland. While the Irish survey had quite independent political and economic roots, the manner and scope of its operation display numerous points of affinity with the Irish natural history. The surveyors were advocates of Baconian natural history, histories of trade and political anatomy. They were thus able to transcend the immediate practical purposes of the survey, to prepare the ground for an elaborate exercise in economic geography. Although the celebrated Down Survey, the dominating feature of this enterprise, owed its triumphant success to the genius of William Petty, it should not be forgotten that the gestation of his scientific opinions occurred during a period of association with the Hartlib circle. Indeed the whole Irish survey took place against a backcloth of growing competition and personal antagonism between Hartlib's friends, Petty and Worsley. Although Worsley has been treated with universal disfavour by historians, he was probably not at variance with Petty on the scope and potentialities of the survey. However he certainly lacked Petty's organisational efficiency. From incidental reports it appears that soon after their arrival in Ireland, 'our loving friends Mr. Worsley and Dr. Petty' were invited by Child to participate in the natural history project. By explaining his interest in whatever 'is naturall, either plants, animals, earth, stones, minerals', or even the 'customes of the Irish and English and Scots and some politick observations concerning the settlement of Ireland', Child hoped to persuade Petty to take up investigations, until they would 'by little and little perfectly understand these parts'. Similarly it was reported that 'Mr. Worsley also is like to engage in the prosecution of these affairs, and this kind of surveying of lands'.[284] These remarks suggest that the natural history was seen very much as an extrapolation of conventional surveying. Child would have realised that a geometrical description of the province would serve as an ideal foundation for a comprehensive economic geography of the kind already outlined by Gerard Boate in qualitative terms. It remained for Petty's genius to organise a geometrical survey and to provide the conceptual insight required for the quantification of the original natural history. Continuity with the work of Boate is emphasised by the involvement of

284. Letters from Child to Hartlib, 29 August 1652, 2 February 1652/3, 28 October 1653, HP xv v. Letter from Hartlib to Boyle, 8 May 1654, Boyle *Works*, vi, p.84.

Miles Symner in the Down Survey. The Boates and many of their associates were involved in Irish land speculation. Accordingly, during the Protectorate, energies became concentrated upon the Irish survey.[285] Wood and Symner hoped that completion of this survey and the emergence of a new class of settlers would add impetus to work on the broader natural history.

When the pacification of Ireland was eventually accomplished, the Republic was faced with the daunting task of assessing the value of estates scattered throughout the province.[286] Accuracy was essential in order to extract maximum value out of the available land. The authorities were assisted to a certain extent by earlier work. They would have had access to some recent estate surveys, and to the records of the more extensive surveys undertaken by Strafford in Ireland; also the nation was well-stocked with surveying handbooks and instruments produced by the accomplished class of mathematical practitioners. A wide range of craftsmen and gentlemen had some knowledge of surveying, through either curiosity or involvement in estate management or property transfer. At first the Irish Council ordered surveys of isolated districts by professional surveyors, but it became apparent that more co-ordinated effort was required to increase the supply of manpower and undertake a general survey of forfeited lands in accordance with the Act of Settlement.[287] Serious concern with this problem is indicated by the appointment of Captain Miles Symner as professor of mathematics at Trinity College Dublin, to serve a strictly utilitarian function, 'forasmuch as there is a great occasion for surveying of lands in this Country, and that there are divers ingenious Persons, Soldiers and others who are desirous to be instructed and fitted for the same'.[288]

The Act of Settlement prompted the mathematical practitioners to intensify their work on surveying. The most substantial contribution came from William Leybourne, who expanded a small tract published in 1650 into a major treatise, *The Compleat Surveyor* (1653). Hartlib noted that Leybourne's first tract, the *Planometria,* would 'give satisfaction to practitioners and for buying and selling of land, in which respect it will bee singularly useful for Ireland'. In the following year practical guides were issued by John Eyre and Henry Osborne, both of whom were surveyors. Osborne's book was designed specifically for the Irish situation. Finally, towards the end of the Irish survey George Atwell issued a small practical work, which was dedicated to Anthony Tuckney, Master of Emmanuel College Cambridge; Atwell praised the mathematical abilities of Hartlib's friend Gualter Frost, the manciple

285. K. S. Bottigheimer, *English Money and Irish Land* (Oxford, 1971).

286. The surveys were initiated by 'An Act for the speedy and effectual Satisfaction of the Adventurers for Lands in Ireland, and of Arrears due to Soldiery there'. Firth & Rait, ii, pp.722–53.

287. Hardinge (133), p.5, describes local surveys by Richard Francis and Thomas Jackson.

288. See above, p.226.

of that college, whose family had influential civil service connections.[289]

Superintendence of the survey was at first the responsibility of Benjamin Worsley, the first parliamentary Surveyor General. Worsley's work in framing the Navigation Acts had probably recommended him for this appointment, but Petty perceptively noted that Worsley's well-known interest in optical instruments was hardly a qualification for his directing a survey.[290] The subsequent detailed history of the survey is not relevant to this chapter, except as an illustration of the important social role of science, and for its value in demonstrating the continuing development of the natural history concept.

It is important to appreciate that Petty's celebrated Down Survey was merely the most important facet of an enterprise which involved at least nineteen different surveys between 1653 and 1660.[291] Worsley's role was less spectacular, but it was nevertheless a valuable adjunct to Petty's work. The 'Gross' (1653) and 'Civil' (1654-6) Surveys undertaken under Worsley's direction came close to *Irelands Natural History* in spirit. By employing the methods of inquisition and estimation stipulated by the Act of Settlement for the sake of speed, these surveys drew up lists of forfeited estates, providing information sufficient for the identification of lands by Petty's officers. The extent of the evidence obtained depended on the terrain, but often considerable topographical and economic information was given. Boundaries were described, the 1641 valuation was given for the whole estate and the acreage devoted to plantation, arable, pasture and waste was indicated. In some cases the assessors provided information of the type valued by Boate, on fertilisers, fishing, industrial sites or local place names. Although Petty was justified in pointing out the limitations of expensive estimation surveys even for immediate purposes, the terriers provided by Worsley's agents have proved to contain vitally important information for historians concerned with seventeenth-century economic geography.[292]

289. John Eyre, *The Exact Surveyor* (London, 1654); Henry Osborne, *A More Exact Way to Delineate the Plot of any Spacious Parcel of Land* (Dublin, 1654); George Atwell, *The Faithful Surveyor* (London, 1658). Osborne's rare work (BM 558*b.29) is not recorded by Richeson or Taylor. Ephemerides 1649. For Frost, see Aylmer (12), p.256.

290. Petty, *History of the Down Survey* (179), p.2.

291. *Petty Papers*, pp.79–81. Apart from the sources listed in note 269 above, the main works on the survey are Petty, *History of the Down Survey* (179); *idem*, *Reflections upon some Persons and Things in Ireland* (211). Hardinge (133) is particularly valuable since it calendars documents subsequently destroyed by fire. See also J. H. Andrews, *Ireland in Maps* (Dublin, 1961); *idem*, 'Ireland in Maps: A Bibliographical Postscript', *Irish Geography*, 1959–63, *4*: 234–43; S. O'Domhnaill, 'The Maps of the Down Survey', *Irish Historical Studies*, 1942–3, *3*: 381–92; E. Lynam, 'Irish Political Geography', *Geographical Journal*, 1932, *79*: 415–18.

292. Hardinge (133), pp.1–20. R. C. Simington, *Books of Survey and Distribution*, Irish Manuscripts Commission: *Roscommon* (1949), *Mayo* (1956), *Galway* (1962), *Clare* (1967); J. G. Simms, 'The Civil Survey 1654–6', *Irish Historical Studies*, 1955, *9*: 253–63. Petty's editor Larcom admits that most limitations in Worsley's work were owing to imperfect instructions. Accordingly it is 'harsh altogether to condemn Mr. Worsley': Petty (179), p.313. Nevertheless Goblet finds no good word to say for Worsley.

After Worsley's initial work it was necessary to prepare definitive estate maps, before the distribution of land to soldiers and Adventurers. This technically difficult operation was boldly undertaken by Petty who gave a promise to complete the first part of the exercise within thirteen months. Overruling Worsley's objections, the Council placed its faith in Petty, who duly completed his initial survey between December 1654 and March 1655. The maps subsequently produced accorded with the most exacting standards; they embraced both forfeited and non-forfeited lands, and they included particularly elaborate detail relating to the degree of profitability of land. The scale of these maps was amazingly large: 40 Irish perches to the inch (c. 1 : 10,080). Subsequently these documents became the source for estate maps issued to soldiers and Adventurers, as well as for generations of manuscript and published maps of Irish baronies and counties.

Petty's survey by the method of 'laying down' as maps, gradually extended between 1655 and 1659 to the whole province. Ultimately the only areas not covered by his work were the counties of Galway and Roscommon, and parts of Mayo. This remarkable mission was accomplished against a background of opposition from Worsley, numerous political critics, jealous professional surveyors, and even the Provost of Trinity College who attempted to prevent the recruitment of surveyors from his student body. Although the survey did not directly involve scientific innovation, Petty's achievement had an important scientific dimension. In the first place, it had required a shrewd understanding of the techniques of surveying, which were rationalised, streamlined and adapted to the Irish situation without sacrifice of accuracy. Secondly, a form of organisation using the principle of the division of labour made the survey a model demonstration of the potentialities of Baconian collaborative enterprise, in which dependence upon individual genius was replaced by the 'united labours of many, though not by any one apart, . . . and in brief which may be finisht by the publick care and charge, though not by the ability and industry of particular persons'.[293]

In this case, Petty persuaded the state to allow him to demonstrate the virtue of the collaborative approach by drawing on the manpower available in the army, from which he established a 'ministery of about one thousand hands'. The ideal interpreters of nature selected by Petty were cast in the Baconian mould—unpretentious, and sometimes only slightly literate soldiers, with previous experience in trades; above all they were capable of withstanding physical hardships. Among other things they were expected to 'wade through boggs and water, climb rocks, fare and lodge hard'.[294] By following the principle of division of labour, Petty believed that his soldiers could survey as successfully as 'persons of gentle and liberall education' equipped with complex rules

293. Bacon, *De Augmentis* (13), p.49.
294. Petty (179), pp.xv, 17–18.

and instruments. Petty followed Bacon's maxim that humble intellects performing simple operations could, if organised efficiently, undertake large-scale scientific enterprises which would have been out of the reach of individual practitioners, however well-educated, skilled, or gifted. The Down Survey provided an ideal test of this form of democratised science, as well as an opportunity to vindicate the aims of the advocates of the Irish natural history.

English surveyors had elaborated complex procedures and a wide variety of instruments, but these were not particularly well suited to inexperienced practitioners or large-scale surveys.[295] Petty's army of surveyors required sturdy, cheap and simple instruments, and methods suitable for the rapid but accurate measurement of varied terrain. The basic surveying instruments selected by Petty were the chain and circumferentor. The former was in universal use and Petty would certainly have opted for the improved decimal chain introduced by Gunter. This chain was not known to Rathborne, but it was advocated by Leybourne. The circumferentor, although known in principle, was less favoured and it was at this time only accorded passing mention in works on surveying. No illustrated description of the circumferentor was included in any English surveying book of the seventeenth century. But as the following description indicates, Rathborne appreciated its potential usefulness:

> 'This Instrument for expedition and portabilitie, exceedeth far the rest, and nothing inferior to any for exactnesse, if care and arte be used; but not so vulgarly used as the playne Table is; the full and perfect use thereof, not lying so open and apparent to all mens understanding.
>
> It is made and framed of well seasoned boxe, contayning in length about eight inches, in bredth halfe as much, and in thicknesse about ¾ of inch. About the middle of the surface thereof, a round hole is to be turned of the depth of halfe an inch, whereof the Diameter to be about 3½ inches, to place a carde and needle therein, to be covered over with cleere glasse. The best carde for this purpose is that, divided in the limbe into 120 equal parts or degrees, with a Dyall according to the Azimuths of the Sunne, wherein the houres are numbred, and the moneths named, serving very aptly to shew the time of the day.
>
> There is also hereunto belonging two sights, double in length, the one unto the other, the longer contayning about seven inches or upwards; the shorter sight of these having one propertie and use,

295. The first comprehensive English monograph on surveying was Aaron Rathborne, *The Surveyor in Foure Bookes*, 1616 (231). To fulfil the need for a more up-to-date treatise, William Leybourne produced *The Compleat Surveyor* (1653), which retained its popularity until the eighteenth century. For minor works see Richeson (244).

in the edge thereof, towards the upper part is placed a small wiyer, representing the center of a supposed circle.

The foot of this Instrument is that with three staves ioynted in the head, and to be taken a sunder in the middle with brasse sockets.'[296]

On the whole professional surveyors preferred complex instruments like the theodolite, the plane-table, or various proprietary hybrids. These were eminently suitable for accurate estate surveys, whereas the method of taking circumferentor readings from the magnetic needle would have resulted in minor inaccuracies. In addition the circumferentor needle was liable to the same irregularities and variations as the mariner's compass. Finally, surveying with a circumferentor necessitated a scrupulous ordering of records and a more indirect method of mapping than that undertaken with the plane-table. Nevertheless, the circumferentor had certain distinct advantages from Petty's point of view. As Rathborne's description indicates, it was extremely simple, being essentially a single strip of wood housing a compass and two sights. Many of the finer points described by Rathborne could be dispensed with to avoid the necessity of inserting metal scales. A simple form of this instrument could readily be mass-produced by Petty's craftsmen. Secondly the circumferentor was more portable than either the plane-table or the theodolite, a factor which also assisted its concealment from suspicious natives! Lastly the minor inaccuracies in readings would be less serious in surveys of large areas. Hence Leybourne had described the circumferentor as the 'most absolute Instrument for the Surveying of any large and spacious business', while John Love recommended this instrument for use in the American colonies. The survival in the United States of numerous early circumferentors suggests that this advice was followed.[297]

Perhaps because of its conventional design, Petty left no description of his circumferentor. In all probability he simplified the instrument known to professional surveyors in order to facilitate its production and use by his staff. This view is supported by the characteristics of an Irish circumferentor and azimuth dial which was made shortly after the Down Survey.[298] Of sturdy construction and simple manu-

296. Rathborne (231), p.129. The description of the circumferentor given by Leybourne followed Rathborne almost verbatim (1674 edn., p.44).

297. Leybourne, *op. cit.*, 1674 edn., pp.233–7. John Love, *Geodaesia* (London, 1688), pp.54–5. S. A. Bedini, *Early American Scientific Instruments and Their Makers* (Washington D.C., 1964).

298. This instrument is located in the History of Science Museum, Oxford. It is signed: 'W.R. Dublin. fe. Latitude 53 20 * 1667 * '. The identity of W.R. has not been established. This instrument is 13.8 ins. long, 5.2 ins. wide at its widest point; it is made from a single piece of wood, 0.8 ins. thick. The sights are 5 ins. high, and unlike the ones recommended by Rathborne, equal in length; each has two apertures, to facilitate back-sighting. The compass dial has 120 divisions and the needle is 4.1 ins. long. Goblet, *op. cit.*, i, pp.255–6, has suggested that Petty's circumferentor was like the example caricatured in the General Map of

facture, this instrument was probably the direct descendant of the instruments used by Petty's soldiers. Further evidence for this connection is provided by the characteristics of the compass-card, which is similar to the cards used on the magnetic azimuth dials manufactured by Henry Sutton in London. Petty is known to have modified the compass-card used in circumferentors in conjunction with Sutton. Sutton provided Petty with squared paper for his surveys and he was probably the London source for the time-scales, protractors and compass-cards mentioned by Petty.[299]

Apart from those parts requiring accurate calibration the army was able to construct its own surveying instruments by pooling resources according to the principle of the division of labour. *Wiremakers* produced chains, *watchmakers* magnetic needles and pins, *woodturners* wooden boxes and circumferentor bases, *pipemakers* circumferentor stands, and *founders* brass fittings. Finally a more versatile workman assembled the parts, balancing needles over the compass cards and adjusting the sights. Thus Petty was speedily able to supply his surveying army with 'circumferentors, chaines, protractors, links for chaines, needles, rulers, royall paper, mouth glew, tents, protracting boards, compasses etc.', at the outset of the Down Survey.[300]

It was then necessary for Petty to organise field operations and detailed cartographical procedures. In instituting a division of labour, Petty was heavily reliant on his senior assistants, particularly the undersurveyors and their more experienced artisans. There is no precise evidence about this organisational structure, but his most active assistants were probably Miles Symner, Henry Osborne, William Webbe, Adam Molyneux and Richard Francis. Symner was probably Petty's most trusted associate; as professor of mathematics at Dublin he was specifically involved in teaching surveying, and reports from Robert Wood indicate his active association with Petty in matters relating to both the distribution of lands and the Irish natural history. Of Henry Osborne Hartlib reported that 'one Osborne that was a Chandler is now a notable mathematician and therefore taken along into Ireland with Colonel Morgan'. Having established himself there, Osborne composed *A More Exact Way to Delineate the Plot of any Spacious Parcel of Land* (Dublin, 1654), published at Worsley's instigation and intended to assist Petty's surveyors; Osborne himself was appointed to direct surveying operations in Cork. William Webbe, a friend of Hartlib

---

Ireland, prefixed to *Hiberniae Delineatio* (1685). However, this is of a continental pattern which is considerably more complex than the English type. Like other illustrations in the same series of maps it was probably selected by the Dutch engravers without any intention of representing the precise type employed by Petty.

299. Petty (179), pp.xiv, 17, 324; Hardinge (133), p.27. For Sutton, see Taylor (278), p.220.

300. Petty (179), pp.xiv, 17, 53.

and a chemist, had been a member of the Common Council of London and a surveyor of episcopal lands in England. Adam Molyneux was the brother of Samuel Molyneux the master gunner who was the father of William Molyneux, the celebrated founder of the Dublin Philosophical Society. Richard Francis had been surveying in Ireland since the time of Strafford; he would have been able to provide local information to assist the more recent arrivals in Ireland.[301]

At a subsidiary level six surveyors were employed by Petty to teach the artisans field techniques. Subsequently these surveyors were probably active in the field; their names occur on the completed surveys listed by Hardinge. Petty adopted the method of traversing boundaries, taking bearings with the circumferentor and measuring distances with the chain. The procedure for registering results in field books and protracting to produce maps, in most respects followed the rules outlined by Leybourne, although Petty claimed to have produced a 'more distinct, methodicall, and comprehensive ffield booke' and a simplified method of estimating the acreage of enclosures, made possible by plotting his maps on squared paper. Each surveyor was provided with a set of clear 'Instructions for surveying and admeasuring the forfeited and other Commonwealth Lands in Ireland' composed by Petty; this would have complemented the instructions on technique derived from the professional surveyors or from Osborne's pamphlet.[302] Each of Petty's teams was involved in two distinct operations, surveying and protracting maps. *Surveyors* either took bearings or measured boundaries; their results were entered into field books, which were used by the *protractors* who prepared maps on large sheets of squared paper. Acreage was then estimated decimally, probably at a central office, which was also concerned with the preparation of barony maps using 'parallelagrames, of which were made greate numbers, and in larger dimensions then perhaps was ever yet seene upon any other occasion'.[303]

Geographers have recognised that the efficient performance of this geometrical operation produced for the first time both a correct impression of the shape of Ireland, and an accurate working estimate of its size. The degree of error of the Down Survey varied greatly, but on average, the land area was underestimated by ten per cent.

Petty's responsibilities had a further important dimension. For the satisfaction of creditors, it was necessary to estimate the value of the forfeited land. The cadastral aims of the survey had been expressed in the original Act, which declared that the 'qualities' and 'quantities' of forfeited lands should be 'certainly and distinctly' known. Surveyors

301. Petty (179), pp.21, 110–11; Hardinge (133), pp.45–104; Ephemerides 1652; letters from Wood to Hartlib, HP XXXIII 1. For further information on Symner, Osborne and Molyneux in connection with the survey, see Barnard (18), Chapter VI. For the Irish land interests of this group, see Bottigheimer, *op. cit.*, Appendices A & B.

302. Petty (179), pp.xv, 17, 46–50, 258. Leybourne, *op. cit.*, pp.233–7.

303. Petty (179), p.xvi. See also Osborne, *op. cit.*

were therefore ordered to distinguish between profitable and unprofitable lands, and furthermore to estimate 'what quantity of Meadow, arrable and profitable Pasture, and what Woods, Bogs and barren Mountains belonging to each of them respectively'.[304] This desideratum was reflected in the instructions given to Petty, which required him to conduct an instrumental survey 'according to the naturall, artificial, and civil bounds thereoff, and whereby the said land is distinguished into wood, bog, mountaine, arable, meadow and pasture'. Petty inserted similar orders into the 'Instructions' given his surveyors.[305]

Through reference to these wider functions, the scope of Petty's survey was extended and his work was brought more closely into line with *Irelands Natural History*. Boate had provided a tentative qualitative economic geography of Ireland, which had been further elaborated in the Gross and Civil Surveys. Its final quantitative expression was the survey conducted by Petty. Besides attention to his official responsibilities, Petty declared that he had a 'far more large and comprehensive' aim. This involved the employment of his surveyors in collecting detailed economic and geographical information on numerous subjects, which was quantified wherever possible.[306] Thus, while observing the categories of analysis described in the original Act, his investigations probed much more deeply, with a scientific, as well as the immediate official aim in mind. This work laid the foundations for his political anatomy of Ireland.

The Down Survey aimed to define 'the quantity, figure, and situation of all the Baronies, parishes and towne or farme land, with the quantity of each, the situation of townes, Castles, bridges, churches, loughes, boggs, mountaines, rivers, highwayes etc'.[307] Apart from their pronounced quantitative bias, Petty's aims were remarkably similar to those expressed on the title page of *Irelands Natural History*. By rigorously pursuing the quantitative aim at every level Petty greatly expanded the scope of Boate's work. Each topic required characteristic analytical procedures. Like Boate, Petty was interested in the production of rope, hemp, flax, wood and honey. In these cases he suggested an average of three years' annual production as a basis for records. When estimating grain crops he aimed at counting the number of seeds produced from each seed planted, or the weight yield per bushel of seed planted. The value of pasture could be assessed by weighing the

304. Firth & Rait, ii, pp.743, 747.
305. Petty (179), pp.9, 13, 46–50.
306. Petty (179), p.123; *Petty Papers*, pp.79–83. S. Masukawa, 'Origin and Significance of Political Arithmetic', *Annals of the Hitotsubashi Academy*, 1956, *6*: 53–79, fully recognises the role of the Down Survey in the evolution of Petty's political arithmetic. This author's *Sir William Petty* (Tokyo, 1967), published only in Japanese, is undoubtedly also highly important. Further work on this subject is being undertaken by Mr. L. G. Sharp of Queen's College Oxford.
307. *Petty Papers*, i, p.79.

hay produced, or by estimating the number of domesticated animals supported on each acre. It was recognised that all data could not be accumulated by the painstaking inductive method used in cartography. Therefore, on the basis of sample information or hypothetical estimates, Petty embarked on a wide range of calculations. He had no direct report of the number of horses in Ireland, but it was assumed that 16,000 families kept 40,000 horses, for work and saddle, while one-third, or 61,000 of the peasantry kept horses for ploughing. Accordingly there were about 100,000 horses, each requiring one acre of pasture, half an acre of meadow and one-sixth of an acre of oatland. Therefore horses claimed 166,000 acres of land in the province.[308]

By relying on shrewd estimates of this kind Petty was able to build up a detailed quantitative picture of the Irish economy. His method of analysis was applied to everything from agricultural products to life expectancy. These procedures involved an element of simplification not tolerated in his cartographical survey, but Petty usually displayed an intuitive awareness of the limitations of his calculations. When estimating the pasture requirements of horses, he realised that an error was introduced because the poor could not provide oats for their animals; therefore a proportionately larger acreage was required for each animal. On the fundamental question of land value, Petty appreciated that value would vary according to the criteria used. Land could be assessed geometrically by area, or by its intrinsic fertility, or by its fertility when improved, or by the accidental factor of rent.[309] His preliminary exercises in political anatomy, undertaken with reference to the Down Survey, revealed the wide potentialities of quantification, but they also underlined the need for clear conceptual analysis in conducting each operation. Petty believed that only by penetrating beyond traditional ideas on estimates of value, to recognise that land values could be estimated according to an objective range of criteria, could any 'intrinsic' relationship between population and land resources be established.

Petty's survey vindicated the belief of the advocates of Baconian natural history that a comprehensive natural history of a region was a both attainable and useful goal. The success of the earlier work had been limited owing to its dependence on the activity of an extremely small group of enthusiasts. In the aftermath of the Civil War this limiting factor was partially removed when Petty was able to employ a large body of disciplined labour for certain fundamental investigations. After 1660, the army was no longer available for service of this kind, and in both England and Ireland regional natural histories were taken up by the new scientific societies. Although the ideal was highly publicised and rich practical rewards were promised, the virtuosi were incapable of commanding the disciplined labour needed for the collection of substantial amounts of well-organised quantitative data or detailed carto-

308. *Petty Papers,* i, pp.79–81; Petty (179), pp.55–8.
309. *Petty Papers,* i, pp.77, 82–3.

graphical records. After 1660 the successful natural histories were basically the work of individual enthusiasts such as Robert Plot. Although Baconian in general spirit, these works tended to reflect the idiosyncratic interests of their authors rather than pursuing the systematic programme adopted by the compilers of *Irelands Natural History*.

The Down Survey was paralleled by a smaller-scale, but equally important development in London, where Petty's friend John Graunt was establishing the science of demography. This is a great claim to make for the humble haberdasher, but it has been upheld by successive generations of critical economists, demographers and statisticians.[310] In view of the profundity of Graunt's work, it is difficult to see why it has attracted so little interest among historians of science. Graunt's *Natural and Political Observations upon the Bills of Mortality*, although presented to the Royal Society and published early in 1662, was obviously the result of many years' preparation. There have been sharply divergent views on the genesis of Graunt's work. It has been argued with considerable ingenuity that Petty played a substantial role in its production, by providing general inspiration, or direct guidance; it has also been asserted that he was partly, or even wholly its author. However, recent commentators have tended to accept that the *Observations* 'were in all essential respects Graunt's work'.[311] In the present writer's opinion this view is fully justified, so that the title page of the *Observations*, which in large print proclaims the author as 'JOHN GRAUNT, Citizen of LONDON', may be taken at its face value. None the less, although Graunt was probably responsible for the original initiative, the basic research, and the composition of the major part of the *Observations*, it is important to recognise that his work was not an isolated phenomenon. It has already been noted that the works of Hartlib and of Petty published in 1648 advocated the collection of medical data. Petty and Graunt became close friends; each was probably fully conversant with the researches, techniques and draft writings of the other. This would explain certain striking resemblances between passages in Petty's *Treatise of Taxes* and Graunt's *Observations*, two works which were published within a few months of one another in 1662. The activities of the two friends were complementary. Petty's geometrical survey gradually extended into a consideration of land values, general economic statistics, and then general estimates of population, whereas Graunt began with population statistics and ended with tentative hypotheses about the relationship between population and land. Both expanded *natural* observations to the point where they could relate to *political*

310. For recent estimates of Graunt see H. Westergaard, *Contributions to the History of Statistics* (London, 1932); W. Willcox (ed.), *Natural and political observations* (Baltimore, 1939), Introduction; M. Greenwood, *Medical Statistics from Graunt to Farr* (Cambridge, 1948); D. V. Glass, 'John Graunt and his Natural and Political Observations', *Notes & Records*, 1964, *19*: 63–100.

311. Glass, *op. cit.*, p.89. The debate is summarised by G. Keynes, *A Bibliography of Sir William Petty and of Observations on the Bills of Mortality* (Oxford, 1971), pp.75–7.

policies. Apart from his friendship with Petty, surprisingly little is known about Graunt's intellectual associations during the 1650s. However, a reference in Hartlib's journal suggests that Graunt was familiar with the work on the Irish natural history. Hartlib wrote in 1652: 'One King of the North of Ireland was brought unto me by Mr. Grant to give me special thanks for publishing the Natural History of Ireland . . . He [King] is very well acquainted with Colonel Hil, Petty, Worsley'.[312] Graunt may have shared with King this acquaintance with Worsley and Colonel Arthur Hill of Lisneygarvey. Although he did not assume important office, Graunt's services to parliament during the Civil War gave him considerable influence in London. He was obviously on good terms with Hartlib and he may well have associated with such economic theorists as Robinson.

In presenting his work to the Royal Society, Graunt stressed that it fufilled the conditions of the third part of Bacon's *Instauratio Magna,* the *History of Life and Death,* which included much comment about longevity at various times in history. Graunt bypassed Bacon's diffuse and anecdotal statements to investigate the population statistics of the capital city in which he had worked since boyhood. The rapid growth of Stuart London brought attendant problems of overcrowded tenements, sanitation, water and food supply; acute epidemics were common experiences. These problems meant that population was a matter for public concern. Graunt decided to test whether common beliefs about London population could be substantiated by an analysis of the Bills of Mortality, which had appeared weekly since the beginning of the century, with annual summaries and categorisation of the causes of death for more recent decades. Superficially Graunt's task was straightforward, involving the collection and simple arithmetical collation of the annual records, whereas Petty had been obliged to collect his own data. However Petty could control the quality of the information collected under his supervision, while Graunt was at the mercy of the 'Old-women Searchers'; in addition, as Graunt realised, there was serious under-reporting of certain important phenomena. Thus he was not able to accept the statistics at face value when searching for underlying quantitative regularities. Judging that there was a constant ratio between the number of women dying in childbirth, which was likely to be accurately reported, and the total number of births, he reached the conclusion that baptisms were seriously under-reported, and the true increase in population consequently disguised. In other cases he recognised that questionable diagnosis rendered figures for certain diseases unreliable; in some instances separate diseases were conflated, while in others a single cause of death appeared under several different headings. But in the case of rickets, he supported the general opinion that this

312. Ephemerides 1652. King was probably John King, a speculator in Irish land; see Bottigheimer, *op. cit.*, pp.185, 205. Col. Arthur Hill was Child's host in Ireland. See also Ephemerides 1653.

disease was of recent origin and was increasing in incidence. He also believed that the records were correct in suggesting a larger number of male births, the disproportion being wiped out by greater male mortality. On the whole, he abstained from complex calculations based on untested assumptions of the kind hazarded by Petty. Perhaps the most ambitious calculation he attempted was an estimation of the total London population. In this case, as in other parts of his work, he supported mortality calculations with independent estimates of the number and sizes of families, as well as qualitative impressions about growth and changes within the city.

As a result of his statistical studies Graunt concluded that population, like land, could be analysed and interpreted quantitatively to expose statistical regularities. The common causes of death exhibited a constant relationship to the number of burials; epidemics had occasionally a spectacular effect, but their long-term influence was less important. In assessing mortality for different age-groups, Graunt detected an extremely high rate of infant mortality, a low average age of the population and a low life-expectancy. He evolved a primitive form of life-table as a means of summarising these conclusions. Finally, although having only very inferior data, he made some preliminary comparisons of mortality figures between London and the rural neighbourhood of Romsey, the home of his friend Petty. Although information on rural areas was extremely inadequate, the evidence seemed to vindicate Bacon's impression that rural populations were more healthy than those in towns. Graunt's work was a spectacularly successful pilot attempt to apply quantitative natural history to population phenomena, at a time when Petty was wrestling with the more complex problem of devising procedures for assembling a regional political anatomy. Both authors demonstrated that scientific methods could be applied to detect a rational order underlying the apparently haphazard phenomena of human societies.

(x) The Full Fruits of Enterprise

From the above description of the work on natural history, it is apparent that, as the Baconians assumed more important public offices, they considerably extended the scope of their scientific activities. They began with modest enquiries about the histories of trade, but very quickly became involved with more general economic issues. This trend was thoroughly consistent with the philosophy of Bacon who had designated for the experimental philosopher an important role in bringing about social amelioration. Acting on hints given by Bacon, the puritan natural philosophers believed their work should extend 'to take in the particular sciences, and the referring or bringing back of particular sciences to natural philosophy; that the branches of knowledge may not be severed and cut off from the stem'.

The new science was applied to an ever-increasing range of subjects. It was thought, by analogy with anatomy, mechanics or Euclidean geometry, that society could be analysed and regulated with scientific precision. Society, like the human body, came to be regarded as a mechanism which could be analysed into a number of discrete elements. Each problem could be investigated scientifically until the entire mechanism was explained in terms of systems of laws, which would enjoy the same status as the generalisations of experimental science. The manner of proceeding adopted depended on individual philosophical affiliations. Hobbes favoured a rigorously *a priori* procedure which used a Euclidean model to outline a comprehensive mechanism of the state. By contrast the Baconians generally adopted a more piecemeal approach; they addressed themselves to specific economic problems, seeking solutions based on detailed inductive investigation. As in natural philosophy no extreme methodological position was followed with absolute consistency. But whatever their views on specific issues all would have agreed with Hobbes that 'the end of knowledge is power; and the use of theorems . . . is for the construction of problems; and, lastly, the scope of all speculation is the performing of some action, or thing to be done'.[313]

The Baconians were extremely optimistic about the relevance of their methods to the social and ecomomic problems of the Puritan Revolution. A few of the advocates of the new philosophy attempted comprehensive reappraisals of political theory; this approach was adopted by Hobbes and Harrington. The Baconians tended to avoid contentious political issues; instead they regarded science as a means of promoting the return of man's dominion over nature, believing that scientific innovation and rational economic organisation would benefit all sections of society.

It has already been noted that Baconian experimental philosophy and the new movement among the economic theorists were two related manifestations of the same mode of thought. Commenting on the level of economic analysis reached in the 1620s, Supple has stated that 'Mun's theory is more logical than the others, and his perception of the operations of exchange rates has a deductive clarity which is very rare in contemporary polemical writings'.[314] The attitudes adopted by Mun were taken up in the next generation by Plattes, Roberts and Robinson. Since they operated from similar premises, the economists and the Baconians tended to reach similar conclusions about the broad range of problems which they had in common. Scientific economics and Baconian philosophy became mutually reinforcing. Indeed the identity of interests and outlook between the various reformers became so close that it is some-

313. Hobbes, *De corpore, Works English,* ed. Molesworth, i, pp.7–8. For excellent studies dealing with economic thought before 1640 and after 1660 respectively, see Supple (275) and Letwin (180). For a recent informative account of economic policy see J. P. Cooper's essay in Aylmer (11).

314. Supple (275), p.217.

what arbitrary to isolate them into separate groups of scientists and economists. Hence it is not surprising that Henry Robinson was drawn into association with Hartlib at the outset of the Puritan Revolution. Robinson took up Hartlib's ideas on social policy and attempted to establish the Office of Address for Accommodations, whereas Hartlib adopted the economist's views on monetary questions and trade. Both subscribed to the view announced in the *Further Discovery,* that it was necessary to embark on a scientific study 'of a whole State and . . . the constitution of all the parts thereof'.[315] This idea was taken up and elaborated by other puritan intellectuals. Gerard Boate intended that his 'true and ample Description' of Ireland would be a prelude to 'the Advancement of Navigation, Husbandry, and other profitable Arts and Professions'. In essentially the same spirit Petty embarked on his quantitative comparison 'between the Body Natural, and Body Politick', with the belief that there was 'a Political Arithmetic, and a Geometrical Justice to be yet further cultivated in the World'.[316] He attached great importance to the biblical text which was frequently quoted in practical economic writings, 'Pondere, Mensura, et Numero Deus omnia fecit: Mensuram et Pondus Numeres, Numero omnia fecit'. Petty regarded the application of algebra to policy as his individual contribution to the development of mathematics. Graunt insisted that his demographic studies had 'both Political and Natural' relevance, 'necessary, in order to good, certaine, and easie Government, and even to ballance Parties and Factions, both in Church and State'.[317] Among the economists, emphasis on quantification is apparent in such works as Roberts's *The Merchants Map of Commerce*. Robinson advocated a central bank for controlling all bullion movements, in order to ensure knowledge of 'the pulse of the ballance of trade'. Only by the accumulation of statistical data could it be known 'what goods each foreigner imports and exports, so here you may see what money he remits or receives, and make a balance'.[318]

Its concern with economic and social issues was probably one of the main factors responsible for the increased appeal of Baconianism to the educated classes. The emergence of Baconianism coincided with a national economic crisis, which affected the fortunes of all classes. Experimental philosophy offered solutions to these problems. It enabled an optimistic tone to be maintained, even during the most depressing moments of the Civil War. It seemed to be one of the main avenues both to improved personal fortunes and to a wider national regeneration.

It is not possible to understand the work of the 'scientists' recruited during the Puritan Revolution without taking full account of their economic motivations. A generation of natural philosophers emerged,

315. Hartlib (136), p.26.

316. Petty, *The Political Anatomy of Ireland* (213) was first published in 1691, but it was composed by 1672, and based on materials gathered before 1660.

317. Petty, *A Discourse Concerning the Use of Duplicate Proportion* (London, 1674), Preface. *Petty Papers,* ii, pp.14–15. J. Graunt (121), sig. A6v, p.151.

318. *CSPD 1650,* pp.182–3.

whose economic and scientific ideas were closely integrated. Such works as Petty's *Discourse Concerning Duplicate Proportion* were characterised by constant cross-reference between mathematical principles and practical problems. The *Discourse* was concerned with such problems as the relationship between sail area and the speed of a ship, the strength of timber, the driving power of animals, the operation of mills, gunpowder and bellows, the comparative prices of commodities, and the power of dams and sea-walls. The versatility shown by Plattes, Hartlib, Robinson, Petty, Worsley, Wood, Potter, Culpeper and Beale, was displayed after 1660 by Collins, Joshua Child, North and Locke.

The utilitarian interests of the Baconians increased their public reputation and commended them as expert advisers on national economic problems. Increasingly they offered advice and increasingly the state was inclined to make use of their services. Baconian inclinations, when combined with political reliability, proved an ideal formula for inspiring the confidence of parliament and the Council of State. As shown above specialised scientific expertise was directly relevant to the problems of mining, metallurgy, coinage or surveying. The Baconians were eager to extend their activities, by applying their methods to a wider range of problems in which scientific analysis seemed to be applicable.

This trend is well-illustrated by the work of the young mathematician Robert Wood. This able pupil of Oughtred was employed by Lincoln College to manage its bursarial accounts. He appreciated the value of decimal arithmetic, and as we have seen soon emerged with a proposal for currency decimalisation. Notwithstanding the absence of official interest in his idea, he pursued his plan to its logical conclusion, proposing that weights and measures should also be decimalised, to secure complete rationalisation of money, weights and measures. During their Irish service, Wood and Petty had first-hand experience of the confusion caused by the co-existence of English and Irish systems of land measurement. For his own purposes of speedy calculation of acreage, Petty adopted a decimal method, while monetary calculations were also made decimally by many accountants as a matter of course. There was widespread dissatisfaction at the lack of standardisation in British weights and measures, so that Petty and Wood were entrants into an already existing debate. Stansfield, for example, in the course of his proposals for economic reform, appealed for 'one constant measure *per universam Anglicam*'. Particularly in the case of grain measures there was great diversity of practice between the market towns and different measures were used even within a single district.[319] In the case of weights and measures, rationalisation was favoured by both scientists and social reformers, whereas it was realised that currency decimalisation might not have served the poor particularly well. Stansfield was merely one of many authors who felt that the diversity of

319. Letter from James Stansfield to Hartlib, 15 December 1656, HP LIII 20.

grain measurements represented a major social abuse. However no effective action was taken to redress this grievance by the administration of the Republic.

Following his work on currency decimalisation, Wood turned his attention to monetary theory, a topic which had been vigorously debated since the time of Mun. During the Protectorate in Ireland monetary issues were considered by a group which included Wood, Petty, Stansfield and Babbington. The last three were primarily involved in designing coinage machinery suitable for use with indigenous metals, while the others were more concerned with monetary theory. All members of the group were especially influenced by factors causing the extremely severe monetary crisis in Ireland. In particular they were concerned to satisfy the popular demand for an issue of farthings, which had also been under continuous debate in the English Committee for the Mint.

An important element in the Irish discussions was an exchange between Wood and William Potter which illustrates the various ways in which science impinged on general economic issues, as well as underlining in this instance the divergent approaches of the academic and the artisan.[320] Both writers were interested in Blondeau's methods of producing a coinage resistant to counterfeiting. Wood traced the inception of his own ideas to journeys 'in progress with my Lord [Henry Cromwell] and casually falling upon the thoughts of preventing the counterfeiting of Farthings &c., they drew on a higher consideration of new mony, which I have since endeavoured to polish by degrees'. When Potter expressed scepticism about the ability of a scholar to produce a practical solution to this problem, Wood replied that a university education was no encumbrance since it taught 'methodizing what others of excellent parts have invented'. Furthermore mathematics sharpened the critical faculties and provided a model of demonstrative reasoning which could be applied to practical problems. After the criticisms of Potter Wood re-examined his own scheme; he subjected his arguments to 'a more serious examination and scrutiny upon them, and considered things more fully and scrupulously, and with some kind of Mathematical exactness and vigor; I wondered to find them . . . so solid, firme and well compacted: and I confesse I was more confirmed in my opinion'. On the proposals for farthings Wood's rational analysis demonstrated conclusions also arrived at by Potter. But on 'Fundamentalls' they were in sharp disagreement, the positions adopted being strongly reminiscent of the debate between Barbon and Locke forty years later. In Wood's view Potter's practical proposals on coinage foundered owing to a basic misunderstanding of the

320. Extensive quotations from Potter's writings are included in letters of Wood to Potter dated 1 December 1658, 15 January 1658/[9], 2 April 1659, 25 May 1659, HP xxxiii 1. Potter's complete texts have not been traced. Quotations in the following sections are taken from these letters. The germ of Potter's ideas can be detected in his *The Key of Wealth,* 1653 (226).

nature of bullion. The inventor adopted the extreme nominalist view that bullion lacked any intrinsic value, being like other commodities devoid of any fixed or inherent value. The values of all commodities were accordingly subject to fluctuation, their worth being determined by custom or man-made law. In Potter's view 'intrinsic value' was equated with 'present price'; any commodity could 'beare a great price at present, that may suddenly be worth little'. Use largely determined values; a commodity in great demand but limited in supply would be valuable, whereas its value would be totally lost if demand ceased. Hence 'if Bullion should cease to be used as Coyne, it would scarce be worth anything'.

Potter was concerned to show that silver and gold were being replaced by copper, brass or even leather for limited purposes; these base substances had proved capable of maintaining their value. He proposed to carry this trend to its logical conclusion, until gold and silver were completely replaced by metals readily available in Britain. Potter's proposal (as quoted by Wood) was that he

> 'would have all metalls (especially those of our owne mines) as well Lead and Iron, as Tin, Brass and Copper to be coyned in great peeces of 5 lb or 10 lb value a peece, according to their true intrinsick value as it is called, to lie in Warehouses or other convenient places for the following uses, and every County to be furnished with a competent quantity thereof; that so if any man demand the making good the aforesaid new money, it may be in the power of the County to pay him, either in Bullion (which this new money, being coyned according to the intrinsick value of the metall, and being a commodity of it selfe worth so much, will at any time procure) or in any such metall so coyned : which metall no person will trouble himselfe to carry away, but leave in the place till he have occasion to assigne the same to some other. Neither can any man except against such coyne of grosse metalls, or will any man sell it for 19s in the pound, it being really worth 20s; & not only so, but currant : Nor will any man esteeme or sell those Tokens at an under-value, that will so easily procure an estate to their full price in a commodity not perishable, &c. as currant money'.

On the basis of the premise that base metals differed from gold and silver only in their currently estimated value, Potter evolved his novel coinage system, which he claimed would increase the supply of money and facilitate trade. Wood was obviously impressed by some of his adversary's arguments, admitting that all commodities were likely to fluctuate in value; in some cases like dress fashions, the variation was considerable, as a result of the whimsy of taste. He also agreed that gold and silver were not valuable according to all criteria; iron was more indispensable for practical purposes, whereas even a clod of earth had unquestionable value by virtue of its ability to support plants. Wood was cautious in selecting arguments to refute Potter; he was sceptical about alchemical views as to the perfection of metals, but less willing to abandon arguments based on 'Antiquity and Universal Consent'. His basic argument related to the physical properties of gold, which ensured its eminent suitability for coinage and guaranteed its value even if it was no longer used for this purpose. Also like precious stones it had an aesthetic appeal and scarcity which would ensure permanent demand and therefore a high value. It was much easier to dismiss Potter's assertions about the current coinage practices in European countries, or about banking and counterfeiting. Finally Wood was able to point to numerous practical disadvantages of the new money, which rendered it not only impracticable but also economically disadvantageous. The new money was to be minted from surplus stocks of metals, but Wood pointed out that such stocks were too small to support currency demands. If newly-mined metals were used, there would be acute national shortages, particularly since enormous quantities of base metals would be required to equal the value of gold and silver in circulation. For instance a £5 iron coin would have weighed 500 lb! Since these coins 'lying dead' in warehouses would be difficult to store and handle, the metal would be much better used for industry or export. Thus the new money had all the disadvantages of the old as well as many additional defects:

> 'In short, if other metalls had been generally made use of for money as well as gold and silver, they would consideratis considerandis have run the like course as those have done . . . I thinke I may suppose, till the contrary be proved, that Gold and Silver when first they were coyned into money, retained the same intrinsick value they had before, which was very high in relation to other metalls and commodities, for the reasons expressed in my former Objections, And their high value . . . inferring allso their Portablenes, made them to be lookt upon in that regard as the fitter materials for money; and consequently other Metalls being much inferiour to them upon that account as well as severall others, and not exceeding them in any other respect, must be concluded lesse fit materials for the generality of the world to make money of.'

Wood succeeded in his primary objective of displaying the weaknesses in Potter's scheme, although his attempt at a systematic defence of bullion was less successful. The debate was additionally significant in exposing the need for a precise definition of such terms as 'intrinsic value'. Both authors recognised the need for a clear unambiguous use of this concept, but they reached diametrically opposite conclusions. Potter believed that bullion had no necessary stable intrinsic value, whereas Wood was convinced that the historical stability of bullion indicated the permanent nature of its intrinsic value. Neither attempted to explain the grounds for according a particular value to gold, silver, or any base metal.

A further stage in analysis was undertaken by William Petty, whose views on monetary theory were perhaps framed in the context of the Potter-Wood debate. He regarded the 'full understanding of the nature of Money, the effects of various species of Coins, and of their uncertain values, as also of raising or embasing them' as 'a learning most proper for Ireland'.[321] Petty's increasing involvement in economic issues followed the logical progression already described for Wood. His mathematical skills and Baconian outlook were utilised in the Down Survey, during the course of which he came to appreciate that settlement could not be undertaken without reference to the relative distribution of profitable and unprofitable lands. Hence Petty became involved in the general question of land valuation, which he recognised was also relevant to the issues of rents and taxation. For the assessment of land value, rent or tax it was not sufficient to rely on 'bargains which a few men make one with another, through ignorance, haste, false suggestion, or else passion or drink'. Rather it was necessary for an underlying intrinsic value to be 'cast up analytically by a distinct particularizing of the Causes'. Geometrical surveying provided the basis for such an assessment. Thereafter, it was necessary to undertake a cadastral survey, estimating the quality of each denomination of land on the basis of the quantity of produce borne. Petty believed that initially commodities should be assessed not in terms of monetary value but by the total weights or measures customarily used for each product. It would have been much simpler to have made direct monetary estimates, but Petty realised that this would not provide an absolute, unchanging value, in line with the mathematical exactness of his geometrical survey. Hay, silver, frogs or mushrooms were subject to fluctuating values; a commodity greatly prized in one region was regarded as worthless in another. However one hayfield could be assessed against another by comparing the average weights of hay produced. Thus the 'intrinsick value' of land could be assessed in terms of the sum total of its various commodities. Finally for the purpose of commercial transactions it was necessary to translate the intrinsic value into a monetary or 'extrinsick value'. Hence Petty was led to the problem which had perplexed Wood: what was the natural relationship between the intrinsic values of bullion and other commodities? Petty proposed an extremely simple but elegant solution: the natural price of a bushel of corn was equal to the weight of silver produced in the course of the same amount of work. Thus by making a quantitative comparison between the productivities of a farm and a silver mine, the real value of a farm could be assessed. Then natural rent could be estimated by taking into account all factors involved in production, as well as accidental features such as distance from markets. Rent was regarded as the surplus left after all expenses were taken into account.[322]

Wood, the Irish civil servant, had shown how mathematical prin-

321. Petty, *A Treatise of Taxes & Contributions* (212), sig.A3r.
322. Petty (212), pp.30–3; see also discussion by Letwin (180), pp.140–6.

ciples could be applied to simplify and rationalise operations in coinage, weights and measures. His attempts at the analysis of more complex monetary questions were not particularly successful. In a similar spirit John Collins, while working at the Excise Office, applied his mathematical abilities to improving and simplifying techniques of accountancy and commercial arithmetic.[323] Petty's economic ideas unfolded during the course of the Down Survey; he proceeded on a more ambitious scale and with greater precision. Although his analysis involved considerable over-simplification, it was comprehensive in scope and thoroughly scientific in nature.

Wood, Collins, Petty and many of their colleagues believed that their scientific and mathematical knowledge was especially pertinent to economic problems. Inevitably they fell short of definitive solutions, but this does not detract from the essentially scientific nature of their programme. This scientific orientation is shown in their inductive approach to problems and in the manner in which they arrived at explanations. It influenced such elementary things as the way in which they kept accounts or organised the work of their assistants; it was relevant to their search for comprehensive data and to their enunciation of rational and comprehensive theories. They believed that society was subject to the kind of regularities which applied to the realm of nature. It was hoped that patient research would ultimately provide an uncontroversial guide to social and economic policies. The economic theorists probably regarded themselves as collaborative contributors to a comprehensive programme, which would benefit all classes and lead to a revival of national fortunes. By this means, the Baconians could become architects of a utopian state resembling the Kingdom of Macaria. Hartlib's *Further Discovery,* Robinson's *Certain Proposals,* Boate's *Irelands Natural History,* Wood's *Ten to One,* Graunt's *Natural and Political Observations,* and Petty's *Treatise of Taxes,* as well as numerous minor documents were complementary contributions towards a detailed social and economic plan.

In framing general programmes, scientific, social, religious and ethical factors became inseparably linked. For instance the schemes for workhouses for the poor were a characteristic manifestation of puritan philanthropy, but they were also conceived as a means to mobilise labour and assemble materials for histories of trade. The Puritans believed that the Jews should be readmitted on millenarian or other religious grounds, but it was also realised that Jews and other aliens were a distinct economic asset, as well as a source of philosophical wisdom and scientific knowledge.

Although they displayed differences in emphasis and disagreed on

323. Collins, *An Introduction to Merchants Accounts* (London, 1652); *idem, The Mariners Plain Scale new plain'd* (London, 1659); *idem, The doctrine of decimal arithmetick* (London, 1685). For a valuable discussion of Collins's later economic writings see Letwin (180), Chapter IV.

certain specific issues, puritan intellectuals were broadly in favour of economic ideas of the kind expressed by Henry Robinson. It has already been noted that Robinson and his colleagues, whose first writings appeared between 1638 and 1641, adopted an approach to economic development which offered an incentive to innovation and scientific planning. Policies framed by Robinson and taken up by Petty's generation were aimed at securing the most efficient deployment of human and material resources. The instigators of this movement reacted against a system which permitted mounting unemployment and neglected industrial and agricultural development. They realised that it was no longer possible to maintain a system based on a monopoly of expensive cloth exports to various parts of Europe. Their economic policies emphasised competitive cheapness, economic diversification and the expansion of trade outside Europe. By adopting these criteria, the machinery of state, which had lost momentum under the Stuarts, would again be revived, by 'setting the wheeles of Trade a running'. The well-regulated state was compared with either a watch or the human body. Full efficiency required the efficient construction and co-ordination of all parts of the economy: 'For if Husbandry, and Trade at home and abroad be well regulated; all hands may be Employed, and where all hands are at work, there the whole strength of a Nation, doth put forth its endeavours for its own advantage'.[324] Another aspect of this analogy was reference to the idea of 'revolution'. Prosperity was not based on the passive accumulation of treasure; the poverty of Spain compared with small trading nations illustrated the dangers inherent in basing wealth on hoarded bullion. A sounder foundation for wealth was provided by an increase in the volume of trade, the greater flow of commodities, and the more rapid circulation of money. Money was compared with blood in the veins; economic vitality depended on the efficient circulation of money; hence the rate of flow of money provided an index of the health of the state. A remarkable precedent for the success of these policies was provided by the Dutch, whose example was followed on general economic questions as well as on numerous aspects of industrial and agricultural practice.

A full account of the economic theories advocated by the Puritans is beyond the scope of this book. For present purposes it is sufficient to note that the close interaction between economic and scientific reform established at the outset of the Puritan Revolution, continued during the Republic. For instance, the urgent requirement to rescue trade from its 'dead state' by relieving the 'famine of money', led to proposals for various types of banking and paper credit, in imitation of the continental banking system. Advocates of industrial expansion and technological innovation were quick to realise the advantages of banking; consequently it is not surprising to find that the banking lobby was

324. Robinson, *Certain Proposalls* (247), p.2; Dymock, *A Discoverie* (94), sig. A2v; Potter, *The Key of Wealth* (226), pp.1–2.

dominated by such figures as Potter, Hartlib, Robinson, Petty, Dymock, Gerbier and Chamberlen.[325]

Schemes for economic diversification were propounded by these as well as other figures. Francis Lodwick outlined a plan of mobilising the army during peace time to carry out public works and agricultural projects. Hartlib's workhouses or Chamberlen's settlements were designed to promote the manufacture of a wider range of textiles using flax and hemp; Hartlib attempted to kindle interest in the breeding of silk-worms. The encouragement of new trades was at the root of Robinson's enthusiasm for naturalisation. Among the foreign settlers, Hartlib's protégés l'Amy and Pruvost were experts in intensive agriculture and fisheries, while Drebbel and his family were skilled dyers. Other foreign workmen dominated developments in glass-working, mining, draining and metallurgy. These foreigners imported both scientific and technical intelligence.

Hartlib saw Petty as the ideal figure to 'invent a hundred new employments or enterprizes' suitable for the employment of the poor or retired soldiers. Petty suggested improvements to the settlement plan announced in Chamberlen's *Poor Mans Advocate*. Among other things, he wished to use his own form of settlement for the compilation of a history of trades. In a statement of policy very reminiscent of Robinson, Petty gave as his aims:

> 'To provide for poore, advance trade and make all manufactures flourish; England should bee endeavoured to bee made the shop of Europe, and it with other countries the markets. To doe this all trades and workmen should bee encouraged and all manner of compendious ways invented wherby they may come to undersel the manufactures and commodities of all other countrys. This would bee better then to strengthen their monopolizing corporations in ignorance and idlenes.'[326]

The promotion of fishing and mercantile fleets was a focal point of the proposals made by the reformers. Fisheries, boat-building and ancillary trades were to provide an extensive source of employment; they would thus exploit valuable food reserves which were available in both summer and winter. This industry would lead to improvements in boat-building, and fishing methods; the English would also become skilled in the secrets of pickling, drying and smoking. The fishing fleet would constitute an apprenticeship for the mercantile fleets which were necessary to secure independence from the Dutch. Exports and entrepôt trade would be increased and trade relations with the colonies would be strengthened. Thus the sea might become an even greater asset to England than to the Dutch, who had hitherto secured the largest interest in the expanded international trade.

325. Horsefield (152), pp.93–5.
326. Ephemerides 1649.

Facilitation of exchange, diversification of industry and an aggressively competitive approach to foreign trade were seen as the means to secure national prosperity, but the final guarantee of success would be the establishment of dominions. It has already been noted that Ireland was regarded as the most immediately accessible base for colonial operations. Even greater expectations were held out for the more distant colonies; it appeared that these, if properly regulated, would ensure Britain's complete economic supremacy. Robinson's summary of this policy illustrates the growing imperialist ambitions of the puritan economic theorists:

> 'that with all possible conveniency wee enlarge our Forraign Plantations, and get farther footing in Barbarie, East and West Indies, with other Countries wheresoever it may be compassed. Not onely that wee may the better provide our selves of Canvas for Sailes, Masts, Timber, with all other things necessary for Shipping within our own Dominions; but also in that a little spot of ground, as England is, with its Dominions, if it doe not enlarge them, in future generations, I feare me, will be found inconsiderable in respect of Spain, Portugall, the United Provinces, or any other European Nation, which shall have arrived to, and be armed with five or ten times a greater strength, power, and riches, either from their Asian, African, or American Dominions.'[327]

Since the days of Elizabeth, intellectuals with scientific interests such as Ralegh, Harriot and Dee had been in the forefront of the movement for the exploitation of colonies and the development of the shipping industry. Their successors during the Puritan Revolution displayed similar inclinations. It was realised that the agricultural and industrial improvements proposed for Britain in the interests of national self-sufficiency, would be assisted by raw materials and seeds imported from the colonies. Alternatively the improvements might be practised with even more success in the colonies themselves, by Britain's surplus population. Besides Robinson, the leading exponent of this point of view was Benjamin Worsley, whose *Profits humbly presented to this Kingdom* succinctly placed Baconian science in its wider economic and ideological context.[328] Worsley believed that his patent industrial process would provide sufficient saltpetre to support various operations in agriculture and fisheries, in addition to its traditional use for gunpowder manufacture. He appreciated that this saltpetre would be used to even greater effect in the more tropical environment of the colonies. By exploiting the use of saltpetre and by taking advantage of advances in husbandry, Britain could be assured of ample and cheap supplies of a wide range of commodities. Hence the nation could become inde-

327. Robinson (247), p.11.

328. This memorandum is given in full in Appendix V below. For the origins of this work, see above, pp.378–81.

pendent of the Dutch who currently controlled British imports. With the establishment of model plantations and the exploitation of trade by Englishmen, the problem of unemployment would be solved and all classes would 'live plentifully and be inriched'.[329] Worsley insisted that an essential precondition for the success of this policy of expansion was 'furnishing these Northerne Regions with the same commodities by our owne shipping from our owne Plantations'. Otherwise the full fruits of enterprise would be dissipated among the Dutch, who were already 'overgrowing us'. But if innovation, plantation and shipping were developed in unison, an economic transformation could be accomplished. Upon the return of prosperity national morale would be restored, providing a 'conducement to valour and great undertakings'. From a position of economic strength Britain would be able to pursue utopian policies at home and become the agency of God's will in foreign policy. Under providential guidance 'wee may sitt as judge and Umpire of al Christian differences, and may draw and ingross the blessings and promises to ourselves that are made Peace makers'.[330]

Gabriel Plattes had already in *Macaria* designated general means whereby science and technology could contribute to economic planning. Worsley, his successor as a utopian planner, working within the context of the Invisible College elaborated a detailed and practicable programme with a similar utopian goal in mind. His memorandum drew together scientific ideas and economic policies within a religious framework which was guaranteed to have wide appeal among the Puritans.

It was of course much easier to frame utopian policies than to secure parliamentary approval for even minor reforms. However evidence from both printed works and unpublished correspondence suggests that a patient and conscientious attempt was made by the reformers to give practical expression to their ideas. Their writings contain valuable information about the state of the economy and are generally regarded as significant contributions to economic thinking. But it is commonly doubted whether the puritan reformers were instrumental in guiding policy, or indeed whether the Republic initiated any distinct shift away from policies of the kind adopted by the early Stuarts. In cases where economic change unquestionably occurred, it is often difficult to know whether this was causally determined by policy. Where it is admitted that there was a mid-century turning point, it is frequently believed that the most significant changes dated from the 1660s rather than from the 1650s. In this case, the economic writings of the 1650s may be regarded as a rehearsal for the practical developments of the following decade.[331] However, although it is extremely difficult to generalise about

329. *Profits humbly presented,* fols. 1r–2r, pp.539–42 below.

330. *Ibid.,* fols. 2r–4r, pp.542–5 below.

331. M. James, *Social Problems and Policy* (158); M. Ashley, *The Financial and Commercial Policies of the Cromwellian Protectorate,* 2nd edn. (London, 1962); C. Wilson, *England's Apprenticeship 1603–1763* (London, 1965). These general works give references to a considerable body of specialist literature.

the complex economic developments of the Puritan Revolution it is clear that each phase was marked by the initiation and enactment of policies which affected many aspects of the economy. At the same time it is the case that long-term objectives were not systematically pursued, and policies often adopted as a matter of expediency in relation to relatively unspectacular local crises.[332]

Thus it might appear that the grandiloquent manifesto of Worsley, Robinson's pragmatic list of reform proposals, or the numerous specialised policy documents produced by the puritan economists, were without influence. However, an examination of specific problems indicates that the pressure groups were able to elicit some response to their schemes, although the results never matched their expectations. The decision to establish the London Corporation for the Poor was clearly influenced by a plethora of pamphlets on poor relief, but the Corporation tended to operate according to traditional practices rather than with reference to the elaborate workhouse schemes developed by Hartlib. Blondeau and his supporters convinced the Mint Committee of the superiority of mill money, but vested interests were able to delay the implementation of the new mechanised methods. On one fundamental monetary question, namely the interest rate, a reduction from 8 per cent to 6 per cent, which was of the kind demanded by Robinson, was introduced. Again, although naturalisation as recommended by Robinson was not allowed, aliens were treated leniently and the Jews were readmitted into Britain.

It is now necessary to determine whether such piecemeal reaction to the reformers' proposals signified any wider interest in their policies. For instance, was Worsley's ambitious *Profits humbly presented to this Kingdom,* described by Hartlib as a 'Work for Parliament', entirely without influence? This document was corrected by Hartlib, circulated privately, and probably intended for publication. Worsley's visit to the low countries was probably undertaken in connection with the proposals contained in *Profits humbly presented.* This experience increased his confidence in the policies advocated in the memorandum. It also furnished him with valuable first-hand information about the economic affairs of Britain's most prosperous neighbours. Worsley's letters from Holland suggest that his advice on economic affairs was taken increasingly seriously both by members of the Council of State and by certain influential politicians. This correspondence also indicates that Hartlib was playing a key role in co-ordinating discussions.

As a logical development of his earlier proposals, Worsley announced a plan for a new plantation to be established in Virginia. He reported that 'there are some Merchants [who] are willing to subscribe a stocke for to send to Virginia, to imploy or transport honest men that are

332. Cooper in Aylmer (11), pp.121–42, provides a detailed study of the period 1649–1653; he points to the complexity of the issues and the dangers of oversimplification.

in want; and that part of it shall be ventured in Tryalls, for planting and introducing new commodities, . . . or for setting up new manufactures'.[333] Although Worsley's intention to promote advanced agricultural and industrial methods by means of colonisation was undoubtedly sincere, he was equally concerned to bring to the administration's attention the unsatisfactory relationship between the American colonies and the mother country. Accordingly Worsley and his backers insisted that their best schemes were currently impracticable because of the royalist affiliations of the governor of Virginia. The plantation proposal was probably introduced as a test-case to attract greater attention to colonial policy from prominent public figures. In the course of his long memorandum on this subject Worsley proposed two main courses of action : first, the replacement of the delinquent government by a parliamentary commission which would act in concert with the English authorities; secondly, implementation of English control of colonial trade, counteracting the efforts made by the governor to deflect trade towards the Dutch.[334] Worsley argued that economic and political factors were inseparably linked, and his view was shared by the politicians and merchants who were among his supporters. Clearly Worsley wished these policies to be applied to all dominions. In all regions it was necessary for 'The Parliaments Authority [to be] instituted and erected, their friends, good men, free preaching of the Gospell, civility and industry countenanced'. Worsley pointed out that the most effective means to enforce parliamentary authority in the colonies was to prevent them from trading with foreign ships. It was therefore requisite for the English government to inspect all ships and personnel entering colonial ports. Worsley claimed that this political measure would bring about considerable economic returns, the 'English bringing goods from English Plantations', while effectively excluding their competitors.

The views expressed by Worsley commanded widespread support among the parliamentarians. His memorandum also ensured that the projects and idealistic notions of the Hartlib circle were drawn to the attention of the merchants and politicians involved in policy making. Although his Virginia colony was allowed to follow his saltpetre project into obscurity, the merits of many of the basic objectives of Worsley and his associates were recognised during the Republic. It has already been noted that the reformers' plans for agricultural and industrial diversification, poor relief, and monetary reform were widely supported. Ideally, they wished to persuade the state to display greater initiative on economic questions by attempting the solution of problems, and the resolution of disagreements, within the framework of general policies established on the basis of the systematic collection and analysis of data.

333. Letter from Worsley to Dury, 17/27 August 1649, HP XXXIII 2.

334. For Worsley's letters and memoranda on Virginia: HP I 2, XXXIII 2, LXI 2.

It was entirely in accordance with the views of the reformers that the decision was taken in January 1650 to establish a Council of Trade. The institution of the Council provided an opportunity to move beyond commercial disputes into a consideration of wider questions of policy and reform. Under the terms of the Act promulgated in August 1650, the Council of Trade was given ample financial resources and a wide range of responsibilities. Its brief included domestic and foreign trade, trading companies, manufactures, free ports, customs, excise, commercial statistics, coinage and exchange, fisheries and plantations.[335] The 'Instructions' to the Council accorded very much with the ideas of the reformers. Its first responsibility was to collect information on all native industries, including new trades and innovations. This provision perhaps reflects an appreciation of the value of histories of trade. The Council was then ordered to consider methods of attracting industries to underdeveloped areas of the country (Instructions 3 & 4), a policy which would probably also have entailed support for Robinson's plans for the improvement of road and river communications. This provision would have appealed to the strong provincial element on the Council. Coincidentally with the wishes of many reformers, the Council was asked to advise on free ports, to accumulate statistics whereby the 'perfect Ballance of Trade may be taken', investigate the parity of English and foreign coinage, and consider the reform of customs and excise (Instructions 5-8). Thomas Violet assumed the role of official investigator of coinage values, while Collins made noteworthy improvements in the management of the Excise Office. The encouragement of foreign trade, and the organisation of merchant companies (Instructions 4, 9 & 10) were hotly debated issues, at a time when the companies were seeking re-affirmation of their privileges against proponents of 'freedom of trade'. The final Instructions (11 & 12) were concerned with the promotion of 'the greate Trade of Fishing' and the reform of the English plantations in America, proposals which had been forcefully advocated by Robinson and Worsley respectively. The Act confidently repeated Worsley's assertion that colonial 'Commodities . . . may be multiplied and improved, as (if it be possible) those Plantations alone may supply the Commonwealth of England with whatsoever it necessarily wants'. The Instructions contained in the Act have attracted very little notice from historians, although one modern student of the seventeenth-century committees on trade and colonisation has correctly observed that 'these statesmanlike and comprehensive instructions are notable in the history of the development of England's commercial and colonial program'.[336] In view of the affinity between these Instructions and the reform literature, it is possible that Worsley and Robinson in particular

335. Firth & Rait, ii, pp.403–6; 1 August 1650. See also *CSPD 1649/50*, pp.4, 17, 140, 462; *CJ*, vi, pp.336, 346–7, 353, 403, 424, 451. Aylmer (12), pp.23, 50, 108.

336. Andrews (3), p.24.

were consulted by the Council of State about the terms of reference of the new Council.

The fifteen-member Council of Trade included a group of Hartlib's supporters. Its chairman, Sir Henry Vane, had been involved in discussions about Worsley's Virginia project and he was a long-standing political ally of Hartlib. Other members of the Council included Vane's brother-in-law, Sir Robert Honeywood, who consulted Hartlib about agricultural and commercial matters; and Honeywood's friend and neighbour from Kent, Sir Cheney Culpeper, who was one of Hartlib's closest associates. The secretary of the Council was Benjamin Worsley, who took on Samuel Hartlib junior as his clerk.[337]

The work of the Council is difficult to assess owing to the paucity of documentary evidence. However during its short span of life the Council appears to have been extremely active; it established specialist sub-committees, and prepared reports on diverse subjects for parliament and the Council of State. Most of the members' time was spent on local disputes and individual trades. On more general issues, measures were discussed to preserve and increase the stock of bullion. That advice on this and other matters was given by Robinson and Violet can be deduced from the printed tracts they issued to reinforce their arguments. A resolution of the debate over the merits of free ports was probably central to the success of the Council of Trade. Worsley, like Robinson, was in no doubt that:

> 'Opening of Free Ports, will conduce to the Quickening of Trade; to the Imploiment of the poor throughout the whole Commonwealth: to the making of all Forreign Commodities more cheap, and more plentiful . . . It will likewise serv to the preventing of Famine, and scarcitie of Corn; to the raising the Exchange, and bringing in of Bullion: to the augmenting of the Revenue of the State: and to the making other Nations more dependent upon this.'[338]

Worsley's expectations may have been inflated, but like his previous writings, *Free Ports* shows an appreciation of the close interrelationship of political and economic policy. Unfortunately free ports proved to be a contentious issue, exposing bitter rivalries between London and the provinces. The discussion of naturalisation foundered in a similar manner. Hence the Council of Trade incurred disapproval from some quarter whenever it showed signs of taking an initiative on matters of economic policy. There was very little protest when, after a year and a half, the Council of Trade was quietly terminated by the Council of State.

The Council of Trade left one important and permanent legacy, the Navigation Act of 1651. The origins, authorship, intentions and influ-

337. Firth & Rait, ii, p.403; see also Cooper in Aylmer (11), pp.133–4.
338. Worsley, *Free Ports* (342); Robinson first advocated free ports in 1641, and repeated his arguments in 1652: (247), pp.11–12.

ence of this Act have been the subject of a protracted debate which is only peripherally relevant to this study. However, while it is generally accepted that Benjamin Worsley and his political and merchant allies played an active part in framing this policy, the nature of Worsley's influence has not been clearly understood.[339] Worsley became the ideologue of this group during the years preceding the Navigation Act. It is apparent from his writings on Virginia that he came to believe that the encouragement of English shipping, even more than free ports, was fundamental to the expansion of England's trade. He recognised that the control of colonial trade would not only be to the advantage of English shipping, it would also impose a political settlement on the recalcitrant American and West Indian colonies. This policy secured the support of both imperialistically inclined politicians and the interloping colonial merchants. Worsley's party exercised considerable influence on the Independent-dominated Commonwealth administration. The initial response to the expansionist position was the Act of 1650, which aimed to reduce Virginia and three other American colonies to conformity by completely prohibiting their trading with foreign ships. In addition a licensing system was introduced to control personnel carried to all English plantations. Finally, the Council of State asserted its authority to control the appointment of governors and other officers in the colonies.[340] This Act was very close to the policy advocated in Worsley's 'A Coppy of my letter to Mr. Strickland' and 'Further Animadversions about Virginia'.[341] The Navigation Act of 1651 represented the logical extension of the policies adopted in 1650. Its intention was to give further incentive to English trade by confining imports from Asia, Africa and America, into England, Ireland and the plantations, to English ships in which the majority of each crew was English. Imports from Europe into England, Ireland or the plantations were restricted to English ships or ships of the country of origin. Various exceptions and special restrictions were introduced and in view of the changed bias, restrictions on colonial trade were less severe. The major concern was the control of imports into England in Dutch ships, especially from the Dutch entrepôt or their herring fisheries.[342] Given the provisions

339. For representative opinions on the Navigation Acts, see L. A. Harper, *The English Navigation Laws* (New York, 1939); J. A. Williamson, *Cambridge History of the British Empire,* vol. 1 (Cambridge, 1929), pp.215–18; Andrews (3), pp.24–48; R. W. K. Hinton, *Eastland Trade and the Common Weal of England in the Seventeenth Century* (London, 1959), pp.90–4 (Hinton reprints Worsley's *Advocate* and *Free Ports*); C. Wilson, *Profit and Power: A Study of England and the Dutch Wars* (London, 1957), pp.48–60; *idem, England's Apprenticeship* (London, 1965), pp.61–4; J. E. Farnell, 'The Navigation Acts, the First Dutch War and the London Merchant Companies', *Economic History Review,* 1963/4, *16*: 439–54; Cooper in Aylmer (11), pp.134–6; C. Hill, *Reformation to Industrial Revolution* (1969 edn.), pp.156–61; R. Brenner, 'The Civil War Politics of London's Merchant Community', *Past and Present,* 1973, No. 58: 53–107.

340. Firth & Rait, ii, pp.425–9; 3 October 1650.

341. HP LXI 2.

342. Firth & Rait, ii, pp.559–62.

of the 1650 and 1651 Acts, the way was paved for full implementation of the policies announced in Worsley's *Profits humbly presented,* which had called for the creation of a profitable English entrepôt upon the basis of a vigorous Anglo-American trade axis.

In view of Worsley's active participation in discussions of colonial policy, it is not surprising that he claimed to have been 'the first sollicitour for the Act for the incouragement of navigation, and put the first fyle to it, and after writt the Advocate in defence of it'.[343] *The Advocate* repeated the arguments of his earlier writings; Worsley pointed out that Dutch economic prosperity had been at the cost of England and the English plantations. He stated four 'unalterable Laws in all Manufactures' controlling the value of manufactured articles. Finally he declared that the English could profitably emulate the Dutch example by improving efficiency in manufactures and establishing an 'Act for the Incouragement and Increas of our Navigation'.[344]

It has been doubted whether the 1651 Navigation Act was fully effective and it has even been suggested that it may have been positively harmful. Nevertheless well-informed contemporary writers believed that this legislation was beneficial to the English economy; for instance Samuel Lambe declared that the 'Act hath breathed some refreshing to the decaying Trade of the English Nation'.[345] For this reason Charles II promptly introduced an act of a similar nature, which closed certain loopholes in the 1651 Act. Thenceforth, Navigation Acts were regarded as indispensable aspects of English policy. But even if as an economic weapon the 1651 Act was not perfectly conceived, it 'marked a vital stage in the evolution of national economic planning'.[346]

The Commonwealth administration proved to be extremely sympathetic to the interloping colonial merchants. Indeed the Venetian ambassador claimed in 1651 that 'the government of the Commonwealth and that of its trade [is] now being exercised by the same individuals'.[347] This comment reflects the close identity of interest which developed between the merchants and politicians within the newly-dominant Independent party. Benjamin Worsley and his associates were extremely active in forging these links and in making use of the expansionist instincts of the Independents to further their own wider social and intellectual aims.

The Commonwealth administration was encouraged to approach economic affairs with a new sense of responsibility. The reformers urged

343. Bodleian, Clarendon MS 75, fols. 300–1.

344. Worsley, *The Advocate* (343).

345. Lambe, *Seasonable Observations* (178), p.3. In 1669 Joshua Child expressed a similar opinion about the Navigation Acts; see Letwin (180), p.8, and *Seventeenth Century Economic Documents,* ed. J. Thirsk and J. P. Cooper (Oxford, 1972), p.74.

346. Wilson, *England's Apprenticeship,* p.63. Similar views are expressed by Hill and Hinton.

347. *CSP Venetian 1647–52,* pp.187–8.

that it was necessary to look beyond the balance of conflicting company interests characteristic of the monopoly system, to frame policies designed to further long-term national interests. While the 1651 Navigation Act avoided direct conflict with the privileges of the established trading companies, it opened the way to freeing the merchants from their control. Hence as a result of this measure the 'freedom of trade' mentioned in the 1650 Instructions to the Council of Trade came within grasp.

The 1651 Navigation Act has been variously attributed to interloping merchants or imperialistic statesmen. The Dutch ambassador believed it was the work of 'some few persons interested in the highest degree in the East Indies and the new plantations of this nation'.[348] Worsley's papers indicate the manner in which the interests of these various parties were reconciled. Worsley's own role, as a negotiator and policy-maker, introduces a further element into the situation. In the spirit of a Baconian natural philosopher, Worsley framed an ambitious plan for national development which took into account the widest range of social and political factors. Wilson has remarked that the 1651 Navigation Act represented the achievement of the 'economics of Leviathan', which were based on economic analysis without reference to a religious ethic. But the works of Robinson and Worsley indicate a continuing integration of religious and economic considerations. Their overriding aim in economic planning was the creation of a Christian utopia. Hence in general terms the 1651 Navigation Act 'realized a Baconian vision towards which men had long been groping'.[349] The Council of Trade and the Navigation Act were the logical outcome of the adoption of policies outlined in *Macaria*. Following this legislative success, the Baconians might have begun to look forward to the day when 'wee shall obtaine our desires, to make England to be like to *Macaria*'.

(xi) The Garden of Eden

In the seventeenth century plant husbandry was widely regarded as the Englishman's most pleasurable labour. It is therefore not surprising that Milton portrayed Adam in his undefiled state primarily as a gardener:

> 'But let us ever praise him, and extoll
> His bountie, following our delightful task
> To prune these growing Plants, and tend thes Flours,
> Which were it toilsom, yet with thee were sweet'.

348. Letter from Beverningk to Nieuwport, 16/26 December 1653, *EHR*, 1893, *8*: 529–31.

349. Hill, *Reformation to Industrial Revolution*, p.157.

Ralph Austen was more specific; he followed Ralegh in believing that Adam kept a 'Garden of Fruit-trees'.[350] In Eden, Adam's primary duty had been that of curbing the natural luxuriance of the earth, by cutting back excessive growth. Yet the biblical texts left the Puritans in no doubt that Adam, even in his undefiled state, was obliged to work—'to till and keep and of the fruit to eat'.[351] Idleness would have been unthinkable, even in Paradise. Since it was necessary for Adam to labour, God appointed him to undertake the most rewarding and productive manual exercise :

> 'God knew that Idleness corrupts the best natures, and therefore Man was imployed in that humble vocation; for though God did at first create the kinds of all Plants, yet doubtless man had and yet hath an honest Allowance to procreate a Diversity of Species by Transplantation, Ingraftings, Innoculatings, and other various Cultivations, which were Incestuous in other Creatures; but as I conceive allowed from the words here *to dress and keep it*.'[352]

Adam was therefore seen as the agent of creative evolution, and by the skilful use of experimental techniques later generations could expect to bring about improvements in the characteristics of cultivated plants.

After the Fall Adam's garden became choked with noxious weeds. Thenceforth, man's burden increased and he was obliged to till the ground—'a lower and inferior labour'. Nevertheless, tending the soil remained one of man's most rewarding tasks, even though it demanded unremitting effort.

The Puritans looked forward to the ultimate fulfilment of the prophecies of the scriptures and of the patristic sources Papias and Lactantius, that the waste places would be reclaimed and become as fruitful as the Garden of Eden.[353]

The actual situation in England contrasted sharply with these utopian expectations. Increases in agricultural productivity failed to keep pace with the growth of the population. Price inflation reduced the purchasing power of the wages of the poor, whose living standards were gradually eroded during the first part of the seventeenth century. The position of the lower classes was particularly difficult during the years of crop failure and pestilence. The most detailed survey of this problem concludes that 'the third, fourth and fifth decades of the seventeenth century witnessed extreme hardship in England, and were probably among the most terrible years through which the country has ever passed'.[354] Yet at the same time there was an amazing sense of optimism

350. Milton, *Paradise Lost,* IV, lines 436–9; Austen, *Treatise of Fruit-Trees* (6), p.12.

351. *Paradise Lost,* VIII, line 320; Genesis 2 : 15.

352. John Pettus, *Volatiles from the History* (209), pp.43–4.

353 Austen (8), sig. ¶1r–2v.

354. J. Thirsk (ed.), *Agrarian History* (280), p.621; see especially Chapters V & IX. See also Supple (275), pp.99–112.

among the enthusiasts for agricultural improvement, who believed that human ingenuity could generate spectacular advances in plant husbandry. Already during the reign of Elizabeth Harrison had reported that 'in comparison of this present, ancient gardens were but dunghills and laistowes . . . for so curious and cunning are our gardeners now in these days that they presume to do in the manner what they list with nature, and moderate her course in things as if they were her superiors'.[355] This optimism was well-founded. Techniques were standardised and improved; the process of innovation began in earnest; information was disseminated in the translations and compendia of such authors as Tusser, Plat and Markham. Native practitioners owed much to the continent; books, plants and even gardeners were imported into England. Increasingly important avenues for the introduction of foreign species, were the voyages to other continents. From the mid-sixteenth century, Europe was inundated with new species which were sometimes of considerable economic importance. Most of these introductions were accessible only to the rich connoisseur, but the challenge of cultivating exotic fruits played an important part in attracting the interest of the aristocracy to horticulture.

Many innovations were only slowly taken up. In 1597 the frontispiece of Gerard's famous *Herbal* portrayed the author holding a sprig of potato. However the cultivation of this plant in England seems to have spread only slowly. Equally, notwithstanding the support of James I, the cultivation of the white mulberry for feeding silkworms was not more than locally successful. However tobacco growing in the Midlands reached such proportions that James I attempted to suppress its cultivation. But it was not these expensive introductions so much as the trickle of improved types of salad crops, the diversification of fruit growing and most of all the large-scale cultivation of cole-seed, root crops and leguminous species which gradually changed the complexion of English horticulture and agriculture.

The ostentatious face of this movement was represented by the gardens of the great houses of the aristocracy. Both in building and gardening this class became caught up in the spirit of emulation and they embarked on extravagant expenditure in an attempt to modify the environment on an extensive scale. Their vision was guided by aesthetic factors, and other philosophical considerations. Bacon and Wotton were the theorists on landscape gardening. The great gardens included extensive buildings and water-works produced by celebrated masons and engineers; as gardeners the aristocrats employed collectors and botanists like John Tradescant. These experts built for Robert Cecil the magnificent gardens at Hatfield, where considerable resources were applied to the cultivation of vines, oranges, lemons and peaches. This

355. William Harrison, *Description of Britain* (London, 1587), Bk. II, Chapter XX.

great garden could be matched by more than a dozen others constructed before 1640, at such places as Audley End, Knowle, Hardwick or Wilton. Successively lower ranks of the gentry imitated this fashion until many improvements entered into general use. Hence when Howell visited a comparatively modest house at Long Melford, he noted that 'for the gardening and costly choice flowers, for ponds, for stately large walks, green and gravelly, for orchards and choice fruits of all sorts, there are few the like in England'.[356] Similarly the visitor to Ware Park was impressed by the degree of activity in 'paling or ditching, plashing of hedges, stocking of trees, catching of moles, or such other kind of husbandry'.[357] In the same garden Wotton was impressed by Sir Henry Fanshawe's subtle understanding of 'the tinctures, and seasons of his flowres'. Fanshawe's garden, or similar examples established by Edward Lord Zouche, or Henry Danvers, Earl of Danby and Sir John Danvers, became repositories for rich collections of plants; they were visited and stocked by able botanists and they took on the character of botanical gardens. Hence it was entirely appropriate that Henry Danvers should establish a formal botanical garden at Oxford in 1621, at which he employed the German Jacob Bobart as the gardener. Such gardens supplied Bacon with much of the original material for *Sylva Sylvarum*. Perhaps more than any other subject, horticulture illustrated for Bacon the potentialities of the search for *magnalia* in nature.

In view of the above developments it is not surprising that the seventeenth century saw the emergence of a marked interest in field botany. This was only slightly reflected in the voluminous but overrated *Herbal* of Gerard (1597), but Thomas Johnson's revision of this work in 1633, represented a new level of sophistication in English botany. Much new information was incorporated into John Parkinson's *Theatrum botanicum* (1640), a work which was as much indebted to gardens as to botanical exploration. This was the last great English herbal, and Parkinson's earlier *Paradisi in sole: Paradisus terrestris* (1629) represented the high-water mark in Stuart gardening literature.

From the above remarks it is apparent that, notwithstanding the failure of agriculture to make large-scale advances, the foundations for substantial progress were laid before 1640. The writings of the agricultural improvers were usually reports on the continuing process of change, rather than prophetic announcements of innovations which were adopted at a much later date. Consequently most of the improvements which are customarily thought to have occurred in the eighteenth century were introduced at an earlier date. Indeed it has been claimed that the germs of the agricultural revolution may be detected as early as 1560; thereafter between 1580 and 1656 the process of change appears to have become greatly accelerated. The major improvements intro-

356. James Howell, *Familiar Letters* (156), pp.106–7.

357. N. E. M. McClure, *The Letters of John Chamberlain*, 2 vols. (Philadelphia, 1939), i, pp.236–7.

duced before 1640 included fen drainage, irrigation, up-and-down husbandry, the more extensive use of fertilisers and the introduction of new crops such as sainfoin, clover, turnips and rye-grass.[358] Even if it is admitted that these improvements were not practised on an extensive scale before 1640, when they are taken together with simultaneous developments in horticulture, gardening, and botany, an impressive pattern of initiative emerges for the years before the Puritan Revolution.

What part did the puritan reformers play in this process? Certainly agriculture became one of their major pre-occupations and their extensive writings came to dominate the literature of this subject. It is also immediately apparent from an examination of the puritan tracts on agricultural reform that this was an area in which they expected to exert considerable influence, partly by promoting legislation, and partly by persuading practitioners to improve their methods. The puritan writings on agriculture have a distinctive quality. Agriculture was brought into line with their work on other aspects of science and the policies which they adopted were similarly dictated by more general social, religious and philosophical beliefs. Hence their writings tended to be on a higher intellectual plane than the traditional literature on husbandry, and in accordance with the spirit of the Great Instauration, their designs were more ambitious. On the basis of their scientific ideas the Puritans were more convinced than any previous generation that agriculture could be revolutionised. They aimed to achieve this transformation by applying Baconian experimental philosophy to an area which Bacon himself had expected to exemplify the great utilitarian value of his methods.

After 1640 an increasingly critical attitude was taken to the previous literature. Old-fashioned authors like Tusser continued to be used, and the genteel gardening and domestic handbooks of Markham retained their popularity; in reaction, the Puritans consciously attempted to inculcate a more scientific attitude to husbandry, as well as to relate their work to current social and economic problems. They made virtually no concessions to the taste of the élite by dwelling on entertaining horticultural novelties. Their basic priorities were the increase of agricultural productivity and the amelioration of the condition of the poorer classes.

The old books were read carefully, and often commented upon in the introductions to the works produced by the Puritans. With reference to the *Maison rustique, or, the Country Farm* Blith commented that books of this type were of 'little use to us'. In the absence of reliable works on husbandry, Blith's friends encouraged him to publish his own book, 'hoping thereby to give either Incouragement to some deeper and sollid Practitioners to hold out their Experienced Principles, or

358. Kerridge, *The Agricultural Revolution* (173), pp.347–8 & *passim; idem, The Farmers* (174), pp.103–29.

else to Exasperate or provoke the offended'.[359] Of books on fruit trees, Austen complained that the old literature was 'full of dangerous and hurtfull instructions, and things notoriously untrue'. Accordingly, Austen aimed to produce 'a plaine sound Experimentall work' of a kind previously unavailable to English pomologists.[360] Much was found to criticise in the earlier writers, but they were not altogether disparaged. Sir Hugh Plat in particular often attracted admiration for his ingenuity and public-spiritedness. One of his works was re-issued during the Republic; it was both successful and reasonably compatible with contemporary writings.[361] The other author regarded favourably by the Puritans was Arthur Standish, whose *The Commons Complaint* (1611) dealt specifically with the problem of timber conservation. This brief tract contained many suggestions which were taken up by the puritan arboricultural enthusiasts. In 1639 John Pell lamented that the simple but valuable recommendations contained in Standish's tract had not been put into effect, while in 1659 John Beale planned to make *The Commons Complaint* the basis for an extensive work designed to promote an interest in forestry among 'true-hearted Common-wealthe-men'.[362]

The prevailing tone of the new agricultural writings is indicated by the above comments of Blith and Austen. They were dissatisfied with earlier writings, not merely because of their unmethodical and misleading advice, but also because they failed to provide a 'rational' and 'experimental' basis for their practices. The reformers felt that it was necessary to replace the traditional compilations of rules of doubtful authenticity and ambiguous phraseology, by systematic guides to the specialist areas of husbandry, couched in 'plaine sound Experimentall' terms.[363] They aimed at basing their advice on the widest possible first-hand experience of current practice, assisted by personal trial whenever possible. Thus a guide to husbandry would be supported by its appropriate history of trade. The reformers were constantly on the look-out for improvements which could be verified by experimental methods and related to general scientific theories. Hence these authors felt an intuitive sympathy for Bacon's experimental philosophy, and they consciously attempted to frame their agricultural writings in Baconian terms. Austen even composed a brief tract based on Bacon's aphorisms about husbandry. He believed that Bacon's 'delight was especially . . .

359. Ephemerides 1650; Blith, *English Improver* (27), sig. (a)3v–4r. The *Maison Rustique* was revised by Markham in 1616 from an English translation by Surphlet, first produced in 1600, which in turn was based on a work originally issued in 1554. For general surveys of the literature, see G. E. Fussell (111), and E. S. Rohde, *The Old English Gardening Books* (London, 1924).

360. Austen, *Treatise of Fruit-Trees* (8), sig. ¶1r.

361. Plat, *Floraes Paradise* (London, 1608); ed. C.B., 1653, 1654, 1659, 1660, as *The Garden of Eden*.

362. Ephemerides 1639; for Beale see below.

363. Austen (8), sig. ¶1r.

in Vegetable Philosophy, which was as it were his darling delight'.[364]

The first pronounced expression of this new tradition of agricultural writing was contained in the series of short tracts published by Gabriel Plattes between 1639 and 1644. Plattes's work gives an immediate impression of originality and vitality. Rather than attempting to compile a handbook of the traditional, eclectic type, he developed further the approach of Standish, concentrating on advice which was relevant to the solution of major social problems. Although Plattes pretended to only a modest education he was certainly not ignorant of previous writings and he was the first agricultural theorist to bear an obvious imprint of the influence of Bacon. But for the most part he bypassed authorities; the scriptures were the only source which he cited frequently. As already pointed out, Plattes had much in common with contemporary puritan economic theorists. As they did with respect to economics, Plattes first described the scientific basis for efficiency in his subject; after which he suggested causes for the current low level of agricultural productivity. Finally, he proposed a series of measures which would reverse this situation. Plattes was particularly concerned to describe improvements which could be undertaken by the poor. He hoped that implementation of his methods would secure the purposeful employment of the poorer classes and enable them to support their infirm brethren. His improved husbandry was also expected to benefit other classes and guarantee the prosperity and political stability of the nation. But he warned ominously that if husbandry, 'the very nerve and sinew, which holdeth together all the joynts of a Monarchy' was not reformed, 'an horrible mischiefe' was bound to ensue.[365]

Little is known about the background to Plattes's agricultural work, apart from his connections with the technician and experienced fen-drainage engineer, William Engelbert, to whom in 1639 he dedicated his first writings, and from whom in the same year he inherited a cartload of inventions. Plattes himself remarked that his writings were based on twenty-four years' experience of agriculture, during which time he must have taken a keen interest in improvements undertaken by fellow practitioners.

In 1639 Hartlib noted that both Plattes and Pell were friendly with Sir Richard Weston who at that time was regarded as 'one of the greatest experimenters and triers of all manner of projectes'. Even before the Civil War Weston was engaged upon enclosures and experiments with new methods of husbandry.[366]

Plattes was criticised by Hartlib for taking insufficient care in perfecting his writings. Indeed he tended to be repetitious, but his work was lively and informative, and his opinions were expressed with trenchant clarity. Although he wrote primarily for those lacking scholastic edu-

364. Austen, *Observations on Bacons Naturall History* (9), sig. A2r.
365. Plattes, *Infinite Treasure* (217), sig. C3v.
366. Ephemerides 1639.

cation, his approach was not unsophisticated. Improvements were explained in detail, and experimental evidence was frequently cited in support of his methods. Finally, his detailed proposals were justified in terms of a theory of plant nutrition, which incorporated a primitive idea of cyclical chemical change. No previous English author had approached this degree of sophistication in the treatment of agriculture. Accordingly, notwithstanding the brevity of his work and the inelegance of some of his explanations, Plattes may be regarded as a pioneer exponent of a scientific approach to agriculture.

Many of the improvements canvassed by Plattes were already in use on at least a small scale, and most had been advocated by one or other of the earlier agricultural writers. Plattes conveniently gathered together a number of extremely useful suggestions into a single tract. The improvements which he included related to forestry and fruit-tree growing, up-and-down husbandry, enclosure, irrigation, pasture maintenance, the mechanisation of sowing, the use of fertilisers, and the diversification of crops under cultivation. He urged that the poor could be supported with ease, if they practised even the most simple and cheap improvements; and he calculated that whole families could subsist on extremely small plots of enclosed land. Plattes promised them that 'Nature is no niggard, but giveth riches to all that are industrious'.[367]

Plattes's *Infinite Treasure* made an immediate impression on Hartlib, who declared that it should be translated and 'set on foot by *praxis*'. Hartlib assisted Plattes and encouraged him to undertake further publications. Hartlib also disseminated the new information about agriculture among his expanding circle of correspondents. Plattes was praised everywhere, and his work encapsulated almost every proposal that was taken up in the later agricultural writings of the Puritan Revolution.

Plattes died in the winter of 1644/5 without having completed his promised 'Treasure House of Nature Unlocked'. Nevertheless the practical optimism of his published tracts and manuscript writings was sufficiently convincing to encourage other agriculturalists to continue his work. A particularly important role was assumed by Hartlib, who increasingly regarded the organisation of effort on agricultural reform as one of the main functions of his Office of Address. He found that many agricultural improvers were willing to adopt the same public-spirited approach as Plattes. It seemed that 'Providence having directed mee by the improvement of several relations unto the Experiences and Observations of Others, I find myself obliged to become a conduit-pipe thereof towards the Public'.[368] Husbandry more than any other subject was used by Hartlib to demonstrate the aims of his Agency to 'do good, in love to the Publick'. He directly maintained poorer practitioners and entered into correspondence with others. He encouraged reticent authors to publish their work and in many cases he took over direct responsibility for

367. Plattes, *Infinite Treasure* (217), p.78.
368. Hartlib, *Discours of Husbandrie* (139), sig. A4r.

organising the publication of their tracts. His English and foreign correspondence was used for collecting information, much of which was noted in his 'Ephemerides'; this material was then incorporated into the successive editions of *Samuel Hartlib his Legacy*, or alternatively made available to other writers. Hartlib never claimed to be more than the co-ordinator of this effort. Nevertheless, this function was valuable in itself. He published important writings by Plattes and Weston which might otherwise have been lost, and his own compilation, the *Legacy*, was one of the most important agricultural writings of the century. His correspondence both encouraged interest in husbandry and facilitated exchanges of ideas among a widely-scattered group of enthusiasts. While the direction of effort was determined by the interests of the practitioners, Hartlib encouraged work on all aspects of husbandry; and the whole enterprise was organised as a contribution towards a Baconian history of the agricultural trades. In this vein Child strongly recommended that their work should contribute towards a '*Systema*, or compleat Book of all the parts of Agriculture'.[369] Austen believed that the impact of Hartlib's work was considerable, accepting that 'the advantages which have of late yeares accrued by your Legacy of Husbandry, (and other pieces made publique by your means, and encouragement), are not small'.[370] In view of the high quality and great contemporary popularity of the writings on husbandry associated with Hartlib it is entirely appropriate that Fussell should characterise the period between 1641 and 1660 as 'The Age of Hartlib'.

The discussions on agricultural reform during the Puritan Revolution were so extensive that a comprehensive list of participants would include a large percentage of the figures discussed in the present book. It is probable that this subject, even when considered in its narrower sense, attracted more sustained attention than any other aspect of science during the Puritan Revolution. The agriculturalists who collaborated with Hartlib were an extremely varied group. His most important associates were the writers; these included the inventors Gabriel Plattes and Thomas Duckett, the remonstrant physician Robert Child who came originally from Kent, Arnold Boate the Dutch physician who had worked in Ireland, Ralph Austen the registrar to the university Visitors at Oxford, Walter Blith the parliamentarian soldier and Warwickshire farmer, Cressy Dymock the inventor and Nottinghamshire farmer, John Beale the clergyman from the West Midlands, and finally a figure outside the puritan and parliamentarian party, Sir Richard Weston of Sutton Court in Surrey. This heterogeneous group engaged in discussions on many technical issues and they collaborated to produce a co-ordinated 'Systema' of agriculture of the kind advocated by Child. This work was greatly helped by advice from many quarters. Agriculture was of interest to a wide group of intellectuals many of whom are not usually thought

369. Hartlib, *Legacy* (142), pp.89–90.
370. Austen, *Treatise of Fruit-Trees* (8), sig. a2r.

of in connection with this subject. Among the enthusiasts were Wilkins, Boyle, Pell, Petty, Wren, Worsley, Wood, Tong and Culpeper. Hence it is not surprising that one of Hartlib's correspondents should comment 'that the Genius of this Age is very much bent to advance Husbandry'.[371]

The puritan agricultural writers represented a continuation and acceleration of the tradition of interest in innovation which extended back to the later sixteenth century. They advocated a number of improvements which had already been tested and found to be effective. However in most cases these innovations had not previously been described or explained adequately, or differentiated from a mass of more adventitious suggestions. The puritan writers took up a more limited number of major themes, and exploited them in depth. The topics which Gabriel Plattes had treated in the briefest terms were reconsidered by Walter Blith, whose *English Improver* (1649) provided an extremely competent survey of current knowledge. Blith's work contains many echoes of the *Discovery of Infinite Treasure*. Each of his major proposals (irrigation, drainage, enclosure, up-and-down husbandry, use of fertilisers, plantation of timber, and diversification of crops) was discussed in a critical and well-ordered manner.

Other authors expanded on Blith's work, particularly with, for instance, fuller information about new crops. Hartlib's edition of Weston's brief essay not only explained the merits of clover husbandry but also described the general advantages of the kind of intensive agriculture practised in the low countries. Numerous crops—sainfoin, lucerne, woad, madder, hemp, flax, etc.—found their champions in the agricultural literature published during the Republic. Very few subjects escaped notice; for example Child advocated the cultivation of potatoes and Hartlib published brief tracts encouraging the more extensive practice of bee-keeping and silkworm breeding.[372]

Perhaps the most obvious distinguishing feature of the puritan agricultural writers was their ability to write competently about subjects which hitherto had been dealt with in only a perfunctory manner. This improvement in the quality of the published work on husbandry was not merely a reflection of the superior abilities or accomplishments of the new authors. Their more systematic and intelligible approach was dictated by a general ethical standpoint which placed considerable emphasis on the efficient dissemination of information to the widest public. Plattes strongly attacked the attitudes of the monopolistic projectors, claiming that 'knowledge that concerneth the publick good, ought not to be concealed in the breasts of a few'. Consistently with this view the puritan writers seriously endeavoured to make their work accessible to the lower classes. Hence Plattes concentrated on simple descriptions of improvements which could

371. Hartlib, *Legacy* (142), pp.110–11.

372. For surveys of the work of the agricultural innovators, see Fussell (111), pp.36–55; Ernle (95), pp.103–29; Jones (161), Introduction & pp.49–79. See especially Kerridge (173), pp.181–325, and Thirsk (280), pp.161–99.

be applied by the poor, and he hoped that his projected *Treasure House of Nature Unlocked* would after earning the guarantee of the imprimatur of a parliamentary committee, meet with universal approval.[373] Similarly since Blith intended his work to be accessible to 'the poorest and plainest Subject' it was written in 'our ordinary naturall country Language, and in our ordinary and usuall home-spun tearmes'. Blith adopted the increasingly held view that ministers should teach the people to exercise their callings more diligently; then the way would be prepared for a 'larger breaking forth of Light and Truth'. Plattes suggested that this educational function could be undertaken by the overseer for the poor in each parish. Austen proposed that recent agricultural writings should be made available for general use in each parish.[374] Others wished to develop the process of vocational education on more formal lines; Snell's 'rural colleges' and Dury's 'mechanical schools' were planned on a national scale; these would have provided the entire agricultural population with general education, and vocational training.[375] A more sophisticated agricultural education would have been given at such agencies as the Literary Workhouses of Petty, or the Noble Schools of Dury. The most ambitious proposals for 'husbandry learning' were made in 1651 by Cressy Dymock. He hoped to gather subscriptions for the erection of a 'Colledge or Society of good Husbandry', which would teach all aspects of agriculture to its students during a seven-year apprenticeship period. The aim of his college would be

> 'the infusing into more sturdy *Husbandmen* of the nation in generall (now too much wedded to their more customary and lesser profitable workings) the more perfect *Principles* of their own *Art*, and such additional *Uses* and Instruments as shall make their *Practises* more *rational, easie*, & really effectual & *beneficial*: so to the advancement and encrease of *publique plenty* and wellfare.'[376]

Dymock's plan for a college to give advanced instruction in agriculture was complementary to the proposal which originally emanated from Plattes, for a college to specialise in agricultural research. Plattes argued that, in view of the supreme economic importance of agriculture, the Commonwealth should support 'a Colledge for Inventions in Husbandrie'. This college was probably envisaged as a loose association of skilled and public-spirited practitioners who were willing to place their services at the disposal of the state. In *Macaria* and later writings Plattes called this

373. Plattes, *The Profitable Intelligencer,* 1644 (220), quoted from Hartlib, *Legacy* (142), pp.173–4. See also Blith (27), p.163.

374. Blith, *English Improver* (27), sig. a2r, a3v, p.1; Plattes, *Profitable Intelligencer* quoted from Hartlib (142), p.207; letter from Austen to Hartlib, 26 Sept. 1653, HP XLI 1.

375. George Snell, *The Right Teaching* (262); Hartlib and Dury, 'Some Proposals', quoted from Webster (320), pp.174, 179.

376. Dymock, *An Essay for Advancement of Husbandry Learning* (91), p.6. See also letter from Hartlib to Boyle, 8 May 1654, Boyle *Works,* vi, p.91.

organisation a 'council of Husbandry' which he hoped would regulate the agricultural arts and 'produce a great perfection in that knowledge which as it is the most ancient of all Sciences, so it is the most excellent and honourable'.[377] Plattes's Council of Husbandry was designed as one of a number of panels of experts which would advise the state on economic matters. This idea was taken up by Hartlib and at all stages in the evolution of his Office of Address, agricultural research and policy-making were accorded central importance.

The educational proposals of the puritan agricultural writers indicate that they were not willing to leave reform to individual initiative. They realised that the treasures of nature would only be revealed by the efficient collaborative enterprise of all sections of society. Active state involvement in education and agricultural development was regarded as an essential prerequisite for the success of this policy of agricultural expansion. Accordingly some of the most important of the agricultural writings were addressed to parliament and the authors did not hesitate to press for ambitious legislative programmes. Hartlib hoped that his services to husbandry would persuade the state to continue its support for his Office of Address. Furthermore he proposed that the state should appoint two 'Publique Stewards or Surveyors', the first of whom would oversee husbandry and the second, forestry. Secondly he urged that protective legislation was needed before tenants would be persuaded to improve their land. He looked forward to the day when all improvements would be enforced by law, stating that 'it were a noble piece of policy and justice if authority should oblige or compel men into it'.[378]

Blith took up these points, and with increasing vehemence he insisted that the improvements described in his book could not be implemented on the extensive scale intended unless tenants were given protection against their landlords; he believed that legislation was also needed to resolve conflicts between rival interests and to encourage specific improvements. He elaborated an extremely ambitious eight-point plan for social reform, which he felt contained the elements necessary to provide the conditions for agricultural expansion. On specific social and economic questions he was very much in sympathy with the ideas of Hartlib and Robinson. Blith believed that, since 'all Lands and advantages thereof are the Common-wealths in general', on questions of improvement individuals should give way to the general interest.[379] The widespread popular agitation against enclosure during the early years of the Republic made the agricultural writers aware that improvement could not be discussed without reference to general questions of social policy. Accordingly Blith and Hartlib's protégés dwelt at length on the intrinsic agri-

377. Plattes, *Infinite Treasure* (217), p.72; *Macaria* (219), p.3; *Profitable Intelligencer,* quoted from Hartlib (142), p.207.

378. Hartlib, *A Discours of Husbandrie* (139), sig. A2r–4v; *idem, The Compleat Husbandman* (145), 'To the Reader'; Ephemerides 1650.

379. Blith (28), sig. Mm1r–3r.

cultural merits of enclosure while at the same time pressing for legislation to ensure that this process would not operate to the disadvantage of the poor. As Austen proclaimed : 'why should not the Poore have their share and proportion, as well as their rich neighbours; . . . yea, let the Poore be first provided for'.[380]

The reformers rapidly evolved the idea that legislation could also be used to control the practices of husbandry. Child proposed that the state should require every farmer to devote up to 1 per cent of his ground to the cultivation of flax or hemp. James Stansfield favoured a law which would enforce the planting of a certain number of fruit trees and other trees per acre. Austen proposed a similar law and wished to include a mechanism for inspection and a time limit, to ensure speedy implementation. Blith pressed for a law to ensure that enclosed land was used equally for tillage, hay production, and pasture. He also proposed that each landowner should be forced to plant each year one oak, elm, ash, walnut, chestnut, and two crabs, on every two or three acres of his holding.[381]

Forestry and fruit-tree growing were subjects which assumed outstanding importance in the puritan writings on husbandry. Accordingly these subjects can be used to illustrate their approach to specific practical problems. It has already been noted that incentive for this development came initially more from Standish and other petitioners concerned about 'timber famine' than from the authors of popular handbooks of agriculture. Then, Plattes took up the call of John Tavener and Standish for the more economical use of land by planting trees in the hedgerows. The plantation of fruit trees was regarded by Plattes as one of the most profitable improvements contained in his book.[382] In the first edition of Hartlib's *Legacy* (1651), Child suggested remedies to counteract the English neglect of woods and orchards. Among other things he advocated legislation to protect existing woods and to enforce replanting where cutting was necessary. Blith devoted only one brief chapter to the improvement of woods and copses in the first edition of the *English Improver* (1649). In the second edition, he added a chapter on orchards, which he decided to curtail after Hartlib had informed him that Ralph Austen 'an artist both learned and experienced' had completed a whole book on this subject.[383] As an advertisement for Austen's book Hartlib

380. Blith (27), Dedication to Parliament, pp.59–99; Austen, *Treatise of Fruit-Trees* (6), Dedication; Dymock, *A Discoverie for Division and Setting out of Land* (94); Plattes, *Infinite Treasure* (217), pp.9–19; Adam Moore, *Bread for the Poor and Advancement of the English Nation* (London, 1653). For the general debate on enclosures, see James (158), pp.106–17; Thirsk (280), pp.200–55.

381. Child in Hartlib (142), p.33; letter from Stansfield to Hartlib, 15 December 1656, HP LIII 20; letter from Austen to Hartlib, 26 September 1653, HP XLI 1; Blith (27), p.72, sig. Mm3r.

382. Plattes, *Infinite Treasure* (217), pp.3, 9–17; *Profitable Intelligence,* quoted from Hartlib (142), pp.208–10.

383. Child in Hartlib (142), pp.14–19, 49–50; Blith (27), Chapter XXI; Blith (28), Chapters XXI and XLIII, and p.258.

issued a brief tract calling for a law to make compulsory general plantation of a wide variety of trees, which would be enforced in each district by two officers named 'Fruiterers' or 'Woodwards'.[384]

Hartlib assisted Austen with the revision of his book, and he superintended its publication and distribution. Five hundred copies were to be printed and Austen asked Hartlib to distribute about half of these to Members of Parliament. Austen's *Treatise of Fruit Trees* (1653) was more literary in tone than most of the puritan writings on husbandry and it was printed together with a meditative work on *The Spiritual Use of an Orchard,* to which Austen attached great importance. Literary embellishments notwithstanding, the central practical section of Austen's *Treatise* was the most systematic and detailed treatment of this subject yet published in England. Particular emphasis was placed on the previously only poorly described techniques of grafting, propagation and pruning. The original edition was quickly exhausted and Austen, again with Hartlib's help, prepared a greatly expanded form of both the *Treatise* and the *Spiritual Use,* which was issued in 1657. This edition included sections on the cultivation of trees in general; on this subject Austen's text was very similar to the relevant chapters of Blith's *English Improver Improved.*

Austen hoped that his activities would be supported by the state within the context of a national programme for tree planting. The Council of State was urged to finance the establishment of plantations under Austen's supervision; these would then 'multiply and expand many thousands of young trees yearly'. With this scheme in mind Austen presented Cromwell with copies of his two treatises, and with a petition addressed to the Council of State which briefly outlined the advantages to the national economy of embarking on an extensive scheme of planting trees both for fruit and timber.[385]

The efforts of Austen's influential academic, clerical and lay supporters to establish public nurseries were not successful. Nevertheless Austen's tireless labours to promote the cultivation of fruit trees attracted widespread attention. His handbook inspired an academic like John Lydall to establish a small nursery at Oxford; other Baconians like Evelyn, Cowley, Aubrey, Boyle, Beale and Sharrock began studying the art of the cultivation and propagation of fruit trees. Soon a considerable group of enthusiasts were engaged in exchanging information and in preparing memoranda on improvements in arboriculture. Evelyn's ostentatious *Sylva,* published after the restoration, has of course become famous, but in many ways it is neither as original nor as perceptive as the earlier work of Austen, Sharrock or Beale. Sharrock's *The history of the propagation & improvement of vegetables* (1660) belongs very much to the

384. Hartlib, *A Designe for Plentie,* 1652 (143).

385. Letters from Austen to Hartlib, 8 February, 10 February 1653, HP XLI 1. His petition is given in full in Appendix VI below. See also letter from Hartlib to Boyle, 15 May 1654, Boyle *Works,* vi, p.91.

tradition of experimental philosophy developed by the Wilkins school at Oxford. Sharrock was more restrained and objective than Austen, and he was also more familiar with theoretical aspects of botany, although possibly less well-informed on current practice.

In contrast to Sharrock, Beale gravitated to the approach of the Hartlib circle. His *Herefordshire Orchards, a Pattern for all England* (1658) was designed to promote the 'publick welfare in the peace and prosperity of this Nation'. Much of this tract was concerned with the propagation and cultivation of fruit trees, and many of Beale's observations resembled those made by Austen; but he was also influenced by the idea of a regional natural history. His 'plain and unpolished account of our *Agriculture* in *Herefordshire*' might be regarded as an application to an English region of the methods pioneered by Boate in *Irelands Natural History*.[386]

Inevitably much of *Herefordshire Orchards* was taken up with descriptions of varieties of fruit trees, and an account of the uses of fruit, with special reference to cider manufacture. Beale claimed that orchards were 'the Pride of our Countrey'. He had been gathering information on this subject for many years; indeed his father was an expert on cider and Beale credited him with the original introduction of the celebrated Redstreak cider apple. However Beale was not merely aiming to compile a handbook of current local practice. At many points he moved towards a scientific explanation and experimental elaboration of his observations. For example, he traced the relationship between the indigenous type of fruit tree, and soil type, concluding that 'some soyle and some air is more agreeable for some kinde of fruit, than for other'.[387] One of his most tenaciously held opinions was that the best cider was produced from apples which were 'more wrethed or wrinckled, or spotted with warts, moles, or freckles, or of a more russet, or yellow colour', growing on trees subsisting in shallow soil on high ground. Some of his most extensive comments related to methods of propagation; these were offered primarily as a corrective to William Lawson's *A New Orchard and Garden* (1618).

After the favourable response to *Herefordshire Orchards,* Beale began work on a version in dialogue form, which has not been preserved. A discourse on cider was also completed at this time, which confirms Beale's detailed and expert knowledge of local practices. In this tract, he argued for the superiority of cider from the point of view of economy, nutritional and medicinal value, and palatability. He believed that the expansion of the cider industry might have considerable economic implications.[388] These ideas attracted the immediate approval of Austen who remarked that 'cider is growne into greate request and its esteeme

386. Beale (23), p.2.
387. *Ibid.,* p.9.
388. Letter from Beale to Hartlib (26pp.), 5 May 1658; 'Extracts of lett[e]
written to Mr. Hartlib' (58pp.), HP LII.

growes more and more, even in those places where they knew not what it was formerly'.[389]

Hartlib sought to further the work on fruit trees by promoting a correspondence between Austen and Beale. There were many minor divergences of opinion between these two authors and Hartlib hoped that their letters would merit separate publication. Beale was a strong advocate of cleft grafting, while Austen preferred tongue grafting; Beale argued for the superiority of the Redstreak in wine and cider manufacture, while Austen favoured pippins or pearmains.[390] But on questions of general policy, the two prima donnas of arboriculture were in agreement. Both believed that the promotion of fruit growing was one of the main tasks of agricultural reform.

After the *Herefordshire Orchards* project, Beale began to assemble material for a more ambitious work on forestry. This was to be entitled: 'The True Interest of the Common-wealth of England. Soliciting a Public Care for the Plantation & Preservation of Orchards, Groves, Woodes, Hedges, Fences & Mounds. For the increase of Fruite, Fuell & Timber with helpefull Directions for the increase of all kind of Foods, namely Corne, Catell, and Foule. First undertaken by Arthur Standish, And further explicated & advanced by severall true-hearted Commonwealthe-men in the way of their Epistolary Addresses To Samuel Hartlib the Elder Esqr.'[391]

In certain respects this miscellaneous collection may be regarded as the complement to Hartlib's *Legacy*. While Hartlib's book concentrated on general husbandry, Beale's collection covered many different facets of forestry and fruit growing. The importance attached to this work is indicated by the care which was taken over the composition of its preface; here Beale was willing to defer to Hartlib, who knew what sentiments would carry the greatest weight with the administration. Nevertheless Beale suspected that Hartlib's republican views would be disapproved of by the numerous 'counterfeit pretenders to commonwealths-men'. The preface began with the general lamentation of the reformers that energies had been consumed in deciding the forms of government, while leaving basic problems of social planning unsolved. The state was warned not to overlook the grave implications of this neglect. On arboriculture, the preface followed the main lines of Austen's petition to the Council of State. The importance of timber as a vital commodity was explained; no nation could exercise internal functions or external power without timber. Nevertheless stocks of timber had been allowed to decline disastrously and no attempts had been made to restore the balance. The nobility in particular were censured, since, instead of pay-

389. Letter from Austen to Beale, 30 July 1658, HP XLV 2.

390. Letter from Austen to Beale, 9 Sept. 1658, 'Concerning Mr. Austens book', HP LII.

391. HP LI. Dated 19 March 1658/9. For a summary of contents, see *HDC*, p.107.

ing attention to serious economic problems, they had dissipated their wealth on ornament and vanities. It was acknowledged that fruit trees had recently been planted in many parts of the country (probably a reference to the influence of Austen's writings) but if equal attention was not given to the planting of timber, the nation's power would be sacrificed to the 'Covetous Dutch-neighbors, or the Spanish Inquisitors'.

From the extremely miscellaneous character of the contents proposed for this collection, it is apparent that Beale had difficulty in obtaining material equal in quality to that available for a work on fruit trees. The book was to open with the text of Standish's pioneering *Commons Complaint*. While Beale felt strong reservations about the quality of this work, he could think of no better introduction to the problem, which he believed had considerably worsened since the time of Standish: 'Hath any such waste ever beene seene or known in England, as hath beene since wee have pretended to a Common-wealth?' The following sections were to include: some miscellaneous observations recommending the experimental planting of a wide range of trees, written by Sir Edward Partridge; a recipe for a wood preservative, a list of the uses of wood, a memorandum between Dawson and Culpeper on the much-discussed topic of protecting trees from the rubbing of cattle, Beale's discourse on willows and sallows, a letter composed by Richard Carew in 1641 (with notes by Beale), on the regeneration of rotten trees; a large treatise on plantations by Dymock, and a concluding section on establishing new woodlands by Beale. The papers relating to this volume indicate that the most substantial, original and systematic work was by Beale himself. The only other contribution of significance might have been the section by Dymock, but this document has not so far been located. However Beale's annotations, his list of the uses of wood, and his notes on the varieties, growth characteristics and uses of various species of sallow and willow contained much accurate and useful information. Finally the conclusions, when taken together with letters on the topics there discussed, provided both an extremely useful digest of current practice and many shrewd botanical observations. Despite lapses into uncontrolled loquacity, Beale's writings show him to have been a perceptive and lucid forestry intelligencer.[392]

Beale's draft conclusions for *The True Interest of the Commonwealth* raised a number of prominent questions relating to arboriculture. He stressed the importance of determining whether each species was raised best by seed, or by vegetative propagation. It was necessary to bear in mind that certain trees were tolerant with respect to soil depth, while others were not.[393] Each species of tree also tended to favour one particular soil type. Finally he noted that, on account of regional variations of soil and climate, the types of tree adapted to, for instance, conditions in Devon, were not suitable for areas such as the Midlands.

392. See especially, Beale's 'Key to the Orchard', [1657], HP LII.
393. See also letter from Beale to Hartlib, 9 April 1657, HP LII.

Like Austen, Beale envisaged a time when planting of trees and shrubs would be undertaken with respect to the most effective land usage; each hedgerow would then yield its store of timber, fuel, fruit, wine and aqua vitae:

> 'When their Ladyes and good Housewifes shall please to emulate their Husbands Rurall Chymistry and convert their bushes into Raspyes, Currants, Gooseberyes, Barberyes, and binberyes or whortleberyes, Heps, Blackberyes, Sloes, Bullaces, Damasins, prunes and thence into Marmalads, Quidenyes, Wines, Brande wines and waters of use, Then will all Passengers confesse and admire it, as a Land of Blessings, in which the Original Curse is Reversed, To whom God hath given the wisdom to Dresse the wildernes into a Paradyse.'

The work on fruit trees and timber of the puritan agricultural writers displayed their ability to contribute significantly to a subject which had been treated only inadequately in the previous literature. They conscientiously collected information about current practices, which was then considered critically and advanced whenever possible by personal observation and experiment. This routine was self-consciously modelled on the methodological axioms of Bacon. A similar approach is evident in other aspects of the work of this group on husbandry. They collected information about the various types of plough in use and they attempted to design new ploughs. Plattes designed an instrument for the mechanisation of sowing corn; this problem was taken up by his successors, each of whom claimed to have produced the most efficient device. In the context of attempts to improve crop yields by the use of fertilisers, experiments were undertaken which were important for the understanding of plant nutrition. Each of these problems related in some way to more theoretical scientific questions. A more detailed assessment of these and other aspects of puritan agriculture must be reserved for consideration in a separate study.

The work on husbandry produced between 1639 and 1660 is cumulatively most impressive. During this period the foundations were laid for a scientific study of the problems of agriculture. But writings however impressive do not constitute an 'agricultural revolution' in themselves. The question remains, was the major improvement in agricultural efficiency, which, it is increasingly felt, dated from the second half of the seventeenth century, related in any way to the work of the puritan agricultural reformers?

The writers who have been discussed above certainly expected their work to have practical effect. Their books were not composed as a contribution towards some abstract problem, or for the attention of a small group of specialists. They believed that agriculture was the area of applied science which could *par excellence* illustrate the practical value of Baconian science. As Blith exclaimed: 'This very Nation might be made the paradise of the World, if we can but bring ingenuity into fashion'.[394] The reformers were not successful in bringing about a major programme of legislation. Indeed the measures which were introduced relating to the preservation of woodlands, enclosure, or fen drainage would undoubtedly have been implemented regardless of the efforts of the reformers. However it is apparent that the agricultural reformers were not merely a small and scattered group of persons out of touch with economic realities. The writers were numerous and their efforts were backed by the work of an even more considerable body of correspondents and collaborators. Furthermore they were extremely well-informed and most were actively engaged in agriculture. Accordingly if each of the figures known to have been involved in this movement acted as an agent of agricultural improvement in his locality, the overall effect of these foci of activity must have been significant. Many of the improvers both in England and in Ireland probably found themselves in the position of Robert Child, who noted that his neighbours were busily reading the work of Blith, Boate and Hartlib. He declared that everyone was trying to perfect husbandry, there being 'scarce any place in Ireland, where men are more active in fencing, drayning, dunging and liming their land'.[395] Interest in improvement was not entirely new; its roots lay in the long-term processes of general social and economic change. Thus the reformers were to a certain extent reporting on a mechanism of change of which they were expert witnesses. But they also realised that husbandry could be improved far more than its practitioners generally appreciated. Hence their writings took advantage of a favourable climate of opinion to disseminate information and encourage wider participation in a movement which could make of England a paradise on earth. At the moment there is no reason to doubt the view of contemporary witnesses, that the work of the puritan agriculturalists contributed towards the acceleration of the pace of agricultural change which was such a conspicuous feature of the second half of the seventeenth century.

394. Blith (28), sig. d3v.

395. Letter from Child to Hartlib, 29 August 1652, Turnbull (290), p.35; & *passim*.

VI

Conclusions

The Puritan World View and the Rise of Modern Science

The scientific movement of the Puritan Revolution is by no means easy to assess. In terms of the activity of the major architects of the 'Scientific Revolution', the period between 1640 and 1660 appears to be something of an interphase. William Harvey lived until 1657, but his old age was spent in somewhat embittered retirement, whereas the impact of the work of Boyle, Hooke, Newton and Ray was not felt until after the restoration. The Puritan Revolution was not rich in its production of scientific classics and, as the statistical surveys conducted by Merton show, this period seems also to have been unproductive in discoveries or inventions of the kind recorded in Darmstädter's encyclopaedic *Handbuch zur Geschichte der Naturwissenschaften und der Technik*. In Merton's view this analysis, supported as it is by circumstantial evidence about the disturbing effects of the Civil War, suggests that a 'low point in scientific output' was reached during the Puritan Revolution. Hence the scientific movement which 'had been gathering momentum for some time previous', was 'repressed by the uncertainties and disorders of the two decades of strife'. In the opinion of both Merton and G. N. Clark, the correctness of this estimate is confirmed by the statements of eye-witnesses and by the apparent flowering of science in the tranquil atmosphere of the restoration.[1]

However Merton was forced to concede that this negative attitude towards the Puritan Revolution could not be upheld without reservation. Indeed paradoxically his analysis of recruitment into science demonstrated that 'the peak of notable seventeenth century scientists in England was reached' between 1642 and 1660.[2] According to these results, the period between 1631 and 1660 was marked by a rapid acceleration in scientific recruitment, while the period of the 'burgeoning' of science after 1660 was marked by the onset of a gradual, but most perceptible tailing-off which continued at a fairly constant rate for the rest of the century. Consequently the great productivity of science after 1660 in terms of Darmstädter's criteria of selection, is largely attributable to the labours of intellectuals whose initiation into science occurred during the Puritan Revolution. Hence Merton concedes that Sorokin may have

1. Merton (188), pp.40–1; Clark, *The Later Stuarts 1660–1714* (Oxford, 1934), pp.27–9.

2. Merton (188), pp.40–3; see also R. T. Gunther, *Early Science in Oxford*, vol. 3 (Oxford, 1925), p.320.

been correct in claiming that revolutions and wars were marked by an '"increase in men of genius"' in areas which include both science and technology. Nevertheless, Merton persisted in believing with reference to the English Revolution that 'times of great social disorder can scarcely yield conditions favourable to scientific investigation'.[3] It is undoubtedly the case that social disruption can impede sustained scientific enquiry, but the present study suggests that English science benefited from the catalytic influence of the revolutionary intellectual and political situation, without there being the kind of traumatic and sustained disorder which would have seriously affected the course of scientific work. It is easy to exaggerate the degree to which the Puritan Revolution was accompanied by wholesale devastation, partly because of the temptation to assume analogies with the consequences of recent revolutions, but also because it is habitual to rely on contemporary royalist commentators who, for propaganda purposes, needed to give an impression of a lapse into barbarism and anarchy during the 'Great Rebellion'.

The Civil War certainly exercised a minor disturbing influence on science. In England however the active military phase of the war was relatively brief and its effects were extremely localised. In London, which was in parliamentary hands from the outset, there was an almost uninterrupted outburst of scientific activity, while even at the deeply partisan universities the recovery of academic momentum was rapid. In Ireland, the disturbance was more general and persistent, but during the 1650s, there was a spectacular recovery in intellectual affairs. The growth in British scientific book publishing was interrupted by the Civil War, but it resumed, and reached an unprecedented level after 1648.

The botanist Thomas Johnson and the astronomer William Gascoigne were fatally wounded while fighting for Charles I. In many other cases professional or academic careers were disrupted by military service and after the war some of those who had sided with the crown suffered ejection from office or went into exile. The aged William Harvey lost many of his scientific papers and the last few years of his researches were consequently undermined. But there were very few cases of this kind and royalist intellectuals like Bathurst, Charleton, Scarburgh, Digby, Oughtred, Morison, Ent, Ward, Ashmole and Towneley quickly accommodated themselves to the new situation. Such factors as financial penalties, loss of estates, exile, and enforced changes of career failed seriously to undermine the course of the scientific work of royalists. It may even be argued that the Civil War caused science to assume greater importance for the dissidents. For those excluded from civil office or political participation, the sciences were an unexceptionable form of recreation. For the impecunious gentry, utilitarian science could offer financial rewards through such avenues as agricultural improvement or technology. Finally, young gentlemen who were debarred from acade-

3. Merton (188), p.43.

mic or ecclesiastical preferment were often deflected into the study of medicine.

As demonstrated in Chapter II, the Civil War brought about a transformation in the position of the puritan intelligentsia. After a brief period of uncertainty the Puritans who had formed the core of the resistance to the Laudian regime found attractive opportunities for advancement in politics, the civil service, the church, the universities and the medical profession. For those outside the official arena there were numerous opportunities of taking part in economically rewarding ventures, such as interloping trade or speculation in delinquents' land. Scientific intellectuals were conspicuously successful in securing positions of advantage, and the success of the older generation of the 'servants of God' encouraged certain less idealistic and more opportunistic members of the younger generation to join their ranks. Younger sons, and youths like William Petty from lower social classes appreciated that the revolutionary conditions offered a means to exploit what had become the advantages of their background, and ascend the social scale. Those who were passing through the later stages in their education during the 1640s came to realise that Baconianism was one of the credentials likely to earn the approval of authority. Accordingly the victorious party in the Civil War may be regarded as directly encouraging that class of its sympathisers who were engaged in scientific research.

Whether viewed from the royalist or the parliamentarian point of view, the two decades of civil war did little to inhibit and much to facilitate the development of the sciences, particularly among members of the younger generation. When this favourable social atmosphere is taken into account, it is not surprising that the various types of new philosophy were cultivated with great enthusiasm in England, and that Baconianism, which was so commensurate with the puritan ethic, was taken up with particular alacrity. In view of this situation it is not justifiable on the ground of social conditions to assume a sharp contrast between the levels of activity within the scientific movements of the Puritan Revolution and the restoration. The Restoration Settlement, accompanied as it was by an unstable political situation, by repressive measures against the Nonconformists and by the civil turmoils caused in the Plague and Fire of London, by no means represented a dramatic return to conditions of tranquillity and civil harmony. The Royal Society and the associated scientific movement in the provinces are therefore to be seen, not so much as a new and spontaneous manifestation of intellectual creativity peculiar to the restoration, but rather as the end-product of a long process of growth and development which had taken place during the decades of the Puritan Revolution.

Because of these considerations it is questionable whether Darmstädter's work has accurately reflected the respective merits of the scientific movements of before and after 1660. In the first place, it will be readily conceded that the information about scientific discovery compiled by

Darmstädter nearly seventy-five years ago, and used subsequently as the basis of Merton's investigations, requires correction in the light of recent historical research. In almost all cases, the inventions and discoveries which Darmstädter attributed to the 1660s are found to be so strongly rooted in the work of the earlier decades, that it is arbitrary to attach particular importance to the formal date of discovery as recorded in traditional lore. There is extreme difficulty in precisely identifying the chronological boundaries of scientific discovery; it is essential to appreciate that in most cases one must take account of a period of gestation and debate, and that in relatively few cases is it possible to conduct the analysis in terms of the sudden insight of an individual. Correction of Darmstädter's work to take cognisance of the observable process of scientific creativity would certainly shift the balance of emphasis of the data to remove the division between the Puritan Revolution and the restoration.

This conclusion is consistent with the valuable evidence about the deflection of energies towards the sciences provided by Merton himself, in the course of his analysis of shifts in vocational interests during the seventeenth century. Figure 1 gives a summary of Merton's findings. He notes that science and medicine followed similar patterns of growth, and suggests that these fields were subject to much the same social forces. His data show that recruitment to science and medicine remained fairly constant until 1626; there followed a process of acceleration,

FIGURE 1

The number of individuals recruited to science and medicine in each quinquennium beween 1600 and 1700. Data derived from Merton (188), p. 32.

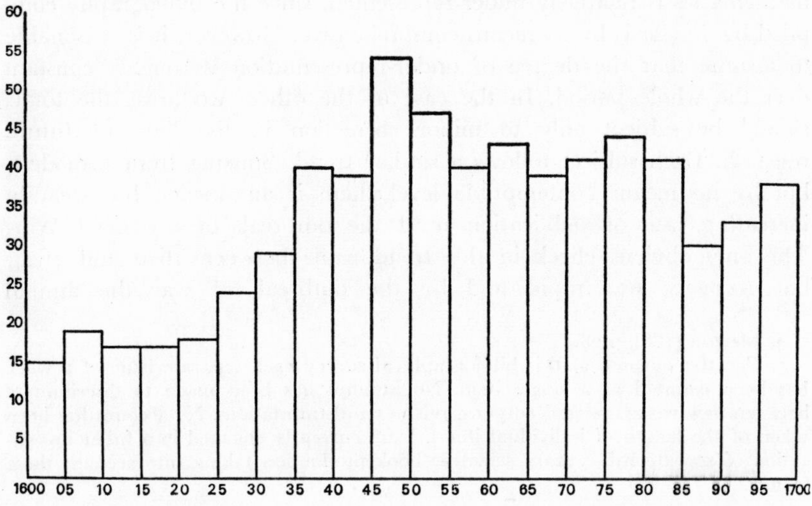

until a peak was reached in 1650. Thereafter a fairly constant level was maintained until 1685. Upon the basis of these findings Merton concludes that during the middle years of the seventeenth century, science 'had definitely been elevated to a place of high regard in the social system of values; and it was this positive estimation . . . which led ever more individuals to scientific pursuits'.[4] He also acknowledges that this social reorientation provided the essential basis for the accelerated rate of advance of the sciences in the latter part of the seventeenth century.

The present study has uncovered much evidence to substantiate Merton's findings, and it is clear that the Civil War exercised only a minor disturbing influence on the groundswell of scientific activity, which had already moved into a phase of accelerating growth during the formative stages of the Puritan Revolution. Hence it is not surprising that a trend towards scientific institutionalisation is found in London among no less than three different groups during 1645 and 1646. Thereafter one may observe a smooth process of growth, diffusion and differentiation, until the formation of the Royal Society in 1660. The university medical schools, always small and vocationally orientated before 1640, were transformed during the later 1640s into much larger and more vigorous centres of research. A similar metamorphosis occurred at the College of Physicians in London, and the mathematicians at Gresham College were successful in reviving the spirit of the early years of this institution.

The general rise in the popularity of the sciences may be judged by the great acceleration in publishing in such important representative areas as mathematics, chemistry, medicine and agriculture after the military phase of the Civil War. This evidence also of course suggests that a considerable amount of scientific work was being undertaken and completed during the period before 1660. As demonstrated in Figure 2, the pattern in publishing followed very similar lines in three representative subjects, mathematics, medicine and agriculture.[5] Of these topics mathematics is relatively under-represented, since the bibliography compiled by Taylor is by no means comprehensive. However, it is reasonable to assume that the degree of under-representation is roughly constant over the whole period. In the case of the other two areas the totals should be subject only to minor correction in the light of future research. Each subject follows a similar trend. Starting from a modest, but by no means contemptible level there is an uneven but steadily increasing rate of publication until the outbreak of the Civil War. The only obvious check in this trend came between 1620 and 1624, but recovery was rapid and by the outbreak of war the annual

4. Merton (188), p.28.

5. For the purpose of this bibliographical survey each separate issue of a work has been counted as a single item. No attempt has been made to discriminate between new works, revised editions, reissues and translations. No account has been taken of the length of individual items. I am currently engaged in a fuller investigation of seventeenth-century scientific book production taking into account these factors.

FIGURE 2

The quinquennial rate of book production between 1600 and 1660 in Agriculture, Mathematics and Medicine.

The data for agriculture and medicine are based on personal findings; the data for mathematics are taken from the bibliography given by Taylor (278).

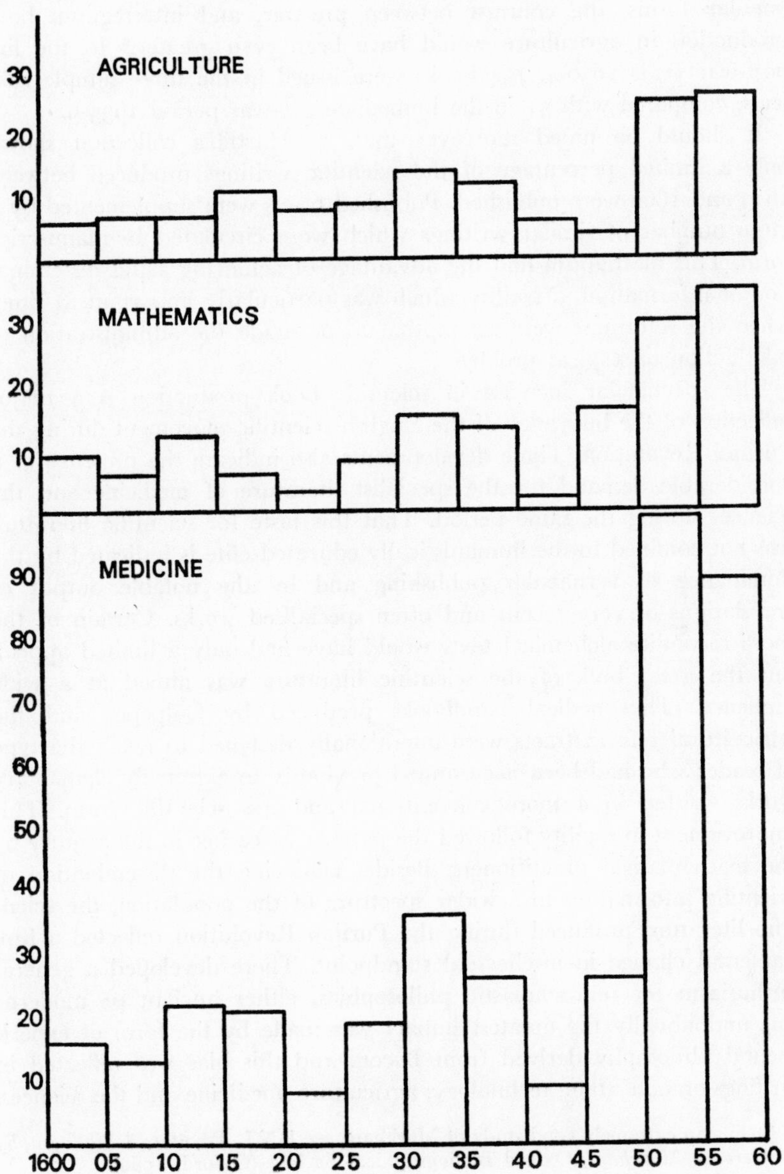

output had nearly doubled in each subject since the beginning of the century. Compared with the thirty-one books published in the three subjects between 1600 and 1604, fifty-one were published between 1635 and 1639. The war initially introduced a severe setback; then there was a rapid acceleration to the high plateau of output between 1650 and 1659. In mathematics and agriculture there was more than a doubling of the annual rate of publication; the increase was even greater in medicine. Had it not been for the great resourcefulness of Gervase Markham (d. 1637) who issued his few writings in many different popular forms, the contrast between pre-war, and interregnum book production in agriculture would have been even greater.[6] In the five post-war years 1650-4, 154 books were issued in the three sample subjects, compared with 51 in the immediate pre-war period 1635-9.

It should be noted moreover that, as Hartlib's collection shows, only a limited percentage of the scientific writings produced between 1640 and 1660 were published. Published tracts were supplemented by a large number of similar writings which were circulated in manuscript form. This mechanism had the advantage of achieving rapid dissemination of information, a facility which was particularly important at times when the reformers were attempting to persuade the administration to take action on topical problems.

The spectacular increase in scientific book production is a major reflection of the buoyancy of the English scientific movement during the Puritan Revolution. These developments also indicate the presence of a considerable demand for the specialist literature of medicine and the sciences during the same period. That this taste for scientific literature was not confined to the humanistically educated élite is indicated by the dominance of vernacular publishing and by the notable output of translations of very recent and often specialised works. Certain of the more recondite alchemical texts would have had only a limited appeal, but the great bulk of the scientific literature was aimed at a wide audience. The medical handbooks produced by Culpeper and the agricultural reform tracts were intentionally designed to reach the type of reader who had been accustomed previously to extremely elementary works written in a more conventional and less scientific form. This improvement in quality followed the pattern set earlier in the century by the mathematical practitioners. Besides achieving the dissemination of scientific information to a wider spectrum of the population, the scientific literature produced during the Puritan Revolution reflected a fundamental change in intellectual standpoint. There developed a general enthusiasm for non-scholastic philosophies, either ancient or modern; but undoubtedly the greatest impact was made by the form of experimental philosophy derived from Bacon, and this bias was reflected in writings on education, technology, agriculture, medicine and the sciences.

6. For an extremely good study of Markham, see F.N.L. Poynter, *A Bibliography of Gervase Markham,* Oxford Bibliographical Society (Oxford, 1962).

Taken as a whole the scientific literature of the Puritan Revolution helped to create a climate of opinion favourable to the philosophical programme of the early Royal Society.

The present study has been concerned with elucidating the work of the puritan element of the scientific community, the emergence of which has been demonstrated in statistical terms by Merton. It has not been my intention to provide a comprehensive guide to scientific discovery in this period, but rather to produce an analysis of the cultural conditions essential to this process. Committed Puritans and parliamentarians were, none the less, the dominant element in the scientific community, and they were responsible for the great bulk of the scientific publications. In addition my treatment of the impact of parliamentary rule on such institutions as the universities and the College of Physicians, has extended the coverage of this study to many individuals who were not sympathetic with puritanism.

The statistical data accumulated by Merton, the historical survey conducted by Christopher Hill in his *Intellectual Origins of the English Revolution* and the reconstruction undertaken in the present book are sufficient to show that the cultivation of science was an important social phenomenon of the mid-seventeenth century. What could be questioned is the relevance of this movement to the main stream of scientific development, as measured by such diverse criteria as Darmstädter's discoveries and inventions, proximity to modern ways of thinking on methodological and metaphysical issues, importance in the generation of a productive approach to specific scientific problems, or contribution to major institutional developments. On all of these criteria the Royal Society and restoration science in general have been accorded supreme importance, while there has been great reluctance to admit that any significant positive role was played by the puritan reformers. It could thence be argued that the statistical evidence relating to the rise of science during the Puritan Revolution is not conclusive, since it may merely reflect the results of largely misdirected effort. The scientific literature produced before 1660 could be regarded as, from a modern standpoint, of uniformly low quality, while the growing body of personnel recruited to science might be thought of as employing its energies unproductively before the restoration.

The dominant historiographical tradition has certainly favoured the view that a dramatic rise in the quality of scientific work occurred after the Puritan Revolution. The restoration natural philosophers are credited with laying the foundations for the best tradition of English inductive science. The image of the dramatic success of the Royal Society was fostered during the early years of the restoration by Cowley, Evelyn, Glanvill and above all by Sprat, and the impression which they gave has been broadly supported by subsequent generations. Apart from certain minor blemishes, which have been ascribed to the tenacity of certain pre-scientific views, or to the participation of dilettantes in the work of the fashionable new society, no difficulty has been experienced by historians in maintaining the reputation of the early Royal Society. While it was readily conceded that the Society was indebted to the pioneers of the new philosophy, on political grounds it was essential for the restoration apologists to minimise the Society's links with the intellectual movements of the Puritan Revolution. Sprat presented the Royal Society as part of a wider scheme to create an English Academy which would reverse the degenerative trends introduced into English culture during the Revolution. Among other things this academy would compile a history of the civil wars 'for there can be no better means to preserve his Subjects in obedience for the future, than to give them a full view of the miseries, that attended the rebellion'.[7] It suited Sprat's ideological commitments to place the Royal Society in the context of the general revival of modern learning. Of all the 'new Philosophers' Francis Bacon was singled out as the 'one great Man, who had the true Imagination of the whole extent of this Enterprise'.[8] The relationship of the founders of the Royal Society to Bacon was seen as a direct one and Sprat acknowledged no debt to the puritan Baconians. Quite the reverse; he argued that the founders had escaped becoming 'engag'd in the passions, and madness of that dismal Age' by retreating into the University of Oxford where they could have 'the satisfaction of breathing a freer air, and of conversing in quiet one with another'.[9] Having achieved this kind of rationalisation Sprat was able to admit that the Royal Society could be traced to antecedents belonging to the Civil War period, while denying that the founders had any significant connection with the dominant religious, political and philosophical parties of that time; they had looked instead for inspiration to the philosophy of the Lord Chancellor to James I.

Later writers have followed Sprat in admitting that a surprisingly large proportion of the leading restoration scientists had been initiated into science during the Puritan Revolution. This applies to almost all of the 'active nucleus' of the Royal Society, and to the vast majority of the 'active members' listed in Chapter II. Of the slightly older generation, very many had been educated in a predominantly puritan environment before 1640. Hence the founders of the Royal Society had been conspicuously exposed to puritan and parliamentarian influences. Regardless of this background, most commentators have been as anxious as Sprat to argue that a considerable intellectual gulf separated the Royal Society pioneers from the exponents of puritan scientific opinion. A fundamental dichotomy is detected within the scientific movement of the 1640s and 1650s, in which the forward-looking scientists of the

7. Sprat (266), p.44.
8. Sprat (266), p.35. A similar point of view was expressed in Cowley's introductory poem to Sprat's *History,* which called Bacon the Moses who had led the Society away from a barren wilderness.
9. Sprat (266), p.53.

Royal Society are rigidly divided from a supposedly ineffectual body of puritan natural philosophers. Sprat's approach has been followed extremely closely by the most recent historian of the early Royal Society. This authority traces the origins of the Society back to John Wilkins, who is eulogised as the architect of the Oxford Experimental Philosophy Club and the principal restorer of Bacon's philosophy. By contrast the major puritan reformers are thought to have been 'temperamentally incapable' of understanding Bacon's conception of science. Compared with the scrupulous, critical, inductive scientists of the Royal Society, Samuel Hartlib and his associates are caricatured as purveyors of 'various practical projects of a limited kind, concerned with such matters as husbandry, methods of school-teaching, and the haphazard collection and dissemination of inventions and discoveries whether proved or merely speculative'.[10]

The intellectual complexion of the founders of the Royal Society is very differently figured by another major authority, who prefers to discover the roots of the scientific achievement of the restoration in the tradition of continental science established by 'highly able, professionally skilled and tough-minded men like Galileo, Kepler and Descartes'.[11] Along with Purver, Hall believes that Hartlib and his colleagues had no real understanding of Bacon's philosophy, being merely concerned 'to pick out the adepts, the inventors, to have rewards offered to them, to assist in perfecting their secrets, and above all to publicise them.'[12] Accordingly, although it is granted that the pre-restoration scientific movement laid the foundations for the work of the Royal Society, modern commentators tend to attribute the greatest importance to the direct influence of Bacon, or to the continental mechanical philosophers, while denying that the puritan intellectual movement played any positive role in this development. The roots of restoration science are thereby disentangled from puritanism and laid instead in the fertile earth of a European philosophical tradition advancing towards the Age of Reason.

It is certainly more congenial to the modern mentality to think of the Royal Society as a manifestation of the progress of the spirit of the disinterested search for scientific truth. But this view is based on a defective interpretation of seventeenth-century natural philosophy, which under-estimates the role of theology and arbitrarily assumes a divorce between social planning and technology on the one hand, and science and philosophy on the other; a dichotomy which cannot be sustained on the basis of the historical evidence. Because of its metaphysical implications, theology must be accepted as a factor directly relevant to the formation

10. Purver (230), pp.206–9.

11. A. R. Hall, 'Science, technology and Utopia in the seventeenth century', in *Science and Society 1600–1900*, ed. P. Mathias (Cambridge, 1972), pp.44–5. For a similar point of view see *idem*, 'Merton Revisited, or Science and Society in the Seventeenth Century', *History of Science*, 1963, *2*: 1–15.

12. Hall, 'Science, technology', p.42.

of scientific concepts, but theological beliefs were important in a much wider context, since no dimension of human speculation or action was untouched by their influence.

According to an equivalent principle, and again on the basis of the historical evidence, it is inadmissible to categorise individuals involved in the investigation of the natural world into such self-contained groups as 'utilitarians', 'technicians' and 'scientists'. Although there was a degree of specialisation of scientific activity, the enthusiasts tended to be involved in science at many different levels, being commonly concerned on the one hand with the theological implications of natural philosophy and on the other with agricultural improvement or mechanical innovations. Conclusions about the independence of scientific activity in the seventeenth century are based not on the impartial and exhaustive examination of evidence, but are rather dictated by the requirements of current ideology, and describe not the relationship which actually existed, but the relationship which it is felt ought to have existed on the basis of present-day opinion about the methodology of science. Elsewhere I have called this the 'restrictive' approach to the history of science, since it presupposes that the sciences developed in a particular manner and that only a narrow range of historical evidence is relevant to the explanation of this phenomenon.[13] This restrictive approach might be acceptable, if it successfully exposed the central mechanism of scientific change, but since it arbitrarily excludes a range of relations fundamental to the understanding of scientific development the technique can only serve to reinforce anachronistic judgements and to obscure the actual pattern of historical change.

The lack of consensus among the orthodox commentators about the philosophical characterisation of the Royal Society suggests that the problem is not amenable to a straightforward solution of the type offered by Sprat. That the Royal Society is difficult to describe in modern terms opens up the possibility that the scientific thinkers of the restoration had more in common with their puritan predecessors than with ourselves. The purist Baconianism described by Purver and the professional experimentalism and mechanical philosophy of Hall are both supported by positive evidence, and both represent legitimate aspects of the work of the Royal Society. On the basis of these and similarly partial approaches, the Royal Society may be portrayed as a body of model Baconians (whatever the model chosen for Baconianism), non-doctrinaire professional experimental scientists, dabblers in natural magic, Hermeticists and Paracelsians, Cartesians or corpuscularian mechanical philosophers, Neoplatonists, etc. All of these elements were present, although no one element was absolutely predominant. Hence a continuous stream of voluble critics from Henry Stubbe and his fellow restoration satirists, to Lynn Thorndike the recent chronicler of the history of magic

13. C. Webster, 'The authorship and significance of *Macaria*', *Past and Present*, 1972, No. 56: 34–48.

and experimental science, has underlined the tendency of the Royal Society from the outset to lapse into the uncritical appraisal of the trivial and the absurd. The Fellows were always aware of this stigma and they were never able to mount adequate defences against their critics, as is indicated by the wavering discussions about the scientific content of Sprat's *History,* or by the inconsequential character of the miscellaneous collection of scientific papers which formed such a large part of the *History.*[14] These mediocre specimens of natural history showed how far the Royal Society had fallen short of the Baconian ideal. It is particularly revealing that Henry Oldenburg, one of the principal architects of the Royal Society's Baconianism, felt embarrassed that Sprat's *History* might lead the reader to doubt 'whether there are performances enough, for a Royal Society, that hath been at work so considerable a time'.[15] It is also notable that the Society chose to defend its scientific reputation with work of an utilitarian bias, and not with specimens of 'modern' scientific discovery.

It is not my contention that there was no serious Baconian motivation within the Royal Society, or that the Fellows made no sustained contribution to such problems as pneumatics or mechanics. But I would like to point out the dangers in assuming too great a uniformity of ethos among Fellows of the Society. Sweeping conclusions have been reached on this subject without any explicit definition of the group to which reference is made. Conclusions about the nature of restoration science depend very much on whether the reference point taken is the entire scientific community, the dominant personnel of the scientific community, the full membership of the Royal Society, the 'active membership' of the Royal Society, or finally the 'active nucleus' of that Society. The Royal Society was initially so large and active that its membership forms the obvious basis for estimates about restoration science, but it is important to appreciate that the Society as a corporate body projected an image which need not necessarily represent the considered viewpoint of more than a small minority of the membership. I have demonstrated in Chapter II that the active nucleus of the Royal Society was extremely diverse in background and philosophical outlook, and the same conclusion applies to the wider categories. Indeed one of the great assets of restoration English natural philosophy both inside and outside the universities and learned societies was its heterogeneity. There was great divergence of opinion on most basic issues and no attempt was made to impose an orthodoxy. The leaders of the scientific movement, such as Boyle, Cudworth, Glisson, Hooke, Oldenburg, Petty, Ray and Willis, represented very different intellectual traditions. Of figures of the second order, many different influences are apparent in the writings of such an eclectic author as Henry Power, while Walter Charleton, very

14. Sprat (266), pp.158–309.

15. Letter from Oldenburg to Boyle, 24 November 1664, Oldenburg *Correspondence,* ii, p.321.

much the intellectual barometer of his age, reflected almost every philosophical point of view in turn, beginning with Helmontianism.

An obvious characteristic, and a further strength, of the English scientific movement was the diversity of interests displayed by individual members. Boyle, Cudworth and Ray were deeply immersed in the theological debate over such questions as materialism, natural law, and God's role in the universe, and on these questions they exerted a long-term influence. Most of the active nucleus of the Royal Society were engaged in a wide variety of scientific researches : many were interested in improvements in medicine, while the dominant element (Boyle, Evelyn, Hooke, Oldenburg, Petty, Wilkins and Wren) were concerned with agriculture, technology, inventions and utilitarian improvements. These 'scientists' were not only actively interested in technology; they were also conversant with the labours of a whole class of technicians and practitioners, whose skills they came to appreciate and imitate. In view of this general concern with innovation and improvement it is not surprising that the Royal Society chose to project itself as a fundamentally Baconian institution, although its Baconian inductivism was neither as exclusive nor as 'modern' as certain modern commentators would have us admit.

It certainly does no justice to the restoration scientists to describe them as 'able, tough-minded, and professional, by no means idealists and dilettantes', in contra-distinction to the 'soft-headed, amateurish or incompetent' utilitarians of the puritan period.[16] Such banal characterisations represent an oversimplification and distortion of the nature of both republican and restoration science, conditioned as they are by a tendency to exaggerate all modern, sophisticated and congenial elements in the later period, while stressing the obsolete, technical and uncongenial elements in the scientific work of the Puritans. The positive scientific achievements of the restoration have been accorded excessive attention, while the scientific work of the Puritans has been almost ignored, on the assumption that it was the product of 'people who wrote about science in general terms [and who] on the whole did little to advance it'.[17] Distinctions of this kind have no real historical foundation.

Looked at from the point of view of the origins of modern science, the picture which emerges of the Puritan Revolution is one in which the puritan intellectuals take on an important but by no means exclusive role in the cultivation of experimental science. From an ideological point of view the scientific community was extremely mixed, each group—Catholic, Anglican, Presbyterian, Independent, separatist (or emergent latitudinarian or deist)—having its own particular bias and priorities, but each contributing its share of the dialogue over the interpretation of the works of nature. Because of their numerical strength, dominant social position, aggressive confidence and scientific awareness,

16. Hall, 'Science, technology', p.45.
17. *Ibid.*

the group falling within the puritan and parliamentarian definition were in a position to make a vital contribution to the rapidly expanding scientific movement. Indeed it would have been extremely incongruous if the Puritans had completely eschewed experimental science, since from a doctrinal point of view they had much in common with those Anglicans who are universally recognised as having been scientifically active. This proximity of outlook is confirmed by the ease with which the two groups merged into a latitudinarian party after the restoration. It has long been appreciated that the latitudinarians played a leading part in the foundation and early work of the Royal Society. In view of the importance of this middle ground there has been some temptation to assimilate the great majority of pre-restoration experimental philosohers, ranging from Hartlib and Dury, to Sprat and Ward, into a diffuse, nascent 'latitudinarian' category, but this has only served to obscure many genuine points of divergence within this group. The introduction of new categories does nothing to diminish the importance of puritanism. If the latitudinarian party is conceived in its widest sense, it becomes largely co-extensive with the puritan movement; whereas if it is conceived in a narrower sense, many intellectuals with unquestionably important scientific interests continue to be categorised as Puritans. In either case puritanism as a general cultural phenomenon, and figures who were puritan and parliamentarian in background, outlook and associations, remain central to the understanding of the English scientific movement.

The introduction of the latitudinarianism issue has however performed one valuable function : it has drawn attention to the dangers of analysing all debates in terms of a basic dichotomy between Puritans and non-Puritans, or between parliamentarians and royalists. For many purposes it is valuable to adopt these classifications, but for purposes of detailed study of the kind undertaken in this book it is necessary to make reference to finer divisions of opinion within the political and religious spectrum. The convention of dividing the spectrum at a central point and terming all individuals to the left of that point 'Puritans' has considerable value as an approximation, but it should not be made to obscure the wide range of variation in the puritan half of the spectrum, or to disguise the affinity between the religious positions on either side of the boundary.

The subjects investigated above show that divisions of opinion frequently arose between the various sections of the puritan community; in most cases, it has been necessary to make reference to the natural groups which occurred within the broader divisions. Each group, whether puritan or non-puritan in primary alignment, tended to develop an attitude towards nature consistent with its social, political and religious position. One cannot observe the workings of the scientific community of this period without noticing the strongly contrasting styles of science which were being evolved in response to different intellectual standpoints.

Thus new entrants into science gravitated towards the group which offered the best opportunity for the realisation of their aspirations, and individuals assumed importance in their fraternity by virtue of their ability to act as effective exponents of a particular ideology. The borderlines between the various groups were never defined rigidly; certain individuals gradually reorientated themselves away from one group and towards another; the pattern of social organisation of science changed in accordance with the pattern of events; nevertheless, at any one point in time it is possible to discern a mosaic of competing groups wedded to different value systems.

The various groups identify themselves both by the type of phenomenon chosen for investigation and by their method of approach. For instance the notable developments in the scientific study of agriculture between 1649 and 1660 were almost entirely the prerogative of a group of Puritans—Hartlib, Blith, Boate, Child, Beale, Culpeper, Austen, etc. On the other hand work in experimental physiology based on the theory of circulation was dominated by Anglicans and royalists—Harvey, Scarburgh, Wren, Willis, Ent, Bathurst, Power, Charleton, etc. In other cases the division occurs along different lines. For instance those Puritans favouring a flexible and decentralised church order (e.g. Dury, Hall, Webster, Dell, Sprigg) were advocates of a science-based education, whereas Puritans sympathetic to the idea of a national church served by beneficed clergy (e.g. Wilkins, Wallis) sided with their Anglican colleagues (e.g. Ward) in opposing the modification of the scholastic curriculum.

In most cases the lines of division are more difficult to draw, but even then noticeable differences in bias are evident. There was for instance extremely widespread interest in the hermetic philosophy; Paracelsus, Comenius and Boehme appealed primarily to Puritans and separatists, whereas the more abstract philosophical authors were taken up by Anglicans. Chemical therapy and the technologically orientated experimental chemistry advocated by Helmont and Glauber respectively were taken up in a highly partisan fashion by Puritans, whereas these authors were given a more restrained and piecemeal welcome by Anglicans.

Puritans as a whole felt that the 'new philosophy' was consistent with the reformed Christian faith. The more radical Puritans cultivated experimental science for its value in utopian social planning, seen in the context of a universal and often animistically conceived regeneration of nature. This group placed a high priority on the search for a systematic control over the works of nature. On the other hand more conservative elements among the Puritans tended to emphasise the value of experimental science as a means to personal enlightenment in a social order which was ordained to be essentially unchanging. In this case they tended to arrive at a more rigidly ordered or even mechanistically conceived construction of the universe. Science became essentially a matter of exposing the immutable pattern of laws bequeathed by divine providence. An ordered body of natural theology became one of the characteristic expressions of this mentality. Those adopting this latter point of view were drawn increasingly closer to Anglican colleagues in their basic conception of nature. Hence although Baconianism provided a common context for puritan science during the Republic, the form of Baconianism favoured by Wilkins and his conservative colleagues took on a different complexion from the Baconianism of the Hartlib circle and the more radical groups. There is therefore considerable justice in Professor Trevor-Roper's characterisation of the former group as the 'High' Baconians and of the latter as the 'Vulgar' Baconians, if High Baconianism is regarded as an expression of the outlook of an élite wedded to traditional social values, and Vulgar Baconianism is seen as the philosophy of a group intent on transforming the social outlook and way of life of the entire population.

Where it has been conceded that some puritan intellectuals made a substantial contribution to seventeenth-century scientific thought, there has often also been a tendency to distinguish absolutely between the parts played by the High and Vulgar Baconians. In general, as indicated above, the former class are regarded as a group of professionals whose contribution was of permanent importance, whereas the latter have been dismissed as amateurs whose work was irrelevant to the central purposes of the Fellows of the Royal Society. There can be no doubt about the importance of John Wilkins as a figurehead in the Baconian movement in the universities, of William Petty as the pioneer of political arithmetic, of John Wallis as a sophisticated mathematician, of Henry Oldenburg as the instigator of a universal scientific correspondence, of Robert Boyle as the major exponent of experimental philosophy in the pre-Newtonian period. Each of these figures, along with many minor associates, spent his formative years during the Puritan Revolution and furthermore, as shown in Chapter II of this book, all were undoubtedly centrally involved in the political and religious affairs of the dominant party during that period. Wilkins, Wallis, Goddard, and Cudworth were from the outset regarded by the parliamentary authorities as persons of unswerving loyalty. They were rewarded for this loyalty and their subsequent compliance earned them great influence and prestige. The younger men William Petty and Robert Boyle associated with the parliamentarian intelligentsia after the first phase of the Civil War; the advance in reputation of both was assisted by their cultivation of influential figures in the parliamentarian party. Oldenburg had begun a similar ascent when the restoration put an end to his expectations of advancement under the parliamentarian regime. Although many of these figures drifted towards a more conservative position, their links with more radical elements in the puritan party were never finally severed. Thus the academics Wilkins, Wallis, Goddard, Cudworth and More began their careers in exactly the same camp as Hartlib, Culpeper and Sadler. Even though the academics recoiled from supporting the utopian policies of the Hartlib group, day-to-day exchanges of information on routine scientific questions continued in a limited but uninterrupted manner.[18] This reinforces other circumstantial evidence suggesting that a state of residual mutual respect was maintained between the two groups. Thus although Ward and Wilkins launched into violent attacks on Dell, Webster and Hobbes for advocating university reform, they tactfully avoided answering the equally severe criticisms of Dury, Hartlib and Hall. Although the intellectual debt of the above-mentioned academics to the Hartlib circle was limited, it is apparent from their interrelationship that there was an area of practical and philosophical interest over which they could feel free to collaborate. When looked at in terms of the full range of their scientific interests, Wilkins and Goddard turn out to have had much in common with Hartlib, Worsley and Beale. Certainly dispassionate examination of the evidence relating to the pre-1660 period would not lead an observer to conclude that the former were operating at a level of sophistication basically different from that of the latter, or that the one group was laying the foundations of modern science, while the other was involved in unrealistic phantasy. Sufficient reasons are not wanting to explain how (for example), even at the end of the Republic Hartlib should regard Wilkins as a suitable head for his Agency for the Advancement of Universal Learning.

The ties of Boyle, Petty and Oldenburg with the Hartlib circle were based on an even more obvious unity of interest and purpose. Boyle's induction into science occurred through the medium of Worsley and the utopian Invisible College. Inevitably this led him in the direction of Hartlib, whose own horizons were expanded by the acquaintance. Worsley and Boyle were to remain among Hartlib's closest scientific coadjutors. Boyle's intellectual maturation occurred in the atmosphere of the Hartlib circle's devotion to Baconian natural history, Glauberian chemistry and Helmontian medicine. Oldenburg and Worsley died within a few days of one another in 1677, and it is interesting that in Lady Ranelagh's affectionate remarks made to Boyle, the two reformers were classed together as two poor men who had 'each of them in their way diligently served their generation, and were friends to us'.[19]

Upon his return from the low countries Petty quickly made common cause with Hartlib, who in turn encouraged Petty's work as an inventor and proponent of educational reform. Hartlib was marginally useful in promoting Petty's career, and Petty found Hartlib a useful source of contacts. But Petty's interest in the Office of Address did not extend to a willingness to subsume his work under its agency. He fully shared the enthusiasm of Boate, Child and Hartlib for social statistics and

18. See for instance G. H. Turnbull (287); C. Webster (319); R. G. Frank (105).
19. Letter from Lady Ranelagh to Boyle, 11 September 1677, Boyle *Works*, vi, pp.531–2. See also letter from Worsley to Sir Thomas Lynch, 30 November 1672, *CSP Col. 1669–74*, p.439.

economic geography, but he preferred to pursue these aims independently, a predisposition which led to a clash of personality with Worsley, who was pursuing largely similar ends in a less well-organised manner. Despite this estrangement, Petty maintained close ties with Hartlib's associates Boyle, Symner and Wood, and he seems to have retained some respect for Hartlib's humanitarian ideals. Unwittingly or not the independently-minded Petty was the main figure to carry into the restoration the ideal of national economic planning and development pioneered by the Hartlib circle.

Henry Oldenburg visited England in 1653 as the diplomatic representative of Bremen. He quickly joined the circle of Lady Ranelagh, Boyle, Hartlib, Dury and Milton; his correspondence before 1660 is dominated by this influential puritan group. Lady Ranelagh and her brother Robert Boyle became Oldenburg's chief patrons; Hartlib took responsibility for the distribution of his letters. John Dury placed his daughter under the guardianship of Oldenburg and his wife; after the latter's death Dury's daughter became Oldenburg's second wife, in 1668. Oldenburg was completely sympathetic with the spiritual outlook of Lady Ranelagh and he felt increasing sympathy with the Quakers. On scientific matters he was impressed by the labours of Hartlib, which he believed 'spelt nothing but the advancement of what is publikely good and privately usefull'.[20] He was at first content to play a modest part in Hartlib's intelligence network, to which he contributed letters from the continent, often composed at as much as weekly intervals and containing the latest information on a broad range of political, diplomatic and scientific matters. Gradually, particularly during the last year of the Republic, Oldenburg's correspondence developed a momentum of its own, as he built up contacts with a wide range of younger scholars who often had little in common with Hartlib. Oldenburg displayed a much greater degree of accommodation than Hartlib to the work of the continental mechanical philosophers. Thus by the time of the foundation of the Royal Society in December 1660 he had effectively taken over from Hartlib as the major English correspondent of continental natural philosophers. Like Boyle he came to take an interest in the physical problems which had for some time dominated the work of the main groups of experimental scientists in France and the low countries. Oldenburg was consequently in an excellent position to supervise the correspondence of the Royal Society, but at no stage did he react against the work of Hartlib, or lose sight of the ultimate humanitarian goals of experimental science.

Thus in a comment which could refer either to Hartlib's group or to other projects under discussion in London, Oldenburg reported to Becher that political affairs in England were moving strongly in the direction of a republican settlement and that he hoped to send details of a plan for a meeting of 'scavans et ingénieux en toutes sortes de

20. Letter from Oldenburg to Hartlib, 21 June 1656, Oldenburg *Correspondence,* i, pp.101–2.

sciences utiles'.[21] Whatever the sentiment in favour of scientific specialisation among his colleagues, Oldenburg consistently expressed the policy of the Royal Society in universalist terms which inevitably remind us of Hartlib's description of the Agency for the Advancement of Universal Learning. For instance, to a new correspondent, Oldenburg wrote of his wish to investigate the secrets of nature for the glory of the Creator and the benefit of mankind (de Naturae Arcanis commercium in Naturae Authoris gloriam, Generisque humani commodum instituere).[22] Similarly he informed the celebrated Hevelius that the Royal Society, with the King's encouragement, was devoted to the improvement of the sciences and arts by observation and experiment for the protection of human life and for social amelioration.[23]

This attitude was carried over into *Philosophical Transactions,* which in many respects may be regarded as an expansion and formalisation of up-to-date collections of information of the kind recorded in Hartlib's Ephemerides until 1660. Indeed through such agents as Boyle, Beale and Oldenburg the Royal Society was able to take over directly not only certain projects begun by Hartlib's group, but also materials from Hartlib's own papers. Oldenburg's prefaces to the *Philosophical Transactions* and his letters to prospective contributors contained exhortations to natural philosophers throughout the world to embark on the systematic exploitation of nature for the benefit of the entire human race. For instance Oldenburg appealed to Stanislas Lubienietzki to report on observations, experiments, mechanical inventions, medical and chemical secrets from Germany and Poland, with a view to assisting the Royal Society's programme to construct a solid system of philosophy which was in a real sense adapted to the necessities of human life.[24] In appealing to John Winthrop to supply information about the mines and agriculture of New England, Oldenburg asked his correspondent to remember that the Society had 'taken to taske the whole Universe' and that their number would achieve 'immortal fame of themselves, and the important benefit of this Island, and whole Mankind'.[25]

The evidence cited above is sufficient to show that the influential group of scientists of the Royal Society who came from a puritan and parliamentarian background had distinct links and in some cases extremely strong bonds of common belief with the Puritans who took up a more radical stance on social and scientific matters. There is therefore nothing in the evidence to support the view that on scientific matters the

21. Letter from Oldenburg to J. J. Becher, 2 March 1659/60, Oldenburg *Correspondence,* i, p.359.

22. Letter from Oldenburg to Peter van Dam, 23 January 1662/3, Oldenburg *Correspondence,* ii, p.13.

23. Letter from Oldenburg to Hevelius, 18 February 1662/3, Oldenburg *Correspondence,* ii, p.25.

24. Letter from Oldenburg to Lubienietzki, 23 July 1666, Oldenburg *Correspondence,* iii, pp.191–2.

25. Letter from Oldenburg to Winthrop, 13 December 1667, Oldenburg *Correspondence,* iii, pp.525–6.

puritan intellectuals can be divided into two distinct and isolated groups only one of which was seriously concerned with the cultivation of science and, thereby, relevant to the rise of modern science. Every step in a more detailed analysis of the situation tends moreover to suggest that puritanism and the period of the Puritan Revolution are more important for the understanding of developments after 1660 than is generally conceded.

It has already been demonstrated in quantitative terms that the rise of the English scientific movement correlates extremely closely with the growth in strength of the puritan party. It is also clear that the Royal Society can be traced back to antecedent associations established by predominantly puritan groups of intellectuals meeting in London during 1645 and 1646. It has as a corollary been proved impossible to drive a wedge between the Puritan Revolution and the restoration in terms of the philosophical context or intellectual sophistication of scientific work. Although much research came to fruition after 1660, the groundwork had been laid in a substantial manner in the previous decades. This is true even if attention is confined to the commonplace case-histories of history of science, while the strength of the scientific movement of the Puritan Revolution is even more apparent if consideration is extended to the range of topics discussed in the main body of the present book. Finally, on the more general questions of philosophical alignment, Baconianism, Neoplatonism, hermeticism or the various forms of mechanical philosophy taken up during the restoration, represent clearly established positions having active groups of exponents during the Puritan Revolution.

The presence of some kind of gulf in scientific activity around 1660 would have made it much easier to claim that puritanism was irrelevant to the explanation of the rise of the English scientific movement. As it is the rise of experimental science correlates almost exactly with the upsurge of puritanism. It has been argued that this is an accidental relationship and that experimental science was successfully cultivated mainly by the non-puritan element in the English church; or alternatively by this group with the assistance of certain reluctant Puritans, and perhaps a narrow conservative segment of the puritan faction. But it is clear that this exclusion principle, however operated, is ineffectual. It is possible to argue at one extreme that the English Catholics (e.g. Richard Towneley, or Sir Kenelm Digby), or at the other, that religious radicals (e.g. Webster, Winstanley, Pinnel, or Sparrow), were highly receptive to the new philosophy or experimental science. What is important from the point of view of the present study is that there is ample evidence to suggest that the entire puritan movement was conspicuous in its cultivation of the sciences, that its members became vigorous proponents of a variety of new approaches to natural philosophy, and that it can be shown that their scientific beliefs were framed with conscious reference to their religious views, each section within the puritan sphere of influence developing a scientific outlook consistent with its doctrinal position. It is reasonable to believe that other religious groups only briefly touched upon in the present study operated in a precisely similar manner. In other words each group at this period of intellectual crisis was involved in readjusting its view of nature with reference to general ideological considerations. What makes the Puritans such an invaluable case study for illustrating this principle is, as already implied, their numerical strength, social importance, their pronounced attention to scientific matters and the explicit manner in which they articulated their ideas about religion, society and the natural world. While it is not contended that an account of the scientific activities of the Puritans embodies everything of significance about the emergent English scientific tradition, it can be claimed to make a vital contribution towards the understanding of the basic motivations of a large group ranging from Worsley, French, Webster and Hartlib to More, Wilkins, Boyle and Oldenburg, and towards the explanation of some of the most important developments in science itself. It is also necessary to bear in mind that the scientific initiative of the Puritans was so productive that the influence of their work and outlook extended to many figures (e.g. Evelyn, Cowley, Digby, Aubrey) with whom they had otherwise little in common.

The contribution of puritan intellectuals is extremely important even if the estimate is made in terms of positive addition to the mathematical and physical sciences, which is the narrowest index used by the historian of science. In this field Boyle and Wallis were supremely important, while in other capacities such figures as Graunt, Petty, Wood, Oldenburg and Wilkins played a notable role, either as subsidiary investigators and intelligencers, or as pioneers of quantification. 'Scientific discoveries' are better seen as the end product of a lengthy phase of research which usually involves collaborative work, the exchange of information by letter, journal, or published monograph, reliance on outside technical expertise, and often reference to formalised agencies for scientific research. Use of this broader, sociological criterion enables a picture to be built up which has a much greater degree of historical validity, but it is also necessary to recollect that experimental investigations and conceptual advances themselves have tended to be treated very selectively by the historian of science. For most scientists educated in the industrialised, urbanised and technologically orientated society of the present century, the greatest value is placed on the history of such recognisable subjects as cosmology, the theory of matter, mechanics, optics and the development of calculus—those subjects which are familiar in terms of contemporary priorities, and prevailing notions about the philosophy of science, a subject which draws its conclusions on the basis of referring almost exclusively to the physical sciences. It should be appreciated that in the pre-industrial period, and in a nation which was largely agrarian, and where the educated élite was largely ignorant of the rudiments of the modern physical sciences, the signs of significant adjustments in intellectual perspective should be sought in subjects high in the contemporary estimation, such as medicine, agriculture and natural history, and in technical subjects relating to the embryonic industries, such as chemistry, metallurgy and mining. Just as it is necessary to recognise the interdependence of philosophical and theological issues, and of the technical and the scientific, so the 'modern' scientific discovery should be looked at in a new perspective, which places it as merely one type of end-product of investigations that can never be completely understood unless reference is made to a wide range of historical factors. Given this order of priorities, it is only consistent to turn away from the classic scientific case-history, to consider such basic issues as the reasons which led a particular society to have a high level of awareness of, and high expectations of understanding, the mechanism of nature. It is also indispensable to know what factors led to dissatisfaction with traditional modes of explanation, and why enthusiasm developed for particular forms of experimental philosophy among such large groups of individuals drawn from many sections of society. Finally it should be considered why energies became directed towards particular problems and what were the determinants of interest in the formal organisation of scientific effort. It may seem that such questions involve excessive attention to factors remote from the end-point of scientific discovery, but this approach is essential if science is to to be seen in its proper historical perspective, and if we are to achieve more than a superficial understanding of scientific change.

In the present study I have sought to explore the relevance of puritanism to the investigation of the natural world in terms of contemporary priorities and with reference to wider contextual factors. The ideas and projects described above illustrate in detailed terms the scientific implications of the world-embracing asceticism which has been described as one of the key manifestations of the social ethic of the Puritans. This question has been treated in general terms by Troeltsch and Weber, and the relevance of the puritan ethic to the rise of experimental science, hinted at by Weber, has been discussed by Merton with particular reference to the seventeenth-century English scientific movement.[26] Somewhat surprisingly none of these commentators has paid more than passing attention to the intellectual movements particularly associated with the Puritan Revolution. They have been chiefly interested in tracing the social implications of Calvinist soteriology, while I have also been concerned to show that eschatology became an important determinant of scientific attitudes. The Puritans were conditioned by the ideal of a dedicated vocational life, which involved the most efficient use of abilities for personal advantage and public service. The glorification of

26. E. Troeltsch, *The Social Teachings of the Christian Churches,* trans. O. Wyon, 2 vols. (London, 1931); M. Weber, *The Protestant Ethic and the Spirit of Capitalism,* trans. T. Parsons (London, 1930); *idem, The Sociology of Religion,* trans. E. Fischoff (London, 1965); R. K. Merton (188), pp.55–111. A slightly different, but extremely valuable approach to this subject is illustrated by the work of Perry Miller (189).

God was thus linked to the idea of the most efficient exploitation of human and material resources. In line with this ethical perspective we find among the Puritans : general dissatisfaction with previous standards, receptivity to alternatives, enthusiasm for efficient education and vocational training, and a ceaseless search for general improvement. The Puritans were dedicated to unremitting exertion, and increasingly they were sympathetic to the virtues of manual labour; successful accomplishment of works provided one of the major means whereby some intimation of election might be obtained, and the sciences, particularly the utilitarian sciences, were one of the avenues whereby substantial works could be performed. The Calvinist God was distant and inscrutable, but the patient and accurate methods of experimental science, penetrating slowly towards an understanding of the secondary causes of things in the search for a gradual reconquest of nature, represented the form of intellectual and practical endeavour most suited to the puritan mentality. Immediate goals were conceived with a proper humility, and progress was necessarily slow, but every step brought further insight into the providence of God, so constantly reaffirming the correctness of the procedure. On the other hand eschatology drew attention to the fact that man had fallen from a position of high attainment, and that in the not-too-distant future he was destined to regain his dominion over nature. Although it was held that this outcome was inevitable, the puritan social ethic precluded any passive reliance on the providential dispensation to bring about this instauration. The eschatological perspective of the Puritans was significantly different from that of many other protestant groups. Calvinists had traditionally believed in the supreme importance of the growth of authority of the church; they were much less concerned with the ideal of the reconquest of nature. Protestant mystics tended to emphasise the virtues of individual illumination through their ideal of the *unio mystica.* The millenarian sects relied on an imminent divine intervention for the punishment of their adversaries and the reward of the elect. By contrast with their protestant allies, the Puritans were convinced that their place among the elect, and the nation's place as the seat of the New Jerusalem, would be assured only if they devoted the utmost energies to the pursuit of a godly life. They believed that not only would they be allowed to progress towards the millennial condition, even before the advent of the last judgement, but that also their rigorous discipline would earn signs of election in the form of personal and national rewards. The Puritans genuinely thought that each step in the conquest of nature represented a move towards the millennial condition, and that each extension of the power of parliament reflected the special providential status of their nation.

Thus the ambitious aims and unflagging zeal which were characteristic of the puritan endeavour to exploit the natural environment for the health and wealth of mankind, were sustained by an enduring expectation of intellectual and social progress. This idea of progress was religious in motivation, but it had the capacity to develop a largely secular expression. The millennial context was important because it carried the guarantee of utopian rewards in the near future, while the puritan social ethic determined that great emphasis was placed on the power of the enlightened elect to bring about their own utopian transformation. Hence the Puritans evolved a system of values incorporating an extremely pronounced belief in social and intellectual progress which, while initially dependent on millenarian eschatology, could persist as millenarianism gradually waned in significance during the later part of the century, and become transmuted into a general secular belief in progress, of the kind which is found during the Enlightenment.[27]

The prevalent social ethic of the Puritans left them in no doubt of their responsibility as agents of the reformed faith to undertake a conscientious and open-minded investigation into the natural world. Such an obligation might be inferred from the theological writings of Perkins, Preston, Ames and their followers, and a whole range of intermediate writings enables us to bridge the gulf between abstract theological pronouncements and practical scientific investigations.[28] In the first half of the seventeenth century the protestant scale of values was such that an implicit obligation was felt to defend all social action and intellectual interests in religious terms. No activity was encouraged unless it was reconcilable with the Christian ethical code, and every human thought and action was thought to bear in some way on personal spiritual standing, or the providential order of things. It was therefore not possible to embark on any course of metaphysical speculation without conscious reference to doctrinal implications, or on any course of practical activity without considering whether it contributed to the life of the Christian Commonwealth.

The pervasiveness of an essentially religious conception of the universe is apparent from the lives and work of the figures discussed in the present volume. It is particularly obvious from the self-conscious attempts to construct a durable Christian philosophy on the part of the Boehmists, Comenius, Boyle, Ray, More and Cudworth. The scientific aspect of the writings of these figures is enveloped in voluminous theological disquisition. Minor authors exhibit the same tendency. It has already been noted for instance that John Wilkins and Seth Ward composed theological apologias for their scientific work at the outset of their academic careers.

27. E. L. Tuveson, *Millennium and Utopia* (Berkeley and Los Angeles, 1949); J. B. Bury, *The Idea of Progress* (London, 1920); C. L. Becker, *The Heavenly City of the Eighteenth Century Philosophers* (New Haven, 1932).

28. I hope to return to this subject in future writings. A substantial basis for the understanding of puritan casuistry is provided by Miller (189). See also G. L. Mosse, *The Holy Pretence: A Study in Christianity and the Reason of State from Perkins to John Winthrop* (Oxford, 1957); H. R. McAdoo, *The Structure of Anglican Moral Theology* (London, 1949); T. Wood, *English Casuistical Divinity in the Seventeenth Century* (London, 1952).

Wilkins and Ward argued very much along the lines established by Preston, who admitted that although the natural faculties had decayed as a result of the Fall, the universe contained such clear evidence of God's handiwork that every man was capable of rectifying his senses to appreciate that the wisdom of God was displayed in the works of creation. This view was neatly summarised by Winstanley who declared that 'To know the secrets of nature, is to know the works of God; And to know the works of God within the Creation, is to know God himself, for God dwels in every visible work or body'. Winstanley was tempted to go much further than Preston, to regard natural religion as the only way to attain 'actual knowledge of the creator', rather than as merely a complement to revealed religion.[29]

This point of view was quite unacceptable to Dell and Webster, who only expressed their positive plans for educational and scientific reform after a period of intensive pamphleteering in the course of which they elaborated their arguments in favour of 'experimental' faith. To them revelation was of supreme importance, the sciences being esteemed primarily for their utilitarian value.

Ralph Austen, the humble registrar to the Visitors at Oxford, used his informative little tract on the growing of fruit trees as a vehicle for a devotional work *The Spiritual Use of An Orchard,* which is in some respects the puritan counterpart of Sir Thomas Browne's *Garden of Cyrus* (1657). Austen believed that 'Fruit-trees and other Creatures doe truely . . . Preach Attributes and perfections of God to us'. This combination of horticulture and theology proved to be successful. The first edition of *A Treatise of Fruit Trees with the Spiritual Use of An Orchard* (1653) devoted 97 pages to the former and 41 pages to the latter subject, whereas in the second edition (1657) both sections were expanded, to 140 and 208 pages respectively. Thus despite the effectiveness and popularity of the practical part, the theological section came to preponderate.

Recognising the importance of puritan casuistry, Hartlib and Dury took great pains to defend their policies for the organisation of intellectual effort in terms of cases of conscience. They were determined to show that their schemes were consistent with the highest codes of Christian conduct. In this context it is interesting to note that John Dury buttressed the published tracts on the practical aspects of the Office of Address with a long manuscript theological treatise justifying the Offices for Communications and Accommodations in terms of the Christian 'dutie of Communication in Spiritual and Rationall Matters'; which was itself justified in terms immediately of the need for the twin reformations of public and private life to go hand in hand, and thence ultimately with reference to the goal of communion with the mystical body of God. Using this chain of reasoning Dury argued that the work of the Office of Address provided an ideal 'Experimentall proof and

29. Winstanley (336), p.50.

trial, or of Scientificall Demonstration . . . that their standing and walking is with God'.[30] Elsewhere Dury and Hartlib developed a similar argument in a more explicitly millennial context, arguing that 'mutual and universal edification', aimed at the spread of 'love and good works' on earth, was an essential part of the preparation for the emergence of the rule of the saints.[31]

In his preface to *Irelands Natural History* Dury followed very much the same line of argument as did Wilkins in the *Beauty of Providence*, giving the most frequently used justification for natural theology, Romans 1 :20, and warning, 'such as respect him not, in the Creation of the World, and in the wayes of his Providence, may be without excuse'. However, whereas Wilkins paid more attention to the value of the study of nature for the purposes of spiritual enlightenment, Dury placed his emphasis on knowledge which was relevant 'to the comforts and Publick Use of a Societie'. In this context husbandry was particularly esteemed in view of its importance as the basis of the economy of plantations. It also followed that one of the most useful forms of activity was 'to have the knowledg of the Natural History of each Nation advanced & perfected'. Once again Dury drew attention to the relevance of the millennium to this scientific programme. He believed that in the autumn of the world perfection of bodily things would prepare the way for the final spiritual enlightenment. Hence the compilers of natural histories would find that in the near future 'when the time of the Restauration of all things, shall come . . . then also the properties and application of the Creature by his means obscured, shall be revealed'.

It has already been pointed out in Chapter I that the Puritans came to accept an extremely literal interpretation of the millennium. An important group, consisting particularly of those with scientific aspirations (as well as the notorious Fifth Monarchists) believed that a utopian state ruled by the elect would be the logical and inevitable conclusion of the struggles of the parliamentarians. This expectation did not lessen during the final years of the Republic. Beale, Hartlib, Culpeper and Worsley seem in their correspondence to make increasing albeit more frantic references to the millennium, as if they were appealing for divine intervention to assist flagging human efforts. For instance in late 1658, Worsley appealed for Potter to take comfort in the assurance that the Lord would usher the millennium 'into the World (and that hee may doe for anything I know in a few, it may be a very few moneths). All the force that can bee made in the World will not be able to resist it'.[32]

Biblicism was one of the most conspicuous elements in English puritanism. Decisions on all issues were approached with explicit and obli-

30. Dury, 'A Further Discoverie of the Office of Address', HP XLVII 10.
31. Hartlib (ed.), *Clavis Apocalyptica* (London, 1651).
32. Letter from Worsley to William Potter, 17 November 1658, HP XXVI 33. For similar comments by Beale, see above, pp.11–12.

gatory reference to the revealed word of God. This bias could have severely limited the expression of the new science in England. The Bible might have been used as an authoritarian scholastic text to implant an inflexible and obsolete view of nature. Indeed some of the protestant textbooks or theological treatises had precisely this effect, by using biblical authorities as a means to enhance scholastic or hermeticist ideas about physics and cosmology. By contrast it is noticeable that the Puritans utilised the scriptures to instil a high regard for the active investigation of nature, through emphasis on natural theology and utilitarianism, and by illustrative reference to the attainments of such figures as Solomon. Typically, Benjamin Worsley pointed out in his long discussion of this problem that God could not be expected, except in certain superficial instances, to reveal directly the essential principles of nature, since this would serve as an incentive towards vanity and sloth; instead the Bible 'in Physicall controversies, . . . hath left men a latitude, to seek (in the free use, exercise, and improvement of their Senses and Reason) to determine them'.[33] Thus Worsley believed that for the purpose of encouraging man to adopt mental attitudes and undertake physical labours conducive to salvation, God had utilised the scriptures as a means of inducing a rational, active and undogmatic approach towards nature. By adopting this standpoint the Puritans could continue to rely on the scriptures to determine their ethical bias, while securing almost complete freedom of action in specific investigations.

The above remarks indicate that Puritans came for a variety of reasons to place a high value on the active study of nature. This was true regardless of whether individual enlightenment or social behaviour was under consideration, and regardless of the importance attached to personal revelation. The God of the Puritans was not only to be admired for the wisdom of his handiwork, or for the creation of an edifice which could be interpreted in terms of a rational system of laws; he was also seen as the architect of an evolutionary process which would lead in the near future to a new level of perfection both in man himself and in nature. The study of nature offered not only a means to intellectual gratification, but also the possibility of immediate and legitimate utilitarian rewards for all social classes. Those who were willing to exploit nature to its uttermost would serve a hard apprenticeship, which none the less promised to earn them almost unlimited blessings in the imminent future.

Puritanism played an active part in promoting other values which were basic to the modern scientific movement. In the period of revived expectations for reformation and the millennium the puritan movement encouraged a critical attitude towards inherited wisdom, an emancipation from scholastic values and an enthusiasm among all social classes for intellectual enlightenment and material progress. Thus there was not

33. Letter from Worsley to Hall, 16 February 1667/8, HP XXXVI 6.

only an acceleration of recruitment into science, and a broadening of its social base of operation, but also a much more fertile exchange of ideas between the social classes and a general rise in the level of mutual co-operation. The sciences became more generally cultivated among the élite, and the greater dignity attached to manual labour encouraged the élite to engage in experimental manipulation and to learn from artisans. Reciprocally the artisans felt encouraged to a new level of intellectual attainment in order that they might take part in more abstract investigations. In this context it is notable that Samuel Hartlib's large group of collaborators contained elevated figures like Boyle and Sir Cheney Culpeper in co-operation with a much larger group who were from more humble backgrounds, and who had no experience of higher education, and would not normally have had access to facilities for the publicisation of their ideas. Through the agency of figures like Hartlib, talented individuals like Plattes, Dymock and Petty were encouraged to exercise their fullest influence. By means of this intellectual and social reorientation, which has been termed the 'marriage' of the craftsman and the intellectual, investigators came to have access to the full range of skills necessary for the examination and solution of complex scientific problems. In addition new areas of investigation such as practical chemistry, metallurgy and agriculture captured the imagination of the élite.

The puritan initiative for the organisation of intellectual activity, related as it was to their ideal of effective employment of vocational talent, was of the utmost importance for the growth of the English scientific movement. This impulse generated a highly professional and committed attitude to personal effort, as well as a feeling that individual gratification should be accompanied by the communication of knowledge to others. Hartlib's tremendous network of communication became the main component in the mechanism for the exchange of information among puritan investigators of technical and scientific problems. Although lacking a completely formal basis, Hartlib's Office of Address achieved the position of a central agency for scientific communication. Before 1660 virtually every new recruit to Baconian science made a point of soliciting Hartlib's assistance. The service for the English Baconians performed by Hartlib was gradually taken over by Oldenburg. Clearly, the tradition of the free communication of scientific information, at the time of its being championed by the Royal Society, was already firmly established among the Puritans. It is notable that such diverse authors as Hartlib, Plattes, Blith and Boyle emphasised that their scientific writings were produced as a means of meeting the obligation to undertake the free communication of knowledge, since knowledge was in any case only obtained by the grace of God. It is also notable that a non-Puritan such as Evelyn, or an ambitious entrepreneur like Petty, found it extremely difficult to accept this obligation to undertake the completely uninhibited release of his scientific 'secrets'. However the correspondence of this period shows that there was a widespread willingness among Puritans to sacrifice proprietorial rights in the interests of disseminating scientific information. This sociological factor is most important for understanding the means whereby such a figure as Boyle was able to attain an encyclopaedic acquaintance with developments in the sciences at a very early stage in his career. It is apparent that Culpeper, Beale, Worsley, Collins, and many other enthusiasts were making an extremely constructive contribution to the scientific movement, although their names are very little known from the published scientific literature of the period. Ideally, the Puritan was to attach a minimum of importance to the personal attribution of scientific knowledge; hence in the publications of the Hartlib circle very little attention was paid to the identification of the authors of either whole tracts or sections of composite works. *Macaria* and *A Further Discovery of the Office of Address* were published anonymously, whereas in other cases tracts issued under such headings as 'published by Samuel Hartlib for the general good of the nation' were actually composed by his associates. Thomason believed that *A Common Writing* (1647) was written by Hartlib, despite the fact that the preface was signed 'F.L.W.' (Francis Lodwick). Initials subscribed to the preface were often the only clue to authorship. Beale wished to present his large agricultural treatise anonymously out of a desire to 'sacrifice my selfe, an unconsiderable member, for the public good'.[34] Such conventions are so alien to the modern mentality that Lord Ernle has mistaken Hartlib's initiative in the dissemination of the work of others for a case of unscrupulous plagiarism.[35]

The Puritans were not content with informal associations; on political, religious and commercial matters bonds of common interest were signified by formal agreements or covenants specifying the conditions and rules of partnership. This tendency extended into the scientific sphere, and it greatly assisted the movement towards scientific organisation. Another factor encouraging this development was familiarity with the attempts made during the Thirty Years War by German protestant intellectuals to establish formal societies, fraternities and academies devoted to the purification of their faith and to the reform of specific areas of knowledge. That this pattern was being applied to promote the advancement of the sciences in England is apparent at the outset of the Puritan Revolution, with such manifestations as Plattes's College of Experience, Comenius's Universal College, and the pact signed by Dury, Comenius and Hartlib, which among other things pledged their support for the reform of education and learning.[36] The growth of scientific organisation among the Puritans has been described in Chapter II above. Puritans like Hartlib, Wilkins, Goddard, Boyle and

34. Letter from Beale to Hartlib, 19 March 1658/9, HP LI.
35. Ernle (95), pp.108–9.
36. 'Foederis fraterni ad mutuam in publico Christianismi', *HDC,* pp.458–60.

Worsley played a leading part in evolving the complex of scientific 'societies', 'colleges' or 'clubs' which emerged in England between 1640 and 1660. Under their aegis, these organisations made rules of membership, evolved programmes of research, organised the distribution of labour and even gathered resources for the employment of ancillary help. Such societies quickly attracted public attention and were a major factor in the rejuvenation of other academic institutions. There was also a notable enlargement of perspective to take into account the value of national and international co-operation. Thus before the restoration the foundations were laid for the establishment of a major scientific organisation in England, and many of the figures who had been active before 1660 were equipped to take the initiative in the creation of scientific societies adapted to meet the requirements of restoration conditions.

As well as promoting widespread participation in experimental science and encouraging its institutional embodiment, the Puritans also played an important part in framing its coherent ideological expression. It has already been noted that puritanism operated as a force in favour of emancipation from scholastic philosophy. There was a general enthusiasm for *philosophia libera,* which implied open-minded examination of all philosophical systems whatever their provenance—ancient or modern. Puritanism gave no sanction to a complete reaction against ancient philosophy, or to any uninhibited acceptance of modern philosophy—no system of values resting on biblical authority could tolerate such a step, and no one codified system, however useful didactically, was likely to meet the needs of the puritan intellect. Hence there developed among the Puritans an omnivorous interest both in neglected ancient sources and in all expressions of the new philosophy. Since puritan theology encouraged both rational and empirical procedures, all philosophical points of view were guaranteed serious consideration by at least some section of the puritan community. John Webster called for 'people professing the Christian Religion to adhere unto that Philosophy . . . that is grounded upon sensible, rational, experimental, and Scripture principles'. The authors whom he recommended as alternatives to the scholastic philosophers included Plato as revived by Patrizi and Ficino; Democritus as interpreted by Descartes, Regius and Holwarda; Epicurus as illustrated by Gassendi; 'Philolaus, Empedocles & Parmenides, resuscitated by Telesius, Campanella . . . ; and that excellent Magnetical Philosophy found out by Doctor Gilbert; That of Hermes, revived by the Paracelsian School', as well as the works of Fludd which he regarded as the most complete philosophical exposition of the Christian point of view available at the time.[37] Pronouncements of this kind about the revival of philosophy were made by numerous authors during the Puritan Revolution, and it is clearly

37. Webster (326), pp.105–6.

extremely misleading to interpret them in terms of a general onslaught of the 'moderns' against the 'ancients'.

During the Puritan Revolution each of the above philosophies found its champion, and each religious group evolved its own conception of the most suitable basis for a Christian philosophy. The Cambridge Puritans followed Whichcote's drift towards Platonism; other advocates of spiritual religion favoured Paracelsus and Boehme. But the figure who exercised the greatest single influence was Francis Bacon, whose programme was able to attract support from reformers of many different philosophical complexions.

Bacon's philosophy seemed to be providentially designed for the needs of the Puritan Revolution. Indeed this suitability was not accidental, considering that the philosopher had an intellectual ancestry largely in common with the English Puritans. Bacon gave precise and systematic philosophical expression to the anti-authoritarianism, inductivism and utilitarianism which were such important factors in the puritan scale of values. The metaphysical aspect of his philosophy avoided the atheistic tendencies which eventually rendered so much of the new philosophy anathema to the protestants. Furthermore Bacon's philosophy was explicitly conceived in the biblical and millenarian framework which was so congenial to the Puritans. One of Bacon's favourite texts affirmed that 'the glory of God is to conceal a thing, but the glory of the king is to find it out'; God had hidden the secrets of nature in such a manner that they would be discovered only by those who took up the call for an active and patient investigation of nature after the example of Solomon. This call had been taken up during the Reformation, and 'that as all knowledge appeareth to be a plant of God's own planting, so it may seem the spreading and flourishing or at least the bearing and fructifying of this plant, by a providence of God, nay not only by a general providence but by a special prophecy, was appointed to this autumn of the world'.[38]

Bacon's view of nature was substantiated and given a didactic impulse by Comenius, with the result that the Puritans entered the revolutionary decades with a philosophical programme ideally suited to their mood for spiritual, social and intellectual reform. Bacon's writings came to have almost canonical authority, and they were used to induce all sections of the population to join together to exploit the potentialities of experimental philosophy. The revolutionaries felt that they were in a position to reap the reward of a national greatness based on the revival of learning, which had been spurned by the corrupt Stuart kings.

Bacon's works were further used to define puritan ideas on the ethical standpoint, methodology and organisation of science. They were also used as a starting-point for specific investigations in specific areas of medicine and agriculture. But the most important legacy of Bacon

38. Bacon, *Valerius Terminus,* in *Works,* iii, pp.220–1.

to the Puritans was his concept of natural history. Bacon's ideas on natural history as framed in his later writings and as applied in a number of fragmentary case studies became the basis for much of the most substantial scientific work of the Puritans. Natural history was attractive to them by virtue of its freedom from authoritarian influence, sound inductive foundation, and great utilitarian potential. It was the form of the new science which could most readily be translated into a positive programme for research to be undertaken by scholars and craftsmen wedded to the puritan ideal of intellectual enlightenment and social service. The systematic compilation of a natural history of the kingdoms of nature was most effectively conducted by John Ray and his colleagues. However the greatest efforts were reserved for the application of this method of natural history to the more unfamiliar areas of economic geography, agriculture and medicine. Boate, Petty and Graunt, Boyle and Sydenham demonstrated the applicability of Bacon's methodology to the areas of utilitarian importance. The long-term natural history research projects begun before 1660 built up into a substantial framework for the scientific effort of the Royal Society, and the Baconianism of the puritan intellectuals was gradually assimilated and adapted to meet the ideological requirements of the dominant groups of restoration scientists. Like their puritan predecessors, they found that Baconian natural history provided an unassailable foundation for experimental philosophy, whereas critics could more readily detect in other forms of natural philosophy the seeds of atheism and subversion.

Thus one of the most direct legacies of the Puritans to the restoration scientific movement was their effective use of the Baconian philosophy as a vehicle to implant in English society an active and exploratory approach towards the natural environment. As a consequence experimental philosophy had before 1660 become firmly established in the system of accepted values, and the foundations had been laid for the substantial scientific achievements of the later part of the seventeenth century. The recent comparative sociological survey undertaken by Ben-David has correctly concluded that Baconianism played the leading part in making 'revolutionary England, of all the countries of the West, . . . the center of the [scientific] movement during the middle of the seventeenth century'. Baconianism prevented natural philosophy from degenerating into a conflict between rival philosophical interests and it provided 'the blueprint of an ever-expanding and changing, yet regularly functioning scientific community'. The Baconianism of the Puritans supplied English science with a valid strategy for conduct and a sense of coherence which were lacking in most scientific groups elsewhere.[39]

A very substantial body of evidence commends the use of the term 'Baconianism' to describe the dominant tendency in English natural

39. J. Ben-David, *The Scientist's Role in Society: A Comparative Study* (New York, 1971), pp.72–4.

philosophy in the middle decades of the seventeenth century. The identification of Bacon himself with the main current in English thought, and the subsequent widespread concurrence with the outlook expressed in the *Instauratio Magna* have been appreciated by numerous commentators since the early nineteenth century, when Bacon first attracted serious historical attention. This conclusion is not likely to be greatly modified in the light of a recent suggestion that in view of Bacon's affinities with the later natural magic tradition, the entire Baconian movement might be more properly designated as part of a 'Rosicrucian' tradition.[40]

The puritan movement which collapsed so completely in 1660 as an ecclesiastical and political force, exercised an enduring effect in the areas of science, technology and agriculture. It would have been injudicious for contemporaries to admit such continuity, and indeed they were obliged to distract attention from it, but the marks of puritanism were indelibly stamped into the fabric of restoration science. The Puritans thus made a notable contribution in respect of the emergence of the modern worldview, but they themselves would not have been satisfied with this result. They had embarked on a more adventurous voyage and the majority of figures discussed in the present study would have felt that their aspirations were realised in only a minor way by such institutions as the Royal Society. Indeed the puritan intellectuals who rehabilitated themselves at the restoration partly shared this conviction. The Royal Society palpably failed to live up to the grandiose pretensions of its charters, and it was not for more than a limited period, and in certain specific areas, the spearhead of the English scientific movement. Henry Oldenburg kept alive the universalist aims of the Society, and William Petty persisted in his plans for the rational planning of the national economy, but circumstances prevented the Royal Society from becoming an effective centre for ambitious scientific enterprises relating to national economic development.

In 1668 Comenius revised his *Via Lucis,* which had been composed at the outset of the Civil War, and dedicated it to the Royal Society in the hope that the institution under its royal patron would pledge itself to the ideals of his utopian *Collegium lucis*. Such expectations were ill-

40. F. A. Yates, 'The Hermetic Tradition' (345); *idem, The Rosicrucian Enlightenment* (346). For my earlier criticism of this point of view see Webster (321).

Wider application of the term 'Rosicrucian' is undesirable for the following reasons:

(a) ambiguity would be created, in view of the quite different meanings of the term used in its narrow and wide senses;
(b) it would tend to attach undue importance to one of a number of seventeenth-century hermeticist myths. Rosicrucianism is best thought of as a peripheral and extreme expression of hermeticism, which never appealed to more than a small group of devotees of the esoteric;
(c) many figures whom Miss Yates describes as Rosicrucian were explicit and active opponents of Rosicrucianism.

founded. Events had moved beyond the point at which millennial hopes of England's becoming the vanguard of a world reformation could be legitimately upheld. Nevertheless, less than thirty years previously Comenius, along with sophisticated thinkers like Milton and learned theologians like Twisse, had believed that God had ordained an imminent transformation which would rescue Europe from the catastrophies of the Thirty Years War and England from the persecutions of the Laudian regime, and which would possibly result in Britain's leading civilisation towards a new level of intellectual attainment and a utopian state of social organisation.

This book has been concerned with describing the ramifications of puritan science in the context of the millennial idea of progress. Millennial eschatology inevitably coloured attitudes towards the natural world. There was little point in engaging in highly abstract metaphysical disputes about the nature of the ether, or entering into long-term scientific investigations at a time when the thousand-year rule of the saints was expected to begin in the immediate future. Instead, it was necessary to arrive at a precise estimate of one's point in the cosmic timetable, and accordingly to make preparations for the onset of the final age. Inevitably the revolutionary conditions aroused expectations which seem to be poorly founded from the point of view of the modern commentator, and correspondingly the intellectual pretensions of the Puritans appear to be absurdly ambitious and optimistic. Nevertheless their eschatological expectations were founded on the biblical exegesis of a group of gifted and critical humanistic scholars and their programme appeared to have the backing of providential authority. The political and military events of the revolution seemed to substantiate the accuracy of their predictions and the spirit of optimism was maintained until the collapse of the Republic made it impossible any longer to sustain it.

Although interest has hitherto been taken chiefly in the question of the permanent influence of puritan science, much greater attention has been paid in the present study to the purely historical aspect of this brief phase of revolutionary intellectual activity, which in many respects forms a complete contrast with the continuous and gradual evolution of knowledge which has occurred since the restoration. It is perhaps only in the most recent phases of acute crisis in science and technology that we have moved into a position whereby a sympathetic estimate of the millenarian worldview can be made. No longer is it possible to look forward without concern to an indefinite period of the unrestricted exploitation of science and technology. Environmental circumstances have necessitated reference to an idea of the social accountability of science, analogous to the view which the Puritans more readily derived from their religious convictions. Consistently with this frame of mind, Bacon insisted that 'all knowledge is to be limited by religion, and to be referred to use and action'. Although the Puritans looked forward to an unprecedented expansion in human knowledge, they realised that it would be necessary to exercise stringent discipline to prevent this knowledge resulting in moral corruption and social exploitation. The essential barrier against such misuse of the favours granted by providence was provided by the puritan ethical code, but it was also felt that the only secure control over the distribution of the fruits of science would be that actively exercised by the godly parliament. From an early stage the puritan experimental philosophers sought to increase this capacity to bring about human improvement by promoting the state supervision of the Great Instauration. In Bacon's *New Atlantis* one of the main institutions of the state was Solomon's House, the agency whereby the health and wealth of the state were maintained. The Baconians believed that this utopian state of affairs could be brought about in England, given a government willing to exercise its solemn obligation to promote the public good. From the time of the publication of *Macaria* the reformers urged the public authority to accept its responsibility to advance piety, learning, and social reform. Their millennial optimism precluded disillusionment when their ambitious philanthropic plans were not immediately implemented. Regardless of the public response the reformers went on conscientiously to fulfil their side of the obligation, to present the state with a comprehensive programme for social welfare, economic advancement and intellectual reform. The scale of this enterprise and the patient perseverance of the puritan reformers in their mission remain impressive. The proposals for a national scientific institution, poor relief, economic planning, and educational reform were worked out in great detail and they were generally conceived in strictly practicable terms, yet the planners rarely lost sight of their utopian objectives. This work has been treated with some respect, but it has too often been regarded as the creation of a group of pious philanthropists who made little direct contribution to the areas for which they sought to legislate, and who totally lacked the capacity to influence events. Their writings have been regarded as of little more real significance than utopian fictions.

The present study has demonstrated that the work of the puritan reformers was of a much more substantial nature. As practitioners, writers and propagandists they contributed considerably towards the remarkable acceleration of experimental science in England; their ideas on education continued to be upheld by an active minority, and their work was conducive to a change in general attitudes to such subjects as economic analysis, agriculture and medicine. The practical successes of the puritan Baconians were sufficiently substantial to persuade their friends and neighbours that a scientific approach towards the natural environment would lead to tangible economic advantages. Puritan projects and pamphleteering were probably instrumental in inducing changes in practices in husbandry and in stimulating industrial initiatives which took effect during the later part of the century, the period which was marked by an obvious upturn in the English economy. Thus the cultural and economic impact of the puritan programme was by no means negligible, although this influence came about through informal mechanisms of publication, example and acquaintance, rather than by legislation and governmental supervision.

The successes of the puritan reformers were not confined to the popular level. It has been shown in Chapter II above that adherence to the experimental philosophy became one of the most acceptable qualifications for intellectuals wishing to seek a career in the universities or in the civil service. The catalogue of puritan natural philosophers holding important offices or performing crucial background services is most extensive. It includes Wilkins, Whistler, Cudworth, Worthington, Sadler, Collins, Graunt, Goddard, Petty, Hartlib, Dury, French, Culpeper, Sparrow, Worsley, Symner, Gurdan and Robert Wood. It is doubtful whether at any other time in English history scientific intellectuals have assumed such importance in the national administration. The Baconians proved themselves to be useful servants of the state and they were rewarded accordingly. It is also clear that they attracted genuine sympathy in parliament and in the Council of State, and their ideas seem to have been acceptable to such leaders as John Pym, Oliver Cromwell, Henry Cromwell, Oliver St. John, Francis Rous, Sir Henry Vane, and John Lambert. Fortunately for the puritan Baconians, the succession of divisions, purges and reorganisations which affected parliament and the Council of State during the revolutionary decades, rarely worked to the disadvantage of the reformers, and in general tended to increase the body of their supporters.[41] Assistance from these quarters was essential for the limited measures of reform which were actually secured. It is fair to claim that the Baconian philosophy and support for science did become part of the official policy of the Commonwealth, despite the fact that such limited headway was made in implementing this policy in its fullest sense.[42] It proved possible in certain directions to overcome the inertia of republican government, and to achieve positive results. Indeed certain measures came to fruition during the later years of the Protectorate when the reformers had almost ceased to hope for success. Between 1656 and 1658 Durham College was established, mechanised coinage was adopted, the Down Survey was completed, sanction was given for the expansion of Trinity College Dublin, and for state aid to the Agency for the Advancement of Learning. But perhaps the most notable achievement came at the outset of the Commonwealth, when the Baconians played an active part in the promotion and estab-

41. Recent discussions of parliamentary politics during this period, although extremely densely researched have largely failed to appreciate the degree to which the Baconian movement throws light on the intellectual predispositions of the politicians: see for instance, D. E. Underdown, *Pride's Purge. Politics in the Puritan Revolution* (Oxford, 1971); B. Worden, *The Rump Parliament 1648–1653* (Cambridge, 1974).

42. Ben-David, *op. cit.*, p.72.

lishment of the Council of Trade and in the framing of the Navigation Acts. Each of these developments was designed to give a substantial impetus to the English economy and to create conditions conducive to the full utilitarian exploitation of scientific knowledge.

According to the scale of values of modern scientists, such achievements may seem to be of minor historical interest; indeed pre-occupation with the technical, utilitarian and ethical dimensions of science is regarded as a severe handicap to serious scientific work. It is certainly true that the integrated worldview of the puritan reformers deflected attention away from many problems which are now regarded as of the utmost importance. But failure by one standard may be estimated as success by another. What is judged scientific achievement in one period is largely discounted in another. The Puritans evolved a comprehensive system of science consistent with their millennial ideology. Modern science has evolved in the context of a quite different, even alien ideology. It is therefore quite understandable that little sympathy has been felt for the priorities and achievements of the Puritans, but this judgement should not be taken as final. Arthur Young regarded Richard Weston as a greater benefactor of civilisation than Isaac Newton. It may turn out that in the scale of values of a future age the utopianism and humanitarianism of puritan science may come to be held in high esteem.

Appendices

The following appendices consist mainly of important original documents relating to major themes discussed above. In transcribing the tracts from manuscript sources, original capitalisation, spelling and italicisation have been preserved. Normal contractions have been expanded and occasionally it has been necessary to clarify the punctuation. Insertions are given in squared brackets and, in the case of longer tracts, page or folio numbers are inserted in the text.

APPENDIX I

University Reform

This appendix reproduces two short unsigned manuscript petitions relating to the reform of Oxford University. The first, Ut felix et fausta fiat Reformatio, was submitted to Samuel Hartlib by Thomas Gilson of Corpus Christi College Oxford, and there is no reason to doubt that he was its author. The petition is dated 1 October [1649]. The text is taken from Sheffield University Library, Hartlib Papers XI. The second, To the Supreame Authority of Parliament, was probably drafted by Hartlib shortly after his receipt of the Latin petition. The text is taken from Sheffield University Library, Hartlib Papers XLVIII 17.

Ut felix et fausta fiat Reformatio Statutorum Academiae Oxoniensis, iis penes quos sit istiusmodi Authoritas haec curae sunto.

Primo. Ut non amplius vel Aristotelis aut Platonis, sed Rationis (nimir. rectae) suprema sit Authoritas in Exercitiis praestandis, quo magis vigeat floreatque Libera Philosophia et ingenua Juventus.

Secundo. Ut Professores et Lectores Publici Studia et Conatus suos egregios, non amplius Interpretationi cujusdam Authoris impenderint (unde Herculis Columnae in Intellectuali Mundo defixae fuerunt, nimir. quia Textum (ut aiunt) transgredi vitii et impudentiae loco habebatur) Potius autem in posterum sudent ad Augmentationem Literarum promovendam Earumque Desiderata supplenda, quaecunque annotata fuerunt ab incomparabili et defaecato Baconis ingenio, aliisque recentioribus ingeniis. Quod gratum Opus ubi semel praestiterint venerabili Convocationis Domui praebeant, et (eorum si contigerit consensus) typis mandare publicis.

Tertio. Ut Custos Archivorum obstringatur selectissima quaeque MS et Opera Reipublicae Literariae utilissima non amplius cum blattis et tineis rixari, sed Venerabili Convocationis Domui praesentare et eorum consensu typis mandare publicis, pariterque Bodleianae Bibliothecae Custos selectiores et rariores Libros eodem modo, et in eundem finem exhibeat.

Quarto. Non amplius pro materia indispensabili habeatur temporis defectus, sed penes Venerabilem Convocationibus Domum sit, sua uti prudentia et consilio, prout emerserit occasio, interim Exercitiis requisitis solide et nervose praestitis. Quo magis acuantur Studiosorum ingenia et ad progressum eminentiorum exstimulari possint.

Quinto. Ut ad minimum Duo Tutores constituantur in unaquaque

Domo, nec plures quam tres, qui viri sint Probi Docti et ad tale munus aptissimi quorum Electio vel sit penes Vice-Cancellarium, vel cujuscunque Domus Praefectum. Eorum autem munus sit Juvenum animos tam Religione vera quam Ratione recta excolere, idque pro virili, usque dum Juvenes 4 vel 5 Annorum spatium in Academia exsolverint.

Sexto. Penes eosdem Tutores sit prudentia et consilio suo uti, de Modo et Methodo instruendi accomodatissima, et sat sit Academiae, si modo laudabiles et pares ei Gradui, quem ambit progressus fecerit Candidatus.

Septimo. Nullum posthac instituatur Juramentum de Rebus Adiaphoris futuris (quibus insidiari posset Conscientia) aut iis, quae absolute in nostra potestate non sunt, nullumque admittatur adaequatum objectum Juramenti, nisi quod fuerit in se simpliciter licitum.

Octavo. Omnes istae Ordinationes Statuta De Concionibus habendis, in unum confluant nervosum et solidum Concionandi genus Expositorium scilicet cujusmodi Conciones bis unaquaque Dominica in Templo Academico habeantur.

[1r] To the Supreame Authority of
Parliament of the Commonwealth
& of England.
The humble petition of Severall
Members of the Universitie of Oxon.

Sheweth.

That whereas wee have not ungroundedly raised our hopes to the expectation of great Things from God through your handes for his glory, the happines of this Nation upon our attentive observation of that Divine superintendency by which you seeme to have beene from heaven constituted the assertors of our Religion Liberty and what ever is dear and that continued gracious and powerfull conduct by which you are still acted and carried on in your councells and undertakings to build up this Christian Commonwealth on its true and sure foundations, wee meane Religion and Common Equity, Both which to promot Effectually you have most Religiously and wisely Designed the promotion and propagation of all pious and Usefull knowledge, to extend Gospell light to the utmost bounds of your Dominions, yea to carry it with other Subservient Learning victoriously into that other Nation soe that although you might excusably at Present bee wholly employed in conflicting with Political Difficulties, having your hands as yet full with Armes, yet you have soe eminently interested the advancement of all good knowledge in your present Actions there, that wee can not but with Rejoicing see true Religion and Learning Conquering superstitions prophanes and barbarisme in all [1v] your Conquests, Not to forget your pious and tender care of your two famous Universities at home both for Augmentation and Reformation for which in the midst of your weighty affaires you continue an Honourable Committee upon all occasions consulting the much desired flourishing State of Piety and Ingenuity here.

We do therefore first as having a Common share with the rest of the Nation in such your Counsells and Resolutions blesse God and pray for their happy Execution and establishment And in particular and above all humbly begg that you would still make it your greatest care (as it is your highest Interest with which you stand charged of God) to advance the power of Godlinesse by protecting and propagating the Truth and puriety of Religion with all fervency and intensnes of Christian zeale and Therefore to goe on to settle and encourage a faithfull Learned and able Ministery in all places throughout the Land.

We hereunto Remembering ourselves more specially concerned in the blessed worke of Reformation here and deeply engaged by God and you not to terminate our desires on this side the highest end as theireof which are (as we judge) after Religion the Reformation and advancement of Learning, We fearre to suffer [2r] any obstruction on our part, of your pious and honourable Intentions towards this worke, thorough want in us of due concurrent readines to accept and pursue them to the best improvement of this Nursery of knowledge and in it the second grand Interest of the State and whole Nation, and therefore with all humble earnestnes beseech you now to erect as you doe the politicke, soe also with as much care and wisdome the literary Republick which of old hath beene soe called, but now expects by you to be soe constituted if you be pleased to consider seriously that raised and refined spirit which Acts this present Age and restlesly impregnates some great mindes with vast attempts, even sufficient to entertaine our thoughts with Expectation if not of new heavens and new Earth, yet of a new world of knowledge and then as becomes your Noble spirits take upon you this designe by your patronage to Command hither, and publiquly encourag such great endeavours to the desired advancement of true Learning.

We can now only mention our allmost Totall deficiency, as to the meanes of Advancement. For the chiefest Thing that is Designed here, or indeed according to the Constitution of our Colledges and [2v] maine end of Learning can or ought to be endeavoured in them, We say the chiefest thing is to Learne and teach the wisdome and inventions of others, and with that Accomplishment to hast to publicke service abroad, whereas advancement and augmentation must be by the united strength of theire men, and of a Consistent growth in Learning that shall be encouraged to make it their calling and the busines of their life. And therefore as you have already most wisely decreed that none shall continue in Fellowship beyond such a convenient time it is our earnest suite that you would compleate your worke by these answerable provisions : First for augmentation of knowledge in the Universitie, and then the new Moulding our constitutions in the severall Colledges to a more ingenious and lesse tedious way of Learning [than] what is already.

1. That in the publicke Academy their may be a greater number of able Professors and all of them enioyned as their owne and proper worke to supply the Defects and make up the Desiderata which are or shall be observed [3r] in the severall parts of Learning and at Convenient portions to print what they shall first read. And because of the eminent usefullnes and great defect of the knowledge of Things and Nature that their may be some speciall provision for skilfull and Industrious men to Read all parts of the Booke of Nature and demonstrate Things themselves to the Senses, That there may be an Examination of old Traditions and strict disquiry made into them, an accurate observation and practicall pursuit of Nature in all Luciferous experiments and soe a repairing or new founding our present Ruinous Fabricks.

2. That their may be a publicke stocke in the hands of Trustees by you thereunto appointed out of the heads and professors of the Universitie for all particular and occasionall Things as the Procuring choice printed Bookes and Manuscripts, Mathematicall Instruments, and Representations of Things, the printing of some few Copies for the Use of Libraries, of more Costly yet usefull Bookes (for want of which the best Workes have never seen the Light) as also the incoragment both of [3v] Forraigne and Domesticke fruitfull wits to disperse their Speculations here and make choice of this place to be delivered of their Inventions.

3. And which must give the Actuating and Empowering forme of the whole Designe of Learning. That the Publicke Library keepers place may be soe augmented and endowed that it may maintaine an Able and faithfull Agent with necessary under officers who by his Correspondency kept with the whole Commonwealth of Learning in all parts under or with the forementioned Trustees shall procure not only instrumentall Bookes and other supplies but men of parts and Ingenuity and continually present you with the Fruit of all humane Industry abroad, And in time manage a perfect Communication and Negotiation, as necessary in Things of Learning as Civill affaires and to the want of which alone wee attribute the Losse of all that single and non united Labour and expense with which many Noble spirits have wasted away themselves both bodyes and Estates and the inefficacy and successles Issue of most Heroicke designes which have either proved abortive births or wholly [4r] dyed with Those that dyed in Travail with them.

Thus much for the enlargment of Learning & farther acquisition which must be in the Publike Academy.

4. The Last particular of this our great request is, that upon this the Statutes of private Colledges (to which the Instruction of the younger sort is hereby Left and reserved as their Taske) may be revived by such whom you shall appoint within a limited time to present to you for the establishment of such constitutions as may together with things of Goverment settle the most profitable and Compendious Course of studies both in Philology and Ancient and Moderne Philosophy in a free

and ingenious way suitable at least to the growing and Thriving state of knowledge and rather preparing the Mind for then prejudically obstructing it against any dawning of reall science.

And now (Most Noble Patriots) as we have judged those desires most reall and necessary, soe we conceive as great hope of obtaining them from you, whose propensions, worthy of such high trust need noe further incentive then the Publike good, but if also the easines and feasablnes of this suite bee considered, surely you will bee willing by some small Liberality [4v] and the exercise of your Authority to perfect and Thoroughly improve what the Magnifency of former Times hath left to your handes and at least set on foot this designe and chalke out and direct the way to future donations and privat benefactors.

We should here commend unto you the important care of the Education of your Children both in your Politicall and naturall Relation in the subordinate schooles that it may be Universall according to Piety and Vertue and in smoother and more successfull wayes and Methods then now obtaine: But you are happily upon this worke already and wee must wholly Leave it to the Tender working of your Fatherly Bowells with much confidence that God by whose signall providence the Supreame Authority hath beene redeem'd into your handes, hath also by his Spirit raysed and heightened your hearts, and with full purpose fastned them upon this Duty to make use of the peacefull Season and greate advantage of Light in this Age, and according to what upon impartiall consultation with your owne Reasons you shall [5r] their behold in cleere and vitall principles to establish a Naturall and every way most exact and well proportioned frame of a weale publicke and Therefore not omit the Repairing and fitting the decayed humane nature to the good of Society by an Universall propagation of all Arts and Sciences in their reality and proper Lustre.

So shall you uphold in your succession, yea exceed the constant and only Splendor of former Common Wealths and Free States to which Goverment Learning ever acknowledged in her Monuments her bravest Spirits and Chiefest acquests. So shall you fulfilling the ends of Magistracy conveigh to the Socyetyes of Men a full Enjoyment of all Gods goodnes in the blessings of this world and as good Stewards give him the due returne of the glory thereof. If you direct and enable men by the right use of their Faculities and the Creatures, mutually to advance the Common good of Mankind and therin to find their owne supplies and particular advantages, Thus shall you at least make men Morrall and Rationall, wise and innocent, and rightly reforme, dealing first and chiefly with the mindes [4r] of Men, you shall truely free us and teach us to know and Relish our Liberty if ingenious Truth make free our better part. Yea so and soe only shall you advance and maintaine the Truth of Religion, sending forth the Light of the Gospell in the hands of other good Learning, And as Reformation from Antichristianisme at first began with the Reformation of Learning which was the Morning

Starr that brought day to Evangelicall knowledge and all progressive Reformations have advanced both in the same proposition, So then shall wee thinke there will be something done in our Reformation, if the Father of Light shall graciously give unto you the hearts and handes of Foster Fathers to beare up alle good knowledge some degrees higher in our Meridian then ever yet it attained, Thus shall those who both misjudge you and see not the neere Alliance of Ingenuity and Freedome, and the joynt Interest of both have all their feares and jealousies Remooved [4v] and your Malitious Enemyes bee Confounded while your name is made pretious and Deare to all the Sonnes of knowledge.

And your Petitioners shall blesse God and pray &c.

APPENDIX II

Durham College

There have been two serious attempts to identify the staff of Durham College, the first by C. E. Whiting, *The University of Durham 1832-1932* (London, 1932), pp. 22-6; the second by G. H. Turnbull, 'Oliver Cromwell's College at Durham', *Durham Research Review*, No. 3, Sept. 1952. In the following table the identifications by these authors are given, followed by my alternative where appropriate.

Name	Status	Identification by Whiting and Turnbull	Revised Identification
William Corker	Schoolmaster—O	Senior Fellow and later Master of Trinity College, Cambridge. Venn, i, p.398 (Whiting).	New College Oxford, BA 1639. Intruded Fellow of Brasenose College Oxford, 1648; Burrows, pp.174, 483; Foster, i, p.329.
John Doughty	Schoolmaster and Fellow—O	Fellow of Merton College; rector of Lapworth, Warwickshire, 1633; royalist. Wood *Athenae*, iii, pp.976–7 (Whiting).	University College Oxford, BA 1640; MA 1642/3. Burrows, p.269.
Richard Frankland	?—L	Christ's College Cambridge, BA 1651/2; MA 1655; vicar of Andrew's Auckland. Later pioneer of Non-conformist academies. Peile, i, pp.520–1 (Whiting).	
Joseph Hill	Preacher and Senior Fellow—O	Magdalene College Cambridge, MA 1649. 1659, minister of St. Oswald's in Elvet and Proctor at Cambridge (Whiting).	

Name	Status	Identification by Whiting and Turnbull	Revised Identification
Philip Hunton	Provost—O	Wadham College BA 1626; MA 1629. 1641, vicar of Westbury, Wilts. *DNB*; *Calamy Revised*, pp.285–6 (Whiting).	
Johann Sibertus Küffeler	Professor and Fellow—O	Son-in-law of Cornelius Drebbel; Dutch inventor and physician (Turnbull).	
John Peachill	Professor and Fellow—O	Magdalene College Cambridge, MA 1653, Fellow 1656. *DNB*; Venn, iii, p.325 (Whiting).	
William Pell	?—L	Magdalene College Cambridge, BA 1655; MA 1658; tutored by Joseph Hill. Rector of Easington 1659. *DNB*; *Calamy Revised*, p.385 (Whiting).	
Georg Ritschel	Schoolmaster and Fellow—O		Given as 'John Richel'. Master of the Royal Grammar School, Newcastle-upon-Tyne, until July, 1657.

Name	Status	Identification by Whiting and Turnbull	Revised Identification
Richard Russell	Schoolmaster and Fellow—O	Student of Christ Church Oxford 1648; BA 1649/50; MA 1652. Translator of alchemical works. Burrows, pp.493, 552 (Whiting).	The translator of alchemical works was probably a different Richard Russell who was brother of William Russell, apothecary to Charles II.
William Spinedge	Preacher and Senior Fellow—O	Fellow of Exeter College Oxford; rector of Poulshot, Wilts. (Whiting).	
William Sprigg	Schoolmaster—O	Steward of New College Oxford. Intruded Fellow of Lincoln College Oxford, 1652. *DNB*; Burrows, pp.354–5, 534 (Whiting, Turnbull).	
Ezerel Tong	Schoolmaster and Fellow—O	University College Oxford, BA 1643, MA 1648. Fellow 1648. Rector of Pluckley, Kent, 1649. *DNB*; Wood *Athenae*, iii, pp.1260–4 (Whiting, Turnbull).	

Name	Status	Identification by Whiting and Turnbull	Revised Identification
Thomas Vaughan	Professor and Fellow—O	Rector of Smarden, Kent 1644. *Calamy Revised*, p.501 (Turnbull).	
Nathaniel Vincent	Schoolmaster—O	Corpus Christi College Oxford, 1648; Christ Church Oxford, 1655; BA 1656; MA 1657. Wood *Athenae*, iv, pp.617–19; *Calamy Revised*, p.502 (Whiting).	
Leonard Wastel	Schoolmaster—O	Rector of Harworth-on-Tees, 1651 (Whiting).	
Robert Wood	Professor and Fellow—O	New Inn Hall Oxford, 1642; Merton College 1642, BA 1646–7; MA 1649. Intruded Fellow of Lincoln College 1650. *DNB*; Wood *Athenae*, iv, pp.167–8 (Whiting, Turnbull).	

O = Original Appointment
L = Later Appointment

APPENDIX III

College of Graduate Physicians

The manuscript 'Proposals' drafted by Rand (Sheffield University Library, Hartlib Papers XLII 10), were sent to Hartlib with a covering letter dated 15 August 1656.

Much honoured friend.

I have sent you the Propositions I told you of, when we were together at my Ladie Ranelaghs. Be pleased to communicate them only to such as you know are averse to the College [of Physicians] and desire that the matter may be kept secret, least we be countermined.

To make you active in the Promotion of this designe, consider that this Societie will gather the most ingenuous spirits about the towne; for the more ambitious, covetous, domineering, and selfish sort of Physitians will evermore joine to the old Colledge. But the more studious, modest, reserved, publick and humble spirited will joine to this new societie. And thinke but what excellent things may be done by the joint Counsel of such a Companie, towards the advancement, not only of Physic, but of all natural Discoveries. Thinke what a thing it will be for you to know where to find a societie of learned men so disposed, to propound any excellent designe unto, or to have their Advice in any busines concerning the public; or to have their Testimonial Suffrage upon occasion of somthing to be presented in public. Sir I leave much more that might be said to your prudent consideration and rest

Your real friend to serve you.
W. R.

Proposals relating to those Graduate Physitians of any Universitie, that have bin there licentiated, and are now resident in London and not incorporated nor desirous to incorporate with the present College.

That being alreadie by Matriculation made Brethren of one or other Universitie, they are obliged to maintaine its priviledges, and amongst the rest to keepe valid its power of licentiateing, against any later and inferior Societie whatsoever.

In order to which. That all Physitians of London so licentiated and not of the Colledge doe associate, unto which association a necessitie may appeare, from the two following Reasons.

1. That in Case the present Colledge shall disturbe them or any of them in their practise, they may by advantage thereof, be in a good Capacitie to defend themselves, assisting one another by Councell and friends; and for the ease and encouragement of particulars, defray the charge of suites and other molestations (to which all are liable) from a Common Stock, ariseing from a light but weekly Contribution.

2. That in Case the Colledge shall move for a Confirmation of their Charter, and possibly the addition of certaine Clauses, that may expressly bring graduate and licentiated Physitians under the restraint and penaltie in their Charter expressed, because not licentiated by them: that in such Cases, Physitians associated as above (being very manie in number in this Cittie of London) will be better able to move for a *salvis Libertatibus Academiarum,* and Exemption from the juristiction of the said Colledge, which is not likely to be denied to Foundations more ancient, comprehensive, and August then the Present Colledge, as all Universities, especially those of our owne Nation are. especially since the ground of the licensing power given the said Colledge, as it is expressed in their Charter and an Act thereto relateing: was, the Avarice and Unskillfulnes in Physic and Chirurgerie, and all other kinds of Learning of such Mechanicks and wicked persons, as without education in literature, thrust themselves upon the Practise thereof; which can no more be charged upon Graduate Physitians of the Universities, then upon the members of the Colledge in London.

Motives hereunto.

1st That Physitians so associated in a friendly Corporation, may assist one another, not only in accidental Consultations, at the charge of Patients, but in all Cases of Difficultie and that seldome occurr in practise, which will be to the Benefit of such as are under their care, the improvement of the facultie of Physic, and consequently the Glorie of Almightie God and deserved Honour of the desired Association. For which purpose meetings may be appointed so often as the said Societie shall judge convenient.

2ndly. That they then may be in a Capacitie of moveing Authoritie, not only for the conservation of their Liberties, but for some further countenance and encouragement, as upon further consideration may be thought fit. Neither is the Erection of two or more Societies for the same end without President even in this nation and Cittie: witnes the two universities and the foure Inns of Court. It may be further urged, that the spaciousnes of London, more then admits it, and that it may be an Induction to the establishment of a third Universitie.

3rdly. The members of this Societie will be upon even termes with the members of the present Colledge and so those disgusts and Animosities, which are frequent at Consultations, to the praejudice often of the patient and Dishonour of both Physitians, will cease, and both of them, like the Sister Universities, accord for the time to come.

APPENDIX IV

Decimalisation

'Ten to One', the undated manuscript proposal for decimalisation is reproduced from Sheffield University Library, Hartlib Papers xxvii 20. From associated correspondence it is clear that the author 'R.W.' is Robert Wood. Wood's tract was completed at Oxford in March 1656 and forwarded to Samuel Hartlib with the following letter.

Honoured Sir,

You being so known a Promotor of any thing that lookes towards the public Good, and having made your inclinations to the carrying on of usefull Designes [as] so universaly appeare in your Communications to this whol Nation; I have adventured to send you this enclosed Proposal, which perhaps you may thinke fitt to publish with some others that are dayly brought to your hands by the wel-wishers to the service of their Country; amongst whom I am ambitious to subscribe my selfe.

Your humble servant
Robert Wood

Lincoln Colledge in Oxford
March 1/11 1655

If you please to print this with any other Papers, I should be glad it might be so done (as easily it may) upon a sheet by it selfe, that I might have 2 or 3 copies thereof.

TEN TO ONE
or
A short and ready way
For the extraordinary Facilitation & Dispatch
Of RECKONINGS.
By meanes only
of Two or Three
NEW DECIMAL COINES
much desired in order to
The Publick Good.
by
R.W.

The End & Design of every useful *Art,* being only *To lessen the Labour & ease the paines of Men,* in relation to the several conveniences of this Life; and every honest man being bound, even by the Law of Nature, *to serve his Generation,* & endeavour what he can the Advancement of the *Public Good*: I shall here point out a *Way,* which if followed will save much trouble I am sure, and consequently prove beneficial to the Generalitie of this Nation, without the least dammage or inconvenience, that by the use of it can be pretended to accrue to any one in particular. Hoping that this my *Proposal* may fall into such Hands (either of His Highness himselfe, or those who under Him, manage the publick Affaires of this Commonwealth; or at least who are conversant with them that doe) as may apprehend the *usefulnes* thereof to be sufficient to excite them to get it put in execution. Of which I have the greater assurance, by reason that the *Design* (though it wholly concern *Money,* yet) requires not the least expence at all to bring it about; if only (as very easily it may) it be but understood aright; which therefore I am now going to make out to any rational Capacity that understands but the first Principles of Arithmetick.

[2] *The ordinary way of Numbering* and most generaly used not only here in England, but for ought I know all the World over (whither the best that might have bin thought upon, I shall not now enquire) is *Decimal,* or from Units to Ten's, from Ten's to Hundreds (that is to say ten Ten's) from Hundreds to Thousands (i.e. ten Hundreds, or ten times ten Ten's) and so onward as farr as you please; every Place from the Unit upwards still exceeding the former tenfold. And in like manner from the Unit downwards, in *Fractions* or Parts of a Unit, the Calculation at this day most received (as being not only the neatest, but farr the most expedite in it selfe, and most conforme to the Other Arithmetick of whol Numbers in all its Operations) is also Decimal: viz. from an Unit to a Tenth part, from a Tenth to an Hundredth part (i.e. a Tenth part of a Tenth) and so to a Thousanth part (i.e. a Tenth part of an Hundredth, or a tenth of a tenth of Tenth part) etc. Every Place downwards being still the Tenth of the former: As they are never so little versed in Arithmetick know well enough.

It is manifest also that *The common way of Counting our English Money is Decimal from a Pound upwards;* viz. 1 lib., 10 lib., 100 lib., 1000 lib. etc; Each following Place being in a continued progression ten times the value of the former; answerable in every thing to that Decimal way of Reckoning in abstracted Numbers, before laid downe. But *under a Pound* we count *not* any longer the Parts or Fractions thereof after any *decimal* kind of Progression, as we doe[3] the Parts of an Unit before mention'd; but after a quite different way from the other, & diverse also in it selfe; viz by Shillings, Pence, Farthings, i.e. by 20th parts of a Pound, 12th parts of a Shilling, 4th parts of a Penny; or by 20th, 240th, 960th parts of a Pound; for so many Shillings, Pence and Farthings doth 1 lib. containe.

This diversitie of stiles or Denominations, viz : Tens, Scores, Douzaines etc causeth distraction of the mind, and consequently pronenes to mistake even in the working of Addition and Subduction; And not only so, but in Multiplying, Dividing and such like, requireth also a world of paines, and besides chargeth the Attention so much, that it soon wearies and weakens it. All which they who are exercised in *Merchants Accounts,* and acquainted with the tediousnes of *Reductions,* will easily acknowledge. Insomuch as many Gentlemen and Merchants that have Accounts to balance or Reckonings to proportion, though they concern their Estates to a considerable value, Yet will rather choose to employ a mercinary hand and hazard the being wrong'd or cozened by others, then engage in so great a trouble themselves; which in the Method I am about to propose they would rather find turn'd to a delightfull recreation.

To save therefore all this unnecessarie labour, and to render the business of Reckoning incomparably more facil, *it were to be wished that besides those sorts of Coines already current amongst us, there might only be allowed by His Highness, Two or Three others, such for value that 10 of the 1st kind, 100 of the 2nd, 1000 of the 3rd, should make 1 lib. sterling:* or [4] which is all one, those of the first sort should each of them be equivalent to the 10th, those of the second to the 100th, and those of the third to the 1000th part of 1 lib. Which therefore I may call, the 1st a Tenth, the second a Hund : and the third a Thous : Though it were easy enough to coyne them other more proper names if need require. A Tenth then is in value just 2 shillings; A Hund : almost 2 pence, and a Thous : a little less then a Farthing, as may easily be estimated. Or if it be judg'd inconvenient for the Commonwealth to have any Coynes so smal in value, as Farthings formerly were; this last sort may be spared, and the other two serve the turne as will, especialy if there were a peece equal to halfe the Hund : or which is all one, to the 200th part of 1 lib. viz that ten of them make a shilling.

And *these Two or Three Coynes are* of themselves *alone sufficient;* for such as will be pleas'd to count by them, *to answer and satisfie all those Ends before laid down;* viz : to remedy all that toyle, and to prevent those troublesome and tedious Reductions from Pounds to shillings, from shillings to Pence etc; and then, after the Operation is performed in Retaile and at large (which might be farr easier don in gross, and with lesse danger of mistake) to bring all back againe to Pounds, as is and must be patiently gon through in the common way : Whereas in this here aimed at; by reason of that continued and everywhere uniforme Decimal Progression upwards and downwards there needs no such confounding ambages, but the worke is performed the shortest, most direct, easy and natural way that is possible. [5] Our Records informe us, and some Footsteps thereof yet remaining among the Common people confirme the Information, That the ancient English way of Accounting was by Nobles, Groates etc. which as it in time gave place to that by Pounds, shillings and Pence, now generally practized, as found by experience somewhat more commodious: So I doubt not but if His Highness would be pleasd to allow some such Coynes as this Paper pleads for, their Convenience would quickly usher in their Use in Reckoning, first with understanding men, and consequently with in a while also among the vulgar. Neither would the Use of these Coynes here designed, render the others of Shillings and Pence unserviceable in Pay or Reckoning, any more then those of Shillings or Pence doe Groats or the rest which we count not by at present. For as now 2 Testons, 3 Groats etc. make a Shilling; so would then 2 Shillings, 4 Testons, 6 Groats, 24 Pence, make a Tenth; and answerably for any of the rest.

Besides the foremention'd advantages of the way here proposed, it carries with it others no less considerable from the helpe of Artificial Numbers or Logarithmes (the most rare and absolute Invention for the dispatch of Arithmetical Operations that ever was or perhaps ever will be discovered) which are applicable only to this decimal way, and doe render it many degrees easier yet and more compendious: as they who understand the nature of Logarithmes cannot but apprehend. And not only this of Logarithmes, but all other Contractions of Multiplication, Division etc. doe pay their tribute and are subservient to this our [6] Decimal Exchecquor; which setting aside those advantages, is of her selfe rich enough to keepe her attendants at farr more ease and without taking a quarter of that paines, which they who sit at the common Beame are necessitated to submitt themselves unto.

I shall adde for a farther confirmation of the advantages of the way here opened, that the more exact Accountants, doe now find it much easier, especialy if the Operation be any thing large, first *to resolve shillings and Pence into decimals of a Pound* (viz. into those here proposed) and so to worke them, and afterwards *to reduce them back againe to shillings and pence;* then to keepe the ordinary road.

In *casting of Accounts,* or *reckoning by Counters,* how easy & ready were the worke, when alwayes *Ten of a lower ranke should make One in the next above it*: which in the way now in use, where sometimes 20, sometimes 12, sometimes 4 doe the same, is not without more intricacy distraction, and difficulty. All which I know will be readily assented unto by such as are a little acquainted with *Decimal Calculation* in general, which is now so universaly entertained for its singular use, that it deserves in an especial manner to be recommended to all that desire to take their past-time in the fair and fruitfull fields of Arithmetick.

If that little Innovation here projected be yet looked upon as too great to be made all at once; it were nevertheless to be wished, for an Essay and tast of the benefitt promised therefrom, That we might have at least *one of the* forementioned *Coynes,* viz: that of 2 shillings value, or *the Tenth of a Pound,* made *current* in this Commonwealth; which as it would prove the greatest stepp to the whol designe, so can it not be imagined any way less convenient either for size, or sayableness (I might maintain it every way more serviceable) then the Halfe crown so much used at present.

All [7] these premisses then considered, why should the *Proposal* here made despaire of success, and since it carries with it so many advantages, and those altogether public; since no privat man can pretend to be damnified by it, since it requires the disanulling or calling-in of nothing now in use, and so can give no offence to any person or partie; since it needs not the least trouble or expence publick or privat to make it practicable, but may be effected as easily as almost any thing imaginable; since in short all that I have here pleaded for, is summed up in this, *That His Highness would be pleas'd to authorize two or three Coynes, which might beare his image and superscription, being for value one the tenth of 1 lib., another the tenth of the former* etc. What hinders I say that such a Designe as this might not be put in execution, surely nothing but the want of its being apprehended arright. To remove which obstacle I hope the same publick spirit which moves me to serve the Commonwealth in the present establishment to the extent of my narrow sphaere, and cast this *Mite* into the *Treasurie,* may stirr up others to offer their *Ten Talents to the Money-Changers;* I say, to make out so cleerly, and inculcat with that force of Demonstration the manifold advantages of the way by me pointed at, that every rational man being satisfactorily convinced, and so the designe here held forth being by the heat of an universal perswasion at length duely ripened, all men may desire with longing to enioy the fruit thereof.

APPENDIX V

Economic Reform

'Proffits humbly presented to this Kingdome' is an anonymous, undated tract, the text reproduced below being taken from Sheffield University Library, Hartlib Papers XV II (23).

No author is given, but the development of general proposals from the basis of a scheme for producing saltpetre, connects the tract with Benjamin Worsley. The first sections overlap with various petitions drafted by Worsley in 1646 to promote his saltpetre project. The later sections, dealing with colonial expansion and navigation, are taken up in Worsley's correspondence composed before the establishment of the Council of Trade in 1649. The tract may have been composed as a result of Worsley's associations within the Invisible College in the early months of 1647, that is shortly before his departure for Holland. Alternatively it might have been written during his Dutch visit. This would explain his jealousy of and respect for the achievements of the Dutch, but a later draft would probably have paid less attention to saltpetre.

Proffits humbly presented to this Kingdome.

[1r] *First.* To exhibitt a way of producing of Salt-petter in greater plentie then ever heretofore and that without diging of houses or Sellars or that great charge and burden generally complained of in the commonwealth.

Secondly. To improove the Hussbandrie of the Land, throughout the whole Kingdom by setting downe certaine wayes to amend some barren grounds. 2ndly of better manuring, and fatning good ground then hath as yet beene used. 3rdly of preparing the seed for the ground. 4ly of ordering the seasons for Tilage, otherwise then before, in preventing of milldewes Blastings and the like inconveniences. 5thly of Tilling, and labouring the ground after a more excellent and ready manner. In a way much differing and more proffitable then the practise now followed. All which things wee have all ready experimented and being once generally assumed, will bee found exceedingly for the increase of all sorts of grayne and fruits proper to this Kingdome.

Thirdly. To better the fishing of this Kingdome. First in great Fishes by using another kind of Salt, which likwise wee will furnish cheaper; by shewing also another course of drying and curing them than hath beene hetherto observed both for the making of them more whollsome and gratefull to the pallate and stomack, and that way more salliable, and also more merchantable in regard of Colour and durance. For whereas Fish, both North Sea,—Codd and newfound-land fish are now soe handled as that diverse of them within a litle whille change their white and Fresh collour, turne black, Heate, and grow strong and moist, nor will endure above a yeare or such a matter, by which the Fisherman looseth much of his price The merchant man of his faime offt times and the common wealth her riches. These may be remedied and the matter soe ordered and provided for as they shall both retaine their colour bee preserved from sweating heating and putrifying one another, and soe last and endure much longer. Secondly for smaller fishes as Herrings by proposing of other kind of nets and another manner of fishing.

Fourthly. To improove the woolls of the Kingdome by a better order and manner of feeding of sheep and preserving them from sickness.

Fifthly. That whereas there are severall commodities both of necesitie and pleasure that wee are forced to fetch out of another Countries; some with ready money and others with the exchange of our proper commodities; as out of Spaine of Italy and Turkey and the rest to the wasteing of the estate of the Kingdome Wee humbly offer to make it most evidently appeare That by such a well regulated plantation as wee shall cleerly and orderly describe with such lawes and constituons in it That the most yea all of those commodities wee now fetch from other partes, may bee had within [1v] our owne dominions and that at very inferiour rates especially those countries we will plant being also ordered and improoved according to the former manner, and government of our praescribed Husbandrie. For those Southern and Westerne partes being by nature, without any art used, richer of themselves, then any groundes in any part of christendome whatsoever Must needes be farr richer being further improoved and Cultivated by a more then ordinarie and excellent way of Industry.

By the putting of all which these into execution; if we may be permitted it will bee soone made appeare these ensuing Benefits will necessarily succeed.

FIRST

It being allready premised The Plantation land to bee richer of itselfe then any other now inhabited in any part of Christendome and to be also after a better way then any countrey yet ever was Husbanded and cultivated, and the Planters themselves according to the constitutions fittest the generall good of this Kingdome disciplined and governed, It must needes follow the commodities it shall beare, whether Wines, Fruyts, Sugars, Drugs and others will bee brought forth farr more abundantly and plentifully and consequently will bee afforded farre more cheape and more reasonable, by many degrees then those from other partes, now brought us, From this first branch and the having of them within our selves These following proffits will naturally spring.

1. Much Bullion, the riches of any Kingdome; now sent for them, may be spared. For it is well knowne, wee buy all our Currantes with ready plate, without the Exchange of Commodity at all to vallew. The Custome of which comming heere to many 1000 lb a yeare wee may give, much a larger allowance to the Principal and yet this is but one among those that are brought in.

2. By this cheapnesse as without soe vast expence of money within the Commonwealth of this Kingdome, will bee exceedingly saved, and preserved. First in privat expences if soe much wine as men now give 7 lb or 8 lb for, they shall hereafter bee certainly furnished with 2 lb or 3 lb. Here will bee halfe the privat expence saved throughout the Kingdome. Besides which it may bee expected when wine shall bee more plentifull, Gallantes will drinke lesse intemperatly. Every man knowing drunkenes rageth least in those Countries where wine is easiest to bee had. Secondly, in Hous Keeping for a privat Gentelman allowing himself 200 lb a yeare for Hous keeping wee cannot esteeme his expences at lesse then 20 lb a yeare in wine, Fruit and Sugar, which is the 10th parte. According to which, we may within compasse vallew the expence of most hous keepers within the Kingdome. If now these Commodities bee afforded at half the rates they now are [2r] accordingly the 20th part of expence in Housekeeping will be saved throughout the whole Kingdome. Now if to this wee shall adde the cheapnesse of graine and Fish by the improovment of our owne Husbandrie and

fishing &c, it will bee impossible to auditt or cast up the proffit of this benefit only.

3. When these commodities are so cheap if there be any extraordinary occasion for monyes, they will easily beare the greater excise, and that with more cherfullnes and lesse trouble to the subjects; a consideration of noe slight vallew.

4. The Ground being richer and the way of managing more excellent it is probable that the commodities thence, especially such druggs as shall be planted there will bee fresher, better and more healthy. Againe wee observe the Raysins to be much fairer in Barbary and Siria then in Spaine and Italy.

5. All the poore in the Kingdome may be this way maintained, all industrious willing laboring mindes in any Art, may by thus set aworke and releeved. Gentelmen and others of Estate undone by the warres may be here succored and not only some but All these may live plentifully and be inriched. Whence also all the inconveniencies comming from having many poore in a Kingdome of Begging—stealing—wandring lazily, and all Habitts of idlenesse will be removed And all Heartes made happy and gladded.

SECONDLY

Whereas the Hollander trading into the same places with us now for those commodities serves not only his owne but other Kingdomes with them as France, Denmark, Poland and all the Easterne and Northern clymats thereby imploying his shipping and stock and ingrossing to himselfe much proffit, being every where able to undersel us by reason of the cheapnesse of his sayling. We furnishing these Northerne Regions with the same commodities by our owne shipping, from our owne Plantations, shall from this second branch gaine these considerable advantages.

(1)

Increase of Trade, and imployment for more shiping.

(2)

Wee shall give a check to prevent the Hollanders over growing us.

(3)

Our Nation receiving the wholl benefitt both of the Commodities it selfe and monopolyzing also the trading for them into their owne hands, it will bee like as but somewhat more, then if Spaine & Italy and those countryes which now vent those commodities [2v] were ours by Conquest and possesion. Because this way we speake of wee can afford their commodities cheaper than wee could by having their countries in subjection. Therefore the Gaine is cleerly greater than would be the conquest of theme.

(4)

Those Commodities will either bring into the Planter, Sayler, Merchant and so to the whole Kingdome, most of all the Bullion in those partes, into which they are traded for, because wee are able now to afford them much cheaper, then they formerly had them, or else it will at least make their commodities much cheaper to us, being bartered at the rates customarily used, which if wee ourselves stand not in need of, wee may the better export to those parts, that doe most want them.

THIRDLY

The enlargment of our Dominions and this encrease and improovment of our Nationall Commodities and trading, will much spread the glory and add to the power and strength of this Kingdome.

1

In Increase of our Shipping which will arise partly through the increase of imployment, partly by the cheapnesse of matterialls, some of which our plantations may afford, and the rest by our trade into the Easte, which will bee also more easily and cheaply procured.

2

By the proffits arising from the tythes or Dutyes which shall be payd from this Plantation and from the Husbandrie and fishing being improoved, may the Royall Navy be much augmented and a continuall great fleet without all charge and burden to the subject maintained By which the Kingdome will not only be secured, but feared and the merchants goodes better then heretofore guarded and defended from the Turkes or other Pyratts abroad.

3

Revenues of the Crowne and commonwealth will by this meanes be vastly accumulated. For the customes will be increased through the increase of trading, and the employment of them toward the repayring or maintaining of a fleet will bee wholly suspended. And therefore they may the more freely to any other Publick use bee disposed and converted, or according to ancient custome Threasurd.

4

From this Plantation in time of warre or of necessitie may this [3r] Kingdome be exceedingly assisted and releeved with shipping men mony and provision like or after the Custome of Confederats. To which advantage wee may add The spirits of men will bee more heightned, and their minds to all generous and greatt actions more fitly disposed, when through these meanes want misery and servitude shall be wholly turned out of doores. And of what conducement to valour and great undertakings the freedome of mens mindes is, Let not only learned Verulam judge, but let the difference between the actions and achivments of the English compared to other Nations, wittnesse.

5

The rates and prices of the Commodities properly apertaining to this Kingdome, as woolles, Cloathes, Tynne Lead &c. will or may easily bee inhaunced, and bettered. For if wee now stand not in need of the commodities of those other countries for the returne and gaine of which wee formerly sent ours thither; it becommeth an obligation to them that wee trade with them, they standing in want of ours: wee noe wayes in necessitie of theirs and therefore seeming to bee noble and charitable to our neighbour or allied kingdomes rather then to seeke a benefit by them, or our owne gaine from them.

6

Standing in the Condition and Relation now named, wee must in the exchange of our owne commodities necessarily, continually import and bring in Bullion. And many occasions being now taken away of wastfull expence of it within the Kingdom and of transporting it againe (as formerly) out of the Kingdom, we may in time become the worlds-cash Koopers.

7

Bullion and money thus Banckt and Hoorded, all thinges may then more and more conveniently bee done, that shall bee thought further to concerne the Splendor, Glory, honour, and wealth of this Kingdom as Ambassodors may bee more Gallantly heere then in other partes entertained or more noblely if welcome, rewarded or our owne more richly and eminently dispatched and attended. But especially new discovering of the Eastherne and Southerne or Polar partes as of Terra Australis, Chyna, Tartary, Japan, Streights of Anian or Northwest passage so often and soe earnestly desired may be againe now seasonably revived and made and the riches of then soe found may bee conveyed. [3v]

8

All commodities in the world being either naturall, or artificiall and the artificiall being framed of the Naturall if then the Naturall be afforded more cheape, and plentifully the Artificiall will be soe also, so that by encreasing and ingrossing of naturall commodities besides the employing and setting of more men on worke we thereby likewise ingrosse Artificiall.

9

The riches wealth and eminency of any Kingdom will strongly invite all sorts of Artists and ingenious men from all places to them; especially if any immunities prifyledges or honours be graunted to encourage them, by which we may as certainly deprive our neighbour Kingdoms of their rich manufactures, as wee have or may doe, of those other naturall commodities, which will yet add more glory and more wealth to the Kingdome, because those manufactures or Arts which togeather with themselves, were strangers, will now togeather with them, become free denyzons, and in the ensuing age natives. And of what exceeding consequences to a Kingdome the affluence and resort of ingenious men, and Artists of all sorts, will be, what riches proffit and advantage if encouraged, they will bring he that is but a novice in Policy, will discerne. Manufacturs being halfe if not the major part of the riches of all Kingdomes. History, and Observation being full of nothing more, then of presidents of countryes, raysing themselves from Nothing to a greattness solely by them. The Gayne of which wee may the better assigne if wee shall consider the income traffique riches and trade, procured to severalls Kingdomes by one ore 2 Arts alone, as of Cloaths and stuffes in our owne land, of Glasse, and paper in Fraunce, and Vennice, of silke in Florence of minemen and Founders in Savoy, Germany, Denmarke and Swethdan advantages of which last, wee have about most, if not above all Kingdomes, were such men encouraged and these Kingdomes and our forraine plantations well searcht and this way improoved.

10

It will follow as a thing of not the least moment, that as wee shall and may thus daily raise and strengthen ourselves so the Kingdoms about us [4r] will, and must necessarily as much decay and weaken. For as wee sending our owne commodities every where abroad and that at gainfull rates, not standing in need of returning others for them, dayly take in without laying out, and soe stil add and improove the wealth and stock of the Kingdome. They contrarily being forced to buy the commodities of others, at greater prices, and either transporting or selling none of their owne, or but at low and meane prices, doe dayly lay out without taking in, and therefore must needes continually decay and weaken. By which meanes as wee shall bee secure from all feare of them soe wee shall bee able to give, and to dictate lawes to them, which advantage may bee turned to a most pious and Christian end in preserving peace Universally amoungst them. For how much the favour and siding of any patent and wealthy Kingdome will ballance and sway the Negotiations of the neighbour Kingdoms, is obvious to the knowledge and observation of every intelligent man, and soe wee may sitt as judge and Umpire of al Christian differences, and may draw and ingross the blessings and promises to ourselves that are made to bee Peace makers.

[11]

If to this wealth and honour thus feasably to bee attained, shall bee annexed a Reformation of laws, and an establishment of rightousnes amoungst us, then to these may wee yet promise to ourselves more glorious thinges as First a Propagation of the Gospell into other unknowne partes wherby Gods name and Love to mankind may be more spread and made manifest. Secondly a Reformation of Education, and soe of all the Unhappinesse hitherto thence springing, by the setting up and ordaining other kind of schools and teaching. Thirdly Advancement of Learning by men appointed and maintained to keep an Universall Correspondency, by erecting of Threasure Houses for the Collection of the History of nature, for experiments both Chymicall and Mechanicall and by increasing of choice and public Libraries. Fourthly endeavoring the conversion of the Jewes a worke as most Divines conceave [4v] shortly to be expected and without doubt at hand, and such as would not only bee a temporall but a true and eternall Honour to them that sought or furthered it. Fifthly The indeavouring an Union and reconciliation throughout all the christian at least all the Protestant Churches.

These being the most Glorious, magnificent and Honourable undertakings that may bee thought of for any Nation But not to bee undergone without much Charge and therefore soe fitt for none, as such a qualified Kingdome as wee speake of and have here set downe. Wee humbly beseech the Father of all mercyes of his infinite love to mankind through his only and true Sonne, by his power and goodnesse, to bring that into perfect Act, that wee have begun to demonstrate in a fayre and easy potentia.

APPENDIX VI

Fruit Trees and Timber

This unsigned petition on the improvement of forestry and fruit-tree husbandry is reproduced from Sheffield University Library, Hartlib Papers LXVI 22.

The authorship is apparent from letters written by Ralph Austen to Hartlib in the autumn of 1658, which refer to his petitioning on this subject. The original title, crossed out in the present copy, is 'To his Highnesse Oliver Lord Protector of the Commonwealth of England, Scotland & Ireland. May it please your Highnesse'. This title was modified by Hartlib to read 'To the Right Honourable The Counsel. The Humble Petition of Ra. Austen of the City of Oxon. May it please your Honours.' This suggests that the document was composed just before Cromwell's death in September 1658 and circulated to the Council of State and Fleetwood thereafter.

It hath a long time beene, and still is, the earnest desire of very many iuditious and good Commonwealths men in this Nation, that the Works of planting and ordering, not only of Fruit-trees, but also of all sorts of other Trees for building, fuell and other uses, may bee set on foot and caried on, for the greater profit of the Nation, then hath beene in former ages: Exceeding great advantages and profits (through the blessing of God) would arise to the whole Nation hereby. For

1. Hereby would bee a supply of all sort of Timber, fit for building ships, which hath beene of late yeares exceedingly wasted and destroyed,

so that unlesse this course for planting more, be taken, and the People put upon it by Authority, wee may clearly see a great scarcity of Timber, for that purpose is like to bee in certaine yeares: and of how great consequence and concernement this is, may also bee foreseene.

2. Secondly: If men did apply themselves to this worke, there would bee a supply not only of Timber for building, but also of Barke for Tanners, which of late yeares is growne very scarce and deare, and some feare they shall bee forced to lay downe their Trade (though so necessary in the Commonwealth) for want thereof. Lether of all sorts is become exceeding deare, upon this Accompt, and like to bee every yeare dearer hereafter, except this course be taken.

3. Thirdly: Hereby also would be a constant supply of all good fuel throughout the Nation, which now (in very many parts) is exceeding scarce and deare: many poore people are almost starv'd in cold long winters, who hereby might have sufficient to refresh themselves.

4. Fourthly: Carpenters, Joyners, Wheelerights, and all Tradesmen, who worke in wood, might hereby have sufficient and of the best, for their severall uses. And so the whole Nation might bee furnished with all sorts of Utensils for all purposes.

5. Fiftly: as concerning planting Fruit-trees, for the further benefit of the Nation (every yard-Land inclosed, as is set forth in the Booke intituled, a Designe for Plenty) the same would be aboundantly profitable many waies.

1. The fruits are good and wholsome food, ordered many waies, both for the sicke and sound, for young and old, rich and poore, all the yeare long.

2. Secondly, the Liquors made of them, Cider and Perry, will bee exceeding profitable; and are found not only by the iudgments of Learned Physitians, but also by Long Experience in those parts where the same are used, to bee very much conducing to health and long-life, two special Earthly blessings, and much desired amongst all men.

3. Thirdly, hereby might be saved the Expence of many thousand Quarters of Mault yearly in the Nation, and of many thousand Lodes of wood in making Mault, and many thousand Acres of Land sowed yearly with Barly, might bee sowed with Bredcorne, or turned into pasture grounds: wee having better Liquors with little or nothing from yeare to yeare, even out of the Fields and hedges.

4. Fourthly: By diligence in planting fruit-trees, there would arise yearly aboundance of fuell for the fire, from the Pruninge of the Trees, and old Trees past bearing.

5. Fiftly: Wee might have speciall Wood for Joyners and other workmen, to make Tables, Chaires, Stooles, and many other usefull Commodities of the Walnut, Peare, and Apple-tree, better then can bee made of Common kinds of wood.

6. Sixtly: By diligent planting of fruit-trees, Timber, and other trees, these Nations (by the good hand of God with us) would become Rich and Wealthy and so be enabled and encouraged to pay all Taxes and impositions, which are necessarily laid on them from time to time. Also by the common use of the foresaid Liquors Cider and Perry, they would bee a strong and healthy People, and Long-lived, able to goe forth to Warre and bee a terror to all our Enemies.

These things are more fully and at large set forth by many who have written of this subject: In Mr. Samuel Hartlibs Legacy of Husbandry: In the Desyne for plenty: In the Treatise Intituled Bread for the Poore: and in a late Treatise of fruit-trees, and many others: Wherefore it is humbly desired that [Your Highness and] this Honorable Council would please to take the same into serious consideration that by a Law (or by a Recommendation of the same to the People) this good worke soe easily effected without prejudice to any, and soe aboundantly profitable to all, may bee promoted.

APPENDIX VII

Gresham College

This appendix reproduces a short, anonymous, untitled and undated document making proposals for the reorganisation of Gresham College. The manuscript is in imperfect condition, but it has been possible to restore most of the missing words. The text is taken from Sheffield University Library, Hartlib Papers XLVII 18.

Although this paper was probably distributed by Hartlib, there is no evidence that he was its author. Indeed, there is little doubt that this brief, lucid and practical project was not his work. Even in the absence of an explicit statement, it can hardly be disputed that the proposals were drafted by William Petty. It is known that Hartlib wished to secure an appointment for Petty at Gresham College, and the proposals were probably composed to encourage the reconstitution of Gresham, along lines approved of by Petty. The direct, logical and unsentimental style is characteristic of Petty, as is the tendency to quantify arguments wherever possible. The practical proposals made are in the spirit of Petty's *Advice to S. Hartlib* (1648) and the lists of technical studies in the concluding section of the text are reminiscent of his natural history schemes. Finally Mr. Lindsay Sharp has confirmed that this document is in Petty's handwriting.

I suspect that Petty's document was composed in the summer of

1649 and that Hartlib may have had this in mind when he reported to Boyle on 24 July 1649 that 'My endeavours are now, how Mr. Petty may be set apart or encouraged for the advancement of experimental and mechanical knowledge, in *Gresham* college at London, of which you shall have a true account also . . .' (Boyle *Works*, vi, p.78).

The Lectures which are usually read in Universities and . . . Gymnasia since they are either but Collections out of bookes already published, or Unpublished Bookes, and since the Readers of them doe not descend to resolve the doubts and difficulties of their Auditors in particulars, may indeed serve to sett forth and make known the Abilities of their Readers, but cannot benefitt the hearers much more then Bookes of the same subjects may doe. And therefore in these times when the use of Printing hath made Bookes treating of almost all Matters in plenty and abundance, There are not the same Reasons for publique Readings as of old, when meetings of many to Heare One Man reade, was a good Remedy against the Want of those Bookes which were read. And consequently Publique Pro[fessors] such as read without interruption or answering particular mens doubts are onely needfull toward such faculties as cannot bee learned by r[easonable] instructions and Explications onely, but require besides some further de[monstration] and also That such faculties as are incapable of ocular demonstration as not being conversant about sensible but rather intellectuall things, doe scarse need such publique Professors.

Having said in what Cases Publique Professors are usefull in generall. W[e] come secondly to consider what professors are most usefull in this Citty of London.

There are already 7 Lectures viz. for Divinity, Civill Law, Rhethorick, Geometry, Astronomy, Physick and Musick sett up and continued by the Memorable Sir Thomas Gresham, But the 3 former of them (if provisions were made for the Juresprudity of their Incumbents) seeme needless to this C[itty] not onely for the generall Reasons afore mentioned, but for others more particul[ar].

[The Professor] of Divinity. The Universities with the many Libraries and helps in them are sufficient to institute Preachers, and those preachers with the maintenance that this citty affords them are sufficient to institute the people in that faculty without a professor thereof at Gresham College, whose but 16 or 17 sermons made there in the whole ye[ar] beare no proportion to those hundreds of others that are daily preached in ordinary Meeting houses and places about this Citty.

For the Civill Law, since the Use thereof is so small in this Commonwealth, and since it is in a Manner discountenanced by the State, what reason of upholding it by a public Profession? The Theory of Rhetorick is sufficiently to be learned in Bookes and the Practise by the sermons of Preachers and the Readings of Lawyers.

So that of the aforenamed 7 lectures, There seems but 4 Usefull to this Citty viz. Those of Physick, Geometry, Astronomy, and Musick, Since as the knowledge of many things concerning within the Compasse of these faculties, are not onely ornamentall to all men, but also Necessary to very Many Usefull Members of the Commonwealth, so beeing all practicall they cannot bee sufficiently taught without personall professors and teachers of them.

In the third place Wee come to consider what particular Subjects and Matters comming within the Compasse or necessary realmes of Physik, Geometry, Astronomy and Musick are most usefull for this Citty, for all either are not, or not so fitt to be taught and professed in this way. As for example.

The Professor of Physick may best employ himselfe about Anatomicall Operations upon the dead Bodies of severall Animalls and in making Experiments concerning the Use of the parts, the motion of the Blood, &c. upon living Brutes. Or else upon chymistry, wherein besides such Operations as respect the Preparations of Medicaments hee may dig[ress upon] other profitable and pleasant Enquiries usually practised by the Studious of that Art. Or lastly upon the demonstration of Plants if the conveniency of a Garden were not wanting.

The Professor of Geometry (omitting the very first Elements of Arithmetick usually taught in every schoole) may teach the Practise of solving questions in logisticall or delineatory geometry, The practise of Measuring of all kinds, Whether surveying of Lands, Measuring of solids, or inaccessible heights and distances &c. with the fabrick and use of Instruments belonging thereunto, and may also descend into Fortification, shewing the practise thereof in the field.

The Professor of Astronomy may at convenient tymes teach Men to know and finde out all the most knowne and remarkable stars and planets, and how to observe their motions distances eclypses &c. and [to] make use of those phenomena or observations either to the examining correcting or new forming of Theories and Systems of the World. Hee may also treate of Dialling, Navigation & Geography, and shew the practise of whatsoever [is] practicall in them.

The Professor of Musick need not so much to teach his Auditors actually to play or make as to explaine the grounds thereof, to teach Men to know the differences and distances of Tones, the Natures of concord and Discords, the Nature of sounds and sounding bodies, the Reasons of the fabric and figure of all Musicall Instruments, Not omitting Enquiries after the Meanes to better hearing answerable to what hath been happily done for the advantage of sight.

[In place] of the 3 Professorships of Divinity, Law and Rhetorick there might be substituted 1, 2 or so many others as might sufficiently treate upon the severall Matters following. Viz.

Upon all Magneticall Experiments as well concerning the attractive, as the directive vertue of the Loadstone, which are very many and wonderful as the best meanes and Cautions for making of Marriners Compasses.

Upon the Effects of concave and convex glasses of what posable figure soever either used alone or with others, dioptrically or catoptrically by sights of sensable sorts, either in reference to Vision, Illumination or Burning, Representing, Colouring &c. and upon the Operations, Tooles and Materialls used in Grinding, polishing and foyling them and upon the meanes of bringing the Workmanship belonging to Glasses nearer to the precepts of the Theory and art.

Upon the Nature of all the Materialls and Ingredients and applications of them One to Others made by Dyers, Tanners, leather dressers, Wool workers, Potters, Metallmen, Timber workers, Soapboylers and such like trades as afford so many and Noble Naturall Experiments.

Upon the Natures of Bowes, Guns, Pumps, Cranes, Mills, fire, furnaces, Ships for burthen and swift sayling, scale beames and Wayes of Weighing Ordinary and more vast weights, skrews, Carts and Carriadges, Clocks, Silkweavers Loomes and harnesses, of founding and moulding in Metalls, Earths, Cements, Wax &c. of Twining Roses, Ovalls and other prater-circular figures, On Schenographicall Pictures and of Weather-glasses and upon all such Trades and practises whereunto are required more Naturall and Mathematicall knowledge then the common Professors of them are usually instructed in, or else do contayne and may yeeld Matter for the best contemplations to Worke upon to their information and benefitt.

APPENDIX VIII

Memorial for Universal Learning

Many variants of this undated and anonymous manuscript exist in the Hartlib papers; a copy is also preserved in BM Additional MS 6269, fols. 23-5. This document was probably written in 1647 and distributed extremely widely by Hartlib. The first known recipient was Joshua Rawlin, who acknowledged receiving the 'Memorial' on 11 May 1648 (HP X 11). The author may have been Hartlib, but the 'Memorial' was perhaps based on a draft by Petty (see above, p. 71).

The text given below is from HP XLVII 4. The main variant (HP XLVII 1) makes essentially the same proposals, but divided up into eighteen instead of eleven sections. More detail is given about the nature of clerical assistance required; gratuities for 'Mechanical men in usant' were requested and funds were to be used for 'the transcribing and printing of whole Tracts and great Workes'.

A Memoriall for advancement of Universall Learning

There bee many wayes and occasions to advance Learning. Some whereof are in season, at one time, and some at another, some in respect of this place or Person, and some of that. Wherefore the only Meanes to procure this advancement will be to contrive how the fairest and best opportunities to that end may be imbraced and made use of in all places and times, when and wheresoever they shall happen: And that the best of them may be chosen, In case of unability to grasp and entertaine all. On the contrary to assigne any summes of Money, allowed by Benefactors, as a yearly Salary to certaine men, of such and such professions, for such and such predeterminate ends and studies will be to narrow a conceipt, to let in the many other unforeseene wayes to doe that busines more effectually. Besides such institutions would quickly bee corrupted and degenerat and that perhaps in the first men, that shall receive those Rewards, who (as it hath beene frequently and Manifestly seene) when their buildings are up pull downe their scaffolds, and besides the allowance of constant regular Salaries will be no oblidgment to Men to deserve well in their charges, though it incourage them to use much paines to procure them.

Wherefore if the Benevolences and Contributions made for the Advancement of Learning shall be bestowed upon the particulars hereafter mentioned (not excluding any other more faire opportunities) without doubt the fruit, which in a short time might be reaped of these seedes would not in all probabilityes delude the hopes, nor frustrate the good intentions of the sowers.

A Remonstrance of Particulars

Whereupon it is likely, the said Trustees may thinke fitt to bestowe the Benevolences and contributions given for the Advancement of Learning and Arts (viz.)

1. Entertainment to an Agent, to find out Men of Parts and Abilities to tender their severall Proposalls for the advancement of Learning to the Trustees, and keepe Correspondences with such as reside in remote and forraigne places, and solliciting of all other businesses subordinate there unto.

2. Entertainment of a Learned Secretary, for Latin and other vulgar Languages one or more, to assist the said Trustees in those Affaires.

3. Rewards for some professed Intelligencers in forraigne Countries, residing in the best and most Centrall places imploying themselves to give notice of any thing singular in the places for Learning or Art.

4. Defraying the Postage of the Intelligencer and Correspondents.

5. The maintenance of some other Schollars of greater abilities to be imployed by way of Translations, Collections, Epitomizing and Methodizing.

6. Defraying the charges of Paper and printing for publick and private Informations.

7. The purchasing and making of Mechanicall modells and workes.

8. The purchasing and making of Naturall experiments.

9. Of rarities and representations of all Common Naturall and Artificiall things.

10. Donations and gratuities for Learned Men in want.

11. Rewards for painting and drawing designes upon all Occasions.

The Benefitt and advantages of all, which as they have beene hitherto altogether lost for want of such persons and meanes, as might incourage them, soe they are soe many and various, as opportunities doe almost daily offer themselves for the promoting of some one of them, and would flowe in more and more, were once a correspondency setled in some way knowne, for theyr being incouraged.

Bibliography

(1) Alsted, Johann Heinrich. *The Worlds Proceeding Woes and Succeeding Joyes. 1. In cruell Warres and Vehement Plagues, 2. In happy Peace and Unity amongst all living Creatures* (London, 1642).

(2) —— *The Beloved City Or, The Saints Reign on Earth A Thousand Yeares; Asserted, and Illustrated from LXV places of Holy Scripture; Besides the judgement of Holy Learned men, both at home and abroad; and also Reason it selfe* (London, 1643).

(3) Andrews, C. M. *British Committees, Commissions, and Councils of Trade and Plantations, 1622-1675* (Baltimore, 1908).

(4) —— *The Colonial Period of American History,* 4 vols. (New Haven, Conn., 1934-8).

(5) Ashley Smith, J. W. *The Birth of Modern Education. The Contribution of the Dissenting Academies 1660-1800* (London, 1954).

(6) Austen, Ralph. *A Treatise of Fruit-Trees Shewing the manner of Grafting, Setting, Pruning, and Ordering of them in all respects: According to divers new and easy Rules of Experience gathered in ye Space of Twenty yeares* (Oxford, 1653).

(7) —— *The Spirituall Use, of an Orchard; or Garden of Fruit-Trees. Held forth in diverse Similitudes between Naturall and Spirituall Fruit-trees, in their Natures, and Ordering, according to Scripture and Experience* (Oxford, 1653).

(8) —— *A Treatise of Fruit-Trees . . .* (Oxford, 1657).

(9) —— *Observations upon some part of Sr Francis Bacon's Naturall History as it concernes, Fruit-Trees, Fruits, and Flowers* (Oxford, 1658).

(10) Aveling, J. H. *The Chamberlens and the Midwifery Forceps* (London, 1882).

(11) Aylmer, G. E. (ed.) *The Interregnum: The quest for settlement 1646-1660* (London, 1972).

(12) Aylmer, G. E. *The State's Servants. The Civil Service of the English Republic 1649-1660* (London, 1973).

(13) Bacon, Francis. *Of the Advancement and Proficience of Learning,* trans. Gilbert Watts (Oxford, 1640).

(14) —— *The New Atlantis by Francis Bacon,* ed. G. C. Moore Smith (Cambridge, 1900).

(15) Baillie, Robert. *The Letters and Journals,* 3 vols. (Edinburgh, 1841-2).
(16) Bailey, Margaret L. *Milton and Jakob Boehme* (New York, 1914).
(17) Barnard, T. C. 'The Purchase of Archbishop Ussher's Library in 1657', *Long Room,* 1971, No. 4 : 9-14.
(18) —— 'Social Policy of the Commonwealth and Protectorate in Ireland' (Unpublished D. Phil. dissertation, Oxford University, 1972).
(19) Barnett, Pamela R. 'Theodore Haak and the Early Years of the Royal Society', *Annals of Science,* 1959, *12* : 205-18.
(20) —— *Theodore Haak F.R.S. (1605-1690). The first German translator of Paradise Lost* (The Hague, 1962).
(21) Barrett, C. R. B. *History of the Society of Apothecaries of London* (London, 1905).
(22) Barrow, Isaac. *Theological Works,* ed. A. Napier, 9 vols. (Cambridge, 1859).
(23) Beale, John. *Herefordshire Orchards, A Patterne for all England* (London, 1657).
(24) Beales, A. C. F. *Education Under Penalty* (London, 1963).
(25) Biggs, Noah. *Mataeotechnia Medicinae Praxeωs. The Vanity of the Craft of Physick. Or, A New Dispensatory. Wherein is dissected the Errors, Ignorance, Impostures and Supinities of the Schools, in their main Pillars of Purges, Blood-letting, Fontanels or Issues, and Diet, &c. and the particular Medicines of the Shops* (London, 1651).
(26) Birch, Thomas. *The History of the Royal Society,* 4 vols. (London, 1756-7).
(27) Blith, Walter. *The English Improver, Or a New Survey of Husbandry. Discovering to the Kingdome, That some Land, both Arable and Pasture, may be Advanced Double or Treble* (London, 1649).
(28) —— *The English Improver Improved. The third Impression* (London, 1652).
(29) —— *The English Improver Improved . . . the Third Impression much Augmented* (London, 1653).
(30) Boate, Gerard. *Irelands Naturall History. Being a true and ample Description of its Situation, Greatnes, Shape and Nature* (London, 1652).
(31) Boehme, Jacob. *De signatura rerum,* trans. John Sparrow (London, 1651).
(32) Boyle, Robert. *Some Considerations Touching The Usefulnesse of Experimental Natural Philosophy,* Second Edition (Oxford, 1664).
(33) Brailsford, H. N. *The Levellers and the English Revolution,* ed. C. Hill (London, 1961).
(34) Bridenbaugh, Carl. *The Beginnings of the American People:*

Vexed and Troubled Englishmen 1590-1642 (Oxford, 1968).

(35) Briggs, Henry. *Trigonometria Britannica: sive de doctrina Triangulorum,* ed. Henry Gellibrand (Gouda, 1633).

(36) Brown, Harcourt. *Scientific Organisations in Seventeenth Century France* (Baltimore, 1934).

(37) Browne, Sir Thomas. *The Works of Sir Thomas Browne,* ed. G. Keynes, 4 vols. (London, 1964).

(38) Brunton, D. and Pennington, D. H. *Members of the Long Parliament* (London, 1954).

(39) Bucer, Martin. *De Regno Christi libri duo ad Eduardum Sextum angliae regem,* in *Scripta Anglicana* (Basel, 1577).

(40) Bullough, G. (ed.) *Henry More: Philosophical Poems* (Manchester, 1931).

(41) Burnet, Gilbert. *History of my own time,* ed. O. Airy, 2 vols. (Oxford, 1897-1900).

(42) Burrows, M. (ed.) *Register of the Visitors of the University of Oxford from A.D. 1647 to A.D. 1658* (*Camden Society,* XXIX, London, 1881).

(43) Calvin, Jean. *The Institutions of Christian Religion* (London, 1561).

(44) Chamberlen, Peter. *The Poore Mans Advocate, or, Englands Samaritan. Pouring Oyle and Wyne into the wounds of the Nation. By making present Provision for the Souldier and the Poor* (London, 1649).

(45) —— *Legislative Power in Problemes, Published for the Information of all those who have constantly adhered to the Good Cause* (London, 1659).

(46) Charleton, Walter. *The Immortality of the Human Soul Demonstrated by the Light of Nature. In two Dialogues* (London, 1657).

(47) Clark, A. *The Life and Times of Anthony Wood,* 5 vols. (Oxford Historical Society, Oxford, 1891-1900).

(48) —— and Boase, C. W. *Register of the University of Oxford,* 2 vols. (Oxford Historical Society, Oxford, 1885-9).

(49) Clark, G. *Science and Social Welfare in the Age of Newton,* Second Edition (Oxford, 1949).

(50) —— *A History of the Royal College of Physicians of London,* 2 vols. (Oxford, 1964-6).

(51) Collier, Thomas. *A Discovery of the New Creation. In a Sermon Preached at the Head-Quarters at Putney Sept. 29 1647* (London, 1651).

(52) Comenius, Jan Amos. *A Reformation of Schooles designed in Two Excellent Treatises* (London, 1642).

(53) —— *A Patterne of Universal Knowledge shadowing forth the largenesse dimension and use of the intended Worke* (London, 1651).

(54) —— *Via lucis vestigata et vestiganda* (Amsterdam, 1668).
(55) —— *The Way of Light,* trans. F. T. Campanac (London, 1938).
(56) —— *The Great Didactic of John Amos Comenius,* trans. M. W. Keatinge (London, 1916).
(57) Cook, John. *Unum Necessarium: or, The Poore Mans Case: Being An Expedient to make Provision for all poor People in the Kingdome* (London, 1648).
(58) Cooper, C. H. *Annals of Cambridge,* 5 vols. (Cambridge, 1842-1908).
(59) Corcoran, T. *Studies in the History of Classical Teaching* (London, 1911).
(60) —— *State Policy in Irish Education A.D. 1536 to 1816* (Dublin, 1916).
(61) Costello, W. J. *The Scholastic Curriculum at Early 17th Century Cambridge* (Cambridge, Mass., 1958).
(62) Covel, William. *A Declaration unto the Parliament shewing impartially the Causes of the Peoples Tumults, Madness, and Confusions* (London, 1659).
(63) Cowley, Abraham. *A Proposition for the Advancement of Experimental Philosophy* (London, 1661).
(64) Cudworth, Ralph. *A Sermon Preached before the Honourable House of Commons March 31 1647* (Cambridge, 1647).
(65) Culpeper, Nicholas. *A Physicall Directory or A translation of the London Dispensatory Made by the Colledge of Physicians in London* (London, 1649).
(66) —— *A Physical Directory: Or a translation of the Dispensatory made by the Colledge of Physitians of London The second edition much enlarged* (London, 1650).
(67) —— *A Physical Directory And in this Third edition is added A Key to Galen's Method of Physick* (London, 1651).
(68) Culverwell, Nathaniel. *An Elegant and Learned Discourse of the Light of Nature* (London, 1654).
(69) Curtis, M. H. *Oxford and Cambridge in Transition, 1558-1642* (Oxford, 1959).
(70) Davis, D. Seaborne. 'The Early History of the Patent Specification', *Law Quarterly Review,* 1934, *50* : 86-109; 260-274.
(71) Debus, A. G. *The English Paracelsians* (London, 1965).
(72) —— *Science and Education in the Seventeenth Century: The Webster-Ward Debate* (London, 1970).
(73) Debus, A. G. (ed.) *Science, Medicine and Society in the Renaissance. Essays to honor Walter Pagel,* 2 vols. (New York, 1972).
(74) de Jordy, A. and Fletcher, H. F. *A Library for Younger Schollers Compiled by an English Scholar Priest about 1655* (Illinois Studies in Language & Literature, *48,* Urbana, Ill., 1961).
(75) Dell, William. *The Building, Beauty, Teaching and Establishment*

of the Truly Christian and Spiritual Church (London, 1646).

(76) —— *The Stumbling-Stone, or, A Discourse touching that offence which the World and Worldly Church do take against Christ Himself* (London, 1653).

(77) —— *The Tryal of Spirits Both in Teachers & Hearers. Wherein is held forth The clear Discovery, and certain Downfal of the Carnal and Antichristian Clergie of These Nations. Testified from the Word of God to the University Congregation in Cambridge* (London, 1653).

(78) —— *The Right Reformation of Learning* (London, 1653); a separately paginated appendix to *The Tryal of Spirits* (77).

(79) Denny, Margaret. 'The Early Programme of the Royal Society and John Evelyn', *Modern Language Quarterly*, 1940, *1*: 481-96.

(80) Dickinson, Francesco. *A Precious Treasury of twenty rare Secrets* (London, 1649).

(81) Doorman, G. *Patents for Inventions in the Netherlands During the 16th, 17th and 18th Centuries* (The Hague, 1942).

(82) Drummond, J. C. and Wilbraham, A. *The Englishman's Food. A History of Five Centuries of English Diet,* New Edition (London, 1957).

(83) Dunlop, R. *Ireland Under the Commonwealth,* 2 vols. (Manchester, 1913).

(84) Dury, John. *A Motion Tending to the Publick Good of This Age, and of Posteritie. Or The Coppies of certain Letters written by Mr. John Dury, to a worthy Knight, at his earnest desire* (London, 1642).

(85) —— *Israels Call to March out of Babylon into Jerusalem* (London, 1646).

(86) —— *Considerations tending to the Happy Accomplishment of Englands Reformation in Church and State* (London, 1647).

(87) —— *A Seasonable Discourse written by Mr. John Dury upon the earnest requests of many* (London, 1649).

(88) —— *The Reformed School* (London, [1650]).

(89) —— *The Reformed-School: and the Reformed Librarie-Keeper. By John Durie. Whereunto is added I. An Idea of Mathematicks. II The description of one of the chiefest Libraries which is in Germanie* (London, 1651).

(90) Dury, John (ed.) *Clavis Apocalyptica: or, A Prophetical Key* (London, 1651).

(91) Dymock, Cressy. *An Essay For Advancement Of Husbandry Learning: Or Propositions For the Erecting a Colledge Of Husbandry: And In order thereunto, for the taking in of Pupills or Apprentices. And Also Friends or Fellowes of the same Colledge or Society* (London, 1651).

(92) —— *An Invention Of Engines of Motion Lately Brought to perfection. Whereby May be dispatched any work now done in England or elsewhere, (especially Works that require strength and swiftness) either by Wind, Water, Cattel or Men. And That with better accommodation, and more profit then by any thing hitherto known and used* (London, 1651).

(93) —— *The Reformed Husband-Man; or a brief Treatise of the Errors, Defects and Inconveniences of our English Husbandry* (London, 1651).

(94) —— *A Discoverie For Division or Setting out of Land, as to the best Form. Published by Samuel Hartlib Esquire, for Direction and more Advantage and Profit of the Adventurers and Planters in the Fens and other Waste and undisposed Places in England and Ireland* (London, 1653).

(95) Ernle, Lord. *English Farming Past and Present,* Fourth Edition (London, 1927).

(96) Evelyn, John. *The Diary and Correspondence of John Evelyn F.R.S.,* New Edition, 4 vols., ed. William Bray (London, 1854).

(97) —— *The Diary of John Evelyn,* ed. E. S. de Beer, 6 vols. (Oxford, 1955).

(98) Ferguson, John. *Bibliotheca Chemica,* 2 vols. (Glasgow, 1906).

(99) Fioravanti, Leonard. *Three Exact Pieces of Leonard Phioravant Knight,* trans. John Hester, ed. William Johnson (London, 1652).

(100) Fixler, M. *Milton and the Kingdoms of God* (London, 1964).

(101) Fortescue, G. K. *Catalogue of the Pamphlets etc. . . . Collected by George Thomason, 1640-1661,* 2 vols. (London, 1908).

(102) Foster, J. *Alumni Oxonienses, 1500-1714,* 4 vols. (Oxford, 1891).

(103) Frank, J. *The Beginnings of the English Newspaper 1620-1660* (Cambridge, Mass., 1961).

(104) Frank, R. G., Jr. 'Oxford and the Harveian Tradition in the Seventeenth Century' (Unpublished Ph.D. dissertation, Harvard University, 1971).

(105) —— 'John Aubrey, F.R.S., John Lydall, and Science at Commonwealth Oxford', *Notes & Records of the Royal Society,* 1973, *27* : 193-217.

(106) —— 'Science, Medicine and the Universities of Early Modern England: Background and Sources', *History of Science,* 1973, *11* : 194-216; 239-69.

(107) Fraser, Antonia. *Cromwell Our Chief of Men* (London, 1973).

(108) French, John. *A New Light of Alchymie written by Michael Sendigovius . . . Also Nine Books of the Nature of Things, written by Paracelsus. . . . Also a Chymicall Dictionary*

explaining all hard places and words met withall in the writings of Paracelsus, and other obscure authors (London, 1650).

(109) —— *The Art of Distillation, or A Treatise of the choicest Spagyricall Preparations performed by way of Distillation, being partly taken out of the most select Chymicall Authors of severall Languages, and partly out of the Authors manuall Experience* (London, 1651).

(110) —— *The Art of Distillation, or, A Treatise of the Choicest Spagiricall Preparations Performed by way of Distillation. Together with the Description of the Chiefest Furnaces & Vessels used by Ancient and Moderne Chymists* (London, 1653).

(111) Fussell, G. E. *The Old English Farming Books from Fitzherbert to Tull 1523-1730* (London, 1947).

(112) Gardiner, R. B. *The Registers of Wadham College Oxford. From 1613-1719* (London, 1889).

(113) Gerbier, Sir Balthazar. *To All Fathers of Families and Lovers of Knowledge and Virtues* ([Dieppe], 1648).

(114) —— *The Interpreter of the Academie for forrain languages, and all noble sciences and exercises. To all Fathers of Families and Lovers of Virtue* (London, 1648).

(115) Gibbens, Nicholas. *Questions and disputations concerning the Holy Scriptures* (London, 1601).

(116) Gibson, Strickland (ed.) *Statuta Antiqua universitatis Oxoniensis* (Oxford, 1931).

(117) Glauber, Johann Rudolph. *A Description of New Philosophical Furnaces, or A new Art of Distilling, divided into five parts*, trans. John French (London, 1651).

(118) *A Glimpse of Sions Glory: Or, the Churches Beautie Specified* (London, 1641).

(119) Goodall, Charles. *The Royal College of Physicians of London, founded and established by Law* (London, 1684).

(120) Goodwin, John. *Imputatio Fidei* (London, 1642).

(121) Graunt, John. *Natural and Political Observations made upon the Bills of Mortality* (London, 1662). Page references are to the Oxford edition of 1665.

(122) Greaves, R. L. *The Puritan Revolution and Educational Thought* (New Brunswick, N.J., 1969).

(123) —— 'William Sprigg and the Cromwellian Revolution', *HLQ*, 1971, *34:* 99-113.

(124) Greville, Robert; Lord Brooke. *The Nature of Truth: Its Union and Unity with the Soule* (London, 1640).

(125) Griffiths, John (ed.) *Statutes of the University of Oxford Codified in the year 1636* (Oxford, 1888).

(126) Hakewill, George. *An Apologie or Declaration of the Power and*

Providence of God in the Government of the World, Third Edition (Oxford, 1635).

(127) Hall, John. *An Humble Motion to the Parliament of England Concerning the Advancement of Learning and Reformation of the Universities. By J.H.* (London, 1649).

(128) —— *The Advancement of Learning by John Hall*, ed. A. K. Croston (Liverpool, 1953).

(129) Haller, W. *The Rise of Puritanism* (Harper Torchbook edn., New York, 1957).

(130) Harder, L. & Harder, M. *Plockhoy from Zurik-Zee* (Mennonite Historical Series, No. 2, Newton, Kansas, 1952).

(131) Harding, John. *Paracelsus His Aurora & Treasure of the Philosophers* (London, 1659).

(132) —— *Paracelsus His Archidoxis, Or, Chief Teachings* (London, 1660).

(133) Hardinge, W. H. 'On Manuscript Mapped and other Townland Surveys', *Trans. Royal Irish Academy: Antiquities*, 1873, *24*: 3-118.

(134) Hartlib, Samuel. *Englands Thankfulnesse, or, An Humble Remembrance presented to the Committee for Religion in the High Court of Parliament* (London, 1642).

(135) —— *The Parliaments Reformation Or a Worke for Presbyters, Elders, and Deacons, To Engage themselves, for the Education of all poore Children, and imployment of all sorts of poore, that no poore body young nor old may be enforced to beg within their Classes in City nor Country* (London, 1646).

(136) —— *A Further Discoverie of the Office of Publick Addresse for Accommodations* (London, 1648).

(137) —— *Londons Charitie, Stilling The Poore Orphans Cry. Providing Places and provision, by the care and indeavour of the Corporation appointed by the Parliament. To cloathe the Naked, feed the hungry, instruct the Ignorant, imploy the Idle* (London, 1649).

(138) —— *Londons Charity inlarged, Stilling The Orphans Cry* (London, 1650).

(139) —— *A Discours of Husbandrie used in Brabant and Flanders. The Second Edition, Corrected and Enlarged* (London, 1652).

(140) —— *Samuel Hartlib his Legacie: or an enlargement of the Discourse of husbandry used in Brabant and Flaunders: wherein are bequeathed to the common-wealth of England more outlandish and domestick experiments and secrets in reference to universall husbandry* (London, 1651).

(141) —— *Samuel Hartlib His Legacie: Or An Enlargement of the Discourse of Husbandry Used In Brabant & Flaunders: Wherein are bequeathed to the Common-Wealth of England, more*

Outlandish and Domestick Experiments and Secrets, in reference to Universall Husbandry. The second Edition augmented with an Appendix (London, 1652).

(142) —— *Samuel Hartlib His Legacy of Husbandry. Wherein are bequeathed to the Common-wealth of England, not onely Braband, and Flanders, but also many more Outlandish and Domestick Experiments and Secrets (of Gabriel Plats and others) never heretofore divulged in reference to Universal Husbandry. With a Table shewing the general Contents or Sections of the several Augmentations and enriching Enlargements in this Third Edition* (London, 1655).

(143) —— (ed.) *A Designe For Plentie, By an Universall Planting of Fruit-Trees* (London, 1652).

(144) —— *Chymical, Medicinal, and Chyrurgical Addresses Made to Samuel Hartlib Esquire* (London, 1655).

(145) —— *The Compleat Husbandman: or, A discourse of the whole Art of Husbandry* (London, 1659). Reissue of the second edition of Hartlib's *Legacy* (141).

(146) Held, F. E. (ed.) *Christianopolis. An Ideal State of the Seventeenth Century* (New York, 1916).

(147) Henfrey, H. W. *Numismata Cromwelliana* (London, 1877).

(148) Herring, Samuel. 'Letter to the parliament 4 Aug 1653', in *Original Letters,* ed. Nickolls (200), pp. 99-102.

(149) Hill, C. *Intellectual Origins of the English Revolution* (Oxford, 1965).

(150) —— *God's Englishman: Oliver Cromwell and the English Revolution* (London, 1970).

(151) —— *Antichrist in Seventeenth Century England* (London, 1971).

(152) Horsefield, J. K. *British Monetary Experiments 1650-1710* (Cambridge, Mass., 1960).

(153) Houghton, Walter E. 'The History of Trades: Its Relation to Seventeenth-Century Thought', *JHI,* 1941, *2* : 33-60.

(154) How, Samuel. *The Sufficiency of the Spirits Teaching, without humane learning* (London, 1640).

(155) Howell, R. *Newcastle-upon-Tyne and the Puritan Revolution* (Oxford, 1967).

(156) Howell, James. *Epistolae Ho-Elianae,* ed. J. Jacobs, 2 vols. (London, 1890-2).

(157) Innes Smith, R. W. *English Speaking Students of Medicine at the University of Leyden* (Edinburgh, 1932).

(158) James, M. *Social Problems and Policy during the Puritan Revolution 1640-1660* (London, 1930).

(159) Johnson, F. R. 'Gresham College: Precursor of the Royal Society' *JHI,* 1940, *1* : 413-38.

(160) Johnson, William. *Lexicon Chymicum. Cum obscuriorum verborum, et Rerum Hermeticarum, Tum Phrasium Paracel-*

sicarum, In Scriptis ejus: Et aliorum Chymicarum, passim occurrentium, planam explicationem continens (London, 1651).

(161) Jones, E. L. (ed.) *Agriculture and Economic Growth in England 1650-1815* (London, 1967).

(162) Jones, R. Foster. *The Triumph of the English Language* (Stanford, Cal., 1953).

(163) ——*Ancients and Moderns. A Study of the Rise of the Scientific Movement in Seventeenth-Century England,* Second Edition (Berkeley & Los Angeles, 1965).

(164) Jonston, John. *Naturae constantia: seu diatribe in qua, per posterium temporum cum prioribus collationem* (Amsterdam, 1632).

(165) ——*An History of the Constancy of Nature. Wherein, By comparing the latter age with the former, it is maintained that the World doth not decay universally* (London, 1657).

(166) Jorden, Edward. *A Discourse of Naturall Bathes and Minerall Waters* (London, 1632).

(167) Jordan, W. K. *Philanthropy in England 1480-1660* (London, 1959).

(168) ——*The Charities of London. 1480-1660* (London, 1960).

(169) ——*The Charities of Rural England 1480-1660* (London, 1961).

(170) Kearney, H. *Scholars and Gentlemen. Universities and Society in pre-Industrial Britain 1500-1700* (London, 1970).

(171) Keeler, M. F. *The Long Parliament, 1640-1641* (Philadelphia, 1954).

(172) Keevil, J. J. *Medicine and the Navy,* vols. 1 & 2 (Edinburgh, 1957 & 1958).

(173) Kerridge, E. *The Agricultural Revolution* (London, 1967).

(174) ——*The Farmers of Old England* (London, 1973).

(175) Keynes, G. *The Life of William Harvey* (Oxford, 1966).

(176) Kittredge, G. L. 'Dr. Robert Child the Remonstrant', Colonial Society of Massachusetts *Transactions,* 1919, *21* : 1-146.

(177) Knowles Middleton, W. E. *The Experimenters: A Study of the Accademia del Cimento* (Baltimore & London, 1971).

(178) Lambe, Samuel. *Seasonable Observations humbly offered to the Lord Protector* (London, 1657).

(179) Larcom, T. A. (ed.) *History of the Cromwellian Survey of Ireland A.D. 1655-6, commonly called 'the Down Survey'* (Irish Archaeological Society, Dublin, 1851).

(180) Letwin, W. *The Origins of Scientific Economics* (London, 1963).

(181) Lyte, Henry. *The Art of Tens, or Decimall Arithmeticke. Wherein The Art of Arithmeticke is taught in a most exact and perfit method, avoyding the intricacie of Fractions* (London, 1619).

(182) Macalister, A. *The History of the Study of Anatomy in Cambridge* (Cambridge, 1891).

(183) McKie, D. 'The Origins and Foundation of the Royal Society of London', *Notes & Records of the Royal Society,* 1960, *15*: 1-37.

(184) Madan, F. *Oxford Books,* 3 vols. (Oxford 1895-1931).

(185) Maddison, R. E. W. *The Life of the Honourable Robert Boyle F.R.S.* (London, 1969).

(186) Malynes, Gerard. *Consuetudo, vel, Lex mercatoria, or The Ancient Law Merchant* (London, 1622).

(187) Mede, Joseph. *The Key of the Revelation, searched and demonstrated out of the Naturall and proper Characters of the Vision* (London, 1643).

(188) Merton, R. K. *Science, Technology & Society in Seventeenth Century England* (New York, 1970).

(189) Miller, P. *The New England Mind: The Seventeenth Century* (Cambridge, Mass., 1939).

(190) More, Henry. *Conjectura Cabbalistica; or, a conjectural essay of interpreting the minde of Moses* (London, 1653).

(191) ——*A Collection of Several Philosophical Writings* (London, 1662).

(192) Morison, S. E. *Builders of the Bay Colony* (London, 1930).

(193) *Motives grounded upon the Word of God and upon Honour, Profit and Pleasure for the Present founding of an university* (London, 1647)

(194) Mullinger, J. B. *The University of Cambridge,* 3 vols. (Cambridge, 1884-1911).

(195) Munk, W. *The Roll of the Royal College of Physicians*, Second Edition, 3 vols. (London, 1878).

(196) Napier, John. *A Description of the Admirable Table of Logarithmes: with a declaration of the most Plentiful, Easy, and speedy use thereof in both kindes of Trigonometrie, as also in all Mathematical calculations,* trans. E. Wright (London, 1616).

(197) Needham, J. *A History of Embryology,* Second Edition (Cambridge, 1959).

(198) Nef, J. U. *The Rise of the British Coal Industry,* 2 vols. (London, 1932).

(199) Newton, A. P. *The Colonising Activities of the English Puritans* (New Haven, Conn., 1914).

(200) Nickolls, J. (ed.) *Original Letters and Papers of State addressed to Oliver Cromwell* (London, 1743).

(201) Norton, Robert. *Disme: The Art of Tenths, or, Decimall Arithmetike, Teaching how to performe all Computations whatsoever, by whole Numbers without Fractions, by the foure Principles of Common Arithmeticke* (London, 1608).

(202) O'Brien, J. J. 'Commonwealth Schemes for the Advancement of Learning', *British Journal of Educational Studies,* 1968, *16:* 30-42.

(203) Oughtred, William. *The Key of the Mathematicks New Forged and Filed: Together with A Treatise of the Resolution of all kinde of Affected Aequations in Numbers,* trans. Robert Wood (London, 1647).

(204) Overton, Richard. *An Appeale from the Degenerate Representative Body the Commons of England* (London, 1647).

(205) Partington, J. R. *A History of Chemistry,* vol. 2 (London, 1962).

(206) Pearl, V. *London and the Outbreak of the Puritan Revolution* (London, 1961).

(207) Peile, J. *Biographical Register of Christ's College,* 2 vols. (Cambridge, 1910).

(208) Peter, Hugh. *Good work for a Good Magistrate* (London, 1651).

(209) Pettus, Sir John. *Volatiles from the History of Adam and Eve* (London, 1674).

(210) Petty, William. *The Advice of W.P. To Mr. Samuel Hartlib For The Advancement of some particular Parts of Learning* (London, 1648).

(211) —— *Reflections upon some Persons and Things in Ireland* (London, 1660).

(212) —— *A Treatise of Taxes & Contributions* (London, 1662).

(213) —— *The Political Anatomy of Ireland* (London, 1691).

(214) Pinnel, Henry. *A Word of Prophesy, concerning the Parliament, Generall, and the Army* (London, 1648).

(215) —— *This Years F[r]uit, From the last years Root* (London, 1655).

(216) —— *Philosophy Reformed & Improved In Four Profound Tractates* (London, 1657).

(217) Plattes, Gabriel. *A Discovery of Infinite Treasure, Hidden Since The Worlds Beginning. Whereunto all men, of what degree soever, are friendly invited to be sharers with the Discoverer* (London, 1639).

(218) —— *A Discovery of Subterraneall Treasure, viz. Of all manner of Mines and Minerals, from the Gold to the Coale; with plaine Directions and Rules for the finding of them in all Kingdomes and Countries* (London, 1639).

(219) —— *A Description of the Famous Kingdome of Macaria; shewing its excellent Government: wherein The Inhabitants live in great Prosperity, Health, and Happinesse* (London, 1641).

(220) —— *The Profitable Intelligencer, Communicating his Knowledge for the Generall Good of the Common-wealth and all Posterity* (London, 1644).

(221) Plockhoy, Peter Cornelius. *A Way Propounded to make the poor of these and other Nations Happy* (London, 1659).

(222) Polemann, Joachim. *Novum Lumen Medicum; wherein the excel-*

lent and most necessary Doctrine of Helmont is fundamentally cleared (London, 1662).

(223) Pope, Walter. *The Life of the Right Reverend Father of God, Seth, Lord Bishop of Salisbury* (London, 1697).

(224) Potter, Francis. *An Interpretation of the Number 666* (Oxford, 1642).

(225) Potter, William. *The Trades-man's Jewel: Or A safe, easie, speedy and effectual Means, for the incredible advancement Of Trade* (London, 1650).

(226) —— *The Key of Wealth; or a new way for improving of trade* (London, 1650).

(227) Prall, S. E. *The Agitation for Law Reform during the Puritan Revolution 1640-1660* (The Hague, 1966).

(228) Price, W. Hyde. *The English Patents of Monopoly* (Cambridge, Mass., 1913).

(229) *Publique Bathes Purged. Or, A Reply to Dr. Chamberlain his Vindication of Publique Artificial Bathes, From the pretended Objections and Scandals obtruded on them* (London, 1648).

(230) Purver, M. *The Royal Society: Concept and Creation* (London, 1967).

(231) Rathborne, Aaron. *The Surveyor in Foure bookes* (London, 1616).

(232) Rattansi, P. M. 'Paracelsus and the Puritan Revolution', *Ambix*, 1963, *11:* 23-32.

(233) —— 'The Helmontian-Galenist Controversy in Restoration England,' *Ambix*, 1964, *12:* 1-23.

(234) Raven, C. E. *English Naturalists from Neckam to Ray* (Cambridge, 1947).

(235) —— *John Ray Naturalist*, Second Edition (Cambridge, 1950).

(236) —— *Natural Religion and Christian Theology*, 2 vols. (Cambridge, 1953).

(237) Rebholz, R. A. *The Life of Fulke Greville, First Lord Brooke* (Oxford, 1971).

(238) Rees, W. *Industry Before the Industrial Revolution*, 2 vols. (Cardiff, 1968).

(239) *The Representative of Divers well-affected persons in and about the City of London 6 Feb 1649* (London, 1649).

(240) Rex, M. B. *University Representation in England, 1604-1690* (London & New York, 1954).

(241) Reynolds, Edward. *A Sermon Touching the Use of Humane Learning* (London, 1658).

(242) Richards, T. *The History of the Puritan Movement in Wales 1639-53* (London, 1920).

(243) —— *Religious Developments in Wales, 1654-62* (London, 1923).

(244) Richeson, A. W. *English Land Measuring to 1800: Instruments and Practices* (Cambridge, Mass., 1966).

(245) Rigaud, S. P. (ed.) *Correspondence of Scientific Men of the Seventeenth Century*, 2 vols. (Oxford, 1841).

(246) Robinson, Henry. *Englands Safety in Trades Encrease. Most Humbly Presented to the High Court of Parliament* (London, 1641).

(247) —— *Certain Proposalls In order to the Peoples Freedome and Accommodation in some Particulars. With the Advancement of Trade and Navigation of this Commonwealth in Generall* (London, 1652).

(248) —— *Certain Proposals in order to a new Modelling of the Lawes, and Law-Proceedings, For a more Speedy, Cheap, and Equall Distribution of Justice throughout the Commonwealth* (London, 1653).

(249) Robinson, H. W. 'An Unpublished Letter of Dr. Seth Ward', *Notes & Records of the Royal Society*, 1950, *7*: 68-70.

(250) Rossi, P. *Francis Bacon. From Magic to Science* (London, 1968).

(251) Rostenberg, L. *Literary, Political, Scientific, Religious & Legal Publishing in England, 1551-1700*, 2 vols. (New York, 1965).

(252) Rushworth, John. (ed.) *Historical Collections*, 7 vols. (London, 1659-1701).

(253) Rutherford, Samuel. *A Survey of the Spiritual Antichrist* (London, 1648).

(254) Schaller, K. *Die Pädagogik des Johann Amos Comenius*, Second Edition (Heidelberg, 1967).

(255) Schenk, W. *The Concern for Social Justice in the Puritan Revolution* (London, 1948).

(256) Schmitt, C. B. *A Critical Survey and Bibliography of Studies on Renaissance Aristotelianism 1958-1969* (Padua, 1971).

(257) Scriba, C. J. 'The Autobiography of John Wallis', *Notes & Records of the Royal Society*, 1970, *25*: 17-46.

(258) Seaver, Paul S. *The Puritan Lectureships. The Politics of Religious Dissent 1560-1662* (Stanford, Cal., 1970).

(259) Shapiro, B. J. *John Wilkins 1614-1672. An Intellectual Biography* (Berkeley & Los Angeles, 1969).

(260) Simon, J. *Education and Society in Tudor England* (Cambridge, 1966).

(261) Smith, John. *Select Discourses*, ed. H. G. Williams (Cambridge, 1859).

(262) Snell, George. *The Right Teaching of Useful Knowledg* (London, 1649).

(263) Spedding, J. *The Letters and the Life of Francis Bacon*, 7 vols. (London, 1862-1874).

(264) Speed, Adolphus. *Generall Accommodations by Addresse* (London, 1650).

(265) —— *Adam out of Eden, or an abstract of divers excellent*

experiments touching the advancement of Husbandry (London, 1659).

(266) Sprat, Thomas. *History of the Royal Society* (London, 1667).

(267) Sprigg, William. *A modest Plea for an Equal Common-wealth Against Monarchy* (London, 1659).

(268) Starkey, George. *Natures Explication and Helmonts Vindication* (London, 1657).

(269) —— *Pyrotechny Asserted and Illustrated, To be the surest and safest Means for Art's Triumph over Nature's Infirmities* (London, 1658).

(270) Stearns, R. P. *Hugh Peter Strenuous Puritan* (Urbana, Ill., 1954).

(271) —— *Science in the British Colonies of America* (Urbana, Ill., 1970).

(272) Stoughton, John. *Felicitas Ultimi Saeculi: Epistola In Qua, Inter Alia, Calamitosus aevi praesentis status serio deploratur, certa felicioris posthac spes ostenditur, & ad promovendum publicum Ecclesiae & Rei literariae bonum omnes excitantur* (London, 1640).

(273) Stubbe, Henry. *Sundry Things from several Hands concerning the University of Oxford, viz. I. A Petition from some Well-affected therein. II A Model for a College Reformation. III. Queries Concerning the said University, and several Persons therein* (London, 1659).

(274) Sudhoff, K. *Bibliographia Paracelsica. Besprechung der unter Theophrast von Hohenheims Namen. 1527-1893* (Berlin, 1894).

(275) Supple, B. E. *Commercial Crisis and Change in England 1600-1642* (Cambridge, 1959).

(276) Syfret, R. H. 'The Origins of the Royal Society', *Notes & Records of the Royal Society,* 1947, *5:* 75-137.

(277) Tatham, G. B. *The Puritans in Power* (Cambridge, 1913).

(278) Taylor, E. G. R. *The Mathematical Practitioners of Tudor and Stuart England* (Cambridge, 1954).

(279) —— *Late Tudor and Early Stuart Geography 1583-1630* (London, 1934).

(280) Thirsk, J. (ed.) *The Agrarian History of England and Wales Volume IV 1500-1640* (Cambridge, 1967).

(281) Thomas, K. *Religion and the Decline of Magic* (London, 1971).

(282) Toon, P. (ed.) *The Correspondence of John Owen* (Cambridge & London, 1970).

(283) Trevor-Roper, H. R. *Religion, the Reformation and Social Change* (London, 1967).

(284) Turnbull, G. H. *Samuel Hartlib. A Sketch of his Life and his Relations to J. A. Comenius* (London, 1920).

(285) —— 'Oliver Cromwell's College at Durham', *Durham Research Review,* 1952, No. 3, pp. 1-7.

(286) —— 'Peter Stahl, The First Public Teacher of Chemistry at Oxford,' *Annals of Science,* 1953, *9:* 265-70.

(287) —— 'Samuel Hartlib's influence on the early history of the Royal Society', *Notes & Records of the Royal Society,* 1953, *10:* 101-30.

(288) —— 'John Hall's Letters to Samuel Hartlib', *Review of English Studies,* 1953, N. S. *4:* 221-33.

(289) —— 'Plans of Comenius for his stay in England', *Acta Comeniana,* 1958, *17:* 7-28.

(290) —— 'Robert Child', Colonial Society of Massachusetts *Transactions,* 1959, *38:* 21-53.

(291) —— 'George Stirk, Philosopher by Fire (1628?-1665),' Colonial Society of Massachusetts *Transactions,* 1959, *38:* 219-51.

(292) —— 'Some Correspondence of John Winthrop, Jr., and Samuel Hartlib', Colonial Society of Massachusetts *Proceedings,* 1960, *72:* 36-67.

(293) Turner, A. J. 'Mathematical Instruments and the Education of Gentlemen', *Annals of Science,* 1973, *30:* 51-88.

(294) Tuveson, E. *Millennium and Utopia* (New York, 1964).

(295) Urwick, W. *The Early History of Trinity College Dublin, 1591-1660* (London, 1892).

(296) Veall, D. *The Popular Movement for Law Reform 1640-1660* (Oxford, 1970).

(297) Vincent, W. A. L. *The State and School Education 1640-1660* (London, 1950).

(298) Violet, Thomas. *The Answer of the Corporation of Moniers to two false Libells printed in London* (London, 1653).

(299) Walker, E. C. *William Dell, Master Puritan* (Cambridge, 1970).

(300) Walker, John. *An Account of the Numbers and Sufferings of the Clergy* (London, 1714).

(301) Wallis, John. *Truth Tried: Or, Animadversions on a Treatise published by the Right Honourable Robert Lord Brook* (London, 1643).

(302) —— *A Defence of the Royal Society in Answer to the Cavails of Doctor William Holder* (London, 1678).

(303) —— 'Dr. Wallis' Letter against Mr. Maidwell 1700', Oxford Historical Society, *Collectanea,* First Series, ed. C. R. L. Fletcher (Oxford, 1885), pp.269-337.

(304) Walzer, M. *The Revolution of the Saints* (London, 1966).

(305) Ward, John. *The Lives of the Professors of Gresham College* (London, 1740).

(306) Ward, Seth. *A Philosophical Essay towards an Eviction of the Being and Attributes of God* (Oxford, 1652).

(307) —— *Vindiciae Academiarum, containing some briefe Animadversions upon Mr. Websters Book, stiled The Examination of Academies* (Oxford, 1654). Introduction by John Wilkins.

(308) Warr, John. *The Corruption and Deficiency of the Lawes of England* (London, 1649).

(309) Warton, Thomas. *The Life and Literary Remains of Ralph Bathurst* (London, 1761).

(310) Watson, F. 'The State and Education during the Commonweath', *EHR,* 1900, *15:* 58-72.

(311) —— *The English Grammar Schools to 1600* (Cambridge, 1908).

(312) —— *The Beginnings of the Teaching of Modern Subjects in England* (London, 1909).

(313) —— (ed.) *The Encyclopaedia and Dictionary of Education,* 4 vols. (London, 1922).

(314) Webster, C. 'Water as the Ultimate Principle of Nature: The Background to Boyle's Skeptical Chymist', *Ambix,* 1966, *13:* 96-107.

(315) —— 'English Medical Reformers of the Puritan Revolution: A Background to the "Society of Chymical Physitians"', *Ambix,* 1967, *14:* 16-41.

(316) —— 'The College of Physicians: "Solomon's House" in Commonwealth England,' *Bulletin of the History of Medicine,* 1967, *41:* 393-412.

(317) —— 'The Origins of the Royal Society', *History of Science,* 1967, *6:* 106-28.

(318) —— 'Henry Power's Experimental Philosophy', *Ambix,* 1967, *14:* 150-78.

(319) —— 'Henry More and Descartes: Some New Sources', *British Journal for the History of Science,* 1969, *4:* 359-77.

(320) —— *Samuel Hartlib and the Advancement of Learning* (Cambridge, 1970).

(321) —— 'Macaria: Samuel Hartlib and the Great Reformation', *Acta Comeniana,* 1970, *26:* 147-64.

(322) —— 'The Helmontian George Thomson and William Harvey: The revival and application of splenectomy to physiological research', *Medical History,* 1971, *15:* 154-67.

(323) —— 'William Dell and the Idea of University', *Changing Perspectives in the History of Science. Essays in Honour of Joseph Needham,* ed. M. Teich and R. Young (London, 1973), pp. 110-26.

(324) Webster, John. *The Saints Guide, Or, Christ the Rule, and Ruler of Saints* (London, 1654).

(325) —— *The Judgement Set, and the Bookes Opened. Religion Tried whether it be of God or of Men* (London, 1654).

(326) —— *Academiarum Examen, or the Examination of Academies* (London, 1654).

(327) —— *Metallographia: or, An History of Metals. Wherein is declared the signs of Ores and Minerals both before and after digging* (London, 1671).

(328) Whichcote, Benjamin. *Moral and Religious Aphorisms to which are added Eight Letters which passed between Dr. Whichcote and Dr. Tuckney* (London, 1753).

(329) Whitelocke, Bulstrode. *Memorials of the English Affairs,* 4 vols. (Oxford, 1853).

(330) Whiting, C. E. *Studies in English Puritanism from the Restoration to the Revolution 1660-1688* (London, 1931).

(331) Wilkins, John. *Mathematicall Magick. Or the Wonders that may be performed by Mechanicall Geometry* (London, 1648).

(332) —— *A Discourse Concerning the Beauty of Providence* (London, 1649).

(333) Wilkinson, R. S. 'The Alchemical Library of John Winthrop, Jr.', *Ambix,* 1966, *18:* 139-86.

(334) Williams, A. *The Common Expositor: An Account of the Commentaries on Genesis 1527-1633* (Chapel Hill, Carolina, 1948).

(335) Wing, D. *Short-title Catalogue of Books printed in England . . . 1641-1700,* 5 vols. (New York, 1945-51).

(336) Winstanley, Gerrard. *The Law of Freedom in a Platform: or, True Magistracy Restored* (London, 1652).

(337) Winter, Salvator. *A New Dispensatory of Fourty Physicall Receipts. Most necessary and Profitable for all House-Keepers in their Families. Besides three other Arts fit for the young Gentlemen* (London, 1649).

(338) —— & Francesco Dickinson. *A Pretious Treasury: or a new Dispensatory. Contayning 70 approved Physical rare Receits* (London, 1649).

(339) Wolfe, D. M. *Leveller Manifestoes of the Puritan Revolution* (New York & London, 1944).

(340) Woodhouse, A. S. P. (ed.) *Puritanism and Liberty* (London, 1951).

(341) Woodward, Hezekiah. *A Light to Grammar, And All other Arts and Sciences. Or, The Rule of Practise Proceeded by the Clue of Nature, and conduct of Right Reason* (London, 1641).

(342) Worsley, Benjamin. *Free Ports: the Nature and Necessity of them stated* (London, 1652).

(343) —— *The Advocate* (London, 1652).

(344) Wren, C. (ed.) *Parentalia, or Memoirs of the Family of Wren* (London, 1750).

(345) Yates, F. A. 'The Hermetic Tradition in Renaissance Science', *Art, Science, and History in the Renaissance,* ed. C. S. Singleton (Baltimore, 1967), pp.255-74.

(346) —— *The Rosicrucian Enlightenment* (London, 1972).

(347) Young, R. F. *A Bohemian Philosopher at Oxford in the 17th Century. George Ritschel of Deutschkahn (1616-1683)* (London, 1925).

(348) —— *Comenius in England* (London, 1932).

(349) Yule, G. *The Independents in the English Civil War* (Cambridge, 1958).

(350) Zilsel, E. 'The Origins of William Gilbert's Scientific Method', *Journal of the History of Ideas,* 1941, *2:* 1-32.

Index